Contents

S0-DZF-348

Preface

The *Manual of Medical Therapeutics* originally was prepared from 1943–1944 by the Department of Internal Medicine of Washington University School of Medicine as a guide for a course in medical therapeutics for fourth-year medical students. Since then the *Manual* has undergone many changes and has enjoyed a much wider distribution among students, house officers, and other physicians and medical professionals.

The emphasis of the *Manual* is on therapeutics, and only those pathophysiologic mechanisms necessary for the understanding of the various medical therapies are discussed. Many topics remain controversial, but we have tried to give the reader a reasonable, conservative, safe approach to such problems. Although the medical therapy outlined here may not represent the only approach to the various disease states discussed, it does reflect the approach employed by the majority of physicians on the staff of Washington University-Barnes Hospital Medical Center. The correct choice of medical therapy will be determined by the individual clinical situation and the medical facilities available.

As in the past, the authors are the chief residents, current fellows, and assistant professors in the Department of Medicine. We, the editors, were chief residents in Medicine in 1982–1983. We are indebted to the many people who helped to bring this edition to publication. Space does not permit the listing of the many members of the Department of Medicine who critically reviewed the manuscripts, but we are most appreciative of their contributions. We are very grateful for the secretarial assistance of Ms. Anita LaTurno, Ms. Karen Roy, Ms. Norma Elder, Ms. Carol Bell, and for the pharmacologic review by Deborah Hahn, Pharm. D. To Ms. Kathleen O'Brien of Little, Brown and Company, we owe thanks for the guidance and understanding that are indispensable in such an effort.

J. W. C.
M. F.

To the **medical house officers** of Washington University School of Medicine, whose concern for excellence in patient care has contributed significantly to the success of the **Manual.**

Manual of
Medical
Therapeutics

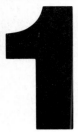

General Care
of the Patient

This chapter is primarily devoted to general topics in therapeutics that are not easily subsumed by traditional medical subspecialties. Although it is beyond the scope of the *Manual* to discuss all the complexities of general patient care, several introductory remarks are in order.

A fundamental principle of patient care is that medical therapy must always be individualized. An approach that is appropriate for one patient may be inappropriate for another with the same disease. Furthermore, the passage of time may dictate varying strategies for the same patient. For example, a stepped-care approach to hypertension is useful as a general guideline; however, the specific antihypertensive program for a diabetic patient with renal impairment may differ markedly from the regimen chosen for a patient with angina or depression.

A second related point is that any medical problem must be viewed in a specific psychosocial context. A therapeutic approach that fails to consider the patient's environmental and emotional background is less likely to succeed than one that takes this background into account. In addition, the management of hospitalized patients is facilitated by the physician's sensitivity to the fact that hospitals may be unfamiliar and stressful for patients. Questions of compliance, family structure, and life-style assume particular importance in the management of outpatients.

I. Hospital orders

A. All orders should be clear, complete, and organized. The importance of writing legibly, especially regarding medications and dosages, cannot be overstated. Initial orders should be written as soon as possible after admission and evaluation and should bear the date, time recorded, and signature of the physician.

B. All orders should be reevaluated at frequent intervals and tailored to the patient's status at that time. If there is a change in an order, the old order should be specifically canceled before the new order is written.

C. Orders for medications to be given prn require careful consideration, especially those concerning the administration of a narcotic. If a prn order for narcotics is written, a definite time limit, not to exceed 48 hours, should be specified.

D. Content and organization of orders. Establishing a routine for writing orders will ensure that no important therapeutic measures will be overlooked. An example of such a routine is as follows:

    1. Admitting diagnosis and patient's **condition.**

    2. Allergies.

    3. Vital signs. Temperature, pulse, respirations, blood pressure, and specific orders (including orthostatic checks, neurologic signs, and changes for which the physician is to be notified).

    4. Diet.

    5. Activity permitted.

6. **Specific nursing instructions.** Intake and output, daily weights, skin or wound care, isolation, postural drainage, etc.

7. **Intravenous fluids,** including composition of fluids and rate of administration.

8. **Medications,** dosage, and frequency and route of administration.

9. **Laboratory tests,** x rays, etc. Open-ended orders, such as "daily CBC," should be avoided to prevent excessive and unnecessary use of diagnostic tests.

10. **Consultations** (e.g., physician specialist, physical therapist, social worker). It is important to specify the reason for the consultation and the questions to which the consultant should direct attention.

II. Drug therapy

A. General comments. Pharmacologic agents should be treated with respect and should only be administered when potential benefits clearly outweigh potential risks. Drugs should not be given merely to satisfy patient expectations.

B. Prescriptions should be written legibly in terms the patient or family can clearly understand. Each prescription should include the patient's name and address, date, name of the drug, dosage, amount dispensed, clear dosage-schedule instructions, number of refills permitted, and signature of the physician. To assist patients in distinguishing among various medications in their possession, it is often helpful to state the reason the drug has been prescribed (e.g., "Hydrochlorothiazide 25 mg, 1 tablet PO daily for high blood pressure").

All prescription containers should be explicitly labeled. Use the generic name whenever possible, write the dosage in metric terms, and never dispense unlimited refills.

C. Adverse drug reactions (i.e., any undesired or unintended drug effects) occur frequently in hospitalized patients and outpatients. The rate increases proportionally to the number of drugs given. Drug reactions may be extensions of known pharmacologic effects (and therefore often dose related), or they may be idiosyncratic. To reduce their frequency:

1. Use as few drugs as possible.

2. Learn the metabolism, routes of execretion, and major adverse effects of the drugs you use. Certain drugs require periodic monitoring of specific laboratory parameters (e.g., gold, penicillamine).

3. Individualize the dose when possible, paying particular attention to the patient's age, size, and metabolic and renal status.

4. Take a careful history of previous drug reactions, and record them conspicuously in the patient's chart.

5. Report unusual drug reactions to the Food and Drug Administration.

D. Drug interactions are complex and embody several different mechanisms (e.g., the interaction between warfarin and phenobarbital). The effect of one drug may potentiate or antagonize the desired or toxic effect of another. Before ordering a new drug, assess the likelihood of a harmful interaction between that drug and those the patient is already receiving. Administer the new drug only if you are reasonably sure that no adverse interaction will occur, or that you will be able to control such an interaction (see P. D. Hansten, *Drug Interactions.* Philadelphia: Lea & Febiger, 1979).

III. Diet and nutrition. This topic, which is so important in general patient care, is discussed in detail in Chap. 11.

IV. Fever

A. General comments. Fever accompanies a wide variety of illnesses, and may be a valuable marker of disease activity. Therefore, under most circumstances, fever should not be treated until its cause is determined. In some cases, however, fever may have deleterious effects, including increased tissue catabolism, dehydration, precipitation or exacerbation of congestive heart failure, delirium, and convulsions (rare in adults). Treatment of fever is indicated when these harmful effects ensue, or when the patient's discomfort is extreme. In addition, heat stroke and malignant hyperthermia are medical emergencies, requiring prompt recognition and treatment (see Chap. 23).

B. Treatment

1. **The antipyretic drugs aspirin** (acetylsalicylic acid) and **acetaminophen** are the treatments of choice in most cases. They are also analgesics and are discussed in detail in secs. **V.B** and **D.**

   In some febrile patients, sporadic use of these agents will cause uncomfortable sweats and chills as the temperature fluctuates. Therefore, these drugs should be given regularly (325–650 mg up to q3–4h) until the underlying disease process has been controlled. Occasional patients are very sensitive to aspirin and may become hypothermic and hypotensive after small doses. Although this is rare, it is wise to use another antipyretic agent in patients whose temperature falls markedly after administration of small doses of aspirin.

2. **Hypothermic blankets** may be effective but require close monitoring of rectal temperatures. Shivering may be a problem. The use of the blanket should be discontinued when the rectal temperature drops to about 38°C, since a further fall usually occurs.

3. **Tepid sponge baths** with water or saline may be used but are less effective in adults than in children.

4. **Ice baths** are reserved for cases of extreme hyperthermia such as encountered in heatstroke (see Chap. 23).

V. Relief of pain

A. General comments. The management of pain must be individualized according to its cause, severity, and chronicity. In addition, the complex interaction between the patient's emotional state, personality, and pain must always be considered, particularly in chronic pain syndromes. Although drugs are the most commonly used therapeutic agents, other nonpharmacologic modalities are frequently appropriate (*Ann. Intern. Med.* 93:588, 1980). Nonopioid preparations should be used whenever possible.

B. Salicylates. Acetylsalicylic acid (aspirin), which has analgesic, antipyretic, and anti-inflammatory effects, is useful for relieving pain originating from many sites. Additional discussion of aspirin appears in the section on rheumatoid arthritis, Chap. 21.

1. **Pharmacologic properties.** The analgesic and anti-inflammatory activity of aspirin probably relates to its ability to inhibit the peripheral production of prostaglandins. Absorbed salicylates are 80% bound to plasma proteins; therefore, higher serum levels of free drug occur in hypoalbuminemia. Salicylates are metabolized by the liver and excreted by the kidneys.

2. **Adverse effects.** Tinnitus, dizziness, and decreased hearing are dose-related side effects. Gastrointestinal distress and GI blood loss (occasionally severe) are frequently encountered. Hypersensitivity reactions (urticaria, bronchospasm, laryngeal edema, hypotension) are uncommon but well recognized (patients with asthma and nasal polyps are especially susceptible).

Small doses of aspirin decrease platelet aggregation and prolong bleeding time. This effect may last up to 1 week. The drug should thus be avoided in patients with bleeding disorders or severe liver disease and in patients taking warfarin. It is desirable to avoid aspirin during the week prior to surgical procedures.

Salicylate overdose is discussed in Chap. 23.

3. Preparations and dosage

    a. Aspirin is the preparation of choice. For relief of pain, the oral dose is 0.3–1.0 gm (5–15 grains) q4h. Rectal suppositories are available but may be irritating to the mucosa and variably absorbed. The rectal dosage is 0.3–0.6 gm q3–4h.

    b. Other salicylate preparations are discussed in Chap. 21. Recent studies indicate that the newer enteric-coated tablets cause less injury to gastric mucosa than buffered preparations or plain aspirin (*N. Engl. J. Med.* 303:136, 1980).

C. Other nonsteroidal anti-inflammatory agents. Except for aspirin, the prostaglandin-inhibiting drugs in this category (e.g., indomethacin, naproxen, tolmetin, ibuprofen, fenoprofen, sulindac) have traditionally been marketed only for the treatment of rheumatologic disorders. However, several compounds in this class are now approved for the treatment of nonrheumatic pain (e.g., zomepirac sodium, naproxen sodium). Some of these drugs compare favorably with codeine-aspirin or codeine-acetaminophen combinations in the treatment of postoperative or dental pain. There are few data to indicate how the nonsteroidal, anti-inflammatory agents compare with each other as analgesics. They are a reasonable choice when aspirin or acetaminophen are inadequate and opioids are to be avoided. They are discussed in detail in Chap. 21.

D. Para-aminophenol derivatives. Acetaminophen has analgesic and antipyretic actions but does not have anti-inflammatory properties. **Phenacetin,** whose major metabolite is acetaminophen, is a constituent in several analgesic combinations, but is generally not used as an isolated preparation. The therapeutic actions of these two drugs are essentially identical.

1. Side effects and toxicity. The principal advantages of acetaminophen over aspirin are the lack of gastric toxicity and the absence of effects on platelet aggregation. The most serious toxicity of acetaminophen is hepatic. Acute overdosage with 10–15 gm may cause fatal hepatic necrosis; management of overdose is discussed in Chap. 23. Toxic hepatitis may also occur in patients chronically ingesting several grams a day. Thrombocytopenia is a rare side effect.

Acute or chronic overdosage with phenacetin may cause hemolytic anemia (especially in patients with glucose 6-phosphate dehydrogenase deficiency) and methemoglobinemia, but these effects are rarely seen with acetaminophen. Chronic phenacetin ingestion of 1–3 gm daily for several years may result in "**analgesic nephropathy**," which is characterized by interstitial inflammation and papillary necrosis. Progressive renal insufficiency may ensue. This syndrome occurs particularly when combinations of phenacetin and aspirin are taken chronically. Acetaminophen, on the other hand, is not firmly established as a nephrotoxin.

2. Preparations and dosage. Acetaminophen is the preparation of choice. For relief of pain, the oral dosage (in tablets, capsules, or elixir) is 325–650 mg q4–6h. Rectal suppositories are also available.

E. Opioid analgesics

1. General comments. In this discussion, the term *opioid* refers to a series of naturally occurring and synthetic drugs that have pharmacologic, but not necessarily structural, similarities to opium or morphine. These drugs are primarily employed as analgesics, but they are also used to suppress severe cough and diarrhea. Common errors that occur with the use of opioids include underestimation of the amount of drug required for pain relief, overestimation of the duration of action, and possibly an exaggerated estimation of the dangers of addiction for medical inpatients.

2. Precautions

    a. Opioids should be used only when other drugs or physical measures will not provide relief of pain. One should give the smallest doses that provide adequate analgesia. **Tolerance** to the analgesic effects of opioids occurs with continued use (i.e., increasing doses are required to maintain the same effect).

    b. Physical dependence may occur with any of the opioid preparations. In most patients, 2 weeks or longer is required for physiologic addiction to develop. However, withdrawal symptoms may be precipitated by the opioid antagonist naloxone after only several days of opioid use. The hazard of addiction should not preclude long-term administration of these drugs to patients with terminal illnesses.

    c. Opioids should be used with extreme caution in patients with hypothyroidism, Addison's disease, hypopituitarism, anemia, reduced blood volume, head trauma, asthma, severe malnutrition, or debilitation. In patients with increased intracranial pressure, opioids may further elevate cerebrospinal fluid pressure. Since these drugs are metabolized in the liver, patients with hepatic disease may be inordinately sensitive to the usual dosage. Phenothiazines, antidepressants, and CNS depressant drugs may markedly potentiate the adverse effects of opioids. If it becomes necessary to use opioids in any of these settings, very small doses should be used initially.

    d. Opioids are contraindicated in certain acute disease states (e.g., suspected surgical abdomen) in which the pattern and degree of pain are important diagnostic signs. Similarly, their administration to patients with acute head injuries may complicate accurate assessment of neurologic changes.

    e. Opioid-induced vomiting may often be avoided by keeping the patient recumbent.

    f. The opioid antagonist naloxone, a short-acting semisynthetic congener of morphine, is used to counteract the symptoms of excess doses of opioids (particularly hypotension and depression of respiration and consciousness). The management of opioid overdose is discussed in Chap. 23.

3. Adverse and toxic effects. Most of the adverse effects of opioids are extensions of their known pharmacologic actions. There are few differences in the adverse effects of various opioids when given in equianalgesic doses, but an individual patient will usually tolerate some preparations better than others.

    a. Central nervous system effects include sedation, mood alteration, euphoria, and pupillary constriction. Nausea and vomiting may be particularly troublesome, even with therapeutic doses.

    b. Respiratory depression occurs in direct proportion to the dose. Therapeutic doses diminish both tidal volume and respiratory rate. Therefore, opioids should be used cautiously, if at all, in patients with pulmonary insufficiency and asthma.

    c. Cardiovascular effects include peripheral vasodilation, hypotension (especially orthostatic), and circulatory collapse.

   d. Gastrointestinal effects include a decrease in propulsive peristalsis in the large and small bowel and an increase in smooth muscle and sphincter tone. Opioids may precipitate toxic megacolon in patients with severe ulcerative colitis.

   e. Biliary tract spasm may be induced, and patients with biliary colic may have an increase in pain. Elevation of serum amylase may result from this mechanism.

   f. Genitourinary effects include increases in ureter, bladder, and sphincter tone. Urinary retention may be provoked, especially in patients with prostatic hypertrophy.

   g. Allergic reactions are rare and include urticaria and other rashes and anaphylaxis, which may account for episodes of sudden death among addicts.

4. Clinical use. When oral opioid preparations are necessary for short-term administration, codeine or oxycodone are the drugs of choice (generally in combination with aspirin or acetaminophen). In situations necessitating parenteral drug administration, we use meperidine or morphine. Oral morphine and hydromorphone are usually given to cancer patients with chronic severe pain (see Chap. 17).

Hydroxyzine hydrochloride, 25–50 mg IM, potentiates the effect of a given dose of an opioid and may reduce the frequency of IM injections. It also has antiemetic properties.

5. Selected preparations and dosage. Information concerning the relative potency of these drugs is given in Table 1-1.

   a. Morphine sulfate. The usual effective IM or SQ dose is 10 mg/70 kg of body weight, although this may vary with the extent of previous administration. In some patients, 5 mg may afford excellent analgesia, while others may require up to 15 mg. The duration of action is roughly 4–5 hours. Morphine may be given cautiously IV (primarily in the setting of acute myocardial infarction or acute pulmonary edema). The usual IV dose is 2–4 mg given slowly over 5 minutes.

   b. Codeine is dispensed as water-soluble sulfate and phosphate salts. Analgesia is enhanced when codeine is combined with aspirin or acetaminophen. The usual analgesic dosage is 30–60 mg PO, IM, or SQ q4–6h. Codeine is also widely used as a **cough suppressant** in a dosage of 15–30 mg PO q4–6h.

   c. Oxycodone is a semisynthetic opioid. In the United States, oxycodone is marketed only for oral use, in combination with acetaminophen or aspirin. The usual dosage is 5 mg PO q6h.

   d. Hydromorphone is a semisynthetic derivative of morphine. The usual dosages are 2–4 mg PO q4–6h or 1–4 mg IM or SQ q4–6h. One should generally start with the lower doses. The drug may also be given IV (over several minutes) and as 3-mg rectal suppositories.

   e. Meperidine is a synthetic opioid. Its duration of action (2–4 hours) is shorter than that of morphine. Meperidine causes less constipation and biliary spasm than a comparable dose of morphine. Adverse effects are otherwise similar to those of morphine except that toxic doses are more likely to cause seizures. The usual dosage is 50–150 mg PO, IM, or SQ q3–4h; IM or SQ injections are locally irritating.

   f. Propoxyphene is structurally related to methadone. In standard doses, its analgesic potency may be no better than that of aspirin, although this varies among individuals. Accordingly, side effects at the usual clinical doses tend to be minimal. The usual oral dosage is 65 mg of propoxyphene

Table 1-1. Analgesic potency of selected opioid drugs

Drug	Oral-parenteral potency ratio[a]	Potency relative to morphine (for equal parenteral doses)[b]
Morphine	1 : 6	1.0
Codeine	2 : 3	0.1
Oxycodone	1 : 2	1.0
Hydromorphone	1 : 5	6.0
Meperidine	1 : 3	0.15
Pentazocine	1 : 3	0.25

[a] For example, morphine is 6 times more potent parenterally than orally.
[b] For example, hydromorphone is 6 times more potent than an equal dose of morphine, when given parenterally.
Source: The figures in this table are approximations based on a variety of references.

hydrochloride or 100 mg of propoxyphene napsylate q4–6h. Combinations of propoxyphene and aspirin or acetaminophen are more effective than either agent alone.

g. **Pentazocine** is a synthetic drug with both opioid agonist and antagonist actions. Its antagonist effect is demonstrated by its ability to induce withdrawal symptoms in chronic users of other opioids. However, the drug is itself antagonized by naloxone. Its unique adverse effects, in contrast to morphine, include hypertension, tachycardia, and hallucinations. Pentazocine originally was considered to have minimal addictive potential, but clinical experience has not supported this contention. Accordingly, the drug confers little advantage over other agents. The usual dosage is 50 mg PO or 30 mg IM q3–4h; SQ administration should be avoided if possible because of local tissue irritation.

Psychoactive Drug Therapy

I. **Sedative-hypnotic and antianxiety drugs**

A. **General comments.** These drugs are among the most widely prescribed medications today, primarily because of the popularity of the benzodiazepines. However, there is reason to believe that the use of these drugs is excessive. Physicians should never prescribe them without fully investigating the source of a patient's anxiety or insomnia.

It is becoming increasingly appreciated that **insomnia** is a symptom that may actually reflect a variety of underlying medical or psychiatric disorders. For example, sleep disturbances may occur secondary to depression, and specific treatment should be directed toward the latter condition. When insomnia occurs as an isolated symptom, behavioral or relaxation techniques should be attempted before resorting to drug therapy.

In general, hypnotics lose their effectiveness within relatively short periods of time. Therefore, their use should be limited to brief periods of a few days or weeks. **Ongoing refills should not be made available.** Many of these medications may interfere with daytime mental functions, and they interact unfavorably with alcohol and other CNS depressants. Most hypnotics change the duration of various sleep stages (e.g., suppress REM sleep), and patients are subject to rebound insomnia when they are discontinued. There is a potential for psychologic and physical dependence with most of these drugs, including the benzodiazepines.

Similarly, use of these drugs for **anxiety** should generally be limited to brief periods of time corresponding to transient anxiety-provoking situations. Patients with chronic nonspecific anxiety rarely experience sustained improvement in symptoms with chronic tranquilizer use; rather, they become entrapped in a situation of psychologic and physical dependence. The management of these patients requires considerable effort by physicians and allied health professionals. Counseling and behavioral techniques may be helpful.

Sedative-hypnotic and antianxiety drugs should be used cautiously and in lower dosage in elderly patients (who may be very sensitive to their effects) and in patients with hepatic insufficiency, pulmonary disease, heart failure, anemia, myxedema, and high fever.

B. Benzodiazepines

1. **Pharmacologic properties and adverse effects.** These drugs have similar actions but differing pharmacokinetics. They are metabolized primarily in the liver and must be used cautiously in patients with hepatic disease. Concomitant administration of cimetidine may increase the therapeutic effect of benzodiazepines. Adverse reactions include excessive drowsiness, paradoxical hyperexcited state, and mental impairment. Withdrawal symptoms occur after prolonged use, necessitating gradual discontinuance of the drug. One should not confuse withdrawal symptoms with an increase in the underlying anxiety itself.

2. **Selected agents**

    a. **Diazepam.** The dosage is 2–10 mg PO tid prn. The half-life is 20–50 hours; metabolites are also active and are slowly degraded into inactive products.

    b. **Chlordiazepoxide.** The dosage is 10–25 mg PO tid prn. The half-life is 6–30 hours; metabolites are also active and slowly degraded.

    c. **Oxazepam.** The dosage is 10–15 mg PO tid prn. The half-life is 3–21 hours; metabolites are inactive. Thus, less accumulation of active drug occurs with prolonged use, as compared with diazepam and chlordiazepoxide.

    d. **Lorazepam.** The dosage is 0.5–1.0 mg PO tid prn. The half-life is 10–20 hours; metabolites are inactive.

    e. **Flurazepam** is specifically marketed for insomnia, although it may be no more effective for this purpose than other benzodiazepines. The dosage is 15–30 mg PO hs. Metabolism is rapid, but the half-lives of active metabolites are 50–100 hours.

C. Barbiturates

1. **Pharmacologic properties.** Both long-acting and short-acting preparations are available. Long-acting barbiturates such as phenobarbital are metabolized slowly in the liver and are cleared primarily by the kidney (partially as unchanged drug). Short-acting preparations (e.g., secobarbital and pentobarbital) are metabolized primarily by the liver and depend minimally on renal excretion. Barbiturates should be given parenterally only in emergency situations such as status epilepticus. The barbiturates have a relatively poor therapeutic index (i.e., a low ratio of toxic to therapeutic dose). Thus, they have been generally supplanted by the safer benzodiazepines for the treatment of anxiety and insomnia.

2. **Adverse effects.** Barbiturates are CNS depressants and accordingly cause drowsiness and mental impairment (but no analgesia). These effects are

additive with other CNS depressants, including alcohol. Barbiturates may paradoxically cause excitement on occasion.

Barbiturates cause **respiratory depression** and are thus contraindicated in patients with pulmonary disease. The induction of the hepatic microsomal system by barbiturates necessitates dosage adjustments of hepatically metabolized drugs such as warfarin. Other adverse effects include hypersensitivity reactions (cutaneous and systemic) and exacerbation of acute intermittent porphyria. These drugs should be avoided in patients with hepatic disease.

3. **Tolerance** to the effects of barbiturates occurs with continued use. **Physical addiction** is a danger when large or even therapeutic doses are taken for more than several weeks. When barbiturates are withdrawn from addicted patients, the decrement in dosage should not exceed the equivalent of 30 mg daily of phenobarbital, to prevent such serious reactions as delirium and seizures. (See T. P. Hackett and N. H. Cassem (eds.), *Massachusetts General Hospital Handbook of General Hospital Psychiatry.* St. Louis: Mosby, 1978.)

4. **Acute barbiturate overdose** or poisoning is a medical emergency (see Chap. 23).

5. **Preparations**

   a. **Long-acting.** Effects are noticeable in 30–45 minutes and last 4–8 hours. Hangovers are frequent. The dosage of phenobarbital is 100–200 mg at bedtime. For daytime sedation, the dosage is 15–30 mg tid prn, but phenobarbital is rarely indicated for this use.

   b. **Short-acting.** Onset of action is 15–30 minutes, and the effects last 2–4 hours. Hangovers are less common. Oral hypnotic doses for pentobarbital, secobarbital, and amobarbital are 100–200 mg hs. These drugs are not used for daytime sedation.

D. **Chloral hydrate** is a rapidly effective hypnotic that seldom produces excitement or hangover and has minimal effect on sleep stages. Sleep usually begins in 15–30 minutes and lasts 5–8 hours. The drug is detoxified chiefly by the liver, and products are excreted by the kidneys. It should not be given to patients with severe hepatic, renal, or cardiac disease. Side effects include gastric irritation, rare skin reactions, and potentiation of the anticoagulant effect of warfarin. Tolerance, addiction, and withdrawal syndromes can be seen with chronic ingestion. Toxic doses cause CNS and respiratory depression. A reduction product, trichloroethanol, may give a positive result for urine sugar with Clinitest tablets. The usual hypnotic dose is 0.5–1.0 gm hs. Single doses or daily dosage should not exceed 2 gm.

E. **Antihistamines**

   1. **Diphenhydramine,** though not marketed as a sedative, may be used for this purpose. Its side effects are principally anticholinergic in nature. The drug is a good choice when a combination of antipruritic and sedative activity is desired. The dosage is 25–50 mg qid prn or 25–50 mg hs.

   2. **Hydroxyzine** is a compound with antihistaminic effects. It is marketed specifically as an antianxiety and antipruritic agent. The drug has sedative and antiemetic effects. Oral preparations include hydroxyzine pamoate and hydroxyzine hydrochloride; the dosage is 25–50 mg qid prn or 25–50 mg hs. Hydroxyzine hydrochloride is also available as an IM preparation. It is often used in combination with meperidine to potentiate the latter's analgesic effect and to provide antiemetic and sedative effects. The usual dosage is 25–50 mg IM q3–4h.

F. **Other agents.** Ethchlorvynol, glutethimide, meprobamate, and methyprylon were all commonly used sedatives until recently. They are relatively toxic compared with the benzodiazepines and are thus not recommended for routine use. Paraldehyde also has few indications. It has generally been replaced by the benzodiazepines in the treatment of alcohol withdrawal. This drug may still have a role in the treatment of status epilepticus (see Chap. 22).

II. Phenothiazines and related antipsychotic drugs

A. **General comments.** These drugs, of which chlorpromazine is the prototype, are commonly used in psychiatric disorders (especially psychoses) and for treatment of nausea and vomiting. Although several dozen compounds are available, the clinician is best served by becoming familiar with a few representative drugs, since they differ widely in their potency and side effects. Addiction does not occur, and overdoses rarely result in death.

B. **Pharmacologic properties.** Although the exact mechanism of action is unknown, the antipsychotic and CNS effects are probably related to dopamine antagonism. These drugs also have anticholinergic, antihistaminic, and antiadrenergic activity in varying degrees. Absorption from the GI tract is rapid but erratic; IM injections yield more bioavailable drug. Their half-lives in plasma are generally in the range of 10–20 hours. Phenothiazines are metabolized by the liver, and metabolites (which are mostly inactive) are excreted in the urine and bile. These drugs should be given cautiously to patients with hepatic disease.

C. **Adverse reactions.** The toxic effects of these agents include those that are extensions of their CNS activity (i.e., sedation, autonomic effects, and extrapyramidal reactions) and those that are idiosyncratic. In general, for the lower-potency preparations such as chlorpromazine (i.e., those that require large doses for a therapeutic effect), autonomic and sedative effects outweigh extrapyramidal reactions; the reverse is true for the high-potency drugs such as haloperidol (see Table 1-2).

1. **Hypotension,** often orthostatic, may occasionally be acute and severe after IM doses.

2. **Anticholinergic effects** include dry mouth, blurred vision, urinary retention, constipation, and tachycardia.

3. **Extrapyramidal reactions**

    a. **Parkinsonian reactions,** which usually occur early in therapy, include the tremor, bradykinesia, rigidity, and abnormalities of gait and posture seen in idiopathic parkinsonism. Treatment with antiparkinsonian drugs, such as benztropine or trihexyphenidyl, may be required if these reactions occur.

    b. **Akathisia,** another early side effect, is a sense of motor restlessness in which the patient has a constant need to move about. It should not be confused with a worsening of the underlying psychiatric disorder.

    c. **Acute dystonic reactions** may occur shortly after starting therapy and are characterized by torticollis, opisthotonos, tics, grimacing, dysarthria, and oculogyric crisis. For severe reactions, diphenhydramine, 25–50 mg PO, IM, or IV, or benztropine, 1–2 mg PO, IM, or IV, are usually effective.

    d. **Tardive dyskinesia** is a late side effect (occurring after months to years of therapy) characterized by involuntary movements of the tongue, lips, jaw, and extremities. The syndrome may emerge during phenothiazine therapy and is frequently unmasked when the dosage is lowered; it may persist indefinitely after the drug is stopped.

4. **Skin reactions** include photosensitivity, urticaria, and maculopapular rashes.

5. **Cholestatic jaundice,** which occurs most commonly with chlorpromazine, is

Table 1-2. Selected phenothiazines and related antipsychotic drugs

Drug	Class	Usual range of total oral daily dosage (mg)	Sedative effects	Hypotensive effects	Extrapyramidal effects
Chlorpromazine	Aliphatic phenothiazine	100–1000	+ + +	+ + +	+ to + +
Thioridazine	Piperidine phenothiazine	100–600	+ + +	+ + to + + +	+
Fluphenazine	Piperazine phenothiazine	2–30	+	+	+ + +
Perphenazine	Piperazine phenothiazine	8–32	+ to + +	+	+ + +
Trifluoperazine	Piperazine phenothiazine	5–40	+ to + +	+	+ + +
Haloperidol	Butyrophenone	2–15	+	+	+ + +
Thiothixene	Thioxanthene	6–60	+ to + +	+ to + +	+ + to + + +

Source: Modified from A. G. Gilman, L. S. Goodman, and A. Gilman. *Goodman and Gilman's The Pharmacological Basis of Therapeutics* (6th ed.). New York: Macmillan, 1980; and from American Medical Association. *AMA Drug Evaluations.* New York: Wiley, 1980.

Table 1-3. Selected tricyclic antidepressants

Drug	Usual total dose on first day (mg)	Usual range of total daily dosage to achieve clinical response (mg)	Sedative effects	Anticholinergic effects
Amitriptyline	50	100–300	+ + +	+ + +
Imipramine	50	100–300	+ +	+ +
Doxepin	50	100–300	+ + +	+ + +
Desipramine	50	100–300	+	+
Nortriptyline	25	75–100	+ +	+
Protriptyline	15	15–60	+	+ +

Source: Modified from A. G. Gilman, L. S. Goodman, and A. Gilman. *Goodman and Gilman's The Pharmacological Basis of Therapeutics* (6th ed.). New York: Macmillan, 1980; and from American Medical Association. *AMA Drug Evaluations.* New York: Wiley, 1980.

a hypersensitivity reaction often accompanied by eosinophilia. Cholestasis usually occurs during the first month of therapy and subsides without residua after withdrawal of the drug.

6. **Hematologic reactions.** In many patients, mild transient leukopenia may develop. Rarely, agranulocytosis may occur, usually during the first 3 months of therapy. Thus, a WBC count should be obtained in patients in whom an infection develops while they are taking these drugs.

7. **Other side effects** include galactorrhea, pigmentary retinopathy or keratopathy, and lowering of the seizure threshold.

D. **Clinical use, preparations, and dosage**

1. **Acute psychotic rections.** Haloperidol is the usual drug of choice in doses of 2–5 mg PO or IM. Doses may be repeated at 1-hour intervals with IM administration until the desired effect is achieved, after which administration tid or qid suffices.

2. **Chronic antipsychotic therapy.** These drugs are useful in schizophrenia, schizoaffective disorders, and organic brain syndromes with psychotic manifestations. Dosages vary tremendously, depending on the clinical setting, response, and side effects; furthermore, individual patients differ widely in their metabolism of antipsychotic drugs. The lowest effective dosages should be employed, especially with elderly or debilitated patients. Initial oral administration is usually tid–qid until the optimal dosage is found; thereafter, the total daily dosage may be given twice a day or as a single dose at bedtime. Fluphenazine is available in a depot form that usually lasts 2–4 weeks. Individual oral preparations, with the usual range of daily dosages and relative side effects, are listed in Table 1-2.

3. **Other uses**

   a. **Treatment of nausea and vomiting.** Prochlorperazine is commonly given in a dosage of 5–10 mg IM or PO qid prn; the dosage as a rectal suppository is 25 mg bid. The incidence of dystonic reactions is relatively high with this drug. Most of the other phenothiazines also have antiemetic properties (thioridazine is an exception).

   b. **Pruritus.** Two preparations used for the treatment of pruritus are trimeprazine, in a dosage of 2.5 mg PO tid–qid, or methdilazine, 8 mg PO bid–qid. These drugs are not recommended as first-line agents in the treatment of pruritus.

   c. **Intractable hiccups.** Chlorpromazine may be given in the lowest effective dosage.

III. **Antidepressants.** In recent years, the use of tricyclic antidepressants has become widespread. However, the mere labeling of a patient as "depressed" is not sufficient reason to begin treatment with these agents. Rather, the clinician should learn to identify the types of depression that may respond favorably to drug therapy. The classification of depression and the indications for treatment are discussed in standard psychiatry textbooks.

A. **Tricyclic antidepressants**

1. **Pharmacologic properties.** These drugs block the uptake of norephinephrine and serotonin by CNS nerve terminals; in addition, they possess significant anticholinergic and antihistaminic properties. Their long half-lives permit once-daily dosage in many instances. Conversion of imipramine to desipramine and amitriptyline to nortriptyline occurs in vivo. All these compounds undergo hepatic metabolism. Individual patients differ significantly in their metabolism of tricyclic antidepressants.

2. Clinical precautions

a. Tricyclic antidepressants are now the leading cause of death by drug overdose in the United States. Because they are given to patients who are at high risk of suicide, **prescriptions should be limited to a total quantity of 1 gm** (without refills) in the early phases of therapy and any other time that the patient appears suicidal. Management of overdose is discussed in Chap. 23.

b. Tricyclics should not be used to treat insomnia when this symptom is not clearly associated with depression.

c. These drugs should be prescribed with extreme caution to patients with cardiovascular disease, prostatic hypertrophy, and glaucoma.

d. Drug interactions. Tricyclic antidepressants negate the antihypertensive effects of guanethidine and clonidine. Anticholinergic side effects may be enhanced with concurrent use of phenothiazines. Alcohol and barbiturates may potentiate tricyclic toxicity.

3. Side effects and toxic reactions

a. Sedation occurs in varying degrees depending on the specific preparation (see Table 1-3). Other CNS effects may include tremor, anxiety, confusion, and lowering of seizure threshold in susceptible patients.

b. Anticholinergic effects include dry mouth, constipation, blurred vision, urinary retention, and tachycardia.

c. Cardiovascular effects include orthostatic hypotension, myocardial depression, tachycardia, dysrhythmias, conduction abnormalities, and ECG changes (prolongation of the QRS or Q–Tc intervals, and ST–T wave changes). **These drugs should be used cautiously in patients with cardiovascular disease.**

d. Hypersensitivity reactions include skin rashes, leukopenia, and cholestatic jaundice.

4. Clinical use, preparations, and dosage

a. For patients with agitated depression who might benefit from sedative drug effects, **amitriptyline** is the agent of choice. When sedation must be avoided, **desipramine** is a logical choice. For these two drugs (and for imipramine and doxepin), the usual starting dose is 50 mg hs. The dosage should be increased every 2–3 days by increments of 25–50 mg until a dose of 100–150 mg hs is reached.

b. Patients usually require 2–4 weeks for a significant clinical response. If no response is obtained during this time period, the dosage may gradually be increased further over several weeks to a maximum of 300 mg daily, although this is rarely necessary. Plasma drug levels should be used to assess nonresponding patients or those with toxic side effects.

c. When good clinical response has been maintained, the dosage should gradually be reduced to the lowest effective maintenance dose. In many patients, the drug can be gradually discontinued after 4–8 months with maintenance of clinical remission.

d. Although single bedtime doses are usually optimal, elderly patients or those with relative contraindications (e.g., cardiac disease) may better tolerate divided doses. Doxepin or desipramine may be less cardiotoxic than other tricyclic agents, although this is controversial.

A list of preparations, doses, and relative sedative effects is given in Table 1-3.

B. Other agents. Monoamine oxidase inhibitors (for depression) and lithium (for manic-depressive or manic disorders) should generally be employed by psychiatrists or other physicians experienced in their use. However, all clinically active physicians should be aware of their major adverse effects.

1. **Monoamine oxidase inhibitors** (phenelzine, tranylcypromine, and isocarboxazid) may interact with tyramine-containing foods or other drugs to produce **hypertensive crisis.** Examples of such foods are certain cheeses, red wines, beer, processed meats, chocolate, yeast, herring, chicken livers, broad beans, and canned figs; drugs include sympathomimetic amines (such as those in cold remedies or diet pills), methyldopa, and levodopa. **Treatment** includes immediate administration of an alpha-adrenergic–blocking drug such as phentolamine. A 5-mg dose is injected slowly IV and may be repeated in 4–6 hours if needed. Levarterenol should be readily available in case an exaggerated hypotensive response to phentolamine occurs.

2. **Lithium** in therapeutic doses may produce goiter (with or without hypothyroidism), nephrogenic diabetes insipidus, and leukocytosis. Symptoms of lithium toxicity (serum levels greater than 1.5 mEq/liter) include nausea, vomiting, diarrhea, drowsiness, tremor, ataxia, seizures, coma, cardiac dysrhythmias, and hypotension. Because lithium is almost entirely excreted in the urine, renal insufficiency predisposes to toxic levels. Loop diuretics and thiazides may promote retention of lithium in the proximal renal tubule, leading to increased serum levels.

Dermatologic Therapy

Prior to initiation of therapy for dermatologic problems, it is important to secure an accurate diagnosis; where applicable, diagnostic procedures (such as fungal scrapings, cultures, biopsies) should be done when the patient is first seen. When possible, therapy should be directed at eradicating a specific etiologic agent. When this is not possible, supportive therapy must include alleviation of symptoms, restoration of proper hydration, cleansing and debridement, reduction of inflammation, protection, and reduction of scaling. If an eruption does not respond in the expected time, the physician should consider the possibility of misdiagnosis or a complication, such as sweat retention, secondary bacterial infection, or contact sensitivity to one of the ingredients of the topical preparation.

I. **General principles**

A. **Restoration of proper hydration**

1. **Dry skin** is a common problem, especially in older patients. Bathing should be kept to a minimum (as infrequently as once a week in severe cases) and should be of short duration.

a. **Soap** should be used only on the face, axillae, crural areas, feet, and obvious dirty areas. Preferably, soap should be minimally defatting and of neutral pH (e.g., Alpha Keri, Basis, Dove, Neutrogena, and others).

b. **Bath oils** should be used routinely; however, patients should be cautioned about slipping in the tub. Commercial products include Alpha Keri, Domol, Lubath, and Lubriderm, among others.

c. **Lubricating emollients** can be applied frequently but should be thoroughly rubbed into the skin to avoid excessive greasiness or sweat retention. Available products include Aquaphor, Eucerin, Nivea, lanolin, hydrophilic ointment USP, white petrolatum, and urea-containing agents (Aquacare, Carmol, Nutraplus, and others).

2. **Excessive moisture** is a problem in intertriginous areas. Drying and ventilation are required. In severe cases, with maceration, exudation, or erosions, moist compresses may be applied, after which the area should be blotted and air-dried. In chronic cases, therapy consists of separation of the skin layers by absorbent cotton and liberal use of drying powders such as talc (cornstarch should be avoided, since it may support microbial growth).

B. **Cleansing and debridement.** Cleansing is particularly useful in weeping, vesiculobullous, pustular, or ulcerated lesions. The ingredients added to the water are less important than proper application. The most universally available and useful solution is saline (mix approximately 1 tsp table salt/500 ml water). Besides promoting cleanliness and debridement, this therapy affords temporary relief of pruritus and reduction of inflammation. Generally, tepid solutions are most desirable, although warm soaks are better for furuncles and cellulitis. A clean, soft, white cloth (such as a diaper) is immersed in the solution, gently squeezed, and applied to the skin; it is reimmersed in the solution q2–3min to enhance debridement and allow for evaporation. This process is continued for 5–15 minutes and repeated as often as q2h, depending on requirements and response. Since wet compresses have a marked drying effect, they should be discontinued before xerosis and fissuring occur. Other commonly used solutions are as follows:

1. **Aluminum acetate** is mildly antiseptic, astringent, and drying. It does not stain. Burow's solution, 30 ml, is diluted to 1–2 liters with water, or 1 tablet or packet may be dissolved in 0.5–1.0 liter of water.

2. **Magnesium sulfate (Epsom salts)** is bacteriostatic. Dissolve 1 tblsp/liter of water.

3. **Silver nitrate** solutions of 0.1–0.5% are bacteriostatic and astringent but cause staining.

C. **Control of itching and burning.** It is important to relieve these symptoms, since uncontrolled scratching by the patient may perpetuate an otherwise limited dermatitis. Itching and burning are only symptoms whose underlying cause should be specifically treated if possible.

1. **Topical agents**

   a. **Camphor** 1–3% and **menthol** 0.25–2.0% provide a cooling sensation.

   b. **Phenol** 0.5–2.0% causes local hypesthesia. Phenol products should not be used on raw or ulcerated skin because of possibly excessive systemic absorption.

   c. **Calamine lotion**

   d. Combinations of the preceding agents are commonly used in an appropriate base. For example, menthol and phenol may be mixed with Eucerin or Nivea.

2. **Systemic agents. Oral antihistamines** are invaluable antipruritic agents. Commonly used drugs include diphenhydramine, 25–50 mg up to q4h, and hydroxyzine, 10–50 mg up to q4h. Other useful agents include cyproheptadine and the phenothiazine trimeprazine. Patients should be warned about the sedative and anticholinergic actions of these drugs.

D. **Control of inflammation.**

1. **Topical corticosteroids** are available in many forms. In order, from most lubricating to most drying, are ointments (water in oil base), creams (oil in water base) and gels, aerosols, and lotions. For example, a lubricating ointment is needed for chronic dry eczema. For an acute weeping eczematous dermatitis, a cream, spray, or lotion would be proper. Lotions and solutions

Table 1-4. Commonly used topical corticosteroids

Creams and ointments
   Low strength
      Hydrocortisone 1%
      Desonide 0.05%
   Medium strength
      Triamcinolone acetonide 0.1%
      Flurandrenolide 0.05%
      Fluocinolone acetonide 0.025%
      Betamethasone valerate 0.1%
      Betamethasone diproprionate 0.05%
   High strength
      Halcinonide 0.1%
      Fluocinonide 0.05%
      Desoximetasone 0.25%
   Lotions and solutions (strengths correspond to those noted above)
      Hydrocortisone lotion 1%
      Triamcinolone acetonide lotion 0.1%
      Fluocinolone acetonide solution 0.01%
      Betamethasone valerate lotion 0.1%

are easy to use in hairy areas, including the scalp. Gels are also effective on the scalp.

2. The **fluorinated steroids** are significantly more effective per unit weight than are hydrocortisone or other nonfluorinated steroids. The potency of these products may be further increased (by means of better penetration) by occlusion with plastic wrap. For occlusion therapy of very limited areas of chronic dermatitis, one may use steroid-impregnated flurandrenolide (Cordran) tape. Excessive occlusion therapy, however, can cause sweat retention, atrophy, maceration, and folliculitis. If extensive areas of abnormal skin are occluded for a long period, pituitary-adrenal axis suppression may result.

3. The **frequency** of application varies with the clinical situation. Topical steroids are usually applied bid–qid, but some patients may require more frequent use initially. Adequate quantities of these preparations should be dispensed; otherwise, applications will be too infrequent or limited. When cream or ointment is used sparingly, 20–45 gm is needed to cover the entire body of an adult once.

4. Strength of preparations. Table 1-4 divides commonly used steroid creams and ointments into three groups. Low-strength preparations are indicated for facial use (stronger preparations may cause facial acne or rosacea). Medium-strength preparations are used in most dermatoses of average severity. High-strength preparations are employed for severe or resistant lesions and for hand and foot involvement. Lotions and solutions are also listed.

E. Protection

  1. Thin, white, **cotton gloves** under rubber gloves may be used to avoid contact with excessive water or chemical irritants. The cotton gloves allow absorption of palmar sweat and may be cleaned frequently.

  2. Barrier creams and ointments (containing silicone) may prevent contact of irritating chemicals with sensitive skin but are not substitutes for mechanical barriers when they can be used.

  3. Sunscreens. For fair-skinned persons or patients with dermatoses exacerbated by exposure to ultraviolet light (UVL), sunscreens are useful adjuncts to long sleeves and wide-brimmed hats; UVB (280–320 nm) is the principal ultraviolet wavelength responsible for sunburn. Certain light-sensitive disorders (e.g., porphyria, phytophotodermatitis) and photosensitizing drugs (e.g., thiazides, tetracyclines, sulfonamides) are responsive to wavelengths in the UVA range (320–400 nm). Sunscreens for UVB are sufficient for routine prophylaxis when sunbathing. Combinations that afford protection against both UVB and UVA are generally required for light-exacerbated dermatoses.

Sunscreens are rated by a "sun protection factor" (SPF 15 is strong, SPF 8 is intermediate, and SPF 5 is mild). Sunscreens should be reapplied after bathing or sweating.

a. **Para-aminobenzoic acid (PABA)** and its esters (padimate O, padimate A) absorb UVB and are ideal for preventing sunburn. It is applied 1 hour before exposure. Numerous preparations are available.

b. **Benzophenone derivatives** (oxybenzone, dioxybenzone) absorb wavelengths from 250–360 nm and, to a lesser degree, from 360–400 nm. They are less effective than PABA in the sunburn range (280–320 nm). Benzophenones are available alone or in combination with PABA and PABA esters.

c. **Titanium dioxide** and zinc oxide are opaque sunblockers that shield against all wavelengths. They would be ideal except for cosmetic unacceptability.

F. **Reduction of scaling.** With few exceptions (e.g., ichthyosis vulgaris), scaling is the result of rapid proliferation of the epidermis. Scaling can be reduced with adequate hydration (see **A.1**), keratolytics, and suppressors of epidermal proliferation. The following are used on intact skin only:

1. **Keratolytics. Salicylic acid** 3–6% comes in an ointment base for general use. Efficacy is increased by occlusion. Salicylic acid 6% gel, used with occlusion, is very effective for focal hyperkeratoses, including those on the scalp. Salicylic acid 40% plaster can be applied to warts and calluses.

2. **Suppressors of epidermal proliferation** are most commonly used in the treatment of psoriasis. Preparations include tars and anthralin 0.1–1.0% ointment, which stains and is irritating (see sec. **II.D**).

II. **Specific therapy of selected disorders**

A. **Acne vulgaris.** Treatment includes topical medications, oral antibiotics, and acne surgery. Routine dietary restrictions are not justified.

1. **Benzoyl peroxide** 5–10% has antibacterial and drying effects and is the mainstay of therapy. It may be applied overnight or twice daily as tolerated by the patient. Initial therapy should consist of a 5% preparation used for limited periods of time, to minimize irritation. Alcohol-based gels (e.g., Benzac, Benzagel, PanOxyl) are more potent than nonalcohol-based gels (e.g., Desquam-X, Persa-Gel).

2. **Retinoic acid** 0.05–0.1% cream or 0.01–0.025% gel inhibits comedone formation but may be irritating (mild facial erythema is to be expected). It is applied once daily and may be alternated cautiously with benzoyl peroxide in patients who do not respond sufficiently to either agent alone.

3. **Topical antibiotic solutions** include clindamycin, tetracycline, and erythromycin. They may be used alone (e.g., in patients who experience excessive irritation with benzoyl peroxide) or alternated with the preceding agents.

4. **Systemic antibiotics** are used for patients with moderate to severe inflammatory acne (usually along with some type of topical therapy). Tetracycline,

250 mg PO qid, is the drug of choice. The dosage is gradually reduced to 250 mg qd or discontinued after improvement has occurred. Erythromycin in the same dosage is also effective.

   5. **Regular drainage** of cysts, nodules, and pustules, removal of closed comedones, and the use of intralesional corticosteroids are necessary for the most effective management of acne.

B. Eczematous dermatitis

   1. **Acute eczematous dermatitis** is characterized by erythema, weeping, and vesiculation. It occurs in **atopic dermatitis, contact dermatitis, dyshidrotic eczema,** and other disorders. It should be treated with wet compresses (see sec. **I.B**), topical steroids applied after each application of a wet compress (see sec. **I.D.1** and Table 1-4), and oral antipruritics to suppress itching (see sec. **I.C.2**). When the dermatitis is extensive or involves the face, as often happens in severe **poison ivy,** rapidly tapered oral corticosteroids may be required (e.g., prednisone, 60 mg on the first day, decreased by 5 mg daily for a total of 12 days of therapy). Oral steroid therapy should last at least 10 days to minimize the possibility of a rebound flare of the rash, but long-term steroid therapy is contraindicated.

   2. **Chronic eczematous dermatitis** (lichenification, scaling, and hyperpigmentation) requires elimination of scratching and other irritating factors. Frequent use of topical corticosteroid creams and ointments (with or without occlusion), topical and systemic antipruritic agents, and emollients are beneficial.

   3. **Preventive measures** are important in the management of eczematous dermatitis. These include elimination of known environmental and contact allergens, avoidance of dry skin (see sec. **I.A.1**), and wearing protective gloves during dishwashing.

C. Intertrigo. The occluding surfaces of skin should be separated to allow drying; wet compresses are useful in severe cases (see sec. **I.A.2**). Topical steroids are helpful, alone or in combination with antimicrobial agents when secondary bacterial or candidal infection occurs. However, combination preparations (e.g., corticosteroids with iodochlorhydroxyquin, nystatin, or antibiotics) should not be used when specific agents suffice. In patients in whom there is a tendency for intertrigo to develop, overzealous cleaning of the areas with soap, iodine, alcohol, etc., should be avoided.

D. Psoriasis

   1. **Most patients have mild to moderate involvement** that is relatively easy to control. Ultraviolet light, including sunlight, is very effective therapy. Topical corticosteroid creams and ointments (of medium to high strength) are applied tid–qid (see sec. **I.D** and Table 1-4). Overnight occlusion of steroids with plastic wrap will hasten the resolution of lesions.

   Some patients derive further benefit when tar compounds are alternated with corticosteroids. The mechanism of action of tars is unknown. Tar gels (e.g., Estar, PsoriGel) are more cosmetically acceptable than other preparations, which include crude coal tar ointment (2–5%) and coal tar solution (liquor carbonis detergens). Tar bath preparations are useful for widespread involvement.

   When there is marked hyperkeratosis, keratolytic agents may initially be alternated with topical steroids. Salicylic acid 6% gel with overnight occlusion and anthralin 0.1–0.4% paste are effective.

   2. **Acute eruptive forms** of psoriasis are cautiously approached to avoid exacerbation into a generalized exfoliative erythroderma. Bed rest, sedation, topical steroids, and lubricating emollients may be used until the process is sufficiently stabilized to permit more vigorous therapy.

3. **The modified Goekerman regimen** is applicable for widespread eruptions resistant to other therapy and is best initiated in the hospital. Crude coal tar 2–4% in petrolatum is applied to the psoriatic lesions at bedtime. In the morning, the patient is exposed to short-wavelength UVL, with daily increments starting from a minimal erythema dose. The eyes must be protected. Next, the patient bathes in water to which a tar bath solution has been added. Tar soap may be used as well. After bathing, steroid creams or ointments are applied regularly, with or without occlusion.

4. **Scalp lesions** can be treated with corticosteroid solutions and tar shampoos. If scaling is severe, treatment may be continued during the night with keratolytic preparations (e.g., 6% salicylic acid gel, 3–5% salicylic acid in acid mantle cream) or anthralin 0.1–0.4% ointment. In the morning, these are washed out with a tar shampoo.

5. Patients with severe generalized eruptions and/or arthritis who are resistant to the preceding treatments and incapacitated by their disease may be treated with **systemic chemotherapeutic agents** such as methotrexate.

6. The combination of systemic psoralens and high-intensity long-wavelength UVL exposure (PUVA) is a recent development in the treatment of extensive psoriasis. The results have been extremely encouraging, but at present the long-term side effects of this treatment are unknown.

   Note. Chemotherapeutic agents and long-wavelength UVL should be administered only by physicians who are very familiar with their use.

E. **Seborrheic dermatitis** is an inflammatory, erythematous eruption with scaling that is frequently oily and slightly yellow. It most often involves the scalp and face. Scalp involvement is most effectively treated by 2.5% selenium sulfide shampoo, applied up to 3 times/week for 5–10 minutes per treatment. Other effective shampoos contain zinc pyrithione, sulfur-salicylic acid, and tar. For more inflammatory scalp lesions, steroid lotion or solution may be applied. A keratolytic gel may be used for areas of thick scaling.

Hydrocortisone cream 1%, applied qd–bid, is effective for treatment of seborrheic dermatitis of the face and other areas. **Fluorinated steroids should not be used on the face.**

F. **Urticaria** (and the related lesion angioedema) is frequently of unknown etiology. However, it may occur secondary to drugs, foods and their additives, dyes, atopy, vasculitis, viral infections, and physical factors, such as pressure, cold, heat, and light. Urticaria accompanied by signs of anaphylaxis is a medical emergency (see Chap. 23).

All identified predisposing factors should be avoided. For established lesions, oral antihistamines are the mainstay of therapy, although topical antipruritic agents may be useful adjuncts (see sec. I.C). For chronic refractory cases, one may have to try a variety of antihistamine preparations, using the maximally tolerated dosages. In cases resistant to these H_1-receptor antagonists, other compounds have been used with varying success. These include H_2-receptor antagonists (e.g., cimetidine), theophylline, and sympathomimetic agents (e.g., terbutaline, ephedrine). Short courses of oral corticosteroids should be reserved only for refractory cases.

G. **Fungal skin infections.** The clinical diagnosis should be confirmed by positive culture, or visualization of fungal forms with a 10% potassium hydroxide preparation, or both.

1. **Candidiasis.** Drying and ventilation are necessary in affected intertriginous areas and in periungual candidiasis.

   a. Nystatin cream, 100,000 units/gm, miconazole 2% cream or lotion, or clotrimazole 1% cream or solution are applied tid.

   b. Periungual candidiasis responds to drying and to thymol 2–4% in 70% isopropyl alcohol, applied bid–tid.

2. **Dermatophyte infections** of small areas of glabrous skin and feet (i.e., tinea corporis, tinea cruris, tinea pedis) respond to miconazole, clotrimazole, haloprogin, or tolnaftate applied tid. Nystatin is not effective.

3. **Tinea capitis, onychomycosis, and widespread dermatophyte infection.** Micronized **griseofulvin,** 0.5–1.0 gm PO daily in divided doses, is the treatment of choice. Therapy is continued until the infection is culture negative and clinically resolved (approximately 4–6 weeks for tinea capitis, 4 weeks for tinea corporis, and 6–8 months for fingernail infection). Toenail infections are often resistant to all therapy, but one may attempt treatment with griseofulvin and topical medications (often for 1–2 years). Headache and gastrointestinal distress are the most common side effects of griseofulvin therapy. As leukopenia and hepatotoxicity may occur, monitoring by CBCs and liver function tests should be done with prolonged therapy. Griseofulvin decreases the anticoagulant effect of warfarin. **Ketoconazole,** a new broad-spectrum antifungal agent, may be effective in resistant cases or in patients not tolerating griseofulvin.

4. **Tinea versicolor.** Regardless of the mode of therapy, this condition often recurs.

   a. Selenium sulfide 2.5% suspension, applied with scrubbing for 15 minutes daily for 1–2 weeks, will clear scaling; pigmentary changes are slow to resolve. Further applications (several times monthly) may help to prevent relapse.

   b. Sodium thiosulfate 25% bid may be applied for several weeks.

   c. Clotrimazole, miconazole, haloprogin, and tolnaftate are effective but are much more expensive.

H. Bacterial skin infections are encountered in a wide variety of clinical situations. Only a few common disorders are discussed here.

1. **Impetigo,** though more common in children, is occasionally seen in adults. The nonbullous type is usually streptococcal in origin; phenoxymethyl penicillin or erythromycin is effective in a dosage of 250 mg PO qid for adults. The bullous type is usually staphylococcal; a beta-lactamase–resistant penicillin (e.g., dicloxacillin) or erythromycin in a dosage of 250 mg PO qid should be used. Frequent warm soaks are useful for debridement of crusts. *ceporex 500 q*

2. **Cellulitis** is usually staphylococcal or streptococcal in origin. Because it is often difficult to identify the offending organism, dicloxacillin, cephalexin, or erythromycin (all at dosages of 250–500 mg PO qid) are used to ensure adequate coverage of both organisms. Patients with toxic symptoms require parenteral therapy (cephalothin, 1–2 gm IV q6h, or oxacillin, 1–2 gm IV q6h).

3. Large **furuncles** (boils) or **carbuncles** should generally be incised and drained. In some cases, frequent application of warm soaks will result in spontaneous drainage. When there is surrounding cellulitis, general toxicity, or the lesion is located on the face, local therapy is supplemented with systemic antibiotics, as discussed in **2** for cellulitis.

   Folliculitis can usually be controlled with good topical hygeine and use of antimicrobial cleansers (e.g., pHisoHex, Hibiclens). However, stubborn, recurrent furunculosis may also require weeks to months of systemic antibiotic treatment (with erythromycin or a beta-lactamase–resistant penicillin).

I. Scabies. Lindane (1% gamma benzene hexachloride) cream or lotion should be applied to the entire body from the chin down, with attention to intertriginous areas, skin folds, and finger webs. It is left on overnight, after which the patient showers and dresses in clothing known to be uninfected. The procedure should be repeated the next evening. All clothes and bed linens recently used must be laundered in very hot water or dry-cleaned. All close contacts should be inspected and treated, if indicated, to prevent reinfestation. Treatment can be repeated in one week if necessary. Alternatively, one may use 10% crotamiton cream or lotion in the same manner. **Lindane is contraindicated in pregnant women and young children.**

J. Warts. Recurrences are not uncommon for most types of warts following treatment.

1. **Common warts.** Liquid nitrogen cryotherapy is the most reliable treatment and may be repeated every several weeks if necessary. Daily treatment with a preparation containing 16.7% salicylic acid and 16.7% lactic acid in flexible collodion is slow but often effective and painless.

2. **Plantar warts.** Salicylic acid 40% plaster cut to fit the lesion exactly may be applied daily under adhesive tape occlusion, followed by removal of macerated tissue. Daily application of 16.7% salicylic acid and 16.7% lactic acid in flexible collodion is also effective.

3. **Condylomata acuminata.** Podophyllin 20–25% in tincture of benzoin is applied by the physician, avoiding normal skin, and is washed off thoroughly 4 hours later. Repeat applications may be necessary on a weekly basis. Liquid nitrogen cryotherapy is also effective.

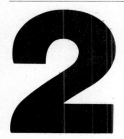

Fluid and Electrolyte Disturbances

Disturbances in acid-base balance and fluid and electrolyte metabolism present physicians with complex diagnostic and therapeutic problems. Proper management depends on a thorough understanding of both disrupted physiology and the potential dangers of therapy. Each patient must be evaluated for preexisting deficits or excesses and continuing losses or gains. The integrity of the patient's hemodynamic and renal function must be determined. Multiple abnormalities may exist simultaneously, making the therapy of each one more difficult. Only after careful consideration of all these factors can the proper therapy be chosen and its rate and route of administration determined.

I. Salts and solutions

A. Commonly used conversions

	mEq of anion or cation/gm of salt	mg of salt/mEq
NaCl	17*	58
NaHCO$_3$	12	84
NaSO$_4 \cdot$ 10H$_2$O	6	161
KCl	13	75
KHCO$_3$	10	100
CaCO$_3$	20	50
CaCl$_2 \cdot$ 2H$_2$O	14	73
Ca gluconate$_2 \cdot$ 1H$_2$O	4	224
Ca lactate$_2 \cdot$ 5H$_2$O	6	154
MgSO$_4 \cdot$ 7H$_2$O	8	123
NH$_4$Cl	19	54

B. IV solutions

	Glucose (gm/L)	Na	Cl	K (mEq/L)	Ca	Lactate
5% D/W	50					
10% D/W	100					
20% D/W†	200					
50% D/W†	500					
0.45% NaCl‡		77	77			
0.9% NaCl‡		154	154			
3% NaCl†		513	513			
Ringer's solution		147.5	156	4	4.5	
Ringer's lactate‡		130	109	4	3	28

*The sodium content of diets is often expressed in grams of Na$^+$ rather than in grams of NaCl; 1 gm of Na$^+$ is 43 mEq, whereas 1 gm of NaCl is 17 mEq. Therefore, a 4-gm sodium diet and a 10-gm salt diet contain approximately equal amounts of sodium.

†Hypertonic solutions should be administered slowly and with caution to prevent circulatory overload.

‡Also available with 5% dextrose.

C. Parenteral additives

	Volume (ml) in ampule	mEq in ampule (not concentration)
7.5% sodium bicarbonate	50	44
42.0% sodium phosphate	15	*
7.5% potassium chloride	20	20
14.9% potassium chloride	20	40
46.0% potassium phosphate	15	†
10.0% calcium chloride	10	14
10.0% calcium gluconate	10	4
25.0% magnesium sulfate	2	4
26.8% ammonium chloride	20	100
		gm in ampule
25.0% mannitol	50	12.5
50.0% glucose	50	25

II. **Maintenance therapy.** This section deals with the need for water, sodium, potassium, and carbohydrate in patients who are temporarily unable to take food or fluids orally but who **do not have** abnormal fluid or electrolyte losses, preexisting deficits or excesses, or inadequate renal function.

    A. Feeding by stomach tube is usually preferable to IV fluid administration when normal alimentation is prohibited for prolonged periods (see Chap. 11, sec. **II.E**).

    B. Parenteral maintenance fluids are indicated when artificial feeding is required for only a short period, or when tube feeding is contraindicated.

        1. The **water requirements** for maintaining fluid balance are the sum of the urine output necessary to excrete the daily solute load plus insensible losses (secondary to evaporation from the skin and respiratory tract) minus the amount of water produced from the endogenous metabolism of fat and carbohydrate. Under normal conditions the body generates approximately 600 mOsm of solute/day. Assuming that a maximal urine concentrating capacity is 1200 mOsm/kg of urine, the minimal urine output is 500 ml/day. If the kidney is incapable of maximal concentration of the urine (e.g., in renal failure or in the postoperative state), or if there is an increased rate of solute production due to catabolism, a urine volume of 1200–1500 ml/day may be necessary. In the afebrile patient living at a comfortable temperature and humidity, 500–800 ml of insensible water losses occurs. Endogenous water production is normally 300 ml. Therefore, normal maintenance fluid therapy consists of approximately 1 liter of water/day. However, under many hospital circumstances the insensible losses may be high (see sec. **III**), and the renal concentrating capacity may be impaired. Therefore, usually larger amounts of fluid (approximately 35 ml/kg/day) are administered.

        2. Sodium virtually disappears from the urine after several days of sodium-free intake, but, in the interval, a mild deficit accrues (in addition, continuing losses may occur in sweat and feces). It is thus customary to supply about 70 mEq Na^+ (4 gm NaCl) daily. As a rule, **potassium** excretion cannot be curtailed sufficiently to prevent significant depletion. A minimum of 20 mEq potassium/day must be given to allow for obligatory urinary losses; usually, 40–60 mEq/day is preferable if renal function is adequate. **Carbohydrate** (100–150 gm/day) is necessary to minimize protein catabolism and prevent ketosis.

        3. Adequate parenteral maintenance may be provided by administering 1000

---

*A 15-ml ampule contains 45 mmols of phosphate (1395 mg phosphorus) and 60 mEq of sodium (see *Ann. Intern. Med.* 89:941, 1978).

†A 15-ml ampule contains 45 mmols of phosphate (1395 mg phosphorus) and 66 mEq of potassium (see *Ann. Intern. Med.* 89:941, 1978).

ml 10% D/W with 20 mEq KCl over 12 hours, and 1000 ml 5% D/W .45% saline with 20 mEq KCl over 12 hours. Calcium, magnesium, phosphorus, vitamins, and protein replacement may be necessary after 1 week of parenteral therapy (see Chap. 11).

III. Replacement of observed abnormal losses. Observed losses of water and electrolytes must be replaced in addition to meeting the maintenance requirements.

A. Insensible and sensible losses. Insensible loss of water (evaporation from the skin and lungs) increases with hyperventilation, fever, high room temperature, and low humidity and should be replaced with 5% D/W.

Sensible loss (sweat), because of its role in body temperature regulation, varies greatly in volume (0–2000 ml/hour). It is extremely difficult to estimate the volume of sweat; in circumstances in which sweat losses may be large, accurate replacement is best guided by changes in body weight. Roughly 500 ml/day may be lost if the body temperature is above 38.0°C. Similarly, baseline water requirements increase by 500 ml/day for each 2–3°C above 32°C of ambient room temperature. Losses should be replaced with hypotonic saline (Table 2-1).

B. Gastrointestinal losses will vary in quantity and concentration of electrolytes. For precise replacement, the electrolyte content of secretions such as diarrheal fluid should be measured. Most laboratories can measure the potassium and sodium in the secretions. If the laboratory cannot determine the electrolyte content of the fluid, the estimates in Table 2-1 are an adequate guide to replacement.

C. Urinary losses. Excessive urinary sodium loss may occur in patients receiving diuretics, recovering from tubular necrosis, experiencing postobstructive diuresis, or with medullary cystic disease or adrenal insufficiency. Urinary potassium loss may be great in patients receiving diuretics or corticosteroids, in the diuretic phase of tubular necrosis, in renal tubular acidosis, or with hyperaldosteronism. In prolonged polyuric states, laboratory determination of urinary sodium and potassium is therefore the only accurate guide to quantitative replacement.

D. Rapid internal shifts of fluid necessitating fluid replacement may occur with peritonitis, pancreatitis, portal vein thrombosis, extensive burns, fulminant nephrotic syndrome, ileus, bacterial enteritis, crush injuries, and, to a variable extent, in the postoperative period.

IV. Salt and water

A. Total body water (TBW) constitutes approximately 60% of the total body weight. Its distribution is illustrated in the diagram (ICF = intracellular fluid; ECF = extracellular fluid; IF = interstitial fluid).

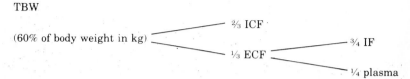

B. Volume depletion (ECF volume depletion) results from loss of sodium and water in various proportions, depending on the pathologic process (see Table 2-1). If the loss is isonatremic, tonicity of the ECF is relatively unaffected, and intracellular volume will change minimally. Loss of water in excess of sodium may occur (sweating, hyperventilation, nasogastric suction, severe diarrhea), resulting in hypernatremia; however, the increased ECF osmolality in this situation will cause intracellular water to move into the ECF and suppress the clinical manifestations of hypovolemia. If the fluid administered contains a lower sodium concentration than the fluid lost, hyponatremia may result. Final

Table 2-1. Electrolyte content of sweat and gastrointestinal secretions

Sweat or gastrointestinal secretion	Electrolyte concentration (mEq/L)					Replacement amount for each liter lost			
	Na$^+$	K$^+$	H$^+$	Cl$^-$	HCO$_3^-$	Isotonic saline (ml)	5% D/W (ml)	KCl[a] (mEq)	NaHCO$_3$[b] (mEq)
Sweat	30–50	5		45–55		300	700	5	
Gastric secretions	40–65	10	90[c]	100–140		300	700	20[d]	
Pancreatic fistula	135–155	5		55–75	70–90	250	750	5	90
Biliary fistula	135–155	5		80–110	35–50	750	250	5	45
Ileostomy fluid	120–130	10		50–60	50–70	300	700	10	67.6
Diarrhea fluid	25–50	35–60		20–40	30–45		1000	35	45

[a]Caution should be used in administering more than 10 mEq K$^+$/hr.
[b]One ampule of 7.5% NaHCO$_3$ contains 45 mEq HCO$_3^-$.
[c]Variable; e.g., achlorhydria.
[d]Administration of more than the observed gastric loss of potassium is often required because of enhanced urinary potassium excretion in alkalosis.

serum sodium concentration will depend on the volume of fluid lost, its electrolyte concentration, the composition and volume of any fluid used for replacement, and the kidney's ability to maintain homeostasis. Hyponatremia and hypernatremia are discussed in **D** and **E**.

The major **causes of volume depletion** include GI losses (vomiting, diarrhea, surgical drainage, ileostomy), diuretic administration, renal or adrenal disease (through abnormal urinary Na loss), and sequestration of fluid (ileus, burns, peritonitis).

1. **Manifestations.** The symptoms of volume depletion include anorexia, nausea, vomiting, apathy, weakness, and orthostatic dizziness or syncope. Signs include weight loss (500-ml fluid loss per pound decrease in weight), postural hypotension, poor skin turgor (best tested on the forehead or sternal region), sunken eyes, and a weak pulse with tachycardia. When the volume depletion is severe, shock and coma may occur.

   There is no practical method of measuring extracellular volume. The serum sodium concentration is **not** a guide to volume depletion (rather, it reflects the relationship between total amounts of extracellular sodium and water); in volume depletion it is often normal. The BUN is usually elevated out of proportion to the serum creatinine; the urine specific gravity is high, the urine sodium concentration is low (except in renal or adrenal salt wasting), and the urine volume is decreased. The hematocrit and serum protein concentration rise; the changes in these values may be useful in approximating the decrease in plasma volume.

2. **Treatment** must be aimed at restoring the contracted ECF volume by administering solutions that replace the lost fluid and electrolytes. Mild degrees of volume depletion may be repleted orally (10-gm salt diet and 2–3 liters of fluid/day). If acidosis is present, part of the sodium should be administered as $NaHCO_3$. Consideration also must be given to potassium and calcium balance. Replacement of ongoing fluid and electrolyte losses and treatment of the underlying cause of those losses are also mandatory.

   If volume depletion is severe, central venous pressure (CVP) or pulmonary capillary wedge pressure may be helpful in gauging the status of volume repletion, particularly if the patient has cardiac decompensation. Because of variability in the measurements, the CVP cannot be interpreted as an absolute value.

C. **Extracellular fluid volume excess.** An increase in total body salt and water occurs in a variety of clinical states, including congestive heart failure (CHF), nephrosis, cirrhosis, and conditions associated with hypoalbuminemia. The underlying disease processes are thought to result in a reduction of the "effective arterial volume," leading to renal salt and water retention. Because the underlying disease process persists, the retained salt and water move into the interstitial fluid or other body spaces (resulting in edema, ascites, effusions, etc.) and thus fail to restore the "effective arterial volume" to normal.

   Acute or chronic renal failure can also be complicated by volume expansion if excessive salt is administered.

1. **Manifestations.** The cardinal manifestation is edema (clinically not apparent until 5–10 lb of fluid have been retained). Manifestations of circulatory overload (dyspnea, tachycardia, venous engorgement, pulmonary congestion) occur in patients with organic heart disease or renal failure who are unable to excrete the quantities of administered salt and water. Ascites is frequently the most prominent finding in patients with cirrhosis.

2. **Treatment** is variable and is directed toward improving the pathologic process. Therapy of the nephrotic syndrome and cardiovascular overload associ-

ated with renal failure is discussed in Chap. 3. Treatment of CHF and cirrhosis are discussed in Chaps. 4 and 12 respectively.

D. Hyponatremia usually results in a reduced serum osmolality and indicates that the amount of sodium present in a given amount of plasma water is less than normal.

The osmolality of the ECF is largely determined by the electrolyte concentration and can be calculated from the formula

$$\text{Osmolality (mOsm/kg)} = 2(\text{Na[mEq/L]} + \text{K[mEq/L]}) + \frac{\text{urea (mg/dl)}}{2.8} + \frac{\text{glucose (mg/dl)}}{18}$$

Normal blood levels of urea and glucose add little to the overall osmolality.

The severity of the symptoms of hyponatremia (confusion, anorexia, lethargy, nausea, vomiting, coma, seizures) depends on the rate of fall of the serum sodium concentration, as well as on the severity of the hyponatremia itself. In general, symptoms do not occur until the serum sodium concentration has fallen below 120–125 mEq/liter.

A useful diagnostic approach to the patient with hyponatremia is through the simultaneous determination of total body salt and water stores.

1. **Hyponatremia with ECF volume excess and edema** (renal failure, nephrotic syndrome, CHF, cirrhosis). In this setting, both total body salt and water are increased but the latter to a greater extent. The mechanism responsible for these hyponatremic states is impaired renal excretion of water. In addition to treatment of the underlying disorder, **water restriction,** usually with diuretic therapy, may be employed to correct the hyponatremia. **Administration of hypertonic saline is hazardous** and seldom of benefit.

2. **Hyponatremia without clinical evidence of dehydration or edema**

    a. **The syndrome of inappropriate antidiuretic hormone (SIADH)** may occur in a variety of settings (most often, in patients with malignant tumors, pulmonary and cerebral disorders, and stress). A variety of drugs have also been associated with SIADH. Initially, the associated hyponatremia is due to water retention, but later is compounded by urinary loss of sodium resulting from volume expansion. The essential criteria for diagnosis of this syndrome are (1) hyponatremia with hyposmolality of serum; (2) urine that is **less than maximally dilute** when compared with plasma osmolality; (3) inappropriately large amounts of urinary sodium; (4) normal renal, thyroid, and adrenal function; (5) no clinical evidence of volume depletion or overload; (6) disappearance of all abnormalities following adequate restriction of water; and (7) the patient should not be taking diuretics.

    When the serum sodium concentration has decreased significantly (below 125 mEq/liter), water intake should be restricted to less than sensible and insensible losses until the serum sodium has returned to normal. Thereafter, water may be given in amounts equal to the sensible and insensible losses plus urine output. Calculation of the water loss necessary to raise the plasma osmolality to normal can be approximated by using the following formulas:

    (1) Current volume body water (L) = 0.6 × current body wt (kg)

    (2) Total body solute (mOsm) = current volume body water (L) × plasma osmolality (mOsm/L)

    (3) Normal volume body water = $\dfrac{\text{total body solute (mOsm)}}{\text{desired plasma osmolality (mOsm/L)}}$

(4) Current volume − normal volume = body water excess (L)

The IV use of potent diuretics (furosemide) to induce a diuresis, followed by hourly replacement of sodium and potassium lost in the urine, can correct severe hyponatremia in 6–8 hours (*Ann. Intern. Med.* 78:870, 1973). Replacement of urinary sodium and potassium losses can be generally accomplished by the use of 0.9% saline (occasionally 3% saline will be required) to which potassium has been added. It should be emphasized that this therapeutic approach is potentially hazardous and is **only** of temporary benefit; it should be reserved for those with severe, symptomatic hyponatremia.

More recently, **demeclocycline** (300–600 mg bid) has been shown to be efficacious in SIADH and may obviate severe water restriction (*N. Engl. J. Med.* 298:173, 1978). This drug has its main use in patients with chronic obstructive lung disease and others who cannot tolerate water restriction. Demeclocycline should be rarely used in patients with liver disease, because its prolonged serum half-life may cause nephrotoxicity. The response to lithium is variable. There are isolated reports that phenytoin (*Ann. Intern. Med.* 90:50, 1979), furosemide (*N. Engl. J. Med.* 304:329, 1981), and oral urea (*Am. J. Med.* 69:99, 1980) may also be effective.

b. The treatment of hyponatremia due to **hypothyroidism, drugs,** or **compulsive polydipsia** involves treatment of the underlying cause as well as water restriction.

c. **Water intoxication,** usually iatrogenic, results from the administration of water to a patient unable to have a water diuresis (e.g., postoperatively or in the presence of renal insufficiency). When water intoxication is chronic or mild, weakness or apathy may be the only manifestation; when it is acute or severe, however, confusion, stupor, muscle twitching, or grand mal seizures may occur.

Restoration of the serum sodium to normal depends on the reduction of body water in respect to sodium. This should be accomplished by restricting water intake. In rare cases of severe, symptomatic hyponatremia (serum Na^+ usually less than 115 mEq/liter), administration of hypertonic saline may be indicated. In this instance, a small quantity of 3% NaCl solution may be used to increase the serum sodium concentration to a level not associated with symptoms; no attempt should be made to restore the sodium concentration to normal by this mode of therapy. The amount of sodium necessary to cause the desired correction in the serum sodium can be calculated by multiplying the difference between the desired and observed sodium concentrations (in milliequivalents per liter) by the TBW volume (in liters). This is potentially a dangerous mode of therapy and can result in severe circulatory overload or CNS symptoms if the sodium concentration is corrected too rapidly. It is rarely indicated.

The method described in **a** (*Ann. Intern. Med.* 78:870, 1973) may also be used when rapid correction of the serum sodium is required.

d. Most cases of hyponatremia are associated with hyposmolality. However, if large concentrations of other osmotically active substances accumulate primarily in ECF, water will diffuse into that space from the ICF and lead to hyponatremia. An increase of 180 mg/dl of glucose, for example, will increase plasma osmolality by 10 mOsm/kg, which in turn will cause a fall in serum sodium concentration of 3.5 mEq/liter. A similar situation is seen after a large dose of IV mannitol. The **treatment** should be designed to decrease the hypertonicity of the ECF (e.g., with the use of insulin in uncontrolled diabetes or by cessation of the mannitol infusion). Hypertonic saline administration should not be used.

3. **Hyponatremia associated with decreased ECF volume** is a state of actual sodium depletion. It occurs when salt and water losses are replaced with relatively sodium-free solutions. These losses can be of renal origin (e.g., osmotic diuresis, salt-losing nephropathy, diuretic phase of acute tubular necrosis, postobstructive diuresis, Bartter's syndrome, diuretic therapy, hypoaldosteronism) or of extrarenal origin (e.g., vomiting, diarrhea, excess sweating, wound drainage, burns). Symptoms are often those of volume depletion (see **B.**1) and can often be confirmed by the demonstration of an orthostatic decrease in blood pressure. The **treatment** is replacement of volume losses with isotonic saline and correction of the underlying disorder.

4. **Pseudohyponatremia.** Hyperlipidemia and hyperproteinemia decrease the proportion of serum that is water. Since sodium is restricted to the aqueous phase, sodium concentration of whole serum is low (if analyzed by flame photometry or indirect potentiometry), even though the sodium concentration and osmolality of serum water are normal. No specific fluid or electrolyte treatment is necessary.

E. **Hypernatremia** may occur if (1) hypotonic fluid losses are replaced by inadequate amounts of water or hypertonic solutions, (2) excess sodium accumulates in the body unaccompanied by adequate water intake, or (3) essential hypernatremia is present. Thirst is protective, and hypernatremia occurs most commonly in patients unable to obtain water.

1. **Manifestations.** Thirst is the major symptom of hypernatremia but may be absent for the very reason that hypernatremia developed (e.g., hypothalamic lesions); water depletion itself may cause confusion and weakness. Urine volume is diminished and specific gravity increased, except when hypernatremia is due to polyuria. The hematocrit may not be increased because of proportionate losses of plasma and red cell water. In hypernatremic dehydration there may be some decrease in skin turgor, mild hypotension, irritability, and slight elevation of plasma proteins, since water has shifted from the ICF to the ECF compartment.

2. **General treatment.** As with hyponatremia, the treatment of hypernatremia is determined by the patient's total body sodium stores. In patients with expanded volume (primary hyperaldosteronism, Cushing's syndrome, or acute salt loads), diuretics and water replacement are indicated. In those with normal sodium stores (diabetes insipidus, states of large insensible water losses), water replacement alone is sufficient. If the serum sodium concentration is less than 160 mEq/liter, water may be given PO; if hypertonicity is more marked, 5% D/W should be given IV. In situations in which both total body salt and water content are low but there is no evidence of circulatory disturbance (renal losses, excess diarrhea, or sweating), hypotonic saline is indicated.

Serum sodium concentration should be determined q6h. One-half the calculated water deficit should be **corrected slowly** over the first 24 hours, correcting the remainder over the subsequent 1–2 days. A more rapid correction of the hypernatremia may result in lethargy or convulsions secondary to cerebral edema. The volume of water necessary to restore the serum sodium concentration to normal may be estimated by the following calculations:

Normal volume TBW (L) = 0.6 × normal body weight (kg)

$$\frac{\text{Normal serum (Na}^+) \times \text{TBW}}{\text{measured serum (Na}^+)} = \text{current TBW}$$

Body water deficit = normal TBW − current TBW

If salt and water deficits are of such magnitude that there is circulatory impairment, isotonic saline should be administered until the hemodynamics are corrected. The patient should be observed for improvement in skin tur-

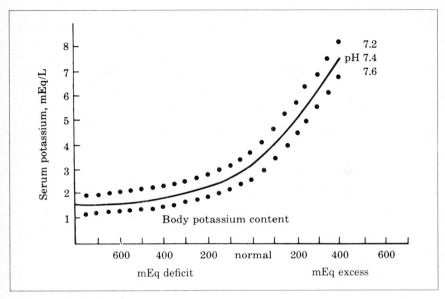

Fig. 2-1. The relationship between serum and tissue potassium. As body potassium rises above normal, the serum potassium concentration rises proportionately. As body potassium falls below normal, however, the decrement in serum potassium concentration becomes less and less. Thus, the serum potassium concentration may not be substantially lower after a deficit of 600–1000 mEq than after a deficit of 300–500 mEq.

gor, blood pressure, pulse, and urinary output. Thereafter, 5% D/W or hypotonic saline may be cautiously administered to correct the hypertonicity (see above).

V. Potassium. The normal daily diet contains 50–100 mEq of potassium. Only about 10 mEq is excreted in the stools and sweat; the remainder is excreted in the urine. Thus, the kidneys normally determine potassium balance. They can increase excretion to adjust to high potassium intake; but, in the absence of potassium intake, they are unable to prevent potassium depletion (5–10 mEq potassium/day may continue to appear in the urine even after a week or more of a potassium-free diet). The serum K^+ concentration (normally 3.8–5.0 mEq/liter) generally reflects total body potassium content, even though only 2% of body potassium is extracellular. It is influenced by the pH of the ECF (serum K^+ concentration is higher in acidosis, lower in alkalosis) as depicted diagrammatically in Fig. 2-1. Changes in the ECF volume also alter the serum potassium concentration but only transiently. The magnitude of potassium depletion cannot be estimated precisely from the value of the serum potassium concentration alone. With moderate potassium deficits, for example, the serum potassium level may even be increased if the patient is acidotic, moderately decreased if the patient has a normal pH, or markedly decreased if the patient is alkalotic.

A. Hypokalemia

    1. Causes

        a. Gastrointestinal loss (urine K^+ < 20 mEq/day) occurs with diarrhea, intestinal or biliary fistulas, ureteroenterostomy, vomiting, or nasogastric suction. In vomiting or nasogastric suction, the potassium deficit may be greater than that which can be explained by measured gastric K^+

losses and is usually due to the enhanced urinary excretion of potassium that occurs in alkalosis and ECF volume contraction (see Table 2-1 for K^+ concentration in intestinal fluids).

   b. **Urinary loss (urine K^+ > 20 mEq/day)** occurs in renal tubular disorders (renal tubular acidosis, diuretic phase of acute tubular necrosis, Fanconi syndrome); in osmotic diuresis (uncontrolled diabetes, mannitol administration); in postobstructive diuresis; in patients receiving diuretics or corticosteroids; and in Cushing's syndrome, primary or secondary hyperaldosteronism, and Bartter's syndrome.

   c. **Inadequate intake of potassium** is an uncommon cause of hypokalemia except in patients whose only intake is potassium-free parenteral fluids; in 1 week they may have a 100-mEq potassium deficit because of continued urinary excretion of potassium.

   d. **Hypokalemia due to a shift of potassium into cells** may result from alkali administration (particularly to acidotic patients) or parenteral administration of glucose or insulin.

2. **Manifestations** rarely develop before the serum potassium has fallen below 3.0 mEq/liter unless the rate of fall has been rapid. They include neuromuscular disturbances (weakness, hyporeflexia, paresthesias, and, rarely, flaccid paralysis or tetany) and cardiac abnormalities (dysrhythmias, increased sensitivity to digitalis, and ECG changes). The ECG abnormalities include flat or inverted T waves, prominent U waves, and depressed S–T segments.

   Additional manifestations include nephropathy (impaired urinary concentrating ability and mild depression of the glomerular filtration rate [GFR]), CNS symptoms (irritability, stupor), GI symptoms (nausea, paralytic ileus), metabolic abnormalities (carbohydrate intolerance, negative nitrogen balance, and alkalosis), and polydipsia.

3. **Prevention.** Patients treated with diuretics or corticosteroids are susceptible to potassium depletion and should be advised to take adequate dietary potassium (e.g., fruits and vegetables). The serum potassium should be measured regularly if therapy is prolonged, and potassium supplements should be prescribed if indicated. Prevention is particularly important in patients taking digitalis, to decrease the likelihood that digitalis toxicity will develop. Patients receiving only parenteral fluids should be given 40 mEq potassium daily unless oliguria or other contraindications are present. Potentially lethal hypokalemia may occur when the serum is made rapidly alkalotic (e.g., in vigorous correction of respiratory acidosis by mechanical ventilation).

4. **Treatment**

   a. **General comments.** Hypokalemia is not usually an emergency; therapy always runs the risk of hyperkalemia, since potassium must traverse the tiny extracellular pool (65 mEq) to replenish cellular stores (3000 mEq). Oral therapy is desirable and is generally adequate.

   The need for potassium repletion with diuretic therapy is discussed in Chap. 7, sec. **II.A.1.**

   b. **Oral therapy.** Dietary supplementation with potassium-rich food often will suffice. It is often more easily tolerated and has fewer side effects than does drug therapy. A well-planned diet can provide an extra 40–60 mEq/day of potassium. There are a variety of **salt substitutes** (*J.A.M.A.* 238:608, 1977) that are cheaper than prescription potassium-salt replacements and contain 10–13 mEq potassium/gm (5 gm equals approximately 1 tsp).

   Table 2-2 lists the ingredients and concentration of most **potassium supplements.** In general (and required in alkalosis), the drug of choice is 10%

Table 2-2. Potassium supplements: products available

Preparation	Ingredient	K^+ (mEq)	Cl^- (mEq)	Per volume (ml)
Liquids				
Kaochlor 10%	KCl	20	20	15
Kaochlor S-F 10% (sugar free)	KCl	20	20	15
Kaon Elixir	K gluconate	20		15
Kaon-Cl 20%	KCl	40	40	15
Kay Ciel Elixir	KCl	20	20	15
Klorvess 10%	KCl	20	20	15
Kolyum	KCl	20	3.34	15
Potassium Chloride Oral				
Solution 5%	KCl	10	10	15
Sugar free 10%	KCl	20	20	15
Potassium Triplex	K acetate, K bicarbonate, K citrate	15		5
Rum-K	KCl	20	20	10
Tablets				
Kaon-Cl Tabs (slow release, wax matrix)	KCl	6.67	6.67	
Slow-K (slow release, wax matrix)		8	8	
Kaochlor-Eff	KCl, K citrate, K bicarbonate, Betaine HCl	20	20	
Kaon	K gluconate	5		
KEFF	KCl, betaine HCl, K bicarbonate, K carbonate	20	20	
Klorvess Effervescent	K bicarbonate, L-lysine monohydrochloride	20	20	
K-Lyte	K bicarbonate, K citrate	25		
PfiKlor-F Effervescent	KCl, K bicarbonate, L-lysine monohydrochloride	20	20	
Powder				
Kato	KCl	20	20	
Kay Ciel Solodose	KCl	20	20	
K-Lor	KCl	20	20	
K-Lyte/Cl	KCl	25	25	
Kolyum	KCl, K gluconate	20	3.34	
PfiKlor for Oral Solution	KCl	20	20	
Potassium Chloride (sugar free)	KCl	20	20	

Source: Adapted from F. G. McMahon. *Management of Essential Hypertension.* Mount Kisco, N.Y.: Futura, 1978. Pp. 94–95.

potassium chloride. It is best administered in a liquid form and should be diluted in juice and given immediately after meals to minimize gastric irritation. **Slow-K** is potassium chloride in a wax matrix that allows for very slow absorption in the small bowel. The rare occurrence of ulcers of the GI tract has been reported with this drug. Many patients who do not tolerate a liquid form will tolerate Slow-K. Potassium acetate-bicarbonate-citrate (Triplex), potassium gluconate (Kaon), potassium bicarbonate (K-Lyte), and potassium chloride (Klorvess) may be more palatable than the 10% KCl solution. An aldosterone antagonist (e.g., spirolactone) may be used if the patient cannot tolerate potassium supplementation or if hyperaldosteronism is playing a major role in the patient's hypokalemia. It should not, however, be used in conjunction with potassium supplements.

   c. **Intravenous therapy.** If the patient cannot take potassium orally or if hypokalemia is severe, parenteral therapy is necessary. The serum potassium level must be known and adequate urine output established before treatment; IV potassium should rarely be given to the oliguric patient.

   The potassium deficit should be estimated (see Fig. 2-1) and the urgency of repletion determined before selecting the dosage and rate of administration of KCl. **Note:** As shown in Fig. 2-1, correction of coexisting alkalosis (if present) decreases the calculated potassium replacement dosage. If the serum potassium level is greater than 2.5 mEq/liter and ECG manifestations are absent, potassium should be given at a rate not to exceed 10 mEq/hour and in a concentration not greater than 30 mEq/liter. Not more than 100–200 mEq/day should be given, even though it may take several days to replace the estimated deficit.

   If urgent treatment is required (i.e., serum potassium level less than 2.0 mEq/liter, presence of ECG abnormalities, or paralysis), potassium may be given (through a peripheral IV line) at rates up to 40 mEq/hour and in concentrations up to 60 mEq/liter. Instances calling for such rapid and potentially dangerous administration of potassium are uncommon. The ECG should be monitored continuously and the serum potassium level checked after the first 50–100 mEq of potassium replacement and q6–12h thereafter until repletion is complete. In critical states, potassium should be administered in saline (unless contraindicated) rather than in dextrose in water, since the infusion of glucose-containing fluids may cause the serum potassium level to fall further.

   d. **Specific therapy.** In patients with hypokalemia due to high levels of mineralocorticosteroids, the underlying disorder should be treated if possible. Indomethacin may be partially effective at raising the potassium levels in patients with Bartter's syndrome.

B. Hyperkalemia

  1. Causes

   a. **Decreased excretion** is common in acute renal failure and in adrenal insufficiency but is uncommon in chronic renal failure unless the patient is terminally oliguric, acidotic, challenged with a potassium load, or has been taking aldosterone-antagonist drugs. Hyporeninemic hypoaldosteronism has been implicated as a cause of hyperkalemia in some patients (often with diabetes and mild renal failure).

   b. **An increased potassium load** may be due to endogenous factors associated with increased tissue breakdown (major surgery, crush injury, rhabdomyolysis, massive hemolysis, or GI bleeding). Exogenous sources include foods high in potassium, potassium-containing salt substitutes, blood transfusions (as much as 30 mEq K^+ liter in plasma when blood is stored for 10 days), and high doses of penicillin (1.7 mEq K^+ million units). It is uncommon for chronic hyperkalemia to develop solely as a result of an increased load if renal function is normal.

c. **With acidosis,** potassium is redistributed from the intracellular space to the extracellular space. Thus, this form of hyperkalemia is unassociated with changes in total body potassium.

d. **Factitious hyperkalemia** occurs when the potassium value in the serum sample is elevated compared with the patient's true serum concentration. The most common causes are a hemolyzed sample, prolonged tourniquet placement, thrombocytosis, and leukocytosis.

2. **Manifestations** may be absent; when they do occur, they are enhanced by concomitant hyponatremia, hypocalcemia, or acidosis. **Neuromuscular manifestations** of hyperkalemia are similar to those of hypokalemia and include weakness, paresthesias, areflexia, and muscular or respiratory paralysis. **Cardiac manifestations** are frequent when the serum potassium level exceeds 8.0 mEq/liter (uncommon at concentrations of less than 6.5 mEq/liter) and include bradycardia, hypotension, ventricular fibrillation, and cardiac arrest. The sequential ECG manifestations are tall, peaked T waves, depressed S–T segments, decreased amplitude of R waves, prolonged P–R interval, diminished to absent P waves, and widening of the QRS complexes with prolongation of the Q–T interval, resulting in a sine-wave pattern.

If the clinical setting suggests the possibility of hyperkalemia, an ECG should be promptly obtained pending laboratory determination of the serum potassium level; ECG changes strongly suggestive of hyperkalemia should dictate the immediate initiation of therapy (see **4**).

3. **Prevention** often depends on prompt recognition of oliguria and subsequent elimination of excessive potassium intake.

4. **General treatment.** Hyperkalemia may be treated by measures that antagonize the effects of potassium, force potassium into cells, or actually remove potassium from the body. Which measures should be used depends on the degree of hyperkalemia, the severity of the clinical manifestations, the ECG findings, and the patient's cardiovascular and renal status. The situation is emergent if the serum potassium is greater than 7.5 mEq/liter or if the ECG shows the changes of hyperkalemia. The ECG should then be continuously monitored during therapy. However, a very high serum potassium level may result in sudden death despite a normal ECG, or a severe dysrhythmia may develop despite only moderate elevations of potassium, especially if the level is rising rapidly. The following is the recommended sequence for the treatment of hyperkalemia:

a. **Calcium** immediately antagonizes the cardiac and neuromuscular toxicity of hyperkalemia, particularly if hypocalcemia is present. (If the patient is receiving digitalis, however, **calcium should be given with extreme caution** because it may induce digitalis toxic rhythms.) Calcium gluconate (5–10 ml of a 10% solution) may be injected IV over a 2-minute period (preferably with constant ECG monitoring). If ECG abnormalities persist, the injection may be repeated after 5 minutes; if this is ineffective, more calcium is unlikely to be of any benefit. Calcium infusions are only temporizing, with a duration of action of approximately 1 hour. Following the calcium infusion, one should immediately initiate one or more of the other forms of therapy discussed in **b–e.**

b. **Sodium bicarbonate** causes rapid movement of K^+ into cells. The onset of action is within 15 minutes, and the duration of action is 1–2 hours. One ampule of $NaHCO_3$ (44 mEq HCO_3^- may be injected IV over a 5-minute period and another injected after 10–15 minutes if ECG abnormalities persist; $NaHCO_3$ may also be added to glucose infusions, as described in **c.** Cardiovascular volume overload and hypernatremia may preclude administration of large quantities of $NaHCO_3$.

c. Glucose infusions in otherwise normal persons will cause a marked elevation in the plasma insulin, which is associated with a rapid reduction in the plasma potassium, due to an intracellular shift of that ion.

Because patients with severe hyperkalemia are often acutely ill, it is difficult to predict whether or not they will have an adequate insulin response to the carbohydrate load. Therefore, 5–10 units of regular insulin should be given IV concomitantly with 1 ampule of D_{50} (25 gm dextrose). This should be given slowly over 5 minutes. The potassium-lowering effect is seen within 30–60 minutes and lasts for several hours.

Alternatively, 1000 ml of 10% D/W with 90 mEq $NaHCO_3$ may be rapidly infused. The first third of the infusion may be given in 30 minutes and the balance over 2–3 hours; 25 units of regular insulin should be given SQ at the same time. If CHF limits fluid and salt administration, the direct IV infusion of D_{50} plus insulin should be used as just described.

d. Cation-exchange resins reduce the serum potassium levels more slowly than the preceding measures but have the advantage of actually removing potassium from the body. Frequently, they are given in combination with one of the preceding measures. Approximately 1 mEq K^+ is removed per gram of resin administered (a heaping teaspoon contains 7–12 gm of resin). A sodium-cycle cation resin, **Kayexalate,** exchanges 1.3–1.7 mEq Na^+ for each milliequivalent of K^+ removed. Thus, it should be administered with caution in patients susceptible to cardiovascular volume overload.

(1) Oral administration is recommended. Since Kayexalate is constipating, it should be given with a poorly absorbed carrier (osmotic agent) such as sorbitol. The recommended dose is 20–50 gm Kayexalate dissolved in 100–200 ml of a 20% sorbitol solution. This dose may be repeated q3–4h up to 4–5 doses/day until the serum potassium has returned to normal.

(2) Rectal administration. If oral administration is not tolerated by the patient, if ileus is present, or if a more rapid effect is desired, Kayexalate may be given as an enema with sorbitol. To 200 ml water, add 50 gm Kayexalate and 50 gm sorbitol and give as a retention enema. If sorbitol is unavailable, Kayexalate may be suspended in 200 ml 20% D/W. Retention of the enema for the desired 30–60 minutes may be facilitated by using an inflated rectal catheter. Occasionally, the prior preparation of the patient with a **Fleet enema** will improve the ability to retain the Kayexalate. Several Kayexalate enemas may be given at hourly intervals thereafter if necessary. A single enema may reduce the serum potassium concentration by as much as 0.5–1.0 mEq/liter, depending on the acid-base status of the patient.

e. Dialysis. Hemodialysis is an effective method of removing potassium, but should be reserved for situations in which more conservative regimens fail or are contraindicated or in which hemodialysis is necessary for other reasons (see Chap. 3, sec. **VI.A**).

5. Specific therapies. For patients with hyporeninemic hypoaldosteronism (type IV renal tubular acidosis) with potassium levels below 5.5 mEq/liter, probably no specific therapy is necessary except dietary potassium restriction. A synthetic mineralocorticoid, fludrocortisone acetate, is often effective for more severe hyperkalemia (*N. Engl. J. Med.* 297:576, 1977). The usual dosage is 0.1 mg PO qd, but up to 0.4 mg/day is occasionally necessary for an adequate therapeutic effect. Sodium retention and hypertension often complicate treatment with this drug. Alternatively, loop diuretics, or oral sodium bicarbonate, or both may be used. Because renal potassium secretion is partially dependent on distal tubular flow, care must be taken to avoid dehydration. Chronic administration of cation-exchange resins is usually

Table 2-3. Rules of thumb for bedside interpretation of acid-base disorders

Disorder	Rule of thumb
Metabolic acidosis	$PaCO_2$ should fall by $1.0-1.5 \times$ the fall in plasma HCO_3^- concentrations
Metabolic alkalosis	$PaCO_2$ should rise by $0.25-1.0 \times$ the rise in plasma HCO_3^- concentration
Acute respiratory acidosis	Plasma HCO_3^- concentration should rise by about 1 mmol/L for each increment of 10 mm Hg in $PaCO_2$ ($\pm$ 3 mmol/L)
Chronic respiratory acidosis	Plasma HCO_3^- concentration should rise by about 4 mmol/L for each increment of 10 mm Hg in $PaCO_2$ ($\pm$ 4 mmol/L)
Acute respiratory alkalosis	Plasma HCO_3^- concentration should fall by about 1–3 mmol/L for each decrement of 10 mm Hg in $PaCO_2$, usually not to $<$ 18 mmol/L
Chronic respiratory alkalosis	Plasma HCO_3^- concentration should fall by about 2–5 mmol/L/decrement of 10 mm Hg in $PaCO_2$ but usually not to $<$ 14 mmol/L

Source: Modified from R. W. Schrier (ed.). *Renal and Electrolyte Disorders.* Boston: Little, Brown, 1980. P. 170.

poorly tolerated. Drugs that may predispose to hyperkalemia (e.g., spironolactone, triamterene, heparin, indomethacin, and possibly propranolol) should be avoided. When hyperkalemia is due to endogenous release of potassium, efforts should be directed at treating the underlying disease process.

VI. Acid-base disturbances

A. General comments. Complete oxidation of carbohydrate and fat yields carbon dioxide and water. Carbon dioxide, when hydrated, yields carbonic acid (CO_2 + $H_2O \rightleftharpoons H_2CO_3 \rightleftharpoons H^+ + HCO_3^-$); the reaction is reversible, and the 22,000 mEq CO_2 produced each day is excreted by the lungs. Thus, under normal circumstances, production of this volatile acid has no effect on pH. Approximately 70 mEq of fixed (nonvolatile) acid is produced per day from the metabolism of sulfur-containing amino acids and of carbohydrates and fats not completely oxidized to CO_2 and H_2O. This acid requires renal excretion.

The lungs, kidneys, and buffers provide defenses against acid-base disturbances. Chemical buffers such as HCO_3^-, phosphate, proteins, hemoglobin, and bone carbonate react quickly with the acid to minimize changes in pH. Respiratory adjustments may also occur. Hyperventilation is a relatively ineffective way of reducing a base excess. The ultimate correction of acid-base disturbances and restoration of buffer is dependent on the kidney. Its role in acid-base regulation is to restore bicarbonate to the blood by reclaiming filtered bicarbonate and generating new bicarbonate to replace that consumed in the buffering process.

Acid secreted by renal tubular cells may be excreted in the urine as hydrogen ions, titratable acid (H^+ buffered by HPO_4^-), or NH_4^+ (H^+ buffered by NH_3). Although the kidney normally can achieve an H^+ concentration in the urine (at pH 4.5, maximal urine acidity) 1000 times that in the blood (at pH 7.4), very little acid can be excreted as free H^+; most of it is excreted as titratable acid (one-third of the total) and ammonium (two-thirds of the total).

B. The simple disturbances of acid-base equilibrium are metabolic and respiratory acidosis and alkalosis. Each of these four disturbances evokes compensatory responses that tend to minimize the changes in pH, but overcompensation does not ordinarily occur (Table 2-3).

In **metabolic acidosis** the primary mechanism is retention of fixed acid or loss of alkali (i.e., a decrease in HCO_3^- or total CO_2); the compensatory response is hyperventilation with a resultant fall in PCO_2. In **respiratory acidosis** the primary mechanism is pulmonary retention of CO_2 (i.e., increase in PCO_2), leading to an increase in volatile acids (H_2CO_3); an increase in renal bicarbonate regeneration is the compensatory response. In **metabolic alkalosis** the primary mechanism is loss of fixed acid or gain of alkali (i.e., an increase in HCO_3^-); the compensatory response is hypoventilation with a slight increase in PCO_2. In **respiratory alkalosis** the primary mechanism is hyperventilation, with a resultant fall in PCO_2; the compensatory response is a decrease in HCO_3^- due to a decreased renal acid excretion and thus bicarbonate regeneration.

The following diagram summarizes the abnormalities that occur in the partially compensated, simple acid-base disturbances. Primary mechanisms are indicated by ⟶, the resultant pH by ⟶, and the compensatory response by ⇢.

	HCO₃⁻	PCO₂	pH
Metabolic acidosis	↓	↓	↓
Respiratory acidosis	↑	↑	↓
Metabolic alkalosis	↑	↑	↑
Respiratory alkalosis	↓	↓	↑

C. **Laboratory diagnosis.** For accurate assessment of acid-base status, **arterial blood samples are mandatory.** Normal **arterial blood gas (ABG) values** are:

pH	PCO₂	Total CO₂
7.38–7.43	35–45 mm Hg	24–29 mEq/L

The syringe should be **coated with heparin** (1000 units/ml) to serve as an anticoagulant and to seal the barrel against air leaks. Free heparin should be expelled from the syringe to avoid the factitious lowering of pH by excess heparin. The sample should be measured immediately, although it can be stored for up to 2 hours in ice. From any two of the three variables (total CO_2, pH, PCO_2), the third may be calculated by using the Henderson-Hasselbalch equation:

$$pH = 6.1 + \log \frac{[HCO_3^-]}{0.0301 \times PCO_2}$$

The PCO_2 may be read from standard nomograms or easily estimated by utilizing the derived equation that follows, thus avoiding the use of logarithm tables.

$$PCO_2 = \frac{[H^+] \times [\text{total } CO_2 \text{ content}]}{24}$$

$[H^+]$ is expressed in nanoequivalents per liter (nEq/liter) and can be derived readily from the pH by remembering that a pH value of 7.4 equals a $[H^+]$ of 40 nEq/liter, and that each 0.01-unit increase in pH is roughly equivalent to a decrease of 1 nEq/liter in $[H^+]$ within the pH range of 7.28–7.45. (For example, a change in pH from 7.47 to 7.30 is accompanied by a rise in $[H^+]$ from 33 to 50 nEq/liter.) The maximal error in PCO_2 calculated by this simplified formula is 7% or less when the pH is 7.10–7.50 (*N. Engl. J. Med.* 272:1067, 1965).

D. **Metabolic acidosis** results from accumulation of fixed (nonvolatile) acid (by ingestion, increased endogenous production, or decreased excretion) or from loss of alkali.

1. **Types of metabolic acidosis.** Metabolic acidosis may be divided clinically into two forms, dependent on the value of the **serum anion gap (AG).**

$$AG = Na^+ - (Cl^- + HCO_3^-)$$

A normal anion gap value equals 12.4 ± 2 mEq/liter.

   a. Increased AG acidosis (AG > 12–14 mEq/liter) generally results from accumulation of organic acids, which can occur with lactic acidosis, diabetic ketoacidosis, uremia, or salicylate, methanol, or ethylene glycol toxicity.

   b. Normal AG acidosis results either from a direct loss of HCO_3^- (e.g., diarrhea, pancreatic fistula, ureteroenterostomies, renal tubular acidosis) or the addition of chloride-containing acids (e.g., NH_4Cl, oral $CaCl_2$ administration, HCl, some hyperalimentation fluids). Discussions of metabolic acidosis and AG can be found in *Medicine* (Baltimore) 56:38, 1977, and *N. Engl. J. Med.* 297:814, 1977.

2. Diagnosis. Definitive diagnosis of metabolic acidosis requires the demonstration of a decrease in the arterial pH as well as the serum HCO_3. The PCO_2 may be decreased because of respiratory compensation. In patients presenting with low serum HCO_3^-, the differentiation between metabolic acidosis and respiratory alkalosis is facilitated by simultaneous measurement of the arterial pH and PCO_2. The compensatory reduction in PCO_2 seen with metabolic acidosis may be marked ($PCO_2 \leqq 10–15$ mm Hg), whereas in primary respiratory alkalosis the reduction in PCO_2 is rarely to less than 25 mm Hg.

3. Treatment. Underlying disorders should receive appropriate therapy. Treatment of ketoacidosis is discussed in Chap. 20.

   a. Therapy of acute acidosis. In an acutely ill patient with an arterial blood pH of less than 7.2, $NaHCO_3$ should be used parenterally. The total HCO_3^- (base) deficit may be estimated from the following formula:

$$HCO_3^- \text{ deficit} = (\text{body weight in kg}) (0.4) (\text{desired } [HCO_3^-] - \text{measured} [HCO_3^-])$$

   The $[HCO_3^-]$ is measured in milliequivalents per liter, and the distribution of HCO_3^- is generally about 40% (0.4) of the body weight. Usually, 2–3 ampules of 7.5% $NaHCO_3$ (44.5 mEq/ampule) are added to 1000 ml 5% D/W. One-half the calculated deficit may be replaced in 3–4 hours if severe CHF is not present. The remainder is replaced by slow IV infusion with continuous monitoring of ABGs and serum electrolytes. **Remember: Correction of acidosis without correction of a potassium deficit may lead to fatal manifestations of hypokalemia** (due to intracellular movement of potassium). Nevertheless, potassium replacement should not be undertaken until the acidosis has been partially corrected and a falling potassium concentration documented. If the patient is hypocalcemic, serum calcium should be monitored and replenished during treatment to avoid tetany.

   Great care must be exercised if the patient with severe metabolic acidosis is placed on a respirator that impairs compensatory hyperventilation, since this may worsen the acidosis.

   b. Chronic metabolic acidosis is most often seen in renal failure when acid ingestion and production exceed excretion. Initially, the acidosis is usually mild (pH = 7.35, and HCO_3^- = 18–23 mEq/liter), but to prevent severe osteomalacia, therapy with sodium bicarbonate may be started as soon as the plasma HCO_3^- begins to fall. Therapy is critical when HCO_3 falls below 15 mEq/liter. **Bicarbonate** (available in 300- and 600-mg tablets) in a dose of 2–4 gm/day (24–48 mEq) is the preferred form of therapy but must be used cautiously to avoid cardiovascular overload and symptomatic hypocalcemia. Some patients find **Shohl's solution** more palatable (90 gm sodium citrate crystalline salt and 140 gm citric acid are dissolved in water to a volume of 1 liter to yield 1 mEq $NaHCO_3$/ml of solution). Shohl's solution is also available as potassium citrate.

Some patients with chronic metabolic acidosis show evidence of phosphate depletion; oral phosphate administration to this group of patients usually will result in increased excretion of titratable acid and improvement of the acidosis (see Chap. 19).

c. Renal tubular acidosis (RTA) may be either hereditary or acquired and can be of three basic types.

(1) Type I (distal) RTA is an inability to maintain a normal H^+ gradient in the distal nephron. Patients with this disorder should receive alkali therapy, since it may improve the often accompanying osteomalacia and nephrocalcinosis. The amount of alkali ($NaHCO_3$) generally needed is 1–3 mEq/kg/day. Not only does alkali therapy improve the acid-base status, but it also stops urinary wasting of calcium and potassium.

(2) Type II (proximal) RTA is due to impaired bicarbonate resorption in the proximal tubule. It is unclear whether adult patients with this disorder require alkali therapy, since they are in acid-base balance (but at a lower serum HCO_3^- level, generally 18–20 mEq/liter), and osteomalacia or nephrocalcinosis does not usually develop. If treatment is undertaken, large amounts of alkali (6–10 mEq/kg/day), in conjunction with potassium supplements (see Table 2-2), are often required. Alkali therapy enhances the renal potassium wasting of this disorder. Alternatively, dietary salt restriction in conjunction with hydrochlorthiazide may be efficacious and better tolerated. With hydrochlorthiazide, the severity of hypokalemia frequently worsens, and potassium supplements (see Table 2-2) are advisable.

(3) Type IV RTA (hyperkalemic acidosis often secondary to hyporeninemic hypoaldosteronism). Treatment of this disorder is discussed in sec. **V.B.5.** Frequently, even with correction of the hyperkalemia with fludrocortisone acetate, a mild degree of acidosis will persist that does not require therapy.

d. Lactic acidosis occurs when there is an abnormal accumulation of some of the more than 1500 mEq of lactic acid produced by the body every day. In most instances, excess lactate is cleared rapidly by the liver through conversion of lactate to pyruvate, a process dependent in part on the redox state of tissue (NADH/NAD ratio). Lactic acidosis is often fatal and must be treated promptly. The most frequent underlying causative factor is **tissue hypoxia**, such as occurs in cardiogenic and septic shock and severe hypoxemia. Lactic acidosis may also occur in uncontrolled diabetes mellitus or as a complication of phenformin administration, excessive ethanol ingestion, severe bacterial infections, pancreatitis, or leukemia. Spontaneous lactic acidosis is an entity in which there is no obvious underlying disorder, but tissue hypoxia must be present.

(1) The **diagnosis** of lactic acidosis should be considered when the clinical manifestations of metabolic acidosis develop in patients with the disease states mentioned. The patients often are comatose, with hyperventilation and shock. The diagnosis is made by measuring excess lactate and excluding other forms of metabolic acidosis with increased AG.

(2) The **treatment** of lactic acidosis should stop excess lactic acid production and reestablish adequate lactate clearance by improving hepatic perfusion. Tissue hypoxia must be corrected, and supportive measures should be promptly instituted. Treatment of underlying sepsis, myocardial or bowel infarction, shock, and ketoacidosis must accompany an attempt to correct the acidosis to a pH of 7.2 with bicarbonate. Frequent evaluation of acid-base status is necessary to ensure that adequate alkali is being given and to prevent alkalosis. Due to the continued generation of acid, more bicarbonate than calculated is often required. In addition, if the blood pH is less than 7.1, the HCO_3^- volume of distribution increases to 80% of body weight. Peritoneal dialysis or hemodialysis may be needed if IV bicarbonate therapy is ineffective or produces CHF or marked hypernatremia. Since many peritoneal dialysate solutions contain lactate, following serum lactate in this situation is misleading. Lactate is not an acid and does not contribute to the perpetuation of the acidosis. Nonetheless, acetate is metabolized predominantly by peripheral tissues instead of the liver, and thus dialysates containing acetate may be preferable to those containing lactate. Because norepinephrine increases lactate production, isoproterenol and dopamine are used to treat shock. Insulin frequently is used in lactic acidosis to treat hyperglycemia and associated ketosis, and its use may increase NAD availability for lactate clearance. Unfortunately, even with such aggressive measures, lactic acidosis carries a high mortality.

4. **Complications of therapy.** Since sodium salts are administered in alkali therapy, volume overload and, occasionally, hypertension may occur. Rapid parenteral administration may precipitate **acute pulmonary edema,** particularly if the patient is oliguric. In that situation, peritoneal dialysis in conjunction with parenteral bicarbonate should be considered. It has been suggested (*Kidney Int.* 14:645A, 1978) that the rapid administration of bicarbonate may, in fact, be deleterious in experimental lactic acidosis. This underscores the need to correct the underlying pathologic conditions while using as little bicarbonate as possible to bring the pH to 7.2.

Patients who can tolerate an increased potassium intake (particularly those with RTA) may be given alkali as the potassium salt instead of the sodium salt.

Tetany may develop if alkali is administered rapidly or excessively. Although tetany may not be entirely due to a decrease in ionized calcium concentration, as is often assumed, calcium administration may be of therapeutic value. To avoid precipitation, calcium salts must not be given in the same infusion as bicarbonate.

Hypokalemia may also occur, since potassium reenters cells as alkali is administered.

E. **Metabolic alkalosis** is diagnosed by noting an elevated serum pH and HCO_3^- concentration.

1. **Chloride-responsive alkalosis** is generally due to vomiting, nasogastric suction, or diuretic use and represents total salt and water depletion (volume contraction). It is the most common cause of metabolic alkalosis. In patients with normal renal function who are not currently taking diuretics, urinary chloride levels are usually less than 10 mEq/liter.

Treatment is aimed at reversal of the underlying (alkalosis-generating) disorder, and NaCl-containing solutions are administered to restore normal volume (since continued volume depletion serves to maintain the alkalosis). Potassium chloride is given to correct the hypokalemia (also see **4**).

2. **Chloride-resistant alkalosis** (urinary chloride > 20 mEq/liter) is generally a result of mineralocorticoid excess states, Cushing's syndrome, Bartter's syndrome, or profound potassium depletion. In the latter situation, hydrogen ions move intracellularly (to maintain electrical neutrality) and augment hydrogen ion secretion by the renal tubule, resulting in severe alkalosis (even in the absence of volume contraction).

Treatment consists of correcting the underlying disorder and replacing potassium deficits with potassium chloride supplements. Occasionally, spironolactone is effective in treating the metabolic alkalosis of mineralocorticoid excess states.

3. **Unclassified causes** of metabolic alkalosis include excess alkali administration or ingestion (especially in renal function impairment) and milk-alkali syndrome.

   Treatment consists of removal of the precipitating cause (excess alkali intake). Sufficient chloride must be supplied so that the kidney can absorb sodium (cation) with the chloride (anion) and allow the excretion of the excess bicarbonate.

4. Rarely, in **severe metabolic alkalosis** (serum pH > 7.6 and serum HCO_3^- > 40–45 mEq/liter), especially when the clinical situation prohibits the use of chloride or potassium salts (e.g., CHF, renal insufficiency) or expeditious replacement is needed (e.g., preoperative stabilization), **cautious** IV administration (via a central line) of acid (isotonic HCl solution, consisting of 150 ml of 1N **HCl** in 1 liter of sterile water) may be beneficial (*Surgery* 75:194, 1974). Alternatives include the administration of 0.1M **NH₄Cl** or **arginine HCl**. However, these agents **may be dangerous** in patients with renal or hepatic failure. Dosage should be based on an apparent volume of distribution of 40% of body weight (kg). The first one-half of the calculated dosage can be replaced over the first 2–4 hours and the remainder, over the next 24 hours (depending on the clinical situation). Acid infusion should be accompanied by frequent measurements (at least q4h) of blood gases, pH, serum electrolytes, and BUN. In patients with volume overload, metabolic alkalosis, and normal renal function, **acetazolamide,** a carbonic anhydrase inhibitor that increases the renal excretion of HCO_3^-, may be efficacious. The usual dose is 500 mg IV or PO.

F. **Respiratory acidosis** is due to inadequate pulmonary excretion of carbon dioxide (inadequate ventilation), with a resultant increase in PCO_2 and hence in H_2CO_3.

   1. The **diagnosis** should be suspected when the ABG results show a decreased pH and an elevated PCO_2 in the presence of any condition known to predispose to the development of respiratory acidosis. Because the normal ratio of dissolved $CO_2:H_2CO_3$ is 1:20, a small rise in dissolved CO_2 (increase in PCO_2) results in a profound fall in pH. Compensatory renal bicarbonate generation (resulting in elevation of the serum bicarbonate concentration) takes several hours to days to develop.

   2. The **treatment** of uncomplicated respiratory acidosis is directed at improving ventilation (see Chaps. 8 and 9). Alkali may actually be harmful, since the low pH is an important stimulus to ventilation in chronic hypercapnia. Potassium and chloride deficiency, often accompanying the metabolic alkalosis superimposed on chronic respiratory acidosis, should be treated by the administration of potassium chloride.

G. **Respiratory alkalosis** is due to a low PCO_2 because of hyperventilation that may result from psychogenic causes (most common), hypermetabolic states (fever, thyrotoxicosis, delirium tremens), gram-negative bacteremia, excessive ventilation by mechanical ventilators (especially in the setting of compensated respiratory acidosis), and hypoxemia. Some degree of respiratory alkalosis may also occur in pregnancy, cirrhosis, and certain cardiac and pulmonary disorders, and CNS lesions, as well as in the early stages of salicylate intoxication (but metabolic acidosis may suddenly intervene, especially in children). Respiratory alkalosis may also result when severe metabolic acidosis is rapidly converted (as in acute renal failure treated with peritoneal dialysis), since a paradoxical intracerebral acidosis then exists with a normal peripheral pH and stimulates further hyperpnea and tachypnea, leading to a fall in PCO_2 or maintenance at the previously low levels.

1. The **diagnosis** should be suspected when ABG results show an increased pH and decreased PCO_2, especially when associated with irritability, light-headedness, paresthesias, tetany, or even syncope in a patient with a disorder that predisposes to the development of respiratory alkalosis. Hyperventilation may not be apparent in patients who have an increased depth of respiration without associated tachypnea.

2. **Treatment** generally is directed at the underlying disorder; as a rule, the alkalosis per se requires no therapy. Tetany or syncope associated with acute hyperventilation (without hypoxemia) may be relieved by rebreathing into a paper bag. If hyperventilation is suddenly terminated (as in the readjustment of a mechanical respirator or rebreathing), acidosis may develop (increase in PCO_2 in the presence of decreased HCO_3^-). When continued hyperventilation occurs (such as in CNS disease or paradoxical CNS acidosis), the use of a CO_2 rebreathing apparatus may be warranted

H. **Mixed acid-base disturbances.** Unfortunately, the clinical situation often is complicated by the presence of simultaneous primary respiratory and metabolic abnormalities. If the physician carefully evaluates the clinical setting and interprets total CO_2, pH, and PCO_2, the actual abnormalities usually will be evident.

If the presumed compensatory changes observed are not consistent with the expected changes shown in Table 2-3, a mixed acid-base disturbance is likely to be present.

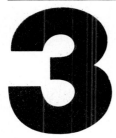

Renal Disease

The biochemical mechanisms underlying most of the clinical manifestations of renal insufficiency are not entirely understood. Many of the signs and symptoms of renal failure are known to reflect alterations in fluid and electrolyte balance, acid-base disorders, and disturbances of calcium and phosphorus metabolism.

I. **Acute renal failure.** Acute renal failure (ARF) is characterized by a sudden reduction in glomerular filtration rate (GFR), limiting the ability of the kidney to maintain the body's internal environment. The hallmarks of the syndrome are rapidly progressive azotemia and oliguria. A less drastic reduction in renal failure with a GFR of approximately 5–10 ml/min and urine volumes greater than 500 ml/24 hours has been termed *nonoliguric acute renal failure.* Progressive azotemia without oliguria may occur in any type of acute renal failure. In general, the nonoliguric variety occurs in 20–30% of cases. Table 3-1 presents a classification of the principal causes of ARF.

After a careful history, physical examination, and urinalysis, the cause of ARF will be apparent in many cases. The presence of RBC casts is indicative of glomerulitis. The characteristic sediment of acute tubular necrosis (ATN) reveals "dirty" brown glomerular casts and epithelial cells, both free and in casts, and is virtually diagnostic. In prerenal azotemia, hyaline and finely granular casts may be present. A benign sediment, i.e., few formed elements present, should raise the possibility of obstruction.

Additional information should be obtained from the composition of the urine (Table 3-2). Low urinary sodium and high urine-to-plasma ratio of creatinine (U/P creatinine ratio) are characteristic of decreased GFR/nephron states as seen in prerenal azotemia and acute glomerulonephritis. In contrast, in conditions with diffuse nephron damage (ATN, chronic renal failure, chronic obstruction) the U/P creatinine ratio is low and urine sodium relatively high. These values taken alone are less reliable in the elderly or in patients with preexisting mild impairment of kidney function. In general, calculation of fractional excretion of sodium (FE_{Na}) provides the most reliable data to distinguish prerenal from intrarenal failure.

A. **Prerenal azotemia**

  1. **Extracellular fluid (ECF) volume contraction** secondary to vomiting, nasogastric suction, postoperative fluid losses, etc., is a common cause of prerenal azotemia. Therapy is aimed at correcting the fluid deficits. Occasionally, it may be difficult to distinguish this condition from ATN, but a careful history, physical examination, urinalysis, and urine chemistry and plasma electrolyte determinations usually lead to the correct diagnosis. However, severe volume contraction may lead to ATN, and, at the stage of "incipient ATN," diagnosis may be difficult. The response to a careful fluid challenge with saline, mannitol, or IV furosemide may be helpful in diagnosing prerenal azotemia; 500–1000 ml of 0.9% NaCl or synthetic ECF* may be

---

*Synthetic ECF is made by mixing 750 ml 0.9% NaCl, 225 ml 5% D/W, and 25 ml NaHCO₃ (3.75 gm/ 50 ml). Each liter provides 137.5 mEq Na⁺, 115 mEq Cl⁻, and 22.5 mEq HCO₃⁻.

Table 3-1. Causes of acute renal failure

A. Prerenal
1. Extracellular fluid volume contraction
2. Congestive heart failure
3. Hypotension
B. Renal
1. Acute Tubular necrosis
   a. Postoperative (especially cardiovascular surgery)
   b. Nephrotoxins, e.g., antibiotics, heavy metals, organic solvents, radiographic contrast agents
   c. All conditions in A above
   d. Pigment release, e.g., transfusion reactions, rhabdomyolysis, crush injury
   e. Eclampsia, septic abortion, uterine hemorrhage
2. Miscellaneous
   a. Acute glomerulonephritis, e.g., poststreptococcal, rapidly progressive glomerulonephritis, Goodpasture's syndrome, systemic lupus erythematosus
   b. Accelerated hypertension
   c. Vasculitis
   d. Uric acid nephropathy
   e. Hemolytic uremic syndrome
   f. Hypercalcemia
   g. Hepatorenal syndrome
C. Postrenal
1. Obstruction to ureters, e.g., clots, papillary tissue, calculi, extrinsic compression
2. Bladder-outlet obstruction, e.g., prostatic hypertrophy, carcinoma

given over 30–60 minutes; or 25 gm mannitol may be given over 15 minutes; or furosemide, 200–400 mg IV, may be tried. An increase in urine flow following these maneuvers may indicate that one is dealing with prerenal azotemia. The increase in urine volume should be replaced parenterally to avoid further volume depletion. There is a danger of rapid volume expansion with saline and/or mannitol if the ECF volume was not contracted. Administration of furosemide may increase urine flow in nonoliguric ATN without any major changes in renal function, or may convert an oliguric ATN to a nonoliguric ATN.

2. **Congestive heart failure (CHF)** is generally not the sole cause of severe renal failure but is often a treatable aggravating factor. It may lead to hyponatremia because of impairment in free water clearance. Physicians should warn such patients not to ingest excessive quantities of water, particularly if they are on salt-restricted diets.

Table 3-2. Laboratory studies in acute renal failure*

Diagnosis	U/P creatinine	U_{Na}	FE_{Na}	U/P osmolality
Prerenal	>40	<20	<1	>1.2
Renal (ATN)	<20	>40	>1	<1.2

U/P = urine-to-plasma ratio; U_{Na} = urine sodium concentration (mEq/L); FE_{Na} = fractional excretion of sodium = (U/P Na ÷ U/P Cr) × 100.
* Reliability of these values can be influenced by residual urine in the bladder, residual bladder irrigation fluid, and prior administration of diuretics.

3. Hypotension, a frequent cause of ARF, must be appropriately evaluated and treated according to its specific origin.

B. Intrinsic renal disease

1. Acute tubular necrosis accounts for approximately 75% of cases of ARF and thus will be discussed in detail along with other selected causes of ARF (see Table 3-1). The clinical course and prognosis vary greatly. Survival is influenced by the precipitating cause, age, associated medical problems, and infection. The principal causes of death are GI bleeding and infection. Acute tubular necrosis is classically divided into three phases: the oliguric, diuretic, and recovery phases.

a. Oliguric phase. Oliguria varies in duration from hours to weeks. Urine volume is usually less than 400–500 ml/day. Complete anuria is rare in ATN and should raise the possibility of obstruction. Since urinary excretion of nitrogenous wastes is negligible, azotemia progresses at a rate determined largely by the rate of protein catabolism. An approach to treatment is as follows:

(1) The **underlying cause** must be identified and treated.

(2) Correction of volume contraction must be done extremely carefully to avoid volume overload.

(3) Diet and fluids. A weight loss of 0.25–0.5 kg/day is anticipated in a starving patient; with increased rates of catabolism, a greater weight loss may ensue. The rate of rise of BUN is related to protein catabolism, and efforts should therefore be directed toward supplying sufficient calories to prevent endogenous protein catabolism (see Chap. 11). The administration of sufficient calories often is limited by the amount of fluid that can be given. Total fluid intake should be limited to insensible losses plus drainage volume and urine output. **Remember:** Metabolism provides about 400 ml water/day. Frequent body weights are imperative in gauging fluid losses and replacement requirements. Appropriate fluid replacement is indicated by loss of 0.25–0.5 kg/day and a normal plasma sodium. Elective hemodialysis can allow more liberal fluid and caloric intake and is particularly useful in hypercatabolic patients who may require parenteral nutrition to reduce endogenous protein catabolism. If conservative management is being tried, one should aim for a diet containing 3000 cal, 40 gm protein, 40 mEq K^+, and 1–2 gm salt. In all diets and fluids administered, attention must be given to electrolyte content, so that intake is not in excess of losses.

(4) Infection is a major cause of mortality in patients with ATN. Prophylactic antibiotics are definitely contraindicated. Instrumentation of the urinary tract and indwelling catheters should be avoided unless absolutely indicated. If an indwelling catheter is required, a closed system should be employed, utilizing topical antibiotic ointment and a rigid sterile technique. Random urine cultures should be obtained frequently. In critical situations there is no contraindication to the use of potentially nephrotoxic antibiotics, provided the dosage is adjusted for renal function and the metabolic status of the patient. Serum antimicrobial levels should be monitored in such patients.

(5) Anemia often develops rapidly over several days following the onset of ATN. It is commonly normochromic, normocytic, and stabilizes at a hematocrit of 20–25%. Depending on the cause and complications of ATN, hemolysis and blood loss become additional causes for anemia. Transfusions are usually reserved for specific indications, such as active bleeding, development of angina pectoris, or symptoms of hypovolemia. Generally, the anemia of renal failure is tolerated well. If transfusion is required, packed RBCs should be used to minimize fluid overload.

(6) Congestive heart failure (cardiovascular overload) often reflects improper fluid and electrolyte management. Restriction of salt and water is indicated. Diuretics are usually ineffective except occasionally in nonoliguric ARF. Digitalis preparations, preferably digoxin, may be administered cautiously. However, the maintenance dose must be reduced, since the renal excretion is reduced (see Chap. 5). **Digitalis intoxication** may be prolonged in these patients, and very little digitalis is removed by dialysis. Furthermore, many patients with ATN and cardiovascular overload do not have intrinsic heart disease and do not respond dramatically to digitalis administration. Volume overload is an important indication for dialysis (see sec. **VI.A.3**).

(7) Acidosis and alkalosis. Treatment is discussed in Chap. 2. Alkalosis is uncommon in ATN unless the patient is losing large amounts of hydrogen ion, e.g., by nasogastric suction. Acidosis almost always develops but does not usually require treatment unless the HCO_3^- is less than 15 mEq/liter. Administration of large amounts of sodium bicarbonate may lead to cardiovascular overload. Dialysis is often necessary in this situation. Tetany and seizurelike movements can be precipitated by rapid correction of systemic acidosis with large amounts of base.

(8) Hyperkalemia and hypokalemia. Hyperkalemia can occur in ATN patients as a result of injudicious dietary intake (e.g., bananas, oranges, coffee), drug preparations that contain K^+, and egress of K^+ from intracellular compartments following trauma, hemolysis, or retroperitoneal hemorrhage. Hypokalemia usually does not develop until the diuretic phase of ATN unless the patient has had substantial diarrhea.

(9) Hypocalcemia, hyperphosphatemia, and hyperuricemia, which may be severe in hypercatabolic states and in rhabdomyolysis, seldom cause symptoms directly. An effort should be made, however, to minimize phosphate retention by restricting dietary phosphate intake and administration of phosphate-binding antacids (see sec. **V.H**). Additional efforts to treat hypocalcemia are usually unnecessary. Serum uric acid levels less than 15 mg/dl serially do not require treatment in the acute situation. For levels greater than 15 mg/dl, allopurinol (200–300 mg qd) is appropriate.

(10) Adjustment of drug usage. Drugs that are excreted by the kidney may have to be given in reduced dosages. (For these modifications, see *Ann. Intern. Med.* 93:62, 286, 1980, and sections in the *Manual* dealing with the drugs in question.)

(11) Convulsions should be treated acutely with parenteral short-acting barbiturates or diazepam with phenytoin sodium being administered concurrently, as discussed in Chap. 22. Drugs dependent on intact renal function for adequate excretion, such as phenobarbital, should be avoided. If hypocalcemia is symptomatic, 10–20 ml 10% calcium gluconate should be slowly injected IV. If water intoxication is suspected (serum sodium < 110 mEq/liter), water should be restricted; rarely, when water intoxication is marked, dialysis is required. Acidosis, if severe, must be partially corrected by administration of sodium bicarbonate, with careful monitoring of the patient for manifestations of hypocalcemia. Most commonly, convulsions are manifestations either of the uremic syndrome or of the disequilibrium syndrome following dialysis. However, convulsions may represent a complication of uremia, such as cerebral hemorrhage or meningitis.

(12) Dialysis. Although many patients without complications can be managed conservatively, perhaps with occasional dialysis for specific indications, the current tendency is toward more aggressive use of dialysis. The advantages of dialysis include more liberal fluid and dietary intake, improved patient well-being, and easier control of fluid balance. The prognosis may be improved by aggressive dialysis. **Specific indications for dialysis** include volume overload, hyperkalemia, severe acidosis, neurologic abnormalities, severe hyponatremia, and hypercatabolism (see sec. **VI.A**).

b. **Diuretic phase.** A progressive increase in urine volume signals the recovery of renal function. The massive diuresis once described is less frequent, probably because of protein restriction, early dialysis, and greater care to avoid fluid overload. However, the regulatory capacity of the kidney remains inadequate during the diuretic phase, and careful attention to replacement of urinary losses is necessary. Daily (or twice-daily) weights and measurement of urine electrolytes are useful guides to fluid replacement. Although urine output is increased, the GFR may remain low for days, and BUN and plasma creatinine may continue to rise. Approximately 25% of deaths occur during this phase of ATN.

c. **Recovery phase.** Renal function continues to improve for 3–12 months and usually returns to a level compatible with normal health. The GFR becomes completely normal in only a minority of patients. Often, some tubular dysfunction remains (e.g., reduced concentrating ability or a mild acidification defect) but is not clinically significant.

2. **Intrinsic renal diseases other than acute tubular necrosis**

a. **Acute glomerulonephritis.** Many of the principles of treatment that follow pertain to glomerulonephritis (GN) from any cause.

(1) **Rest.** Bed rest is indicated during the acute stage, associated with hypertension and positive sodium and water balance. During the 4- –8-week period of rapid improvement, graduate ambulation should be allowed. One will note a significant increase in the microscopic hematuria or quantitative proteinuria after ambulation; this usually subsides somewhat with bed rest. However, no specific evidence exists to support an improved prognosis with prolonged bed rest.

(2) **Diet.** Rigid salt restriction (1–2 gm daily) may be required during the acute phase of edema formation and hypertension. There is no evidence that protein restriction affects the prognosis unless the patient is acidotic from severe impairment of renal function.

(3) **Hypertension.** Hydralazine, methyldopa, clonidine, prazosin, diazoxide, and sodium nitroprusside may be effective antihypertensive agents, since they do not ordinarily produce decreases in renal blood flow or GFR (see Table 7-1).

(4) **Edema and congestive heart failure.** Salt restriction is the cornerstone of therapy and, along with bed rest, usually suffices unless pulmonary vascular congestion develops. Marked fluid and salt overload may require dialysis. Less frequently, a mild natriuresis may occur with furosemide, even with a marked reduction in GFR. Phlebotomy or plasmapheresis is also reliable therapy in this situation. Digitalis can be employed when indicated; however, maintenance doses must be adjusted appropriately.

(5) **Antibiotics.** Although it is generally felt that antibiotic therapy probably does not prevent development of poststreptococcal acute GN, a course of therapy is warranted to remove the potential immunologic source from the pharynx, skin, or both.

(6) **Corticosteroids.** Routine administration of glucocorticoids during acute GN has not been effective in arresting the symptoms or shorten-

ing the course; furthermore, the hypertension and edema secondary to corticosteroids may aggravate the underlying disease.

(7) Cytotoxic drugs are not indicated in poststreptococcal acute GN.

(8) Uremia. If uremia develops, therapy should be modified in accordance with the basic principles outlined in sec. **1.a.**

b. Acute vasculitis may present with glomerulitis and ARF; one should be alert to involvement of other organ systems in diagnosing these entities. Systemic lupus erythematosus often is responsive to high-dose prednisone, $60-100$ mg/24 hr/M^2. Cyclophosphamide and prednisone may be useful in periarteritis nodosa. Wegener's granulomatosis may respond dramatically to cyclophosphamide (see Systemic Lupus Erythematosus and Necrotizing Vasculitis, Chap. 21).

c. Hepatorenal syndrome is a unique form of functional renal failure that develops in patients with severe liver disease (especially following diuretic therapy, paracentesis, or GI bleeding). It is usually associated with portal hypertension, jaundice, and ascites. The most common finding is a strikingly low urinary sodium concentration, often less than 5 mEq/liter, with a high U/P creatinine ratio. This syndrome is often difficult to differentiate from prerenal azotemia, and careful assessment of cardiovascular function and ECF volume is essential. A judicious trial of volume expansion may be required. In general, although several maneuvers may result in transient increases in urine output, no treatment of clinical value has been devised. However, the placement of a peritoneojugular (LeVeen) shunt may reverse the oliguria in selected cases (*Arch. Intern. Med.* 137:1248, 1977).

C. Postrenal azotemia (obstructive uropathy). Obstruction to urine flow can occur at any level of the urinary tract and **must always be included** in the differential diagnosis of ARF. Presentations include total anuria, fluctuating urine output, polyuria, urinary tract infection, pain, or unexplained renal failure. When obstruction is suspected, patency of the urinary tract must be proved, but needless instrumentation of the urinary tract should be avoided. Sonography and computed tomography scanning are the methods of choice in the diagnosis of obstruction. In some cases, retrograde pyelography will be necessary to demonstrate patency of at least one ureter.

1. Postobstructive diuresis describes the clinical state that can occur after relief of severe urinary tract obstruction. Marked polyuria associated with the excretion of large amounts of sodium and potassium may occur. Although self-limited (may last several days), the diuresis may be of such degree and duration as to cause marked contraction of ECF volume and peripheral vascular collapse. Effective therapy requires the prompt quantitative replacement of urinary losses of water, sodium, and potassium. This replacement must be milliequivalent for milliequivalent and milliliter for milliliter, with frequent measurements of urine volume and serum and urine electrolytes.

2. Uric acid nephropathy. Administration of cytotoxic agents to patients with hematologic and other disorders may result in rapid lysis of cells and potentially severe hyperuricemia. This disorder also may develop in other hyperuricemic patients. Acute renal failure results from intrarenal or extrarenal deposition of uric acid crystals, leading to obstruction to urine flow. Therapy should include allopurinol (preferably prophylactically), diuresis, and alkalinization of the urine. A total of $600-900$ mg/day of allopurinol in divided doses is often required to reduce the serum uric acid level. Acetazolamide, 250 mg PO qid for a few days, may be used to alkalinize the urine. Dialysis, especially hemodialysis, can be extremely effective in the treatment of hyperuricemia. Lower urinary tract obstruction (e.g., uric acid stone) should be treated in the usual way (see sec. **IV.C.1**).

II. Glomerulopathies. Disorders of the structure and function of the glomerulus constitute one of the main clinical problems of nephrology and are the most common cause of end-stage renal failure requiring dialysis or transplantation. Classification of these disorders may be according to clinical features, morphology of biopsy sections, or presumed pathogenic mechanisms. No one classification is suitable for every purpose; the reader is referred to L. E. Early and C. W. Gottschalk (eds.), *Strauss and Welt's Diseases of the Kidney* (3rd ed.). Boston: Little, Brown, 1979, for a detailed discussion of the various categories. The principles of treatment to be outlined are presented by general category of glomerular disease. For **indications for treatment of the following disorders with corticosteroids and/or cytotoxic agents,** see **B.**

A. Types of glomerulopathies

1. Minimal-change nephrotic syndrome (lipoid nephrosis or nil disease) presents with proteinuria and often with the nephrotic syndrome and accounts for abut 20% of all adult cases of nephrosis. It is characterized by a normal histologic appearance on light microscopy, negative findings on immunofluorescence, and foot-process fusion on electron microscopy.

A response to glucocorticoid therapy (1 mg/kg/day) is obtained in 75–85% of adult patients. Corticosteroids are usually given over 3 months. The response may be a lasting remission, an initial response with frequent relapses, or a corticosteroid-dependent response (i.e., proteinuria recurs if glucocorticoid therapy is withdrawn). Frequent relapses, or corticosteroid dependence, and glucocorticoid nonresponders may all respond to cyclophosphamide (2 mg/kg/day) alone or in combination with glucocorticoids. However, if proteinuria does not remit within 2–3 months, it may be necessary to repeat the biopsy to reassess the diagnosis (see **2**).

2. Focal glomerulosclerosis is regarded by some as a variant of lipoid nephrosis, with which it may be easily confused in its early stages. Focal glomerulosclerosis may be responsible for the "nonresponders" among patients with an apparent lipoid nephrosis and is usually associated with a progressive decline in GFR, the nephrotic syndrome, and hypertension.

3. Membranous glomerulopathy is commonly associated with the nephrotic syndrome. Although this disease may occur at any age, the majority of patients are over 40 at the time of diagnosis. The onset is insidious, with hypertension and azotemia occurring late in the course of the disease. The most comon form of the disease has no known cause and is therefore termed *idiopathic membranous glomerulopathy.* However, the same morphologic picture also may be seen in association with systemic disease (e.g., carcinoma, lymphoma, systemic lupus erythematosus, malaria) or with the ingestion of heavy metals or penicillamine. The course is indolent and slowly progressive and may be punctuated by spontaneous remissions. Sudden deteriorations in renal function or worsening of the nephrotic syndrome may indicate the occurrence of **renal vein thrombosis.**

4. Proliferative glomerulonephritis encompasses a variety of glomerular abnormalities characterized by proliferation of mesangial and endothelial cells. It is not clear whether the wide variety of appearances seen on biopsy represent distinct clinicopathologic entities or merely stages of the same type of structural damage. The usual presentation is with proteinuria and hematuria and often the nephrotic syndrome. Problems of classification make it difficult to predict the course of diseases of this type. In general, the course is one of progressive decrease in renal function leading to renal failure.

5. Membranoproliferative (mesangiocapillary) glomerulonephritis may present as acute or subacute nephritis, nephrotic syndrome, or asymptomatic proteinuria, usually accompanied by hematuria. Decreased GFR occurs in half the patients and, if present at the onset of the disease, usually is indicative of a poor prognosis.

In general, the course is a slowly progressive one, leading to renal failure within 10 years in 50% or more of the patients. A shorter course is usual if GFR is reduced at the time of diagnosis.

B. Therapeutic considerations in the treatment of glomerular disease. The mainstays of treatment for GN are **glucocorticoids** and **cytotoxic agents** (cyclophosphamide, azothiaprine, chlorambucil). However, the results of treatment of glomerular diseases with these agents have been extremely variable, perhaps because morphologic changes in the glomerulus may represent a common pathway for different pathogenetic factors. Thus, groups of patients with apparent similarities on morphologic grounds may be pathogenetically heterogeneous and thus have variable clinical courses, making assessment of the results of therapy difficult. One approach to this problem, which is the current practice at our institution, is to plot the logarithm (and/or the reciprocal) of the serum creatinine of patients against time (see Fig. 3-1). It has been shown that the rate of progression of renal disease can be quantitated in this fashion using simple linear regression analyses (*Kidney Int.* 11:62, 1977; *Lancet* 2:1326, 1976); there is a straight-line relationship in most cases. A mathematically defined reduction in renal function (i.e., positive slope on the graph) constitutes an indication for treatment. The response to therapy can also be assessed by noting whether a change in the slope of the line occurs during treatment, and, if so, whether or not this change is favorable. This provides the advantage of having each patient serve as his or her own control. An example of this approach is illustrated in Fig. 3-1.

If a progressive decline in renal function is observed, treatment should be attempted. If deterioration is relatively slow ($T^{1/2} > 12$ months), treatment with prednisone (60 mg/day) should be initiated. If no benefit is apparent after 12 weeks, cyclophosphamide (2 mg/kg/day) should be added to the regimen. When rapid deterioration is evident ($T^{1/2} < 12$ months), therapy with prednisone ($1-2$ mg/kg/day) and cyclophosphamide (2 mg/kg/day) should be given initially. Some patients may benefit from the addition of antiplatelet agents (dipyridamole, aspirin), particularly if membranoproliferative GN is present on renal biopsy. Recent experience suggests that plasmapheresis, together with immunosuppressive agents, may be beneficial in the rapidly progressive GN of Goodpasture's syndrome. (A review of therapeutic modalities for the treatment of glomerular disorders can be found in *Med. Clin. North Am.* 62:1157, 1978.) The complications of glucocorticoid and cytotoxic therapy are discussed in Chap. 21.

III. Nephrotic syndrome. Nephrotic syndrome (i.e., proteinuria >3 gm/day, serum albumin <3 gm/dl, edema, and hyperlipidemia) may be a manifestation of many pathologic processes. Appropriate investigation to discover the underlying cause of the nephrotic syndrome should be followed by specific therapy when possible. If the diagnosis of a proteinuric state (especially, nephrotic syndrome) is not known, renal biopsy should be considered.

The principles of **general management** of the nephrotic syndrome include the following:

A. Diet. Because of considerable urinary protein losses, the diet should be rich in protein of high biologic value ($100-150$ gm/day unless the patient is azotemic). Total caloric intake should be $25-50$ kcal/kg/day.

B. Infections and general medical problems, including hypertension, should be treated promptly and vigorously.

C. Salt restriction and diuretics. With currently available diuretics, stringent salt restriction is usually unnecessary in the control of edema of mild or moderate severity. An intake of $2-4$ gm sodium chloride is compatible with successful

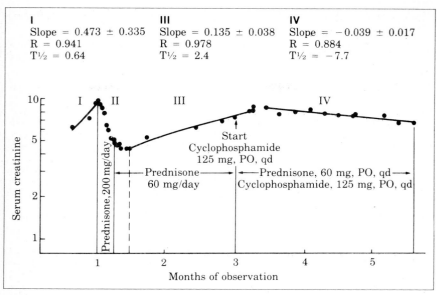

I
Slope $= 0.473 \pm 0.335$
R $= 0.941$
T½ $= 0.64$

III
Slope $= 0.135 \pm 0.038$
R $= 0.978$
T½ $= 2.4$

IV
Slope $= -0.039 \pm 0.017$
R $= 0.884$
T½ $= -7.7$

Fig. 3-1. Course of a patient with glomerulosclerosis illustrated by a plot of the logarithm of serum creatinine against time. Deteriorating renal function (I) underwent a reversal on treatment with high-dose prednisone (II). Continuation of prednisone at 60 mg/day was associated with gradual deterioration of renal function (III) with a positive slope on the plot. The addition of cyclophosphamide to the regimen was associated with a negative slope (IV), indicating an improvement in renal function. T½ is the time required for renal function (GFR) to decrease by 50% (or for serum creatinine to double) and is calculated from the regression line for the serum creatinine values. (Courtesy of Dr. Phillip Hoffsten, Washington University, St. Louis, Missouri.)

therapy in most cases. When edema is severe, sodium in the diet can be reduced to 10 mEq/day, with diuresis achieved by drug therapy. Furosemide is extremely useful, although its diuretic effect is often reduced in the nephrotic syndrome. Additional measures that may be used in patients in whom diuresis is difficult to achieve include keeping the patient recumbent, giving aminophylline at night, using combinations of diuretics, e.g., thiazide, furosemide, and spironolactone (do not use the latter if the GFR is less than 25 ml/minute because of the danger of hyperkalemia), and, in selected cases, infusions of salt-poor albumin followed by 40–80 mg furosemide IV. The possibility of inducing hypotension and ARF by vigorous salt depletion in patients with low plasma proteins should be kept in mind.

IV. Nephrolithiasis. Nephrolithiasis is a significant medical problem, accounting for approximately 2 in every 1000 hospitalizations in the United States.

    A. Clinical manifestations of stones are variable and, except for the passage of a stone, are nonspecific. Affected patients may present with hematuria (gross or microscopic), urinary tract infections, incidental findings on x-ray study, pain, or, rarely, oliguria and uremia (requires bilateral ureteral obstruction or obstruction of a solitary functioning kidney in patients with previously normal renal function). Pain may be located in the back, abdomen, or groin; it varies from mild discomfort to excruciating pain lasting for a variable period. Nausea and vomiting often occur, and tenderness is often present in the area of the kidneys or ureters. The pain is not colicky in most instances, even though the term *renal colic* is commonly used.

B. Investigation. After a careful history and physical examination, the following measures should be taken:

1. Any stone passed or recovered at operation should be sent for analysis (stones may be sent to Louis C. Herring and Co., P.O. Box 2191, Orlando, Fla. 32802).

2. Since calcium is present in 85–90% of all stones, investigation of **calcium homeostasis** is important. On a normal calcium and phosphate intake (800–1000 mg calcium and 1000 mg phosphate), 24-hour urines should be collected for determination of calcium, magnesium, creatinine clearance, and tubular resorption of phosphate. Urinary calcium over 4 mg/kg/day (for both sexes) is considered hypercalciuric. Since many patients with stones ingest a self-imposed low-calcium diet, a common pitfall is to measure calcium excretion on their usual diet (low calcium) and thus possibly miss a diagnosis of hypercalciuria. If hypercalciuria is found, one should exclude the causes of increased calcium excretion, e.g., hyperparathyroidism, milk alkali syndrome, vitamin D intoxication, renal tubular acidosis, sarcoidosis.

3. **Urinary excretion** of uric acid should be measured (>800 mg/day is abnormal).

4. Several determinations of **serum calcium** should be obtained in the fasting state (avoid venous stasis in collecting the sample). Ionized calcium should be measured where facilities are available.

5. An **IVP** should be obtained, particularly if the patient presents with renal colic or hematuria or has a history of urinary tract infections.

6. **A urine culture** should be obtained.

7. To uncover incomplete forms of renal tubular acidosis that may be a cause of nephrocalcinosis, a **urinary acidification evaluation** should be undertaken if there is depression of plasma bicarbonate or nephrocalcinosis or in the absence of other definite diagnostic criteria.

8. Measurements of immunoreactive parathyroid hormone, 25-hydroxy vitamin D, and 1,25-dihydroxy vitamin D may be helpful.

C. Treatment. During the acute phase of renal colic, therapy is directed toward relieving pain, maintaining a brisk rate of urine flow, and treating complications or predisposing factors if known. The urine must be strained through a gauze sponge and the stone sent for analysis. Many stones will pass spontaneously; others will require removal by appropriate urologic procedures. **Recurrent stones** often present difficult management problems and cause high morbidity. Identifiable predisposing factors, such as hyperparathyroidism, excessive milk ingestion, hyperuricemia, and renal tubular acidosis, must be treated. It is traditional to encourage "recurrent stone-formers" to ingest large volumes of fluid, but the results with respect to preventing new stones have been discouraging.

Specific therapy is important in certain situations, as follows:

1. **Uric acid stones.** Allopurinol should be administered in a dosage of 100 mg tid or as a single tablet (300 mg/day) in the presence of hyperuricemia or hyperuricosuria. Bicarbonate, 50–100 mEq/day, should be given until hyperuricemia is corrected. Actual dissolution of uric acid stones can be accomplished by maintaining an alkaline urine.

2. **Idiopathic hypercalciuria,** i.e., elevated urinary calcium in the absence of any identifiable cause, accounts for almost 50% of cases of recurrent nephrolithiasis. Hypercalciuria is the final common pathway for a number of underlying pathogenic mechanisms, including intestinal hyperabsorption of calcium, increased bone resorption, and impaired renal tubular resorption of calcium or phosphate. Since these basic mechanisms may occur in combina-

tion, diagnosis is difficult. In general, administration of a **thiazide** (hydro-chlorothiazide, 50 mg bid) or chlorthalidone, 50–100 mg/day, reduces urinary calcium and decreases stone formation. Modest salt restriction should also be imposed to maintain the reduction in urinary calcium. If hypercalcemia develops during treatment with thiazides, the patient should be re-evaluated for hyperparathyroidism, sarcoidosis, or other causes of hypercalcemia. Dietary calcium should not be restricted to less than 600–800 mg/day, since this results in increased oxalate excretion and reduced pyrophosphate excretion. Cellulose phosphate may be a useful treatment in patients with proved intestinal hyperabsorption of calcium. Allopurinol should be used with coexisting hyperuricosuria.

3. **Cystine stones.** Human urine normally does not contain cystine in excess of its solubility. Thus, the presence of cystine stones usually indicates congenital cystinuria. Increasing the urine pH to about 7.8 doubles the solubility of cystine. Maintaining urine output in excess of 3 liters/day (should include 2 glasses of water before retiring and 2 glasses at 2 A.M.) results in decreased cystine stone formation and, at times, actual stone dissolution. D-Penicillamine, 1–2 gm/day, is effective therapy for this condition. Complications of D-penicillamine are discussed in Chap. 21.

V. **Chronic renal failure.** Many chronic progressive renal diseases result in the irreversible loss of the majority of nephrons from the functional nephron population. Often, these patients are unaware of the presence of renal disease until severe renal failure has developed, in which case they must be differentiated from patients with ARF. Of help in this differentiation is renal size, which can often be determined by a flat film of the abdomen or by laminography. Most patients with advanced chronic renal disease (end-stage kidney disease) have small, contracted kidneys (exceptions may include patients with diabetic nephropathy, amyloidosis, myeloma kidney, collagen disease, and malignant hypertension), and extensive diagnostic evaluation is not indicated.

Management of chronic renal failure (CRF) is directed toward maintaining the functional integrity of the residual nephrons. With appropriate management, the majority of patients will remain almost symptom free until the GFR has fallen below 10 ml/minute, and many will remain so until it has fallen to 5 ml/minute. Reversible decreases in renal function contribute significantly to morbidity and mortality in these patients; **the correctable processes** of volume contraction, obstruction, CHF, hypertension, presence of a renal toxin, and infection must always be excluded if azotemia worsens. Satisfactory treatment often will result in return of the BUN and GFR to levels present before the acute insult. In addition, control of hypertension and infection slows the relentless and progressive nephron destruction. Accurate measurement of GFR is important in following these patients. For clinical purposes, creatinine clearances are adequate even though they overestimate the true GFR at levels of function below 20 ml/minute.

A. **General measures.** Patients should be encouraged to remain as active as possible to improve their quality of living and minimize protein catabolism. Multivitamins should be given routinely if the patient is being dialyzed (the soluble vitamins are readily dialyzable) and if dietary intake is poor. Folic acid supplements are also necessary for patients on dialysis.

B. **Diet** is an important component of the therapy of CRF and is all too often ignored.

1. **Protein restriction** is not indicated until the GFR falls to a level at which symptoms and signs of uremia either are present (BUN usually > 100 mg/dl) or can soon be expected to appear (BUN > 75 mg/dl). Dietary management should be appropriate for the degree of renal failure, and stringent protein restriction should be avoided until clearly indicated. Most patients should receive from 0.50–0.75 gm/kg of protein of high biologic quality. Greater degrees of protein restriction are necessary if the patient is severely acidotic

and has symptoms of uremia. As the frequency of dialysis is increased, a greater amount of protein can be added to the patient's diet. Additional protein loss resulting from proteinuria, peritoneal dialysis (10–30 gm/24 hours), and hemodialysis (approximately 12 gm/6 hours) should be replaced with protein of high biologic value, such as eggs or meat. With all low-protein diets, high caloric intake is critical if catabolism is to be minimized and positive nitrogen balance maintained (unless obese, patients should ingest 50 kcal/kg/day). Patients with slowly progressive forms of chronic renal disease and very low levels of renal function may experience a gratifying reduction in their symptoms with proper dietary management.

2. **Salt.** Uremia per se is not an indication for salt restriction. Most patients with chronic renal disease should be given a 4- –6-gm salt diet (essentially a normal diet without added salt), since they are unable to excrete sodium-free urine. Occasionally, this salt-losing tendency may be more marked. Infrequently, other patients may excrete a urine almost free of sodium. Dietary salt management will be more precise if 24-hour urinary sodium excretion is measured while the patient is on a known salt intake prior to discharge from the hospital. The patient should be kept volume expanded as indicated by trace edema, unless precluded by cardiac decompensation, since slight volume expansion will maintain a maximal GFR. Contraction of ECF volume and marked deterioration of renal function often develop in patients with CRF placed on needless salt restriction. In the rare patient requiring more than 8–9 gm salt/day, bouillon can be used as a palatable source of salt (one cube contains about 2.5 gm of salt). Some patients will require $NaHCO_3$ for acidosis and will be able to tolerate the increased Na^+ load without fluid retention and weight gain; if these occur, however, the intake of salt should be decreased by 1.5 gm (25 mEq Na^+) for each 2 gm of $NaHCO_3$ (24 mEq Na^+) given. Patients should be instructed to weigh themselves every day. They should be aware that rapid changes in weight reflect salt and water balance and should modify their salt intake accordingly.

3. **Fluids.** Because of relatively fixed urinary osmolalities in chronic renal disease, the range of water excretion (either conserving it or excreting it) is markedly impaired. To remain in solute balance, the uremic patient should pass 1.5–2.0 liters of urine/24 hours. Prolonged periods of fluid deprivation with obligatory solute excretion will result in negative salt and water balance, dehydration, and a further reduction in renal function. During intercurrent illnesses with fever, nausea, vomiting, or diarrhea, supplemental (often parenteral) fluids will be necessary to maintain a proper ECF volume.

C. **Management of CHF** has been discussed in sec. **I.B.1.a.(6).** Furosemide will produce a diuresis even when the GFR has fallen below 20 ml/minute, although the natriuretic effect is significantly reduced after the GFR drops below 10 ml/minute. The use of high doses has been associated with hearing loss. This effect appears to be reversible for furosemide but may be irreversible for ethacrynic acid (which should not be used in CRF). Diuretic agents and digitalis (dose modified for level of renal function), coupled with careful salt and water restriction, may result in marked improvement.

D. **Hypertension** is common in CRF. Volume expansion is more often a major contributing factor than is increased renin production. When controlling hypertension by salt restriction, it is important to avoid deterioration of renal function due to excess volume contraction. Antihypertensive agents are usually required in addition to salt restriction. **Hypertensive crises** can be managed with diazoxide and sodium nitroprusside (see Chap. 7).

E. **Hyponatremia** may be dilutional or represent a true sodium deficit associated with signs of ECF volume contraction and deteriorating renal function. In the latter situation, urgent correction with synthetic ECF (and $NaHCO_3$ if indicated) is necessary. For a more detailed discussion see Chap. 2, sec. **IV.D.1–4.**

F. Hyperkalemia and hypokalemia. The ability to maintain K^+ balance usually is preserved until very late in the course of chronic progressive renal disease, at which time restriction of dietary K^+ becomes necessary. Marked hyperkalemia, however, more often occurs secondary to acute endogenous K^+ loads (catabolic illnesses, hemolysis, GI and soft-tissue hemorrhage, or severe acidosis) than to renal failure alone. Triamterene, spironolactone, or amiloride may result in lethal hyperkalemia and should not be used in renal failure. Some drugs are marketed as the K^+ salt and can be the source of significant amounts of K^+ when given in massive doses (penicillin has about 1.7 mEq K^+/million units). In a few patients with CRF, hyperkalemia out of proportion to the reduction in GFR develops because of relative aldosterone deficiency; such patients respond to mineralocorticoids (0.1–0.2 mg 9-fludrocortisone/day). Acute management of hyperkalemia is discussed in Chap. 2, sec. **V.B.4.**

Hypokalemia resulting from anorexia, vomiting, or diarrhea may require careful administration of K^+ supplements.

G. Acidosis per se is not treated unless the serum or plasma bicarbonate concentration is less than 15–16 mEq/liter or symptoms are present. Occurrence of acidosis of this degree in CRF usually is associated with an acute acid load that can be endogenous (increased catabolism related to an intercurrent infection) or exogenous (administration of drugs such as methionine, NH_4Cl, and aspirin). Dietary indiscretions with increased protein intake may result in further uremic decompensation with acidosis. Prior to correction of acidosis, the patient's cardiovascular, Ca^{2+}, and K^+ status must be evaluated (see Chap. 2, sec. **VI.D.3.a**). Treatment of acidosis may be important in the prevention of osteodystrophy.

H. Hypocalcemia and hyperphosphatemia are the rule in CRF once the GFR falls below 25–30 ml/min. However, secondary hyperparathyroidism probably exists long before renal function falls to this level. The elevated serum phosphate is lowered by reducing phosphate intake and administering phosphate-binding gels **(Basaljel, Amphojel, Dialume).** Because of potential hypermagnesemia, magnesium-containing antacids (e.g., Maalox, Gelusil, Creamalin, Aludrox, Mylanta) should not be used.

The serum phosphate ideally should be kept at 4–5 mg/dl; lower levels may result in osteomalacia. Once the serum phosphate is controlled, supplementary calcium becomes mandatory, (to maintain normal calcium balance), especially in patients on a restricted protein diet (low-protein diets usually contain only 350 mg calcium). Elemental calcium, 1.0–1.5 gm, should be ingested daily (e.g., **Os-Cal,** 500 mg tid, or **calcium carbonate,** 1 gm qid).

I. Renal osteodystrophy. Bone disease in uremia results from secondary hyperparathyroidism, decreased 1,25-dihydroxy vitamin D production with consequent calcium malabsorption, long-standing acidosis, and abnormal bone collagen metabolism. Treatment should be undertaken, preferably after definitive diagnosis by biopsy, and should include phosphate-binding antacids, calcium supplementation, careful use of vitamin D or its metabolites, and parathyroidectomy when necessary. The treatment of renal osteodystrophy with potent metabolites of vitamin D may give rise to serious complications and should preferably be undertaken by persons with expertise in the field.

J. Hyperuricemia develops when the GFR falls below approximately 30 ml/minute and may progress if the GFR falls further; however, the serum uric acid rarely exceeds 10–12 mg/dl. Frank gouty attacks are uncommon in patients without a previous history of gout. Uric acid stones are uncommon. Although allopurinol in the usual dose will lower serum uric acid without decreasing GFR, it is **rarely necessary.**

K. Pruritus, hiccups, and nausea may respond to phenothiazines (e.g., 5 mg prochlorperazine PO q6h) but are usually resistant to such therapy. Intractable pruritus often is associated with severe secondary hyperparathyroidism and often disappears after parathyroidectomy. Aquaphor cream has been advocated for symptomatic relief.

L. Dialysis and transplantation. A detailed discussion of chronic hemodialysis and transplantation is beyond the scope of the *Manual,* and only selected comments will be made here. The indications for and complications of dialysis are discussed in further detail in sec. **VI.** Patients with what appears to be "end-stage" CRF and who are not candidates for chronic dialysis should not be denied acute dialysis if potentially reversible factors may have resulted in a deterioration of renal function. Often, such a dialysis will allow the patient to regain a level of renal function compatible with a comfortable life for several months. Chronic dialysis is an acceptable form of therapy, and its use can return many patients with end-stage renal failure to society as functioning members. The current 5-year survival of patients on chronic dialysis is 62%. Complications include infections (15% of deaths), especially viral hepatitis; cardiac complications (30% of deaths), which include CHF, myocardial infarction, and pericarditis; cerebrovascular accidents (17% of deaths); and bone disease with metastatic calcification secondary to hyperparathyroidism.

Renal transplantation represents a significant advance in the management and rehabilitation of the patient with CRF. The graft survival rate for an A-match, living-related homograft at 2 years is 90%, while that of cadaver grafts is 60%. The techniques of chronic dialysis and transplantation are complementary and are employed together in many centers.

M. Drugs. It is important to be aware of the function of the kidney in eliminating drugs and their metabolites from the body, and in prescribing a drug for a patient with renal impairment, great care must be taken because of potential renal or extrarenal toxicity (*Ann. Intern. Med.* 93:62, 286, 1980).

VI. Indications for and complications of dialysis

A. Indications for dialysis. Most indications for dialysis are relative, and often other modes of therapy are available. In general, these indications apply both to acute and chronic renal failure.

1. Hyperkalemia usually can be controlled without dialysis, especially if the potassium load is not increased and potassium exchange resins can be given. Some patients are hypercatabolic, or acidotic, or have large endogenous or exogenous potassium loads and need dialysis to control life-threatening hyperkalemia. Rarely, peritoneal dialysis will be ineffective in controlling massive hyperkalemia; hemodialysis then must be employed.

2. Metabolic acidosis often accompanies renal failure and, when severe, is usually associated with an acute acid load or a loss of base. When volume overload precludes administration of significant amounts of sodium bicarbonate, dialysis can effectively treat both disorders.

3. Cardiovascular overload can be corrected readily by dialysis. Commercially available peritoneal dialysis fluids contain 1.5 or 4.5 gm/dl dextrose, giving them an osmolality of 372 and 525 mOsm/liter respectively. The hypertonicity of these solutions provides an effective osmotic force for removing salt and water from the patient. Hemodialysis can correct hypervolemia by ultrafiltration of blood in the dialyzer.

4. Pericarditis. This serious complication of uremia all too often results in death from cardiac tamponade. It may develop insidiously, with fever as the only clinical manifestation. Usually, these patients have been poorly dialyzed or have greater degrees of hyperparathyroidism than do unaffected patients. Dialysis is the treatment of choice, but **regional heparinization is mandatory** because of the potential for tamponade from pericardial hemorrhage if systemic heparinization is used. Whereas frequent hemodialysis is the recommended therapy for uncomplicated uremic pericarditis, pericardiectomy is recommended for pericarditis complicated by effusion and impairment of cardiac function (*Surgery* 80:689, 1976).

5. **Uremia.** The clinical manifestations of the uremic syndrome, especially uremic encephalopathy, can be corrected readily by dialysis. Because of the lower clearance of most substances, peritoneal dialysis takes 3–6 times as long as hemodialysis. It is preferable to institute dialysis before clinical uremia and its associated complications develop.

6. **Combinations of acid-base and/or fluid and electrolyte abnormalities** are often present in a single patient with renal failure. The situation may be made more complex because of coexistent hyponatremia, water intoxication, hypocalcemia, or hyerkalemia. Dialysis provides a safe and effective means of reversing this spectrum of abnormalities.

B. **Hemodialysis versus peritoneal dialysis.** Since both methods have inherent advantages and disadvantages, the preferable dialysis technique depends on the individual patient's needs.

1. **Peritoneal dialysis** is technically less complicated than hemodialysis and can be done on almost any hospital ward. Peritoneal dialysis of most substances is one-third to one-sixth that of hemodialysis but, given enough time, is equally effective in most circumstances. The peritoneal cavity should be relatively intact and generally should not be used in the presence of undiagnosed abdominal disease, extensive adhesions, or immediately after certain abdominal operations. Peritoneal dialysis, however, is inadequate for most patients with drug intoxication and may be inadequate in renal failure associated with markedly catabolic states.

2. **Hemodialysis** is more efficient than peritoneal dialysis, causes less discomfort to the patient, and can be carried out frequently and indefinitely. Hypotension, severe intrinsic heart disease, or a hemorrhagic diathesis may preclude the use of hemodialysis or markedly impair its effectiveness.

C. The **complications of peritoneal dialysis** are frequently related to acid-base or fluid and electrolyte abnormalities. They can often be prevented by careful monitoring.

1. **Volume depletion.** A technically effective peritoneal dialysis may remove several hundred milliliters per exchange from the patient and result in hypotension. Water removed in excess of electrolytes can result in **hypernatremia**, especially if hypertonic dialysate is being used. The physician must monitor the patient's blood sugar and electrolytes. Careful determinations of input, output, and weights are essential. Undesired fluid loss must be replaced with hypotonic solutions.

2. **Volume overload** may result from two causes. First, if the patient is severely hyponatremic, Na (and H_2O) will move from the dialysate into the intravascular space; this may result in cardiovascular overload. Second—and more commonly—inadequate drainage of dialysate will promote its absorption. If shortening the dwelling time of the fluid and repositioning the patient and/or the dialysis catheter fail to correct the patient's positive fluid balance, hemodialysis may be required. Hypertonic dialysate should not be used if the peritoneal dialysis is not functioning properly.

3. **Infection.** The danger of peritonitis (5–10% incidence in most series) demands sterile techniques, closed sterile drainage systems, and frequent cultures of peritoneal drainage. It is desirable to limit the duration of peritoneal dialysis to 36–48 hours. Prophylactic antibiotics should not be given. If bacterial peritonitis occurs (positive fluid culture, unexplained fever, cloudy fluid, abdominal tenderness with or without rebound), after appropriate cultures are taken the dialysis may be continued with the addition of appropri-

ate antibiotics to the dialysate (e.g., cephalothin, 100 µg/ml; gentamicin, 8 µg/ml; ampicillin, 50 µg/ml; and/or carbenicillin, 200 µg/ml) coupled with full therapeutic parenteral dosages adjusted for renal insufficiency. This procedure may also be followed for peritonitis occurring during continuous ambulatory peritoneal dialysis.

4. **Metabolic alkalosis** may develop, especially if the peritoneal dialysis is prolonged. Dialysates contain 45 mEq/liter of sodium lactate or acetate, and both are metabolized ultimately to bicarbonate. Bicarbonate cannot be used in the fluid because it precipitates dialysate calcium.

5. **Hyperglycemia** may become marked, especially in diabetic patients or patients receiving hypertonic dialysates. Hyperosmolar coma and death have been reported, indicating the necessity of monitoring the blood sugar. If hyperglycemia develops, the hyperosmolar fluid must be discontinued (at least temporarily) and the blood sugar controlled with insulin. Suspect hyperglycemia whenever a patient on peritoneal dialysis complains of thirst or becomes obtunded.

6. **The disequilibrium syndrome,** manifested by nausea, vomiting, headache, vascular lability, visual blurring, leg cramps, peripheral paresthesias, mental clouding, anxiety, hyperventilation, convulsions, coma, and, occasionally, death, occurs in some patients coincidentally with the rapid correction of severe uremia. This syndrome is more common after hemodialysis than after peritoneal dialysis. Anticonvulsants may be required, but the best treatment is prevention by gradual correction of severe uremia.

7. **Digitialis intoxication** represents a frequent, serious complication. Predisposing events include lowering of the serum K^+ by simultaneous correction of hypocalcemia, hyponatremia, and acidosis. Patients who have received digitalis must be carefully monitored clinically, chemically, and by ECG. The digitalis dosage must be reduced appropriately in uremia. The serum levels of cardiac glycosides are not affected by routine dialysis treatment.

8. **Miscellaneous problems** include excessive abdominal discomfort, embarrassment of respiration in patients with severe pulmonary disease, hemorrhage, perforation of a viscus, pneumonia, and atelectasis. Some of these problems are related to elevation of the diaphragm by the artificial ascites and can be lessened by using more frequent and smaller exchanges.

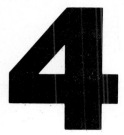

Coronary Heart Disease

Angina Pectoris

Angina pectoris is chest discomfort associated with myocardial ischemia. The discomfort typically is described as a retrosternal dullness or heaviness that may radiate to the arms or neck. It may be precipitated by exertion, emotion, or environmental factors (e.g., cold) that increase myocardial oxygen demand. This discussion will be oriented toward coronary occlusive disease and will not cover other causes of cardiac ischemia, e.g., bridging, aortic stenosis.

The **diagnosis** of angina is suggested by the history. In men and older women, a history of typical angina is good evidence (>90% probability) of coronary artery disease. This is especially true when risk factors, such as smoking, hypertension, hyperlipidemia, obesity, diabetes, type A personality, and a positive family history, are present. Consequently, diagnostic procedures in this group are indicated predominantly to assess therapeutic options. Patients with chest pain that is unlikely by the history to be anginal and with few risk factors have a low incidence (<25%) of coronary artery disease. Noninvasive diagnostic tests frequently are falsely positive in this group. Thus, noninvasive diagnostic evaluation is valuable only if the tests are normal. **Patients with a history suggestive of, but not classic for, angina constitute the group in which both positive and negative noninvasive evaluations are of high predictive value.**

The **treadmill stress test** provides more information than simple positivity or negativity. Other important variables include exercise tolerance, time to angina, degree of S–T depression, and duration of the abnormal S–T response, as well as changes in hemodynamics determined by physical examination. Exercise **thallium imaging** or exercise **radionuclide ventriculography** is valuable when evaluating patients unsuitable for treadmill testing (e.g., patients with conduction defects or taking digitalis). The use of a stress test with a radionuclide procedure augments sensitivity and specificity somewhat and thus may be helpful if the presence of disease is not determined by the treadmill test.

The definitive diagnosis of coronary artery disease is made by **coronary angiography.** Coronary angiography is comparatively safe, with an acceptable mortality of 0.1–0.2%, and should be utilized when the presence or absence of coronary artery disease cannot be determined by other means and/or to evaluate patients for invasive therapy. In addition, this technique provides prognostic information, since mortality is best correlated with the number of coronary arteries significantly obstructed and with left ventricular function.

The **therapy** of angina must be tailored to the individual patient. **Patient and family education is essential.** Risk factors and situations known to precipitate symptoms should be modified. Cessation of smoking, weight reduction, exercise, diet and/or pharmacologic therapy for hyperlipidemia (see Chap. 20), and the removal of stressful physical and emotional stimuli may enhance survival. Basic CPR should be taught to family members. Effective pharmacologic treatment is based on improvement in coronary blood flow, reduction in myocardial oxygen requirement, and alteration of precipitating environmental factors.

Table 4-1. Nitrates

Drug	Onset (min)	Duration of action (hr)	Dosage	Schedule
Nitroglycerin				
Sublingual	1–2	1/2	0.3–0.6 mg	prn
Sustained release	60	8–12	1.3–9.0 mg	q8–12h
Ointment	15	4	1/2–2 in.	q4–6h
Transdermal	Variable (as rapid as 30 min)	24	Variable	Daily
Isosorbide dinitrate or tetranitrate				
Tablets, sublingual	2–5	1–2	2.5–10.0 mg	q3–4h
Tablets, oral	15–30	4	20–60 mg	q6h
Tablets, sustained release	60	6–12	40–80 mg	q8–12h or hs

I. **Drug therapy.** Patient compliance in drug therapy (see Tables 4-1–4-3) is aided by simple regimens, minimal side effects, and a widely spaced dosing schedule. In addition to a beneficial symptomatic response, objective evidence of a therapeutic response, such as changes in heart rate or blood pressure or performance on the treadmill, should be documented. Drug levels are frequently helpful.

A. Sublingual **nitroglycerin** is the cornerstone of therapy (Table 4-1). The primary antianginal effect is an increase in venous capacitance, leading to reduced ventricular volume and pressure and improved subendocardial perfusion. Coronary vasodilatation, improvement in collateral flow, and afterload reduction augment this primary effect. However, if hypotension is induced, the therapeutic effect is lost because of reduced coronary perfusion coupled with reflex tachycardia and increased inotropy. Sublingual nitroglycerin is available as 0.3-, 0.4-, and 0.6-mg tablets. Therapy should be initiated with a small dose to avoid headache, postural hypotension (especially in the elderly), and reflex tachycardia (more common in the young). Other effects, such as burning of the tongue or a sensation of warmth or flushing, often occur; lack of these effects suggests outdated or ineffective medication. Peak action occurs within 2 minutes and continues for 15–30 minutes. Nitroglycerin may be repeated twice at 5- –10-minute intervals if pain is not relieved promptly. Patients should be informed of (1) possible side effects, (2) the benefit of tolerating a full dose (0.3.–0.6 mg), (3) the rarity of tolerance to the drug, (4) the precaution of taking the drug while sitting or lying (necessary in some patients), and (5) the need for storage in an airtight amber bottle, with replacement every 2 months. The patient should be counseled to take nitroglycerin at the first indication of angina and prophylactically before situations known to precipitate angina and to come to the hospital if it does not relieve chest discomfort.

B. **Long-acting nitrates** (Table 4-1), given PO in low doses, are ineffective because of rapid hepatic degradation. Thus, sustained, delayed release (as a capsule or ointment) and large oral doses are recommended.

1. **Nitroglycerin** is available as 1.3-, 2.5-, 6.5-, and 9.0-mg long-acting, sustained release oral preparations (Nitro-Bid, Nitrospan, Nitroglyn). Doses may be given q8–12h. A 2% nitroglycerin ointment also is available and may be applied to tape (as a measure of dose) and attached cutaneously. An average dose of ointment usually covers 1–2 in. of tape. The dosage should be titrated q4–6h to relieve angina without causing headache. Both dosage

Table 4-2. Beta blockers

Drug	Selectivity at low doses	Lipid solubility	Dosage (mg/day)	Dosage schedule
Atenolol	+	+	100	Daily
Metoprolol	+	+ +	150–300	q12h
Nadolol	0	+	80–240	Daily
Pindolol	0	+	10–40	q6h
Propranolol	0	+ + +	120–400	q6–12h
Timolol	0	+ +	15–45	q12h

0 = none; + = mild; + + = moderate; + + + = potent.

forms are beneficial at bedtime when sustained release over the night is important.

2. **Isosorbide dinitrate** and **tetranitrate** conjugers are available in 2.5-, 5-, and 10-mg tablets for sublingual use (Table 4-1). Antianginal effects are short lived (≤1 hour). The oral administration of these agents in high dosages (e.g., 20–60 mg qid) exceeds hepatic metabolism and produces therapeutic blood levels. Administration and withdrawal of high-dose oral therapy must be monitored, because either nitrate tolerance or dependence may occur. Short-acting and extended-release oral preparations are available.

3. Another **transdermal** application utilizes an adhesive patch containing nitroglycerin that releases a constant amount into the skin; thus plasma levels depend on cutaneous blood flow. Recommendations for conversion from other forms of nitrate are not available.

C. **Beta-adrenergic–blocking agents** (Table 4-2) reduce the heart rate and contractile response to dynamic or isometric exercise or environmental stimuli. Thus, these agents ameliorate angina by diminishing myocardial oxygen consumption. Their effect on coronary flow is controversial, but they may constrict the coronary vasculature.

There are several **different forms** of beta blockers. Beta-1 selective agents at low dosages are less apt to exacerbate pulmonary or peripheral vascular disease or to mask symptoms of hypoglycemia. At high dosages, selectivity is partially lost. Less lipid-soluble agents may have a lower incidence of CNS side effects and impotence. Agents with intrinsic sympathomimetic activity (e.g., Pindolol) dilate peripheral vessels and have less effect on resting heart rate. There is no clear difference among beta blockers in their antianginal efficiency.

The **dosage** is adequate if the heart rate is 55–60 beats/minute at rest and does not exceed 90 with exercise. Asymptomatic bradycardia is not a reason to stop treatment. Increasing dosage increases antianginal effects but also causes more side effects. When dosage is increased, the physician should observe the patient for evidence of congestive heart failure (CHF). Most beta blockers can be administered on a twice-a-day basis because of a longer biologic than plasma half-life. Atenolol and nadolol may be administered once daily.

Contraindications to beta blockade are severe CHF, atrioventricular (AV) block, marked resting bradycardia, and Wolff-Parkinson-White (WPW) syndrome with atrial flutter or fibrillation. If CHF is mild, concurrent treatment with digoxin may permit the use of beta blockers. Frequent **side effects** may include bronchospasm, nausea, diarrhea, postural hypotension, claudication, impotence, fatigue, headache, nightmares, depression, hallucinations, subtle deterioration in intellectual capacity, salt retention, and potentiation and masking of hypoglycemia and hyperglycemia. Abrupt withdrawal may be associated with angina, dysrhythmia, myocardial infarction, and even death. When

Table 4-3. Calcium-entry blockers

Action, dosage, and side effects	Verapamil	Diltiazem	Nifedipine
Vasodilatation	+ +	+	+ + +
Effect on hemodynamic performance	Slightly negative	No change	Improved
Blocks reflex sympathetic effects	+	+ +	0
Affects AV conduction	+ + +	+ +	0
Dosage (mg/day)	240–480	120–360	30–120
Dosage schedule	q8h	q8h	q6–8h
Side effects	AV block, constipation, heartburn, nausea, flushing; can precipitate left ventricular failure	AV block, hypotension, flushing; rarely, precipitates left ventricular failure	Palpitations, hypotension, nausea, flushing, edema

+ = Mild effect; + + = moderate effect; + + + = potent effect.

beta blockers must be stopped, they should be tapered if possible. For surgical procedures, the preoperative discontinuance of beta blockers is rarely necessary.

D. **Calcium-blocking agents** (Table 4-3) constitute a diverse group of compounds that alter calcium flux in cardiac and vascular smooth muscle and electrophysiologic structures (e.g., the AV node). Although these agents experimentally reduce ischemic injury and may terminate supraventricular dysrhythmia (see Chap. 6), their antianginal efficacy is mediated predominantly by their effects on vascular smooth muscle. These agents improve the efficiency of myocardial performance, i.e., reduce oxygen demand at any given level of performance, and also improve coronary perfusion. Their direct negative inotropic effects are balanced by peripheral arterial vasodilatation. Changes in venous tone are unusual and have been reported only with nifedipine. These agents are particularly effective in reversing **coronary vasospasm.** They have a role in the treatment of many patients with stable, variant, or unstable angina, either alone (especially in patients unable to tolerate nitrates or beta blockers) or in synergism with other agents.

Nifedipine improves hemodynamic performance to a greater extent than verapamil or diltiazem, but lacks their noncompetitive sympathetic antagonism and thus is associated with side effects, such as dizziness and flushing. **Verapamil** is most likely to exacerbate CHF if it is severe. **Diltiazem** has minimal side effects and is unlikely to perturb resting hemodynamics.

E. **Sedatives, tranquilizers, and antidepressants.** In most patients whose angina is adversely affected by emotional stress, tension, or depression, the judicious use of sedatives, tranquilizers, or antidepressants may be considered. Diazepam, 2–5 mg PO tid–qid, or phenobarbital, 15–30 mg PO tid–qid, may benefit these patients (see Chap. 1). Antidepressant drugs, such as nortriptyline and amitriptyline, should be used for depression as appropriate. They have antidysrhythmic properties but occasionally cause tachycardia and elevation of blood pressure.

F. Digitalis and diuretics are useful when angina is associated with CHF or hypertension. Digitalis may exacerbate angina in the absence of CHF.

G. Antidysrhythmic drugs. Angina may be precipitated by dysrhythmia, a relationship that may be demonstrated by Holter monitoring or graded exercise testing.

II. Invasive therapy. Percutaneous transluminal angioplasty (PTCA) and coronary artery bypass surgery (CABG) are invasive procedures with the goal of improving regional coronary blood flow.

A. Coronary bypass surgery (CABG) is beneficial in patients with angina refractory to medical management, patients with symptomatic left main coronary artery disease, or patients with severe angina unable to tolerate antianginal therapy even if single-vessel coronary artery disease is present. Substantial controversy exists concerning other benefits. Recent data suggest that stable chronic angina, even with three-vessel coronary artery disease, can be managed aggressively with medical treatment with a 2–3% yearly mortality. However, many of the data supporting surgical treatment of stable angina in patients with three-vessel coronary disease compare surgical mortality with a medical group mortality in excess of this 2–3% figure. Nonetheless, many believe that survival is improved by CABG in patients with three-vessel disease. Controlled trials in unstable angina also have been unable to demonstrate unequivocal benefit on mortality or work status. The fact that these controversies persist is indicative that even if beneficial, the effects of CABG on mortality are marginal. This does not imply that only patients with refractory angina should be considered surgical candidates. Each patient must be considered individually in terms of life-style, evidence of silent ischemia, the severity of ischemia (e.g., degree of ST–T change, the presence of hypotension or chronotropic incompetence), and the extent of the coronary artery lesions as well as the amount of myocardium subtended by the most critical lesions. In addition, certain types of patients have diffuse disease (e.g., patients with hyperlipidemia) and thus may be less successfully grafted or are at a higher risk than other groups (e.g., women).

Prior to surgery, a careful search for signs of infection (e.g., genitourinary, oral, and cutaneous sites), the early discontinuance of antiplatelet drugs, and discontinuance of anticoagulants the day prior to surgery will reduce the incidence of operative complications. Postoperatively, antiplatelet agents (aspirin plus persantine or sulfinpyrazone) may aid graft patency, presuming no contraindications exist to their use.

B. Percutaneous transluminal angioplasty (PTCA) is accomplished by positioning a specially designed balloon catheter adjacent to a coronary artery lesion and inflating the balloon to increase luminal diameter. The lesions that are most amenable to this procedure are noncalcified proximal coronary lesions. **All patients undergoing PTCA should be candidates for CABG, since CABG may be necessary if PTCA fails or if complications occur.** At present, this promising technique is still in its infancy and requires further development prior to widespread application.

Unstable Angina

Unstable angina pectoris is a clinical syndrome characterized by either the new onset of severe angina or a changing pattern in previously stable angina, i.e., increased frequency, severity, duration, or occurrence at rest. It has been regarded as a sign of impending acute myocardial infarction, but if it is properly managed, less than 10% suffer myocardial necrosis. Most patients with this syndrome will demonstrate transient S–T segment or T wave changes with episodes of chest pain without evidence for myocardial infarction.

Optimal therapy and long-term management of these patients is controversial; mortality among surgically or medically treated patients is comparable. Surgically treated patients have a higher initial incidence of myocardial infarction, but medically treated patients have a greater incidence of severe, persisting angina over the subsequent year. However, the prognosis in patients with significant disease of the left main coronary artery is better with surgical therapy. The majority of patients with unstable angina can be stabilized (preferably in a coronary care unit) with **aggressive medical management** using long-acting or IV nitrates and beta blockers. Calcium-blocking agents are effective in such patients and may eventually become first-line agents. The treatment of other underlying medical problems and aggressive therapy of CHF is essential. Frequently, hemodynamic monitoring with a Swan-Ganz catheter will allow for a more rapid resolution of CHF and permit rapid administration of large doses of nitrates and beta blockers. Patients who fail to respond to aggressive medical management are uncommon but should be considered for emergent cardiac catheterization and surgery. Coronary angiography is warranted for all patients with unstable angina because the incidence of left main coronary disease may be 20%.

Variant Angina

The role of coronary vasospasm in ischemic heart disease has become increasingly recognized. Vasospasm has been implicated as a contributor to sudden death and may play a role in the pathogenesis of unstable angina and acute myocardial infarction. Chest pain due to vasospasm occurs spontaneously, especially while at rest or awakening. These episodes are not initiated by increases in myocardial oxygen demand but result from spontaneous constriction of a major coronary vessel, leading to segmental ischemia, reduction in left ventricular dP/dT, S–T segment elevation or depression, and finally subjective recognition of chest pain. As many as 50% of ischemic episodes may not be associated with symptoms. Episodes are frequently accompanied by dysrhythmia (ventricular tachydysrhythmias or heart block). Changes in the ECG usually identify the region of ischemic myocardium supplied by the vasospastic vessel. Vasospasm may occur in normal coronary arteries but is usually superimposed on fixed atherosclerotic lesions.

The **diagnosis** of variant angina is established most definitely by coronary angiography. In the absence of high-grade fixed coronary obstruction, ergonovine maleate can be given to provoke vasospasm if variant angina is suspected. Holter monitoring serves as an important noninvasive screening test for the diagnosis. The documentation of transient S–T segment elevation with or without symptoms, heart block, or dysrhythmia supports the diagnosis. Exercise stress testing and thallium-201 scintigraphy provide alternative means of evaluation.

Although nitrates, calcium-entry blockers, and beta blockers (high dosages only) may be effective, the **treatment** of variant angina remains empiric. Nitrates or calcium-blocking agents are the drugs of choice. Some patients may have more symptoms with beta-blocker therapy. Coronary artery bypass surgery is beneficial only when severe fixed coronary artery disease is present.

The **prognosis** in patients with this syndrome is variable. Some patients experience asymptomatic intervals of varying duration or even permanent resolution, while others progress to myocardial infarction or sudden death. Although variant angina is a clearly defined clinical entity due to vasospasm, it is only one element in the spectrum of vasospastic disease.

Myocardial Infarction

Myocardial infarction (MI) is an emergency requiring careful management. Two-thirds of the deaths from ischemic heart disease occur from ventricular fibrillation early after the onset of symptoms. Thus, mortality can be reduced by minimizing delays in transport to the hospital and cardiac care unit (CCU). Infarction usually occurs in patients with high-grade occlusive coronary disease but can occur in normal coronaries as a result of spasm, embolism, intimal hyperplasia, or thrombosis (especially in women taking oral contraceptive agents).

I. Diagnosis. The diagnosis of myocardial infarction formally requires at least two of the following criteria: (1) a history of characteristic chest pain; (2) evolutionary changes on the ECG, and (3) elevated (cardiac) enzymes. Current convention is to rely most heavily on enzymatic changes.

   A. Chest pain may be characteristic or atypical for ischemia. The distinction between chest pain associated with myocardial ischemia and that associated with necrosis is often impossible on clinical grounds.

   B. Electrocardiographic changes. Q waves occur in association with myocardial necrosis only 65% of the time. Q wave sensitivity is better with anterior infarction (75%) than with lateral and posterior infarction (40%). The presence of Q waves designates the infarction as transmural electrocardiographically (not pathologically). Transmural infarction is associated with a high incidence of total thrombotic coronary artery occlusion (75–80%) and a 15–20% hospital mortality. Survival is related predominantly to the extent of acute necrosis, with an overall 10% mortality during the first year. The diagnostic use of ST–T changes increases sensitivity, but nonspecificity prevents their use as a definitive diagnostic marker of infarction. When infarction occurs with only ST–T changes, the infarction is termed *nontransmural* and is generally associated with partial coronary artery occlusion and a 7–10% hospital mortality in the absence of extension. However, the subsequent course of the illness in such patients is frequently complicated by recurrent infarction ($\approx$ 20% by 9 months), and the 5-year prognosis is equivalent to that in patients with transmural infarction.

   C. Enzymes and isoenzymes. Elevated activity of total plasma lactate dehydrogenase (LDH) or creatine kinase (CK) provides good diagnostic sensitivity but can occur in a variety of conditions other than infarction, such as after IM injection, trauma, surgery, and pulmonary embolism. Specificity has been markedly improved by the measurement of isoenzymes.

   In patients suspected of MI, plasma LDH and CK isoenzymes should be measured routinely. Blood should be collected on admission, 3–4 times thereafter for CK (q8–12h), and twice thereafter for LDH (q12h).

   1. Creatine kinase comprises three plasma isoenzymes: MM, MB, and BB. Elevated plasma MB CK activity is virtually specific for myocardial injury. Elevation occurs within 4–6 hours of chest pain, reaches a peak in 12–20 hours, and returns to normal in uncomplicated cases sooner than total CK (36–48 hours versus 72–96 hours). The sensitivity and specificity of elevated MB CK measured within 24–36 hours of chest pain are greater than 95% with careful biochemical techniques. Total CK levels may increase after cardioversion, defibrillation, cardiopulmonary resuscitation, or cardiac catheterization; however, the MB fraction will not be detectable in these situations unless some degree of myocardial cell death has occurred. The activity of MB CK may be elevated in the absence of ischemia with vigorous exercise, hypothyroidism, polymyositis, and prostatic and bronchogenic carcinoma. Plasma MB CK determinations are useful in the diagnosis of postoperative MI after noncardiac surgery but are not diagnostic following cardiac surgery because myocardial injury is induced by the procedure itself. Infarct size, which can be estimated from plasma CK and MB CK release, is the most important prognostic factor for survival.

   2. The heart is rich in LDH isoenzymes, especially LDH_1. When MI occurs, plasma elevations can be measured within 12 hours of chest pain and reach a

peak in 24–48 hours; LDH remains elevated for 10–14 days. An LDH_1/LDH_2 ratio greater than 1 is considered evidence of myocardial injury. The diagnostic sensitivity and specificity of LDH isoenzymes for MI is reduced somewhat by the release of LDH_1 and LDH_2 isoenzymes when renal, brain, gastric, or red cell damage occurs.

D. Plasma myoglobin levels have not yet proved useful in the routine management of patients suspected of acute MI due to lack of specificity. Myoglobin is released within 3–4 hours of the onset of symptoms, reaches peak levels in 10–16 hours, and rapidly returns to normal within 24 hours.

E. Radioisotopic diagnosis

1. **Technetium (^{99m}Tc)-labeled pyrophosphate** accumulates in dead myocardial cells and can be detected externally by a gamma camera. When necrosis is present, images are usually positive within 24 hours of the onset of infarction. Imaging should be done at 48–72 hours to optimize sensitivity. This technique is highly sensitive (>90%) in the detection of transmural infarction but is less reliable for the detection of nontransmural infarction. Positive scans may not be obtained in some patients until 5–7 days after MI, and thus optimal sensitivity may require repeat imaging at this time. Pyrophosphate imaging is the technique of choice for patients admitted several days after the onset of infarction or when CK or LDH isoenzymes cannot be obtained. **False-positive images** due to noncardiac disease generally can be avoided if multiple views are obtained. However, positive images in the absence of infarction have been reported in patients with aneurysms, calcified valves, and pericarditis. Positive images in patients with unstable angina usually imply an element of myocardial necrosis. The prolonged **persistence** of an abnormal image after infarction occurs frequently in patients with large MIs ($\approx$25%) and is an adverse prognostic indicator.

2. **Thallium-201 imaging** is useful for the detection of ischemia after exercise and remote infarction. Patients admitted with cardiac symptoms that are due to unrecognized ischemic heart disease may exhibit perfusion defects. In general, the presence of a defect in the appropriate clinical circumstance suggests coronary disease but does not give any information about the time of occurrence of the insult. Serial thallium images can be used to assess the progression or resolution of ischemia but lack sensitivity and specificity for the diagnosis of MI. Although thallium defects occur in patients with cardiomyopathy, the size of the defect and the clinical circumstance can clarify the origin of such defects.

3. Technetium (^{99m}Tc)-labeled red blood cells are used for blood pool imaging. **Radionuclide ventriculography** (RVG) provides a noninvasive measurement of right and left ventricular ejection fraction and documentation of regional-wall abnormalities. In critically ill patients, this technique, coupled with hemodynamic data from a Swan-Ganz catheter, provides a helpful assessment of ventricular function.

II. **Management.** Following the introduction of CCUs, in-hospital mortality in patients with MI dropped from 30–40% to 10–20%. This reduction was predominantly due to detection and treatment of potentially lethal ventricular dysrhythmias. A mortality of 10–20% has persisted as a result of massive myocardial damage and pump failure. When 40% or more of the left ventricular myocardium is necrotized, death is likely. Myocardial infarction evolves over several hours, with the extent of myocardial damage related to the anatomic defect in the coronary artery and to myocardial oxygen consumption. Reducing myocardial oxygen demand by decreasing heart rate or blood pressure in patients with acute MI may be associated with a reduction in infarct size. Although therapeutic approaches to modification of infarct size are not yet ready for routine application, the major objective of routine therapy in patients with MI should be directed toward reducing oxygen demand.

Patients with transmural infarction have a high incidence of total thrombotic occlusion, and thrombolysis with reperfusion of the ischemic area is possible in some of these patients. This complicated technique may benefit patients who can undergo lysis early after the onset of symptoms (3–4 hours) and who present with S–T segment elevation suggesting evolving transmural infarction. The appropriate subsequent medical or invasive management of these patients is undefined at the present time.

A. Electrocardiographic monitoring and an adequate IV line should be established as soon as possible. Nursing personnel should be properly trained to recognize and treat dysrhythmias; however, prophylactic therapy is indicated.

B. General measures. Rest is of prime importance. The room should be quiet, and visitors should be limited to members of the immediate family. Visits should be brief. Oral rather than rectal temperatures should be recorded. Patients with uncomplicated infarction generally spend 5 days in the CCU. Should a complication arise, the stay must be extended until the patient's condition is stabilized.

C. Control of pain will reduce oxygen consumption and levels of circulating catecholamines and should be achieved promptly with adequate doses of effective drugs. **Morphine** is the drug of choice and should be given slowly IV in doses of 1–4 mg. The pain of infarction is often short lived. Pain persisting beyond 24 hours may indicate extension of the infarction, pericarditis, or pulmonary infarction. When the pain is refractory to morphine and mild tranquilizers, other measures must be considered. Beta blockers are important second-line agents for the control of pain. Propranolol can be given IV in 1-mg aliquots. The use of nitroglycerin until recently has been considered relatively contraindicated in patients with MI, due to the potential for hypotension. However, if the patient is carefully monitored and hypotension is avoided, sublingual or IV nitroglycerin may be useful. The administration of low-dose nitrous oxide may also be helpful in the control of pain.

D. Sedation is important, but analgesics should not be used for this purpose. Instead, a mild sedative (chlordiazepoxide, diazepam, phenobarbital, or chloral hydrate) usually suffices (see Chap. 1).

E. Oxygen therapy at 2–3 liters/minute by nasal prongs is indicated during the initial stages of MI. Blood gases should be obtained on admission and oxygen administration adjusted accordingly to keep PO_2 above 70 torr (a lower PO_2 may be indicated if there is coexisting chronic lung disease). Oxygen therapy is not indicated when the PO_2 is in the physiologic range.

F. Rehabilitation. Although tissue repair may require 6 weeks, the length of hospitalization should be adjusted to the individual patient. Generally, the patient is hospitalized for 2 weeks, unless there are complications. There is evidence that patients, even those at "high risk," benefit if allowed to sit in a bedside chair with legs extended for a short period several times daily. Advantages include increased mental and physical comfort, easier ventilation, prevention of shoulder-hand syndrome, decreased risk of peripheral venous stasis with thromboembolism, and decreased incidence of hypostatic pneumonia, urinary retention, and constipation. The patient should be assisted from bed to chair. Although the precise schedule of ambulation must be tailored to the clinical progress of each individual patient, the following general outline is suggested:

1. The bedside commode is preferable to a bedpan.

2. Patients should be instructed to move the toes and feet actively while in bed to prevent venous congestion.

3. Patients with an uncomplicated course should be encouraged to begin sitting in a chair within 24 hours after admission.

4. In uncomplicated cases, patients may begin to help themselves with regard to shaving, feeding, and toilet on the first day.

5. Walking in the room should be encouraged beginning on the fifth to seventh day, preferably with monitoring.

6. Patients should be fully ambulatory by 10 days and, generally, discharged from the hospital by 14 days.

7. Patients usually may return to their jobs within 2 months.

8. After returning to work, the patient should be instructed regarding rehabilitation. Progressive exercise programs, such as jogging or walking, should be instituted under close supervision.

G. Diet. For the first day, the diet should be liquid or soft, low in salt, and easily digestible. Very hot or cold food and beverages should not be given during the first few days, since they may cause vagal stimulation and cardiac dysrhythmias. As the patient improves and appetite increases, a more liberal diet may be allowed.

H. Bowel care. Constipation is a common problem and should be prevented by the routine administration of stool softeners and mild laxatives.

I. Anticoagulant therapy. Definitive criteria for anticoagulation do not exist, and evidence at present indicates that it does not modify the actual process of atherosclerosis or minimize the amount of myocardial damage. Recent data suggest that patients with anterior myocardial infarction are at high risk (33%) for the development of a mural thrombus, especially if apical dyskinesis is present. Although the incidence of embolism is unknown, patients with anterior MI should, if possible, be evaluated for the presence of mural thrombus (two-dimensional echocardiography is the preferred technique) and, especially if they have a complicated course, should be considered for anticoagulation. The duration of such therapy if initiated is undefined. Documented systemic embolism, regardless of the locus of infarction, is an indication for full-dose anticoagulation. The role of antiplatelet therapy in acute MI has not yet been clearly defined. To reduce the incidence of peripheral venous thrombosis, **all patients should receive subcutaneous heparin** (5000 units q8h) unless a contraindication to such therapy is present.

III. Complications

A. Dysrhythmias, both tachycardia and bradycardia, often occur in the first 24 hours after MI. Ventricular dysrhythmias are particularly dangerous, since they may lead to ventricular tachycardia and fibrillation. Dysrhythmia also may decrease cardiac output and coronary perfusion and increase myocardial oxygen consumption. Prior to initiating treatment, potential exacerbating agents, such as other drugs, should be discontinued, and coexisting conditions, including hypoxia, acidosis, and electrolyte imbalance (especially potassium) should be corrected. Left ventricular failure or hypotension predisposes to dysrhythmia. The type and urgency of treatment of dysrhythmia in the setting of an acute MI may differ from those outlined in Chap. 6. Emphasis is placed on the **prevention** of potentially lethal dysrhythmias (e.g., ventricular tachycardia).

1. Ventricular dysrhythmias

a. Ventricular premature depolarizations (VPDs) occur in virtually all patients with acute MI and may herald ventricular tachycardia or fibrillation. However, in the majority of patients, ventricular tachycardia or fibrillation are not heralded by "warning dysrhythmias."

(1) Prophylactic therapy reduces the incidence of ventricular fibrillation from 6.5% to 0.3%. Although this dysrhythmia is generally promptly

Myocardial Infarction 71

detected and corrected in a well-staffed CCU, both the dysrhythmia and its treatment are associated with potential morbidity. For this reason, prophylactic lidocaine therapy is recommended for patients under 65 years of age. **Lidocaine** should be administered as an initial bolus of 75–100 mg and an IV infusion begun at 2 mg/minute. Since the half-life of lidocaine is prolonged by CHF, hypotension, and hepatic disease (see Chap. 6), a lower bolus dose and an infusion rate of 1 mg/minute should be used in such patients. Prophylactic therapy is indicated only during the first 24 hours.

If prophylactic therapy has not been initiated, VPDs should be treated if they occur (1) in the vulnerable period of the cardiac cycle (at or near the peak of the T wave), (2) in salvos of two or more, (3) frequently (more than 5/minute), or (4) with multiple forms. Ventricular tachycardia or ventricular fibrillation may originate with late as well as early VPDs. Thus, the frequency of VPDs is a better indicator for treatment than their coupling interval. Multiple boluses of lidocaine are needed to maintain levels when urgent therapy is initiated (see Chap. 6).

(2) If lidocaine therapy is ineffective, IV **procainamide** may be employed. Procainamide therapy should be initiated with a loading dose of 750–1000 mg, administered in 100-mg aliquots q6min, with careful monitoring of the QRS duration, Q–Tc interval, and vital signs.

b. Patients who experience recurrent malignant ventricular dysrhythmias resistant to other therapy may be benefitted by **bretylium.** Since bretylium may cause hypotension (especially in patients receiving other vasoactive therapy), the drug should be given cautiously at a dose of 5 mg/kg diluted 1:4 in normal saline and infused over 8–10 minutes. For at least 6 weeks following discharge from the CCU, patients who experience recurrent VPDs or have ventricular fibrillation associated with an acute MI should be maintained on oral quinidine, procainamide, or disopyramide at a dosage known to establish a blood level in the therapeutic range.

c. Should **ventricular fibrillation** occur, immediate **defibrillation** with 200–300 watt-sec is indicated. Defibrillation should be repeated if the initial attempt is unsuccessful. Subsequently, CPR should be initiated and defibrillation repeated at 360 watt-sec after bicarbonate and epinephrine have been administered. The precordial thump is appropriate only when it does not delay defibrillation attempts. Patients who experience ventricular fibrillation should be maintained on antidysrhythmic therapy as indicated in **b.**

d. **Ventricular tachycardia** necessitates **cardioversion** unless it responds promptly to IV therapy.

e. Ventricular irritability refractory to the preceding measures may be treated by **overdrive pacing.** Ventricular pacing at a rate of 100–110 is preferred. Some ventricular dysrhythmias, e.g., torsade des pointes, also can be treated with atrial pacing.

f. Patients who manifest recurrent sustained malignant ventricular dysrhythmias or ventricular fibrillation after the acute phase of infarction should be considered for **invasive electrophysiologic study.** Such a study is designed to establish the drug therapy most apt to obviate the dysrhythmia. If such therapy cannot be devised, mapping and excision of the ectopic focus can be done in specialized centers. If such facilities are not available, group I antidysrhythmic agents (see Chap. 6) should be utilized to achieve a high therapeutic plasma level. Surgical therapy is not recommended during evolving MI.

g. Accelerated idioventricular rhythm is common in MI and often is an escape rhythm (rate 60–100/minute), manifesting itself when the sinus rate slows below 60/minute. Its course is usually benign, with a duration of less than 48 hours. Specific treatment may not be necessary. Injudicious use of atropine to keep the heart rate high in an effort to suppress the dysrhythmia should be discouraged. However, patients with this rhythm should be monitored closely, since deterioration to ventricular tachycardia and fibrillation can occur.

2. Atrial dysrhythmias

a. Sinus tachycardia, a common dysrhythmia, frequently is associated with some degree of heart failure but also may be due to hypoxia, pain, anxiety, fever, or drugs. Treatment is directed at the underlying cause. If prominent or persistent, the judicious use of propranolol may be indicated after contributing abnormalities have been corrected, especially when hypertension is present in patients with anterior infarction (see **D**). Persistent tachycardia during the course of MI is an adverse prognostic sign.

b. Sinus bradycardia should not be treated when hemodynamic or electrical disturbances are absent, because increasing the heart rate increases myocardial oxygen requirements and may exacerbate ischemia. When therapy is necessary, atropine sulfate, 0.5–1.0 mg IV, is often effective. Temporary pacing is preferred to multiple doses of atropine and is required for refractory symptomatic bradycardia.

c. Atrial premature depolarizations may be a forerunner of supraventricular tachycardia, but treatment is usually not warranted unless they are frequent, precipitate tachycardia, or occur in runs. Treatment is outlined in Chap. 6.

d. Paroxysmal supraventricular tachycardia (PSVT) is frequently associated with heart failure. If the patient's condition is **unstable** (hypotension, chest pain, dyspnea), cardioversion is the treatment of choice. Although ventricular irritability is an occasional sequel to **cardioversion,** it should be considered for all supraventricular tachycardias (except sinus tachycardia) to prevent exacerbation of myocardial ischemia.

If the patient's condition is **stable,** vagotonic maneuvers may be tried. If these are unsuccessful and the PSVT utilizes the AV node as part of a reentrant circuit, **verapamil** may be used unless severe CHF is present. Cautious IV administration (1–2 mg/minute) of 0.075 mg/kg is necessary (see Chap. 6).

Alternatively, a patient whose condition is stable may be treated with digoxin, 0.25–0.5 mg IV initially, followed by an additional 0.125–0.25 mg IV or PO q4–6h until the full loading dose is reached. Maintenance therapy is then continued at 0.125–0.25 mg PO or IV daily. Propranolol, 1–3 mg IV or 10–40 mg PO, has also been used acutely instead of digoxin. Vagotonic drugs (edrophonium) and sympathomimetic drugs (phenylephrine and metaraminol) are best avoided, because the former can produce hypotension and the latter can cause an abrupt increase in afterload, cardiac work, and oxygen consumption. Rarely, PSVT in this setting is due to digitalis toxicity (particularly if block coexists) and should be treated as outlined in Chap. 5. Recurrent episodes may be treated with rapid atrial stimulation (see Chap. 6).

e. Atrial flutter often responds poorly to pharmacologic measures. If the patient's condition is unstable, **cardioversion,** beginning at low energy levels (10–40 watt-sec), is the treatment of choice. This may convert the rhythm to sinus rhythm or to atrial fibrillation (see **f**). Rapid atrial stimulation may also be helpful. If the patient's condition is stable, **verapamil,** 0.075 mg/kg given IV at 1–2 mg/minute, may be helpful. Digoxin, 0.5 mg

IV, or propranolol, 1–3 mg IV or 10–40 mg PO, also may be useful when verapamil can not be given (see Chap. 6). These therapies frequently will produce atrial fibrillation. If there is no slowing of ventricular rate in an hour, or if CHF or hypotension develops, cardioversion becomes the treatment of choice. If atrial flutter is recurrent, digitalis may be used to control the rate, with a group I agent added to reduce atrial ectopy.

f. **Atrial fibrillation** is deleterious to ischemic myocardium because the ventricular response is usually rapid and the atrial contribution to ventricular filling is lost. **Cardioversion** is generally the initial treatment of choice, starting at 25 watt-sec. Digitalis or propranolol may be used to control the ventricular rate. Dosages are the same as in **e**. Cardioversion may not be indicated if the ventricular response is slow (e.g., 100/minute). (**Note:** Supraventricular rhythms in the setting of MI are often transient and may not require long-term therapy.)

3. **Junctional tachydysrhythmias**

   a. **Accelerated junctional rhythm** is usually a benign escape rhythm in patients with sinus bradycardia.

   b. **Paroxysmal junctional tachycardia** (rate 120–180/minute) has the same significance and requires the same treatment as PSVT (sec. **2.d**), but carotid massage and the Valsalva maneuver are less likely to be successful. At times, lidocaine is helpful. Vagotonic and sympathomimetic drugs should not be used.

   c. **Nonparoxysmal junctional tachycardia** has a slower rate (70–130/minute) than the paroxysmal type. Onset and termination are gradual. This rhythm is usually associated with cardiogenic shock or digitalis intoxication. Treatment is directed toward the underlying condition.

4. **Atrioventricular block** may be first degree (prolongation of P–R interval), second degree, or third degree (complete heart block). Second-degree block includes Mobitz type I (Wenckebach) block, in which there is gradual prolongation of the P–R interval and a narrow QRS complex prior to a nonconducted beat (the block is located above the bundle of His in most instances), and Mobitz type II block, in which dropped beats are not preceded by P–R prolongation and the QRS complex is wide (the block is usually situated below the bundle of His). In third-degree heart block, the atria and ventricles have independent pacemakers, and there is usually a slow ventricular rate. Most patients have either bilateral bundle branch block or trifascicular block.

The implications of AV block are more ominous with anterior than with inferior infarction. In **anterior infarction,** complete AV block may develop abruptly, often being preceded only by first-degree AV block or some form of intraventricular block. In this setting, AV block is usually associated with a large area of infarction and high mortality. In **inferior infarction,** heart block occurs progressively, i.e., complete AV block is usually preceded by first-degree or second-degree block. The ventricular or junctional escape rate is rarely slow enough to cause symptoms. When third-degree block occurs, the escape rhythm is often from high in the bundle of His (rates of 55–60/minute are common), and the QRS remains normal in width. Usually, AV block in inferior infarction is transient, although the mortality in inferior infarction with complete AV block is 25%. The treatment for bradycardia occurring with heart block is **ventricular pacing.** Sequential AV pacing may benefit patients with pump failure. **Indications for pacing** in MI include:

   a. Third-degree heart block. Patients with anterior MI in whom third-degree heart block develops should undergo permanent pacing regardless of whether or not the third-degree block resolves.

   b. Mobitz type II second-degree heart block with anterior infarction.

   c. Bifascicular block with or without P–R prolongation developing as a result of infarction.

   d. Any degree of block associated with symptomatic bradycardia.

B. Congestive heart failure, a common complication of MI, is associated with increased mortality. Detection and prompt therapy are essential. The use of radionuclide ventriculography to assess left and right ventricular function in patients with acute infarction will aid markedly in detection. If heart failure does not clear totally and rapidly, a Swan-Ganz catheter should be placed to allow for more aggressive therapy. The following approach to the treatment of CHF is recommended:

   1. Diuretics are the first line of treatment for mild CHF (e.g., S3 gallop, basilar rales) but must be used cautiously, since overdiuresis can lead to hypovolemia. If the severity of CHF increases, or if it is severe initially, inotropic support or vasodilator therapy is indicated.

   2. Inotropic support

   a. Parenteral therapy usually necessitates **hemodynamic monitoring.** A thermodilution Swan-Ganz catheter should be positioned in the pulmonary artery via the median basilic vein by cutdown or percutaneously via the femoral vein, because complications associated with jugular or subclavian insertion may have severe consequences in patients with acute infarction. Scrupulous sterile technique during insertion and subsequently is mandatory. In the setting of infarction, long-term monitoring is rarely necessary, and the Swan-Ganz catheter generally can be removed within 48 hours. Careful evaluation for complications of catheterization, such as thrombosis with pulmonary infarction, hemorrhage, knotting, dysrhythmia, endocarditis, sepsis, fracture, or balloon rupture, is essential.

   End-expiratory pressure measurement of right atrial pressure (RA), pulmonary artery end-diastolic pressure, and pulmonary artery occlusive pressure (PAOP) are most accurate if the catheter is positioned below the left atrium (i.e., the lower lobes posteriorly). Cardiac output can be measured by thermodilution but is prone to a multiplicity of mechanical and technical errors. If cardiac output measurements are not available or if confirmation of a change in cardiac output is necessary, serial changes (not absolute values) in the mixed venous oxygen saturation drawn from the pulmonary artery can be utilized acutely to reflect changes in tissue perfusion. **All measurements should be evaluated in terms of the clinical response and viewed critically if they fail to correlate.** Total peripheral resistance (TPR) in dyne · sec · cm^{-5} can be calculated by the following formula:

   $$TPR = \frac{MAP - CVP}{CO} \times 80$$

   where MAP = mean arterial pressure, CVP = central venous pressure, and CO = cardiac output.

   Once the patient is hemodynamically stable, **attempts to "improve the numbers" may do more harm than good.** In general, patients with infarction (1) require high filling pressures (PAOP ≈ 18–20 mm Hg) to maximize cardiac output; (2) TPR <1200 is within the normal range; (3) when a large V wave is present in the PAOP tracing, the post–A wave pressure correlates best with true left ventricular end-diastolic pressure.

   b. Dobutamine, a beta agonist, is the preferred parenteral ionotropic agent. Cardiac output is increased and filling pressure decreased at doses that do not cause significant increases in heart rate, blood pressure, frequency of dysrhythmias, or infarct size. The **starting dose** is $1-2$ μg/kg/minute, which should be increased until hemodynamic improvement occurs or a dose of 10.0 μg/kg/minute is reached. The onset of action is rapid (seconds); the plasma half-life is 2½ minutes. Tachycardia constitutes the major side effect and usually resolves with dosage reduction. Tapering the drug over several hours will help mitigate the reduction in hemodynamic performance seen when the drug is discontinued.

   c. **Dopamine,** the second-choice inotropic agent, increases cardiac output but also heart rate and blood pressure. It does not decrease elevated filling pressure. Therapy should be initiated at a low infusion rate ($1-2$ μg/kg/minute) and slowly increased until the desired hemodynamic response is obtained. At low dosages ($0.5-2.0$ μg/kg/minute), dopamine causes renal vasodilation, but higher dosages (>10 μg/kg/minute) may induce an undesirable rise in TPR. There is no evidence for synergism when dopamine is combined with dobutamine.

   d. **Digitalis** has little value as an inotropic agent in CHF due to MI during the first $48-72$ hours. Digitalis has a delayed onset of action, a relatively long half-life, and may induce dysrhythmias. Its only value is when CHF persists $4-5$ days after MI, when an oral agent is required, or when persisting chest pain is associated with cardiomegaly.

3. **Vasodilator therapy** with IV nitroprusside or nitroglycerin may be useful in the treatment of CHF. (For details on the use of these agents see **D.5** and **6.**) Although neither agent has been approved for this use, they are particularly useful in patients with high peripheral resistance and pulmonary congestion. Careful monitoring is essential, since hypotension may occur if preload is lowered excessively. Patients with severe CHF and hypotension (systolic blood pressure <100 mm Hg) may not tolerate afterload reduction unless their TPR is very high.

4. **Combination therapy.** In patients in whom an inotropic agent is required to increase cardiac output and whose TPR remains high, the combination of dobutamine with nitroprusside or nitroglycerin IV may be beneficial.

C. **Cardiogenic shock** is a severe form of pump failure that usually signifies a $35-40\%$ loss of functioning myocardium. The mortality from the syndrome is nearly 80%, despite aggressive intervention.

   1. The **diagnosis** requires the following criteria:

      a. Hypotension (systolic blood pressure <80 mm Hg or mean <60 mm Hg).

      b. Oliguria (<500 ml/24 hours).

      c. Elevated filling pressure. Hypotension and shock can be seen when a decreased cardiac output is due to relative hypovolemia. Fluid administration alone may correct the hypotension in this situation.

   2. **Treatment** of this disorder is outlined in **B.1–4.** The only additional therapeutic interventions that have been proposed are intraaortic balloon pumping and external counterpulsation. Intraaortic balloon pumping acts by reducing cardiac work via impedance reduction during systole and by increasing diastolic pressure and thus coronary flow. Unfortunately, the use of circulatory support in patients with cardiogenic shock has achieved variable success. At present, treatment with intraaortic balloon pumping should be reserved for the support during cardiac catheterization of patients in whom a surgically correctable lesion is suspected.

D. Control of **hypertension** reduces myocardial oxygen demand and infarct size. The following approach is recommended:

   1. **Bed rest, relief of pain, and sedation** are frequently all that are required for mild hypertension.

2. If mild hypertension persists, **diuretic therapy** is recommended unless hypovolemia is suspected.

3. If the diastolic pressure remains mildly elevated (<105 mm Hg), **oral agents** (e.g., methyldopa) may be utilized. Treatment of more severe hypertension necessitates **parenteral therapy,** usually with hemodynamic monitoring.

4. If hypertension is present in association with tachycardia, normal central pressures for patients with MI (PAOP <18 mm Hg), high cardiac output, and normal or only moderately elevated peripheral vascular resistance, **beta blockade** is the therapy of choice. This hemodynamic syndrome can occur in patients with anterior transmural infarction and will respond to 1-mg aliquots of IV propranolol to a maximum dose of 0.15 mg/kg. Subsequent oral therapy with beta blockers can be initiated. Other patients with severe hypertension usually manifest reduced cardiac output and high systemic resistance. These patients require IV nitroprusside or nitroglycerin.

5. **Sodium nitroprusside,** a short-acting, balanced vasodilator, reduces systemic vascular resistance and venous return. Fresh solutions should be administered in 5% D/W through shielded IV tubing (the drug is light sensitive) via a constant infusion pump. The **initial dosage** is $10-15$ μg/minute. This dose can be increased by increments of $5-10$ μg q5–10min. The dosage needed for therapy depends on the clinical circumstance; heart failure in general responds to lower dosages (frequently 50 μg/minute), whereas hypertension may necessitate up to 100 μg/minute. Increases in heart rate imply inadequate filling pressure.

Nitroprusside is metabolized to cyanide by red blood cells and subsequently to thiocyanate by the liver. If high doses are utilized (>10 μg/kg/minute) or renal dysfunction is present, these metabolites accumulate. Thiocyanate serum levels should be monitored in these circumstances and should not exceed 10 mg/dl. The first sign of toxicity may be metabolic acidosis, although fatigue, nausea, anorexia, hypothyroidism, hiccups, disorientation, and psychosis can occur. This drug should be used only for the treatment of severe hypertension or severe CHF. Nitroprusside may adversely affect ischemia and mortality in patients with acute infarction.

6. **Intravenous nitroglycerin** has effects that are similar to those of nitroprusside in patients with CHF but with a more marked effect on venous capacitance. In patients without CHF, the effect on afterload is less marked. In addition to improving CHF, IV nitroglycerin may be beneficial in the therapy of severe hypertension; however, studies are limited. Intravenous nitroglycerin improves ischemia and may reduce infarct size in many of these patients.

In most studies, the **initial dose** (10 μg/minute) and dose-titration schedules (increased by 10 μg q5–10min) were developed with noncommercial products. Newer preparations will likely necessitate lower dosages. Adverse hemodynamic effects usually stimulate tachycardia; however, vagal responses with hypotension alone or with concomitant bradycardia can occur and require treatment with atropine. In contrast to patients with unstable or variant angina or recurrent angina after infarction, the pain associated with acute infarction responds less well to IV nitroglycerin.

E. **Hypotension** may occur for a variety of reasons.

1. **Autonomic abnormalities,** including vagotonic reactions with hypotension, are common in the early hours of infarction, especially with inferior infarction. Hypotension associated with an inappropriate heart rate response should be treated with atropine (0.5–1.0 mg IV). Such patients frequently need saline administration.

2. Persistent hypotension mandates central hemodynamic monitoring. **Cardiogenic shock** (see **C**) or **hypovolemia** (relative or absolute) may be respon-

sible, especially in patients with right ventricular infarction (see **H**) or in patients receiving diuretic therapy.

F. Extension of the infarction occurs in ≈17% of patients following MI. Patients with infarction require enzymatic evaluation if chest pain and ECG changes recur. Chest pain and ECG changes are sensitive markers of extension but lack specificity. Patients with subendocardial infarction have a far greater risk of in-hospital extension. Most extensions occur 7–10 days after infarction; accordingly, early discharge, especially in patients with subendocardial infarction, is not recommended.

G. Ruptures of the interventricular septum or papillary muscle are manifested by a loud systolic murmur and the concomitant onset of intractable CHF. Ventricular septal defect (VSD) is more likely to be associated with a precordial thrill. A Swan-Ganz catheter is frequently helpful for diagnosis. A step-up in oxygen saturation may be observed from the right atrium to the right ventricle in VSD. In papillary muscle rupture, the pulmonary artery occlusive pressure (PAOP) may reveal a large V wave. Neither of these above findings, however, is specific. Patients with mitral valve dysfunction or VSD should have hemodynamic monitoring, and, if function is severely compromised, therapy with intraaortic balloon pumping (IABP) and afterload reduction should be initiated. Subsequent cardiac catheterization and, if possible, surgery should be attempted. Although the longer the interval from acute MI the lower the surgical mortality, the prognosis is generally poor.

H. Right ventricular (RV) infarction is common in patients with inferior MI and may predominate over infarction in the left ventricle. In such a situation, RV failure is out of proportion to LV failure, and hypotension is common. At times, severe RV infarction may be confused with pericardial tamponade. The diagnosis can be made by right heart catheterization with a Swan-Ganz catheter that demonstrates the steep Y descent in the right atrial tracing, the dip and plateau (constrictive or restrictive pattern) in the RV tracing, and normal or only mildly elevated PAOP. In response to fluid therapy, right-sided pressure increases disproportionately to left-sided pressure. The preferred therapy consists of judicious fluid administration and dobutamine.

I. Ventricular aneurysm. Dyskinesis is observed in many patients with acute MI and frequently improves with time. Ventricular aneurysms may be suspected on the basis of the ECG findings (persisting S–T segment elevation 6 weeks after infarction), intractable heart failure, or poorly controlled ventricular dysrhythmias. The diagnosis may be suggested by fluoroscopy, two-dimensional echocardiography, or radionuclide ventriculography (RVG), but definitive diagnosis is made by cardiac catheterization. Intractable CHF, symptomatic low cardiac output, unmanageable ventricular dysrhythmias, and systemic emboli constitute indications for surgery. Anticoagulation should be maintained before, during, and after the operation. An important variant of ventricular aneurysm, with a more dire prognosis, is **pseudoaneurysm**, actually a form of cardiac rupture in which pericardial extravasation of blood is restricted locally by the pericardium, and an aneurysm with a narrow connection to the LV cavity develops. These aneurysms occur after transmural MI and have a propensity to rupture. Thus, they usually necessitate surgery.

J. Pain and a precordial rub due to **pericarditis** are common during an acute infarction. When treatment is necessary, aspirin is the drug of choice. Other nonsteroidal drugs may also be useful. Corticosteroids may retard myocardial scar formation and should not be administered.

K. Post–myocardial infarction syndrome is a relatively infrequent syndrome characterized by pericarditis, pleuritis, pneumonitis, fever, leukocytosis, elevated sedimentation rate, and elevated levels of antimyocardial antibodies. This syndrome may mimic angina or infarction, and the ECG may show diffuse, marked S–T segment elevation. Occurrence is usually between the second and eleventh weeks after infarction. The course may be lengthy, with frequent remissions and exacerbations. Therapy is symptomatic and includes anti-inflammatory agents, such as salicylates or indomethacin (25–50 mg PO tid–qid). If symptoms are severe, corticosteroids, e.g., prednisone, 1 mg/kg PO qd, may be used initially. Corticosteroids should be tapered slowly to minimize exacerbations. Administration of anticoagulants should be discontinued unless the clinical situation clearly dictates their continuance (e.g., documented pulmonary embolism), since hemorrhagic pericarditis with tamponade can occur.

L. Recent investigations suggest that therapy after acute MI (**secondary prevention**) may reduce morbidity and mortality. Patients should be evaluated for evidence of postinfarction ischemia by an exercise or a radionuclide stress test. Patients with positive stress test findings and patients with subendocardial infarction are at high risk of subsequent cardiovascular morbidity. The response of specific subgroups to therapy has not been studied; however, beta blockade is highly effective in reducing mortality in studies containing all postinfarction patients. Oral antiplatelet agents (aspirin, 300–1500 mg daily alone or with persantine, 75 mg tid, or sulfinpyrazone, 200 mg qid alone) may produce a similar, though less pronounced, benefit. Accordingly, unless contraindicated, **secondary prevention therapy with beta blockers or antiplatelet drugs is indicated at least for patients at high risk.**

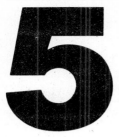

Congestive Heart Failure

Heart failure is usually defined as an inability of the heart to pump sufficient blood to meet the metabolic demands of the body. This definition is of little assistance to the clinician, since there is no simple objective method to measure this inability. In practice, the most common and obvious abnormalities related to heart failure are signs and symptoms of circulatory congestion and thus the designation *congestive heart failure* (CHF). For practical purposes CHF is diagnosed and designated as left sided, right sided, or biventricular if the respective atrial pressures are elevated.

The principal **compensatory mechanisms** utilized by the failing heart include (1) the Frank-Starling phenomenon, (2) myocardial hypertrophy, (3) increased catecholamine release, and (4) tachycardia. These compensatory mechanisms and their ultimate failure are responsible for three basic **physiologic alterations,** which can occur individually or in any combination and are responsible for the following symptoms of CHF: (1) **Decreased cardiac output** causes hypoperfusion, resulting in confusion, weakness, and cold, clammy extremities. (2) **Elevated left atrial pressure** causes pulmonary venous congestion, leading to exertional dyspnea, nonproductive nocturnal cough, orthopnea, and paroxysmal nocturnal dyspnea. (3) **Elevated right atrial pressure** is associated with systemic venous congestion, manifested by pedal edema, abdominal discomfort (secondary to hepatic congestion), abdominal distention (secondary to ascites), and anorexia. Nocturia is present with pulmonary or systemic venous congestion.

The presence of CHF is usually established on the basis of a typical history, physical findings (rales, S3 gallop, edema), and a chest radiograph. Additional noninvasive (e.g., echocardiographic) or invasive (e.g., pulmonary artery catheterization) studies may be necessary in selected patients.

Once the presence of CHF has been established, a specific **underlying cause** should be sought. Common underlying causes include (1) hypertension, (2) coronary artery disease, (3) valvular heart disease, (4) congenital heart disease, (5) pericardial disease, (6) toxins (ethanol), (7) endocrinopathies (thyroid disease), (8) inflammatory disorders (myocarditis), (9) infections, and (10) infiltrative disorders (amyloidosis, hemochromatosis). **Precipitating factors** should also be identified. These include (1) physical, environmental, or emotional stress, (2) fever, (3) systemic infection, (4) anemia, (5) dysrhythmias, (6) pulmonary emboli, (7) renal disease, (8) sodium-retaining agents (nonsteroidal anti-inflammatory drugs) or cardiac depressant drugs (disopyramide, beta blockers), (9) increased sodium load (dietary or parenteral), (10) pregnancy, (11) superimposition of another underlying cause, and (12) noncompliance with a medical regimen.

Specific therapeutic measures to correct the underlying and precipitating causes should be instituted whenever possible. Thereafter, management involves supportive measures, enhancement of contractility, relief of congestive symptoms, vasodilator therapy, and other therapies (see Table 5-1).

The following discussion is oriented toward the therapy of left ventricular or biventricular failure with normal or decreased cardiac output.

Table 5-1. Stepwise therapy of patients with congestive heart failure

Functional class	Intervention
I. Symptomatic only with greater-than-ordinary activity II. Symptomatic during ordinary activity	Identify and correct underlying and precipitating causes of CHF. Modify physical activity and modestly restrict dietary sodium. Administer digoxin and/or a diuretic.
III. Asymptomatic at rest; symptomatic with minimal activity IV. Symptomatic at rest	Restrict activity and dietary sodium further. Intensify diuretic therapy; combination regimen frequently required. Consider chronic vasodilator therapy. Parenteral vasodilators, parenteral inotropic agents, and specific additional interventions (see sec. **V**) are utilized in selected patients.

I. **Supportive measures.** In the presence of overt cardiac decompensation, patients are restricted to bed or chair. The head of the bed is elevated (30–45 degrees), and oxygen is administered to correct hypoxemia. The increased risk of thromboemboli associated with CHF and bed rest can be reduced by minidose heparin (5000 units SQ bid), passive leg exercises, and elastic stockings. The duration of bed rest should be as short as possible to minimize deconditioning. Patients with compensated CHF are encouraged to maximize their functional capacity; supervised dynamic exercise training is permitted, but isometric exercise is avoided.

II. **Enhancement of contractility**

A. **Digitalis** is the only agent with significant positive inotropic effect suitable for chronic therapy of CHF. However, the response to therapy is often less than desired. The inotropic effect appears related to reversible inhibition of a sarcolemmal Na^+, K^+–adenosine triphosphatase (ATPase), with subsequent enhancement of calcium availability to the contractile proteins. In addition to its positive inotropic effect, digitalis has a vagotonic effect and direct effects on the electrophysiologic properties of cardiac membranes.

The latter two properties render digitalis **most effective** in the treatment of patients with CHF and atrial fibrillation (or flutter) with a rapid ventricular response. The drug is **effective** in CHF resulting from hypertensive, valvular, ischemic, and congenital heart disease. It is **helpful, but probably less effective** in patients with CHF secondary to myocarditis, high cardiac output states, cor pulmonale, and congestive cardiomyopathy. Digitalis is **not effective** in patients with isolated mitral stenosis, restrictive cardiomyopathy, and pericardial constriction or tamponade, except when atrial flutter or fibrillation with a rapid ventricular response is also present. Digitalis is **contraindicated** in patients with (1) hypertrophic cardiomyopathy and dynamic outflow tract obstruction (unless supraventricular tachyarrhythmias occur that are unresponsive to propranolol and verapamil); (2) second-degree, or greater, atrioventricular (AV) block in the absence of an electronic pacemaker; and (3) Wolff-Parkinson-White syndrome with antegrade accessory pathway conduction during atrial fibrillation/flutter.

Increasing the dosage of digitalis increases the positive inotropic effect; however, the therapeutic index is low, and the incidence of toxicity increases as dosage increases. Safe administration is complicated further by the lack of a discrete therapeutic end point. Several series have reported a 6–23% incidence of toxicity in hospitalized patients on digitalis. **Some physicians initiate** therapy of mild CHF with sodium restriction plus a diuretic, rather than digitalis, to avoid potential toxicity.

1. **Prior to initiating therapy**

   a. Determine if the patient is currently taking a digitalis preparation. If the history is unclear, obtain a serum digitalis level (see **3**).

   b. Obtain an **ECG** before therapy and again when digitalization is complete. Digitalis can induce repolarization changes suggestive of ischemia. A baseline tracing is also useful if toxicity is suspected at a later date.

   c. **Evaluate renal function and serum potassium concentration. Thyroid function, arterial blood gases,** and serum **calcium** or **magnesium** concentrations should also be evaluated if an abnormality is suspected. Whenever possible, abnormalities, particularly hypokalemia, should be corrected prior to initiation of therapy.

2. **Pharmacology**

   a. **Preparations. Digoxin is the preparation of choice.** Ouabain is available only for IV use. It has a slightly more rapid onset of action than IV digoxin but not to a clinically significant degree. The long serum half-life of digitoxin can increase the incidence and duration of toxicity. When digitoxin is discontinued in favor of digoxin, therapy should be interrupted for 3 days; otherwise, the combined effects produce toxicity. All further discussion will be restricted to digoxin.

   b. **Pharmacokinetics.** Digoxin in tablet form is 75–85% bioavailable. This figure approaches 100% for pediatric elixir. Small bowel disease may impair absorption, as may certain drugs (cholestyramine, Kaopectate, magnesium trisilicate, sulfasalazine, and neomycin). **Intramuscular digoxin is absorbed erratically; IV administration is recommended when parenteral therapy is indicated.**

   Following IV administration, digoxin's onset of action is 15–30 minutes; the peak effect occurs at 1½–2 hours. Following oral administration, the onset of action is at 2 hours, and the peak effect is at 6 hours.

   Digoxin's volume of distribution approximately equals lean body mass. Myocardial digoxin concentrations are several times greater than serum concentrations, and this ratio is highly variable. This is one reason why serum digoxin levels do not reliably predict therapeutic efficacy or toxicity.

   Digoxin is eliminated primarily by glomerular filtration. When the glomerular filtration rate (GFR) is normal, the serum half-life is approximately 36 hours. **When GFR is reduced, the serum half-life is prolonged.** Digoxin undergoes enterohepatic circulation, and a small amount is normally lost in the stool. However, in 10% of patients, enteric flora metabolize digoxin, interrupt its enterohepatic circulation, and shorten its serum half-life by 10–50% (*N. Engl. J. Med.* 305:789, 1981).

   c. **Administration.** The following recommendations are general guidelines. Therapy should be individualized in all cases. When in doubt, always begin with the lower dosage.

   Total body stores of digoxin are 0.75–1.25 mg when steady-state serum levels are in the therapeutic range. These body stores can accumulate in one of two ways: (1) A **loading dosage** (0.75–1.25 mg PO or IV over 12–24 hours in three to six divided doses) **is administered when the clinical situation requires a prompt therapeutic effect.** The loading dosage depends on lean body mass and route of administration but is independent of GFR. The initial dose is 0.25–0.5 mg; subsequent doses should not exceed 0.25 mg. The peak effect of each dose must be observed before the next dose is given. (2) **Initiate therapy with a standard daily maintenance dose when the situation is less urgent.** When this method is used, serum levels reach 90% of steady state after 3.3 half-lives (5 days with a normal GFR, 15 days with end-stage renal disease).

The usual **maintenance dose** is 0.125–0.25 mg PO qd; rarely, as much as 0.5 mg PO qd is required. The maintenance dose selected depends on the GFR; lean body mass and route of administration are of less importance. Patients with diminished renal function will require smaller maintenance doses (e.g., 0.125 mg PO qod with GFR < 30 ml/minute).

Note: Rapidly administered IV digoxin increases peripheral and coronary resistance by central mechanisms. This potential source of adverse clinical effects is avoided if IV digoxin is administered over several minutes.

3. **Serum digoxin levels** are measured by radioimmunoassay (RIA). Digitoxin levels are determined by a different RIA. Unfortunately, there is no constant relationship between serum level, therapeutic effect, and risk of toxicity. The same serum level may be therapeutic at one time and toxic at another, even in the same patient. Clinical evaluation of the patient and the ECG are of paramount importance when assessing digoxin therapy. Serum digoxin levels are an adjunct.

Serum levels are measured at their nadir, or at least 6 hours after the last dose. The therapeutic range is 0.5–1.8 ng/dl, although occasional patients manifest toxicity at such levels. Levels greater than 2.0 ng/dl are associated with a substantial risk of toxicity. Doses and levels required to control the ventricular response in patients with atrial fibrillation may be somewhat higher than those usually required to treat CHF.

Serum levels are most useful when (1) renal function is changing, (2) a known drug interaction is occurring, (3) the therapeutic effect is not apparent (to detect noncompliance or reduced bioavailability), or (4) toxicity is suspected. Critically ill patients receiving multiple medications have a particularly high risk of digoxin toxicity, and their serum digoxin levels should be obtained at regular intervals.

If the digoxin level is high, dosage should be reduced unless required to control the ventricular response in atrial fibrillation. If the digoxin level is low and the clinical response adequate, dosage need not be altered. Attempts to obtain a "high therapeutic level" frequently result in toxicity.

4. **Factors affecting the response to digoxin**

   a. **Drug interactions**

      (1) **Quinidine** administration usually causes a doubling of serum digoxin levels. When quinidine therapy is initiated with a maintenance dose, digoxin levels increase rapidly over 48 hours and reach a new steady state after 4–5 days. If a patient is loaded with quinidine, digoxin levels increase rapidly over 24 hours, and a steady state is established after 2 days. The mechanism of this drug interaction, though not well defined, apparently involves a reduction in digoxin's volume of distribution and rate of elimination. In this setting, increased serum digoxin levels correlate with an increased risk of toxicity. Accordingly, the digoxin dose should be reduced by one-half when quinidine is initiated. Careful ECG and clinical evaluation is conducted until a new steady state is reached; a serum digoxin level is obtained at that time. Whenever the dose of quinidine is altered, additional changes in the dose of digoxin should be made.

      (2) **Verapamil** administration consistently produces a 60% increase in serum digoxin levels. Digoxin's volume of distribution and excretion

are both reduced. This interaction is clinically significant, although verapamil may provide some protection against digoxin-induced automatic rhythms. The combination can also precipitate high-grade AV block (*Clin. Pharm. Ther.* 30:311, 1981).

(3) Antibiotics can increase serum digoxin levels by 10–40% in patients whose enteric flora interfere with digoxin's enterohepatic circulation. A number of drugs may impair digoxin absorption (see **2.b**).

b. **Factors predisposing to digoxin toxicity** include (1) hypokalemia (e.g., diuretic induced), (2) hypomagnesemia, (3) hypercalcemia, (4) acid-base imbalance, (5) hypoxemia, (6) increased endogenous or exogenous sympathetic tone, (7) decreased GFR, (8) hypothyroidism, (9) increased age, and (10) drug interactions (see above).

Selected patients are extremely sensitive to digoxin; in amyloid heart disease this is probably secondary to altered cardiac binding (*Circulation* 63:1285, 1981). Patients with ischemic heart disease and patients in Functional Class III–IV also have an increased susceptibility to digoxin toxicity.

c. **Factors contributing to resistance to digoxin's effect** include (1) malabsorption, (2) impaired enterohepatic circulation, (3) hyperthyroidism, and (4) hypocalcemia.

5. **Digoxin toxicity is a clinical diagnosis;** there are no pathognomonic features. When toxicity is suspected, digoxin should be withheld until the situation is clarified. The response to discontinuance of therapy is critical to the diagnosis. An elevated serum digoxin level provides supportive evidence.

a. **Noncardiac manifestations** of digoxin toxicity occur in at least 30% of patients. **Gastrointestinal symptoms** include anorexia, nausea, vomiting, abdominal discomfort, and diarrhea. **Psychic disturbances** may occur, such as fatigue, drowsiness, nightmares, restlessness, agitation, and psychosis. **Visual disturbances** include altered color perception (especially red green), scotoma, flickering color forms, and yellow halos. Ingestion of large quantities of digoxin (e.g., suicide attempts) can inhibit skeletal muscle Na^+, K^+–ATPase, resulting in massive release of intracellular potassium and life-threatening hyperkalemia.

b. **Cardiac manifestations.** Although most types of cardiac dysrhythmias have been reported with digoxin toxicity, certain rhythm disturbances are considered characteristic. **Disorders of impulse conduction** include AV block (first-degree, Wenckebach, and third-degree) and sinoatrial exit block. **Disorders of impulse formation** are secondary to enhanced automaticity of atrial, junctional, and ventricular tissues. Typical **supraventricular automatic rhythms** include atrial premature depolarizations (APDs), paroxysmal atrial tachycardia (usually with AV block), and junctional tachycardia (occasionally with Wenckebach and/or AV dissociation). Common **ventricular dysrhythmias** include ventricular premature depolarizations (VPDs), especially multiform VPDs and bigeminy. Ventricular tachycardia, bidirectional tachycardia, and ventricular fibrillation are also seen.

Note: Patients with atrial fibrillation require careful evaluation for evidence of regularity of the ventricular rate that may indicate digoxin-induced junctional rhythm. "Relative regularization" is a more subtle finding, often due to junctional rhythm with Wenckebach periodicity.

c. **Treatment.** When digoxin toxicity is suspected, **stop administration of the drug and evaluate the role of predisposing factors.** Certain rhythm disturbances require specific treatment.

(1) Patients with **AV block** require **observation** in a monitored setting. Hemodynamically significant bradycardia may be treated initially with **atropine** (0.5–1.0 mg IV). A **temporary transvenous pacemaker** is indicated if the response to atropine is incomplete or high-grade (Mobitz type II and third-degree) AV block is present. **Potassium impairs AV nodal conduction, and supplemental therapy is contraindicated in the presence of high-grade AV block unless an electronic pacemaker is in place.** Isoproterenol is relatively contraindicated because of its tendency to induce ventricular ectopic activity.

(2) Complex **ventricular ectopy** requires therapy.

   (a) Serum potassium should be maintained in the high-normal range (4.0–4.5 mEq/liter). The total body potassium deficit and type of dysrhythmia determine the dosage and route of administration of supplemental potassium; more than 10 mEq/hour IV is rarely indicated.

   (b) When additional therapy is required, **lidocaine** is the drug of choice. An initial bolus of 100 mg IV (or 1.0 mg/kg) is followed by a second bolus of 0.5 mg/kg in 5 minutes. A continuous infusion of 1–4 mg/minute should be started at the time of the initial bolus.

   (c) Phenytoin is an alternative antidysrhythmic agent. The initial IV dose is 250 mg diluted in normal saline and given slowly over 10 minutes. Additional doses of 100 mg may be given over 5 minutes, but the total loading dose should not exceed 10 mg/kg. Maintenance therapy is rarely necessary in this setting because of phenytoin's long serum half-life.

   (d) Procainamide should be used only if the above agents fail, because CHF and AV block can be exacerbated. Administer 50 mg IV q2–3 minutes to a maximum of 1 gm or until hypotension or a 25% increase in the QRS duration or the Q–Tc interval occurs. The loading dose may be followed by a continuous infusion of 2–6 mg/minute.

   (e) Propranolol, also a second-line agent, can be effective but should be used with great care; CHF and bronchospasm can be exacerbated. The drug is contraindicated in the presence of second- or third-degree AV block unless an electronic pacemaker is in place. Administer 1 mg IV every 3–5 minutes to a maximum of 0.15 mg/kg while carefully monitoring heart rate and blood pressure.

   (f) If drug therapy is not successful, a temporary pacemaker for **overdrive suppression** is indicated.

   (g) Certain measures are relatively contraindicated. Quinidine will increase serum digoxin levels. Although good results occasionally have been reported with **bretylium**, it produces an initial release of catecholamines that can be deleterious. **Cardioversion** can restore sinus rhythm but, in the presence of digoxin toxicity, can also precipitate fatal ventricular dysrhythmias. Diuretics, carbohydrates, and insulin can decrease serum potassium levels and aggravate the rhythm disorder.

(3) Supraventricular dysrhythmias, including paroxysmal atrial tachycardia with block and junctional tachycardia, are usually stable and require only **observation. Potassium** supplementation is indicated if serum levels are low and second- or third-degree AV block is not present. When drug therapy is necessary, **phenytoin** is the agent of choice. In addition to suppressing ectopy, AV conduction is often enhanced. Alternative agents include procainamide and propranolol (in the absence of AV block). Lidocaine, verapamil, and cardioversion are not effective in this setting.

B. Parenteral inotropic support with beta-1–adrenergic agonists is reserved for patients with acute, severe heart failure, as may be seen in the perioperative or periinfarction period. It is also useful in patients with poor baseline cardiovascular function (Class III–IV) who present with a subacute or acute deterioration.

    1. Dobutamine is the inotropic agent of choice. However, if total peripheral resistance (see sec. **IV**) and blood pressure are low, **dopamine** ($\geqslant$ 10 µg/kg/minute) is preferred because of its alpha-adrenergic effects (see Chap. 4 for dosages). Hypertensive patients and those with markedly elevated total peripheral resistance are more effectively treated with parenteral vasodilators.

    2. Aminophylline has weak inotropic and diuretic properties and may be a useful adjunct to the therapy of refractory pulmonary edema. The loading dose is 4–5 mg/kg over 20 minutes. The maintenance dose in patients with CHF is 0.2–0.5 mg/kg/hour by constant infusion. Adverse effects include nausea, dysrhythmias, and seizures.

III. Reduction of congestive symptoms. The principal symptoms in most patients with CHF are related to venous congestion, not hypoperfusion. When congestive symptoms are initially detected, total body water is increased by at least 2–3 liters, and total body sodium is increased proportionately. Congestive symptoms may be minimized by appropriate dietary modification and diuretic therapy.

A. Dietary sodium restriction plays a lesser role now than in the past because of the availability of potent diuretics. Compliance with a salt-restricted diet requires a highly motivated and adequately instructed patient. In such a setting, dietary modification can be an effective tool.

The average American consumes 10–15 gm of sodium chloride daily. (For comparison, 1 liter of normal saline contains 9 gm of NaCl, 3.6 gm of Na^+, or 2¼ tsp of table salt.) A hospital "no added salt" diet contains 6–8 gm of NaCl and is appropriate for patients with mild to moderate CHF. For patients with an acute decompensation or advanced CHF, a 3- –4-gm salt diet is practical. More stringent salt restrictions are useful temporarily but long-term compliance is poor.

At the time of hospital discharge, it is of utmost importance that patients be on a diet to which they can adhere. Salt-restricted diets may be made more palatable by using **salt substitutes.** With the exception of Morton Lite Salt, which is equal parts NaCl and KCl, the commonly available salt substitutes (Adolph's Salt Substitute, Co-Salt, Diasal, Morton Salt Substitute, and Nu-Salt) are basically KCl. They contain 12–15 mEq K^+/gm (60 mEq K^+/tsp) and are less expensive than prescription potassium supplements (*J.A.M.A.* 238:608, 1977). Salt substitutes should be recommended to patients with the same care as prescription KCl. Daily use should be relatively standardized and serum potassium monitored. Renal insufficiency and use of potassium-sparing diuretics are relative contraindications to potassium supplementation.

B. Fluid intake of 2–3 liters/day is permissible for most patients. Fluid is restricted to 500–1500 ml daily when dilutional hyponatremia is present.

C. Diuretics complement therapeutic regimens that already include dietary modification and, in most cases, digoxin. Their use is potentially hazardous; inappropriate administration can result in serious electrolyte and acid-base disturbances and in intravascular volume depletion with impaired cardiac output and renal hypoperfusion. Complications not directly related to their diuretic action may also occur. Attention to the guidelines that follow will reduce the incidence of adverse effects.

1. **Principles of treatment**

   a. **Obtain a baseline weight.** Thereafter, obtain daily weights (using the same scale), intake and output, or both. Postural changes in blood pressure and pulse should be monitored during therapy.

   b. Obtain baseline and periodic serum **electrolytes, BUN,** and **creatinine.**

   c. Begin with a small dose of a **mild diuretic** unless renal insufficiency is present or the patient is acutely ill.

   d. Edema fluid can be mobilized at a rate of approximately 1 liter/day; pleural fluid and ascites are mobilized more slowly. **Weight loss exceeding 1 kg/day is likely to result in intravascular volume depletion.** Postural changes in heart rate and blood pressure or a rise in the BUN-creatinine ratio are sensitive indicators of overly aggressive diuresis.

   e. Patients taking digoxin and a kaliuretic diuretic normally receive **supplemental potassium.** Potassium supplementation for patients with cardiac disease not receiving digoxin is recommended if serum potassium is less than 3.5 mg/dl or if symptoms of hypokalemia are present.

2. **Diuretic agents.** See Table 5-2.

   a. **Thiazide diuretics** are preferred for use in mild to moderate CHF. They are well absorbed, induce a modest diuresis, and are generally well tolerated. Chlorothiazide, hydrochlorothiazide, and chlorthalidone differ only in their duration of action. The dose-response curve for thiazide diuretics reaches a plateau; dosages exceeding those in Table 5-2 will not augment the diuretic response. The effectiveness of thiazide diuretics can be diminished by increased resorption of sodium in the distal nephron; however, addition of a potassium-sparing diuretic restores responsiveness. **Thiazides are not effective when the GFR is less than 30 ml/minute.**

   Side effects related to their renal actions include hypokalemia, hyponatremia, metabolic alkalosis, hyperuricemia, hypercalcemia, and exacerbation of hepatic coma. Other rare side effects include skin rash, thrombocytopenia, leukopenia, vasculitis, and acute pancreatitis. Hyperglycemia may also be seen, typically in patients with glucose intolerance.

   b. **Metolazone,** chemically a thiazide diuretic, is unique in that it has significant effects on the proximal tubule as well as the cortical diluting segment. Small doses are frequently effective in patients refractory to other diuretics. Metolazone retains its efficacy in patients with renal insufficiency. Side effects are the same as with other thiazides.

   c. **Furosemide** is a potent, fast-acting diuretic and retains its efficacy in patients with renal insufficiency. The dose-response curve is linear. Intravenous administration promptly induces venodilation, and cardiac filling pressures fall even before diuresis begins. This action makes it particularly useful for the therapy of acute CHF.

      (1) **Oral therapy** is usually initiated with a 20-mg dose. In the hospital, this may be doubled and repeated q6–8h until satisfactory diuresis ensues. Combination diuretic therapy is indicated in patients unresponsive to a 200-mg dose.

      (2) The response to **IV therapy** is more marked than to oral therapy. For equal effect, an IV dose should be one-third to one-half less than an oral dose. Young patients without a history of diuretic use should receive 10 mg initially. The initial dose may be doubled and repeated q1–2h as needed. Individual doses of 500 mg may be required for patients with renal failure.

Table 5-2. Diuretic agents

Agent	Primary site of action	Maximum Natriuretic effect (%)[a]	Route of administration	Average daily dose (mg)[b]	Onset of action	Duration of action
Thiazides						
Chlorothiazide	Distal tubule	5–10	PO	250–500	2 hr	6–12 hr
			IV	500	15 min	
Hydrochlorothiazide	Distal tubule	5–10	PO	50–100	2 hr	12 hr
Chlorthalidone	Distal tubule	5–10	PO	50–100	2 hr	24 hr
Metolazone	Proximal and distal tubule	5–10	PO	2.5–20.0	1 hr	24 hr
Loop diuretics						
Furosemide	Ascending limb, loop of Henle	20–25	PO	20–80[c]	1 hr	6–8 hr
			IV	10–80[c]	5 min	2–4 hr
Ethacrynic acid	Ascending limb, loop of Henle	20–25	PO	50–100	30 min	6–8 hr
			IV	50	15 min	3 hr
Potassium-sparing diuretics						
Spironolactone	Distal tubule	2–3	PO	50–200[d]	1–2 days	2–3 days
Triamterene	Distal tubule	2–3	PO	100–200[d]	2–4 hr	12–16 hr
Amiloride	Distal tubule	2–3	PO	5–20[d]	2 hr	24 hr

[a] As percent of filtered load.
[b] The dose given and frequency of administration are determined by the patient's clinical response.
[c] Larger doses may be required in patients with renal insufficiency.
[d] Commonly given in divided doses.

(3) The most common **side effects** include hypokalemia, hyponatremia, hyperuricemia, and hypochloremic metabolic alkalosis. Inappropriate use can induce profound volume depletion, hypotension, and prerenal azotemia. Rarely reported side effects include hyperglycemia, gastrointestinal upset, thrombocytopenia, neutropenia, and skin rash. Transient hearing loss has been reported after large IV doses; administration over several minutes minimizes this risk.

d. Ethacrynic acid is comparable to furosemide with respect to potency and mechanism of action. Side effects, including ototoxicity, are also similar.

e. Spironolactone is a competitive antagonist of aldosterone, and, in the absence of elevated aldosterone levels, its effects are extremely limited. It is administered for its potassium-sparing effect or to augment the effect of other diuretics. Its onset of action is delayed, and its duration of action is 2–3 days. Therefore, dosage changes should be made only after several days of therapy. Because of its potassium-sparing effects, the drug is **contraindicated** in patients with renal insufficiency. Special caution is required when treating either diabetic patients (who may have type IV renal tubular acidosis) or patients receiving captopril. Potassium supplements (including salt substitutes) are relatively contraindicated. Serum potassium levels must be followed carefully. Because spironolactone antagonizes androgen activity, gynecomastia, diminished libido, impotence, and irregular menses can occur.

f. Triamterene and amiloride are potassium-sparing diuretics. They act more rapidly and predictably than spironolactone, and their effectiveness is aldosterone independent. Contraindications and precautions are the same as for spironolactone.

3. Selecting a diuretic regimen. The net effectiveness of a diuretic regimen depends on the severity of CHF, renal function, and sodium intake. If renal function is normal, and the patient has mild to moderate CHF, therapy is initiated with a thiazide diuretic. Spironolactone, triamterene, or amiloride may be added for its potassium-sparing effect, or for additional diuresis, or for both.

If the clinical response is inadequate, furosemide should be used. When 160–200 mg of furosemide daily is not effective, a thiazide diuretic or metolazone may be added. A loop diuretic plus metolazone is the most potent diuretic regimen currently available.

Maintenance therapy is usually administered once daily; however, patients with persistent nocturnal symptoms benefit from a twice-daily regimen. The second dose should be administered 5–6 hours before bedtime to allow uninterrupted sleep.

IV. Vasodilators. Vasodilator therapy is indicated when patients with chronic CHF remain in Functional Class III–IV **despite optimal therapy with digoxin and diuretics.** Vasodilators are also useful in patients with Class II CHF and hypertension, mitral regurgitation, or aortic regurgitation. Appropriately selected patients usually can be improved by at least one functional class. Subjective and objective evidence of improvement is demonstrable at rest and during exercise. Preliminary results suggest survival may be improved in patients with congestive cardiomyopathy who respond to vasodilators.

Vasodilators alter preload and afterload without effecting contractility. **Preload** is the myocardial wall stress during diastole. **Afterload** is the myocardial wall stress during systole. Preload and afterload are intimately related and cannot be manipulated independently.

Left ventricular **preload** is estimated clinically by measuring pulmonary artery occlusive pressure (PAOP) or, if equivalent, pulmonary artery end-diastole pressure (PAEDP). Optimal ventricular filling pressure, usually 16–18 mm Hg, is determined by two opposing factors. First, the Frank-Starling relationship dictates that as ventricular filling pressure increases, stroke volume increases. However, unless left ventricular compliance is markedly reduced (e.g., in aortic stenosis), the Starling curve reaches a plateau at a PAOP of 18–20 mm Hg, and additional increments in PAOP do not augment stroke volume. Second, a PAOP in excess of 20 mm Hg results in accumulation of pulmonary interstitial fluid. Pulmonary congestion may develop at a lower pressure if capillary permeability or plasma oncotic pressure is abnormal.

The PAOP may be lowered with diuretics or vasodilators. When left ventricular function is markedly depressed, even cautious diuretic therapy has an increased propensity to deplete intravascular volume and reduce cardiac output. In this setting, vasodilators can reduce preload and congestive symptoms without untoward effects. However, **excessive preload reduction (PAOP <10–14 mm Hg) can compromise stroke volume and cardiac output, resulting in tachycardia and hypotension.**

The best estimate of **afterload** for clinical purposes is total peripheral resistance:

$$TPR = \frac{MAP - CVP}{CO} \times 80$$

where MAP = mean arterial pressure, CVP = central venous pressure, and CO = cardiac output. The normal range is 900–1350 dyne·sec·cm^{-5}. Mean arterial and central venous pressures can be estimated noninvasively; however, accurate determination of cardiac output requires invasive methods.

The normal left ventricle can maintain cardiac output despite increased afterload; the failing left ventricle cannot. Neuroendocrine mechanisms activated in patients with CHF increase TPR. There are two ways to reduce TPR in this setting. First, positive inotropic agents reverse the sequence of events that produced the initial reflex elevation. However, in most instances, available inotropic agents do not entirely normalize ventricular function, and TPR remains abnormal. Furthermore, certain inotropic agents directly increase TPR (e.g., dopamine, >10 μg/kg/minute). Second, an arteriolar dilator directly lowers TPR, which permits increased stroke volume (and cardiac output) without increasing stroke work or significantly decreasing MAP.

Patients with markedly elevated TPR (>1800 dyne·sec·cm^{-5}) almost uniformly respond to an arteriolar dilator with an increase in cardiac output. A favorable response occurs occasionally in patients with modestly elevated TPR. There are no reliable criteria to predict which patients with modestly elevated TPR will respond favorably (although patients with mitral or aortic regurgitation usually do), nor is there a value to which TPR can be routinely lowered without adverse effects. Some patients continue to improve until TPR is reduced to 500–600 dyne·sec·cm^{-5}; The condition of others deteriorates when TPR is still above normal. Therefore, therapy must be individualized, and patients should be monitored closely. **Excessive TPR reduction is manifested by hypotension, tachycardia, and diminished cardiac output.**

Any vasodilator that reduces afterload also reduces preload. An unrecognized excessive decrease in preload is frequently responsible for the failure of afterload reduction therapy.

A. Guidelines for vasodilator therapy in patients with Class III–IV CHF

1. Vasodilator therapy should be initiated and titrated in the hospital.

2. An optimal regimen will be obtained most reliably with the aid of invasive monitoring. A **thermodilution pulmonary artery catheter** is strongly recommended when parenteral vasodilators are used, or if systolic blood pressure is

less than 100 mm Hg. In these situations, blood pressure should be monitored frequently, if not continuously.

3. Vital signs should be obtained supine and erect in ambulatory patients, especially 30–90 minutes after each dose, when the peak effect generally occurs.

4. If mean arterial pressure decreases or heart rate increases more than 10–15%, therapy should be reevaluated. When a pulmonary artery catheter is in place, the PAOP should be maintained at 14–18 mm Hg.

5. Begin with low doses and increase stepwise. If a pulmonary artery catheter is in place, the dosage may be increased q4–6h. Otherwise, changes should be made only once daily. When combinations of vasodilators are used, adjust only one agent at a time.

6. **Venodilators** (e.g., nitrates) are most useful in patients with a relatively normal cardiac output and congestive symptoms. They principally reduce preload. Afterload is reduced to a lesser degree, and cardiac output increases slightly.

7. **Arteriolar dilators** (e.g., hydralazine) are useful for the treatment of patients with increased TPR and decreased cardiac output. Preload is also modestly reduced, and fluids may be required to maintain an adequate filling pressure (14–18 mm Hg). Inappropriate use produces hypotension, tachycardia, and increased myocardial oxygen consumption, which can exacerbate ischemic heart disease.

8. **Balanced vasodilator therapy** (e.g., nitroprusside, prazosin, nitrates plus hydralazine) is desirable when pulmonary congestion and diminished cardiac output coexist.

9. **Significant left ventricular outflow tract obstruction is a relative contraindication to vasodilator therapy.**

B. **Parenteral vasodilators** are very useful for the treatment of selected patients with CHF and hypertension or increased TPR. Patients receiving these agents must be carefully monitored in an ICU to minimize the incidence of hypotension. A thermodilution pulmonary artery catheter is recommended in all cases. Blood pressure is monitored frequently, if not continuously. Parenteral vasodilators are infused through a separate IV line, and the infusion rate is controlled by an automated device. When therapy is being discontinued, the infusion rate should be tapered gradually to prevent "rebound" exacerbation of CHF.

1. **Indications** for therapy include acute pulmonary edema, perioperative or periinfarction CHF, acute mitral or aortic regurgitation, severe CHF in patients requiring cardiac catheterization or surgery, and an exacerbation of CHF in patients whose baseline function is poor (Class III–IV). A brief trial of parenteral therapy, to document responsiveness, may be useful in potential candidates for chronic vasodilator therapy.

2. **Agents**

   a. **Sodium nitroprusside,** a potent, balanced vasodilator, decreases PAOP and TPR and can substantially increase cardiac output. Its serum half-life is 1–3 minutes, allowing rapid titration of dosage and effect. A standard preparation contains 50 mg in 250 ml 5% D/W (200 μg/ml). The solution and IV tubing must be protected from light. Therapy is initiated with 10–15 μg/minute and increased by similar increments q5–10min, as indicated by the clinical and hemodynamic response. (The PAOP should be maintained at 14–18 mm Hg, heart rate should increase ≤10%, and serial determinations of cardiac output and TPR should be made.) The maximum dose is 5–6 μg/kg/minute.

Hypotension is the most common **side effect.** Adverse effects related to nitroprusside metabolites can also occur. Nitroprusside decomposes nonenzymatically in the blood, releasing cyanide that is converted rapidly to thiocyanate by a hepatic enzyme system. Thiocyanate is then excreted by the kidneys. Impaired conversion of cyanide to thiocyanate results in metabolic acidosis. Thiocyanate can cause fatigue, nausea, confusion, hyperreflexia, and convulsions. Toxicity is rare when dosages of ≤ 3 μg/kg/minute are used for less than 72 hours; nevertheless, extreme caution is required when treating patients with hepatic or renal insufficiency. In these settings, IV nitroglycerin is preferred. If prolonged therapy is required, serum thiocyanate levels are monitored and should remain at 10 mg/dl or less. Thiocyanate is dialyzable. Life-threatening cyanide toxicity may be treatable with thiosulfate or sodium nitrite and may be prevented by simultaneous infusion of hydroxycobalamin (*N. Engl. J. Med.* 298:809, 1978).

b. Intravenous nitroglycerin is a potent venodilator with modest effects on arterioles. The serum half-life is 1–3 minutes, permitting rapid titration. A standard preparation contains 50 mg in 250–500 ml 5% D/W (200 or 100 μg/ml). Because of avid adherence to polyvinylchloride, the solution is prepared in a glass bottle, and polyethylene tubing is used. Treatment is initiated with 5 μg/minute and increased by 5–10 μg/minute q3–5min as indicated. The maximum dosage is usually 200 μg/min.

Hypotension is the most common complication but is usually preceded by a drop in PAOP. Therapy of the hypotension includes stopping the infusion and volume expansion. Rarely, a pressor is required. Paradoxical bradycardia occasionally accompanies drug-induced hypotension. When this occurs, IV atropine is frequently required.

Nitroglycerin is preferred to nitroprusside when selective preload reduction is desired. It may be superior in the setting of myocardial ischemia (see Chap. 4).

c. Phentolamine, a rapid-acting alpha-adrenergic–blocking agent, primarily dilates arterioles. Its serum half-life is 2–4 minutes. The initial infusion rate is 100 μg/minute, which may be increased by 100 μg/minute q5min to a maximum of 2 mg/minute. Phentolamine administration is frequently associated with tachycardia and gastrointestinal side effects. Because of these adverse effects and its high cost, it is rarely used.

Note. When the stock solution of a parenteral vasodilator is changed, the rate of infusion should be reduced by 10–15% and then retitrated to the appropriate dosage. This reduces the risk of hypotension related to in vitro degradation of the old stock solution or variation between preparations.

C. Chronic vasodilator therapy. See Table 5-3.

1. Nitrates. All nitrates have similar hemodynamic effects and differ principally in their duration of action. The dosing interval for chronic therapy should be 4 hours or longer to facilitate compliance. Oral isosorbide dinitrate, oral sustained-release nitroglycerin, and transdermal nitroglycerin preparations fulfill this requirement. Their onset of action occurs approximately 30 minutes following administration; a parenteral or sublingual preparation should be used in acute situations.

Headache is the most common side effect but usually resolves after several days of therapy. Methemoglobinemia is an extremely rare complication. Tolerance is not a common clinical problem. Therapy should be tapered rather than discontinued abruptly.

2. Hydralazine is predominantly an arteriolar dilator; preload is also modestly reduced. Hemodynamic guidelines for selecting patients who respond favor-

Table 5-3. Long-acting vasodilators

Agent	Site of action		Dose		Interval between doses (hr)
	Venous	Arteriolar	Initial	Maintenance[a]	
Nitrates					
Isosorbide dinitrate (sublingual)	++++	+	2.5 mg	10–15 mg	1–3
Isosorbide dinitrate (PO)			10 mg	20–80 mg	4–6
Sustained-release oral nitroglycerin			2.5 mg	9–27 mg	6–8
Transdermal nitroglycerin					
2% Ointment			0.5 in. ($\approx$ 10 mg)[b]	1–3 in.	4–6
Nitrodisc			8 cm^2 (16 mg)[b]	8–16 cm^{2c}	24
Nitro-Dur			5 cm^2 (26 mg)[b]	5–30 cm^{2c}	24
Transderm-Nitro			10 cm^2 (25 mg)[b]	10–20 cm^{2c}	24
Hydralazine	+	++++	25 mg	50–100 mg	6–8
Prazosin	+++	++++	1 mg	2–7 mg	6–8
Captopril	++	++++	25 mg	50–150 mg[d]	8
Minoxidil	+	++++	2.5 mg	5–20 mg	12
Nifedipine	++	++++	10 mg	10–30 mg	6–8

[a]Maintenance dosage depends on the clinical response.
[b]Numbers in parentheses indicate quantity of nitroglycerin in the reservoir. The nitroglycerin in 2% ointment, Nitro-Dur, and Transderm-Nitro is 20% bioavailable; 70% of Nitrodisc's nitroglycerin is bioavailable.
[c]Represents the reservoir sizes available rather than dosage range recommended.
[d]Dosage reduction required with renal insufficiency.

ably are not well established. Patients with markedly elevated TPR, or hypertension, or both are good candidates. Patients with significant left ventricular enlargement may be more likely than others to respond favorably (*N. Engl. J. Med.* 303:250, 1980).

The **dosage** required for patients with CHF is usually 75–100 mg PO qid; occasional patients may require doses 3–4 times larger. High-dose therapy (≥400 mg/day) is associated with a substantial (10–15%) risk of a drug-induced lupus–like syndrome. Patients receiving such dosages should have a significant and well-documented response to therapy. Other less common side effects include headache, nausea, vomiting, abdominal pain, peripheral neuropathy (responsive to pyridoxine, 50 mg PO qd), and skin rash.

Adverse hemodynamic effects may result from excessive reduction of TPR or PAOP and include hypotension, tachycardia, decreased cardiac output, and exacerbation of ischemic heart disease.

3. **Prazosin** is a postsynaptic alpha-1 adrenergic–receptor blocker with a balanced vasodilator effect. The initial dose is 1 mg, preferably at bedtime in ambulatory patients, although first-dose syncope is rare when CHF is present. The hemodynamic response is triphasic. Cardiac output increases most after the initial dose, decreases over the next several days, and then increases again. Significant attenuation of prazosin's chronic hemodynamic effect may occur in 10–20% of patients (see **Note** below).

4. **Additional vasodilators.** The following agents have been studied less extensively than nitrates, hydralazine, and prazosin or have more serious side effects:

   a. **Captopril,** an angiotensin-converting–enzyme inhibitor, is a balanced vasodilator that can be useful in the treatment of CHF. Blood pressure usually decreases with captopril, especially after the initial dose. Hypotension can be profound if PAOP is low. Cardiac output improves gradually over several days.

   The initial dosage is 25 mg PO tid; larger doses prolong the duration of action without increasing the peak effect. Captopril is excreted by the kidneys, and dosage should be reduced in patients with renal insufficiency.

   Side effects include rash, angioedema, fever, ageusia, agranulocytosis, and membranoproliferative glomerulonephritis. The latter usually resolves when the drug is discontinued. Baseline and periodic urinalyses and WBC counts with differential should be obtained. Because captopril lowers serum aldosterone levels, hyperkalemia can result when it is used in combination with potassium-sparing diuretics.

   b. **Minoxidil** is a potent direct-acting vasodilator similar to hydralazine. It markedly increases sympathetic activity in patients with hypertension but not in appropriately selected patients with CHF. Nevertheless, particular caution is necessary in patients with coronary artery disease. Significant fluid retention frequently accompanies its use and may require an increased diuretic dosage.

   Major side effects include hypertrichosis and reversible T wave changes. Headache is seen rarely. Pericardial effusion may occur.

   c. **Nifedipine,** a calcium channel–blocking agent, has potent vasodilating properties and may be useful for the treatment of CHF. Its use in this setting remains investigational.

Note: Attenuation of the initial beneficial effects of vasodilator therapy occurs in a small percentage of patients. Attenuation is most common with prazosin but may occur with other vasodilators. Increasing the vasodilator dosage is not helpful.

However, attenuation is often associated with increased fluid retention secondary to hyperaldosteronism and resolves with the addition of **spironolactone** to the therapeutic regimen. If this is not helpful, a different vasodilator should be substituted.

D. **Vasodilator therapy for the treatment of cor pulmonale** has had variable results. Currently available agents predominately effect the systemic rather than the pulmonary circulation. This differential effect can increase in patients with pulmonary vascular disease. Effects on the systemic circulation may cause hypotension, tachycardia, or increased cardiac output. If cardiac output increases more than pulmonary vascular resistance decreases, pulmonary artery pressure will actually increase. There are no guidelines to select patients who will respond favorably, and severe adverse reactions, including death, have occurred in some patients. If vasodilator therapy is attempted, extreme caution should be employed, and a thermodilution pulmonary artery catheter must be used. The use of vasodilators for the treatment of cor pulmonale remains investigational.

V. Additional therapeutic options

A. **Thoracentesis and paracentesis** may be performed for diagnostic or therapeutic purposes. When dyspnea and large pleural effusions are present, gradual removal of up to 1 liter of fluid can yield prompt relief. Removal of excessive quantities of pleural fluid occasionally results in ipsilateral pulmonary edema. Paracentesis (≤1 liter) is useful therapeutically if tense ascites compromises respiration. Depending on its cause, removing large quantities of ascitic fluid can lead to rapid reaccumulation and precipitate intravascular volume depletion.

B. **Morphine sulfate** and **rotating tourniquets** may be indicated in the treatment of pulmonary edema. **Phlebotomy** is useful in refractory cases.

C. **Ultrafiltration** is occasionally required in patients with severe fluid overload refractory to diuretic therapy.

D. **Intraaortic balloon counterpulsation** is a potent method of mechanically reducing afterload. **Indications** for the balloon pump include (1) intractable heart failure secondary to acute mitral regurgitation, ventricular septal rupture, or ventricular aneurysm and (2) intractable angina pectoris. The balloon pump is utilized only after maximal medical therapy has failed to stabilize the patients adequately for cardiac catheterization and surgery. Balloon counterpulsation may be combined with vasodilator or inotropic therapy. However, administration of pressors will antagonize its effect. **Contraindications** include aortic dissection or aneurysm and aortic insufficiency. Serious complications occur in 10–20% of patients, including vascular dissection and lower extremity vascular insufficiency.

Cardiac Dysrhythmias

Cardiac dysrhythmias result from abnormalities in impulse initiation (automaticity) or abnormalities in impulse propagation (conduction). The nature of these abnormalities and their response to antidysrhythmic agents vary, depending on the part of the cardiac conduction system involved and the underlying cause.

Antidysrhythmic agents available in the United States are divided into five groups based on their electrophysiologic properties in isolated cardiac muscle and Purkinje fibers (Table 6-1). Continued modification of this classification scheme will be required as new antidysrhythmic agents are marketed and as more information becomes available regarding the interaction of these agents with specific ionic currents responsible for cellular depolarization and repolarization.

I. **Group I antidysrhythmic drugs: disopyramide, quinidine, and procainamide.** These agents are effective in suppressing **atrial** and **ventricular** premature depolarizations (APDs and VPDs) and repetitive dysrhythmias of diverse causes. In isolated tissues, these agents induce concentration-dependent increases in action potential duration, effective refractory period (ERP), and diastolic threshold potential; and reductions in maximal diastolic potential, action potential amplitude, maximal upstroke velocity of phase 0, membrane responsiveness, and spontaneous phase 4 depolarization. These alterations result from effects on both active and passive membrane properties and collectively decrease conduction velocity, excitability, and automaticity. Alterations in conduction velocity and excitability are in part due to a direct depression of the mechanism controlling the voltage and a time-dependent increase in sodium conductance. These effects are enhanced by hyperkalemia. Specific interactions between these agents and the ionic currents responsible for repolarization and spontaneous phase 4 depolarization have not been completely elucidated. They do not appear to affect the slow inward calcium current significantly.

The magnitude of action potential prolongation induced by these agents depends on the location of the fiber within the conduction system. The change is more pronounced for fibers with short action potential durations and less marked for those with longer durations. These changes effectively diminish the disparity in cellular recovery, resulting in more homogeneous repolarization throughout the ventricular conduction system. These agents exert a greater depressant effect on diseased or partially depolarized fibers than on normal fibers.

The electrophysiologic alterations induced by these agents are important in explaining their **toxicity.** As serum concentrations increase, the QRS and Q–Tc intervals widen, reflecting progressive reduction in conduction velocity and prolongation of cellular repolarization respectively. **Toxic doses** of these agents may paradoxically enhance Purkinje fiber automaticity, giving rise to bizarre ventricular dysrhythmias. Torsade de pointes and ventricular fibrillation (VF) have been reported with each of these agents. At high plasma concentrations, sinoatrial block or arrest, high-grade atrioventricular (AV) block, or asystole may occur. Toxicity is additive with other group I antidysrhythmic agents.

These agents may cause deleterious effects in patients with atrial fibrillation or flutter. They slow intraatrial conduction and reduce the number of impulses pene-

Table 6-1. Comparative effects of antidysrhythmic drugs

Effects	Group I: procainamide, quinidine, and disopyramide	Group II: phenytoin and lidocaine	Group III: propranolol	Group IV: bretylium	Group V: verapamil
ECG					
Sinus rate	→, ↑	↑, ↓	↓, →, ↓	↓	→, ↑
P–R interval	→, ↑	→	↑	↑	↑
QRS duration	↑	→	→	↑	→
Q–Tc*	↑	↑	→	↑	→
Hemodynamic					
Blood pressure	→, ↓	→	↓	↑, then →	↓
Cardiac output	↓	→	↓	→	↑
Contractility	↓	→	↓	→	→
Left ventricular end-diastolic pressure	→, ↑	→	↑	→, ↑	↑
Major toxic effects	Cardiovascular	CNS	Cardiopulmonary	Cardiovascular, Renal	Cardiovascular
Metabolism and excretion	Hepatic and renal	Hepatic	Hepatic	Renal	Hepatic and renal

↓ = decrease; → = no change; ↑ = increase.
*Q–Tc = QT/√RR (normal = 0.38–0.42).

trating the AV node. As a result, concealed conduction of atrial impulses in the AV node is decreased. This effect, coupled with their direct vagolytic effect on the AV node, may markedly increase the ventricular response to atrial fibrillation or flutter.

Finally, these agents are **myocardial depressants** and peripheral vasodilators. They may induce hypotension, particularly when given IV, and may have additive effects with other myocardial depressants or peripheral vasodilating agents.

A. Disopyramide

  1. **Absorption and excretion.** Oral doses of disopyramide are 80–100% absorbed and reach a peak plasma concentration in 2 hours. Protein binding is concentration dependent and ranges from 5–65%. With an oral dose of disopyramide, 40–60% is excreted unchanged in the urine. The remainder undergoes hepatic degradation, and some metabolites are excreted in the urine. In healthy subjects, the serum half-life ranges from 4–10 hours, with a mean of 7 hours. The half-life increases in patients with acute myocardial infarction and with reductions in creatinine clearance. Changes in urinary pH do not affect disopyramide excretion. **Serum levels** of 2.8–7.5 µg/ml correlate with clinical efficacy.

  2. **Clinical utility**

     a. **Suppression and prevention of VPDs and ventricular tachycardia (VT).**

     b. **Suppression and prevention of APDs and supraventricular tachydysrhthmias** (at present not FDA approved for this use). European studies have shown disopyramide to be comparable to quinidine and procainamide in converting atrial fibrillation or flutter to sinus rhythm and in maintaining sinus rhythm following cardioversion. Disopyramide is also effective in reentrant supraventricular tachycardias (SVT) associated with accessory bypass tracts.

  3. **Toxicity and precautions**

     a. Disopyramide should not be administered to patients with prolonged Q–Tc intervals and should be discontinued if an increase of more than 25% occurs in the Q–Tc interval during therapy.

     b. Disopyramide should not be administered to patients with preexisting second- or third-degree AV block without a temporary or permanent pacemaker and should be used with caution in patients with bundle branch block or sinus node dysfunction. The drug should be discontinued if an increase greater than 25% occurs in the QRS duration.

     c. Disopyramide should not be administered to patients with atrial flutter or fibrillation unless the ventricular response has been controlled.

     d. Disopyramide should not be used in patients with severe congestive heart failure (CHF) or shock.

     e. Anticholinergic effects include dry mouth, urinary retention, constipation, blurred vision, abdominal pain, exacerbation of glaucoma, and drying of bronchial secretions.

     Note: Toxicity is more common in patients with renal or hepatic dysfunction.

  4. **Drug interactions**

     a. Coumadin enhances the effect of disopyramide.

     b. There is no interaction with digitalis preparations.

  5. **Preparations and dosages.** Available forms include 100- and 150-mg capsules. The usual maintenance dosage is 100–300 mg q6–8h. In patients with

hepatic dysfunction, CHF, or moderate renal insufficiency (creatinine clearance <40 ml/minute), dosage should not exceed 100 mg q6h. In patients with marked renal impairment, the recommended dosage regimen is a 200-mg loading dose followed by 100 mg q10h, q20h, or q30h for creatinine clearances of 15–40, 5–15, and 1–5 ml/minute respectively.

B. Quinidine

1. **Absorption and excretion.** Absorption of an oral dose is virtually complete, with peak serum levels achieved in 2 hours. Parenteral administration results in peak serum levels in less than 1 hour. The serum half-life is 5–7 hours, with 50–80% of the drug in plasma being protein bound. The drug is metabolized primarily in the liver and then excreted in the urine. The serum half-life is not significantly altered in patients with renal dysfunction or CHF but increases with age and in the presence of hepatic dysfunction. Serum levels of 1.3–5.0 μg/ml correlate well with clinical efficacy.

2. **Clinical utility**

   a. **Suppression and prevention of APDs and VPDs.**

   b. **Ventricular tachycardia.**

   c. **Automatic and reentrant supraventricular tachycardias (SVTs).**

   d. With maintenance doses of quinidine, **conversion of atrial fibrillation or flutter** to sinus rhythm occurs successfully in approximately 20% of patients. Quinidine is also effective in the short-term (up to 6 months) prevention of recurrence of atrial fibrillation or flutter after conversion to sinus rhythm; however, long-term prevention has not been demonstrated.

3. **Toxicity and precautions**

   a. Quinidine should not be administered to patients with prolonged Q–Tc intervals and should be discontinued if an increase of more than 25% occurs in the Q–Tc interval during therapy. On rare occasions, however, syncope and sudden death have occurred without evidence of Q–Tc prolongation.

   b. Quinidine should not be administered to patients with preexisting second- or third-degree AV block without a temporary or permanent pacemaker and should be used with caution in patients with bundle branch block. Quinidine should be discontinued if an increase of 50% or more occurs in the QRS duration (25% in patients with underlying interventricular conduction delays).

   c. Quinidine may exacerbate CHF and should not be used in patients with severe CHF or shock.

   d. Quinidine should not be administered to patients with atrial flutter or fibrillation unless the ventricular response has been adequately controlled.

   e. Gastrointestinal reactions include diarrhea, nausea, and vomiting. These symptoms are usually mild and can be controlled by symptomatic treatment without stopping the drug.

   f. Cinchonism (salivation, tinnitus, vertigo, headache, visual disturbance, confusion).

   g. Hypotension (usually associated with parenteral administration) is due to both the weak alpha-blocking properties of the drug and the decrease in myocardial contractility.

   h. Other reactions include thrombocytopenia, rash, hepatitis, hemolytic anemia, proteinuria, fever, and angioedema.

4. Drug interactions

  a. In patients on long-term digoxin therapy, serum digoxin levels increase about twofold when therapeutic doses of quinidine are given.

  b. Antacids delay drug absorption.

  c. Coumadin effects are potentiated by the drug.

  d. Phenobarbital and phenytoin reduce the serum half-life significantly.

5. Preparations and dosages

  a. Quinidine sulfate is available in tablets or capsules of 200 and 300 mg. The usual dosage is 200 mg q6h, with a maximum dose of 2.4 gm/day. Extentabs (Quinidex, 300 mg) are given q8–12h.

  b. Quinidine polygalacturonate (Cardioquin) is available in tablets containing the equivalent of 275 mg of quinidine sulfate. This form causes less gastric irritation and may be given q8–12h.

  c. Quinidine gluconate (Quinaglute) is available in sustained-release tablets of 324 mg, which contain 200 mg of the base drug. The drug may be administered q8–12h. **Parenteral formulations** are available. When given IV, the drug should be diluted (800 mg into 50 ml 5% D/W) and given at a rate of 1 ml/minute, with careful observation of blood pressure and ECG. The maximum dose should not exceed 500 mg. Intramuscular administration is rarely indicated.

C. Procainamide

1. Absorption and excretion. Absorption of an oral dose is rapid and 75–95% complete. Peak serum concentration is reached 1 hour after an oral dose and 25 minutes after IM injection. Initial effects are seen within 20–30 minutes following oral ingestion, 5–10 minutes after IM injection, and immediately after IV administration. At therapeutic concentrations, 15% of the drug is protein bound. Procainamide is eliminated by both hepatic metabolism and renal excretion. Normally, 75–95% is eliminated in the urine; 30–60% appears as unchanged drug and the remainder as metabolites. The major metabolic pathway is hepatic acylation to N-acetylprocainamide (NAPA). The serum half-life is approximately 3 hours, but in patients with CHF or severe renal dysfunction, it may be as long as 5½ and 16 hours respectively. **Serum levels** of 4–12 µg/ml correlate with clinical efficacy.

2. Clinical utility

  a. Suppression and prevention of APDs and VPDs.

  b. Ventricular tachycardia.

  c. Reentrant and automatic SVTs.

  d. Conversion of atrial fibrillation or flutter to sinus rhythm. Procainamide is comparable to quinidine.

3. Toxicity and precautions

  a. Prolongation of the Q–Tc interval occurs less frequently with procainamide than with quinidine or disopyramide. Nonetheless, the drug should not be administered to patients with prolonged Q–Tc intervals and should be discontinued if Q–Tc prolongation occurs during therapy.

  b. Procainamide should not be administered to patients with preexisting second- or third-degree AV block without a temporary or permanent pacemaker and should be used with caution in patients with bundle branch block. Procainamide should be discontinued if the QRS duration increases more than 25%.

c. Myocardial depression is especially associated with IV administration. The drug should not be used in patients with severe CHF or shock.

d. Procainamide should not be administered to patients with atrial flutter or fibrillation unless the ventricular response has been controlled.

e. A lupuslike syndrome (fever, serositis, arthritis) may be seen in as many as 33% of patients on chronic therapy. This syndrome usually spares the kidney and abates when the drug is stopped. Serologic abnormalities, such as positive antinuclear antibodies, frequently in high titer, may develop in 75% of patients with chronic administration.

f. Other reactions include fever, rash, nausea, vomiting, diarrhea, confusion, and agranulocytosis.

Note: Due to the additive toxicity of the pharmacologically active metabolite NAPA, both NAPA and procainamide serum levels should be monitored routinely during therapy. Toxicity is more common in patients with renal dysfunction.

4. **Drug interactions.** Coumadin and digitalis preparations do not interact with procainamide.

5. **Preparations and dosages**

   a. **Oral.** Capsules of 250, 375, and 500 mg are available. For patients with ventricular dysrhythmias, a total oral daily dosage of 50 mg/kg of body weight administered in six to eight divided doses results in therapeutic serum levels. To obtain a therapeutic level initially, a loading dose of 750–1000 mg is frequently necessary. For atrial dysrhythmias, an initial dose of 1.25 mg may be followed in 1 hour by 0.75 gm if there have been no ECG changes. A dose of 0.5–1.0 gm may then be given q2h until the dysrhythmia abates or the limit of tolerance is reached. The suggested maintenance dose is 0.5–1.0 gm q4–6h. A sustained-release preparation (Procan SR) in 250-, 500-, and 750-mg tablets is available that permits q6h dosing intervals.

   b. **Intravenous.** To avoid hypotension, the drug should be infused as a continuous infusion of 30–50 mg/minute until the dysrhythmia is suppressed or a maximum loading dose of 1 gm has been administered. Vital signs should be checked q5min during the infusion. A maintenance infusion of 2–6 mg/minute may then be used (2 gm of procainamide diluted in 500 ml of 5% D/W will give a mixture in which 1 ml/minute = 4 mg/minute).

   c. **Intramuscular.** The IM dose is 500–1000 mg q6h. Dosage adjustment may be necessary because of variable absorption.

II. **Group II antidysrhythmic drugs: lidocaine and phenytoin.** These agents are effective against both automatic and reentrant **ventricular dysrhythmias** but are relatively ineffective against supraventricular dysrhythmias. Lidocaine and phenytoin are also the drugs most effective against digitalis-induced dysrhythmias. In isolated Purkinje fibers, these agents depress phase 4 automaticity but have no significant effect on sinus node automaticity. Preliminary studies indicate that these agents also counteract abnormal forms of automaticity, such as depolarized, stretched Purkinje fibers or digitalis-induced afterdepolarizations. Alterations in action-potential variables depend on the tissue studied and the extracellular potassium concentration. In normal Purkinje fibers, these agents increase diastolic threshold potential and decrease action potential duration and ERP but do not significantly alter membrane responsiveness. The greatest change in action potential duration is seen in areas of the His-Purkinje system having the longest action potential duration. These agents tend to reduce the dispersion of cellular recovery throughout the ventricular conduction system. In ischemic, partially depolarized fibers, these agents markedly slow conduction velocity by depressing membrane responsiveness and the time course of reactivation. These effects are enhanced by hyperkalemia. Alterations in conduction velocity and excitability are in part due to a direct depression of sodium conductance, whereas shortening in action potential duration appears to be mediated through enhancement of the potassium current responsible for cellular repolarization. These agents can abolish ventricular reentry by either improving or impairing conduction. If unidirectional block is due either to tissues depolarized by stretch or to heterogenous recovery times, these agents can improve conduction by causing hyperpolarization and more uniform recovery respectively. If unidirectional block occurs in depolarized, ischemic tissues, these agents abolish reentry by producing bidirectional block.

At therapeutic concentrations, group II agents do not have significant electrophysiologic effects on sinus, atrial, or AV nodal tissue. However, in **high doses,** they can produce sinus arrest and heart block in patients with underlying abnormalities of impulse generation and propagation.

Finally, group II agents are **myocardial depressants** and should be used with caution in patients with severe left ventricular dysfunction.

A. Lidocaine

1. **Absorption and excretion.** The onset of action is immediate following IV administration. The distribution half-life of a single IV dose is 8–17 minutes. After tissue loading has occurred, the half-life range is 87–108 minutes. When given IM, antidysrhythmic blood levels are usually obtained within 5–15 minutes and persist for 60–90 minutes. About 30% of the drug is protein bound, and 90% is metabolized by the liver, with less than 10% excreted unchanged in the urine. The serum half-life is prolonged in patients with hepatic dysfunction, CHF, shock, and in patients over 70 years of age. **Therapeutic serum levels** are 2–6 μg/ml (equivalent to an infusion rate of 3–4 mg/minute), but adverse reactions have been observed at lower levels.

2. **Clinical utility**

   a. Lidocaine is the **drug of choice** for emergency treatment of VPDs or VT, particularly in the setting of acute myocardial infarction. Many investigators recommend prophylactic lidocaine use in patients with acute myocardial infarction.

   b. The drug should be used on a **prophylactic basis** if ventricular dysrhythmias are anticipated during cardioversion.

   c. Lidocaine is frequently effective in slowing the rapid ventricular response in patients with atrial fibrillation or flutter and antegrade conduction over an accessory bypass tract.

3. **Toxicity and precautions**

   a. Central nervous system effects include convulsions, confusion, stupor, and (rarely) respiratory arrest. These generally resolve when the drug is stopped, but seizures may require treatment with IV diazepam.

   b. Negative inotropic effects are usually seen only with high dosages.

   c. Induction of dysrhythmias may occasionally occur, including sinus arrest, AV block, and augmentation in AV conduction or atrial rate in patients with atrial flutter or fibrillation.

   Note: Toxic effects are common in patients over the age of 70 or in those with CHF, shock, or hepatic dysfunction.

4. **Drug interactions**

   a. Decreased metabolism occurs with isoniazid, chloramphenicol, propranolol, and norepinephrine.

   b. Increased metabolism occurs with phenobarbital, isoproterenol, and glucagon.

c. Large doses may enhance the muscle-relaxant effects of succinylcholine.

5. Preparations and dosage. Lidocaine is supplied as a 1% or 2% solution or in ampules for IV bolus therapy (50 or 100 mg/ampule). It is also available in single-use vials of 1–2 gm for preparing IV infusions. **Initial therapy** should consist of an IV bolus of 1 mg/kg. To obtain and maintain therapeutic levels, this bolus must be followed by a second bolus of 0.5 mg/kg in 5 minutes. At the time of the initial bolus, **maintenance therapy** should also begin, with an IV infusion at a rate of 1–4 mg/minute (20–60 μg/kg/minute). This can be done by removing 50 ml from a 500-ml bag of 5% D/W and adding 2 gm (50 ml of a 4% solution) of lidocaine; at this dilution, 1 ml of solution contains 4 mg of lidocaine. The initial bolus and maintenance dose should be reduced by 50% in patients with CHF, shock, or hepatic dysfunction and in patients over 70 years of age. Intramuscular administration should be used only when IV administration is impossible. The recommended initial dose is 300 mg, although in the early hours of acute myocardial infarction, higher doses may be necessary.

B. Phenytoin

1. Absorption and excretion. Absorption after oral administration is variable and incomplete. The onset of action after IV administration is prompt. Phenytoin is hydroxylated in the liver and then excreted in the urine; however, the rate of hepatic metabolism is variable. Approximately 70% of the drug is protein bound. The serum half-life after oral administration is 22–24 hours. Cardiac tissue levels decline more slowly than do serum levels. **Serum levels** between 10–20 μg/ml correlate with therapeutic effectiveness. Serum levels are essential because of wide variations in hepatic metabolism and the risk of significant toxicity at levels greater than 20 μg/ml.

2. Clinical utility

    a. Digitalis-induced dysrhythmias (supraventricular or ventricular).

    b. Phenytoin is of little benefit as a primary agent in the treatment of dysrhythmias not due to digitalis. Its secondary role is in combination with other antidysrhythmic agents (e.g., with a group I drug in a patient in whom Q–Tc prolongation has occurred without suppression of the dysrhythmia).

3. Toxicity and precautions

    a. Nystagmus, nausea, vertigo, ataxia, and cerebellar dysfunction.

    b. Hypotension, sinus bradycardia, and respiratory depression may occur with rapid IV administration. These effects may be mediated by the IV vehicle (alcohol propylene glycol) and can be minimized by slow administration (50 mg/minute).

    c. Induction of a lupuslike syndrome.

    d. Gingival hyperplasia, megaloblastic anemia, rash, adenopathy, serum sickness, and vomiting.

    e. Due to the acidity of the parenteral drug, sterile abscesses (IM route) and thrombophlebitis (IV route) may occur.

Note: Toxicity is common in patients with hepatic dysfunction.

4. Drug interactions

    a. Increased metabolism can be seen with administration of any drug that induces hepatic enzymes.

    b. Decreased metabolism may result from concomitant use of coumadin, isoniazid, glucocorticoids, insulin, chloramphenicol, disulfiram, amphetamines, and phenylbutazone.

c. Coumadin metabolism is accelerated.

d. Vitamin D inactivation is increased, and chronic use may lead to osteomalacia.

e. Hepatic toxicity with halothane is increased.

5. **Preparations and dosage**

   a. **Oral.** The drug is available in 100- and 300-mg tablets. A **loading dose** of 1 gm is required to initiate therapy, followed by 500 mg on days 2 and 3 and then a once-daily maintenance dose of 300–400 mg (4–6 mg/kg/day).

   b. **Intravenous.** The **loading dose** is 250 mg diluted in normal saline (crystallization occurs in dextrose-containing solutions) and given slowly over 10 minutes. Subsequent doses of 100 mg may be given q5min as needed. Digitalis-induced dysrhythmias frequently respond to the initial 250-mg dose and rarely require large amounts of the drug. Frequent monitoring of the ECG and blood pressure and examination for signs of nystagmus are necessary in patients receiving this drug IV. A continuous infusion should not be utilized.

   c. The **IM dose** is 50% greater than the usual oral dose, but this route is rarely utilized because of sterile abscess formation.

III. **Group III antidysrhythmic drugs: propranolol.** The principal effects of propranolol result from its competitive beta-adrenergic–blocking action. Beta-adrenergic stimulation causes a marked increase in automaticity in isolated Purkinje and sinus node tissues and can induce abnormal automatic rhythms due to catecholamine-dependent, slow responses and afterdepolarizations. Beta stimulation enhances AV node conduction and shortens refractoriness. As a result, beta blockade is **effective in decreasing automaticity and abolishing reentrant dysrhythmias involving the AV node.** In **ventricular tissue,** propranolol has little effect on action potential characteristics of ventricular muscle but significantly shortens action potential duration and the ERP of Purkinje fibers, resulting in a more homogeneous recovery throughout the ventricular conduction system. In **high concentrations,** propranolol is a direct membrane depressant, similar to the group I agents. Finally, propranolol can favorably influence dysrhythmias by its effects on myocardial oxygen supply-demand relations.

The beta-blocking effects of this agent also account for its cardiac **toxic effects.** The negative inotropic and chronotropic effects of sympathetic blockade may exacerbate sinus bradycardia, inhibit AV node conduction, and cause myocardial depression.

A. **Absorption and excretion.** Propranolol is rapidly and completely absorbed from the GI tract. More than 90% of circulating propranolol is bound to plasma protein. Hepatic extraction is high (50–80%), so that little free compound is available to the circulation after a single oral dose. The major metabolite, 4-hydroxypropranolol, is equally as potent as propranolol as an antidysrhythmic agent but has a shorter half-life. Variations in hepatic metabolism and blood flow may cause marked variations in serum levels for a given dose. The serum half-life of small oral doses of propranolol is 2–3 hours; however, with larger doses and long-term administration, the half-life ranges from 3–6 hours. The serum half-life is not markedly prolonged in patients with diminished renal function. Propranolol may decrease its own elimination rate by decreasing cardiac output and hepatic blood flow. Following IV administration, beta blockade occurs almost immediately. Given IV, 1 mg is approximately equal to 10 mg administered PO during long-term administration. **Serum levels** in the range of 100–150 ng/ml are generally associated with clinical beta blockade.

B. Clinical efficacy

1. **Atrial fibrillation and atrial flutter.** Propranolol reduces the ventricular response and may be effective when digitalis has failed. Propranolol also enhances the responsiveness to vagal stimulation.

2. Termination and prevention of both **automatic and reentrant SVTs,** particularly SVTs that utilize the AV node as part or all of the reentrant circuit.

3. Ventricular dysrhythmias are less responsive to propranolol than to group I drugs, except those that are clearly catecholamine related. Propranolol may be helpful when used in combination with other antidysrhythmic agents, particularly those in group I.

4. **Digitalis-induced dysrhythmias,** in the absence of high degrees of AV block, may respond to propranolol. However this indication applies only after potassium and phenytoin have been tried.

5. Sinus tachycardia rarely requires treatment and frequently is needed to maintain cardiac output. When treatment is indicated, as in patients with a metabolic disturbance, propranolol is the drug of choice.

C. Toxicity and precautions

1. In patients with severe **CHF** or **shock,** propranolol should be used only if the failure or shock is secondary to a tachydysrhythmia. Concomitant digitalis administration may permit the use of small doses of propranolol. The myocardial depressant effects of propranolol can be treated with inotropic agents, such as dopamine and dobutamine.

2. **Negative chronotropic effects** will slow the heart rate and exacerbate conduction disturbances of the AV node.

3. **Cardiac dysrhythmias** or **angina** may be precipitated by the abrupt withdrawal of this agent. Whenever possible, the drug should be tapered over several days.

4. Hypoglycemia may be induced by propranolol therapy, and propranolol's beta-blocking properties may mask the symptoms of acute hypoglycemia.

5. Propranolol should be used with caution in patients with asthma, chronic obstructive pulmonary disease, and allergic rhinitis.

6. Other side effects include nausea, vomiting, light-headedness, depression, rash, fever, paresthesias, and visual disturbances.

D. Drug interactions.
Propranolol may accentuate the chronotropic effects of digoxin and the negative inotropic effects of other antidysrhythmic agents.

E. Preparations and dosage

1. **Oral** propranolol is available in 10-, 20-, 40-, and 80-mg tablets. The dose may vary considerably, but 20–80 mg q6h is usually adequate for antidysrhythmic efficacy.

2. **Intravenous.** When needed emergently, propranolol should be given in 1-mg aliquots diluted in normal saline; 1–3 mg is generally sufficient. The maximum acute dose is 0.15 mg/kg.

3. **Metropolol, nadolol, and atenolol** are three new beta blockers currently approved for the treatment of hypertension but not for the treatment of cardiac dysrhythmias.

IV. Group IV antidysrhythmic drugs: bretylium tosylate.
Bretylium has direct electrophysiologic effects as well as important interactions with the autonomic nervous system. In Purkinje fibers, bretylium has no direct effect on normal phase 4 depolarization. However, automaticity transiently increases after drug exposure because of the initial release of norepinephrine from adrenergic nerve terminals.

Bretylium produces a marked prolongation in action potential duration and ERP in Purkinje fibers and ventricular muscle. In ventricular muscle from dogs surviving experimental infarction, bretylium prolongs action potential duration and ERP in normal Purkinje fibers more than in fibers from the infarcted zone. This differential effect reduces the disparity in ERP between normal and infarcted zones. Bretylium has no consistent effect on resting membrane potential, rate of phase 0 depolarization, membrane responsiveness, or conduction velocity. The drug's efficacy in terminating reentrant dysrhythmias is probably related to marked alterations in refractoriness or stabilization of sympathetic tone.

The **toxicity** of this agent is primarily due to its interaction with the automatic nervous system. Bretylium accumulates in peripheral adrenergic nerve terminals, resulting in an initial release of norepinephrine, producing a sympathomimetic effect. The initial release of catecholamines may exacerbate digitalis-induced dysrhythmias. Subsequently, bretylium inhibits the release of norepinephrine by producing adrenergic neuronal blockade and may cause hypotension.

A. **Absorption and excretion.** The onset of action is prompt with IV administration, **although maximum efficacy may require 15–20 minutes.** When given IM, the drug requires 30 minutes to reach therapeutic levels. The serum half-life varies from 4.2–16.9 hours. Myocardial binding is intense, and serum levels may not reflect pharmacologic efficacy. After 24 hours, 70–80% of bretylium is excreted unchanged in the urine. Detailed evaluation of **serum levels** and their correlation with therapeutic and toxic effects has not been accomplished.

B. **Clinical utility**

   1. **Refractory ventricular dysrhythmias,** including VT and VF, constitute the primary indication for the use of this drug. It may be effective in cardiac arrest, even if VF has been present for long periods and is refractory to other maneuvers (e.g., lidocaine, defibrillation).

   2. Ventricular dysrhythmias associated with digitalis intoxication may respond to bretylium, but conventional agents (potassium, phenytoin) should be tried first.

C. **Toxicity and precautions**

   1. Supine and orthostatic **hypotension** may occur.

   2. Initial elaboration of catecholamines may exacerbate digitalis dysrhythmias.

   3. Other side effects include nausea, vomiting, parotid pain and swelling, lightheadedness, rash, emotional lability, and renal dysfunction.

D. **Drug interactions**

   1. Bretylium's effectiveness may be reduced when used with other antidysrhythmic drugs.

   2. Bretylium may heighten the response to infused catecholamines.

   3. The hypotensive effects of diuretics or vasodilator drugs may be augmented during bretylium administration.

E. **Preparation and dosages.** Parenteral bretylium is available in 500-mg ampules.

   1. **Ventricular fibrillation.** An initial IV bolus of 5–10 mg/kg is followed by either a continuous maintenance infusion of 1–2 mg/minute or repetitive IM or IV doses of 5–10 mg/kg q6–8h.

   2. **Ventricular tachycardia.** Dilute 500 mg of bretylium in 50 ml of 5% D/W (10 mg/ml). An initial IV bolus of 5–10 mg/kg should be given over an 8- –10-minute period, followed either by a maintenance infusion of 1–2 mg/minute or repetitive boluses of 5–10 mg/kg IV or IM q6–8h. Intramuscular adminis-

tration may be associated with local tissue necrosis unless the dose is divided and injection sites rotated.

V. **Group V antidysrhythmic drugs: verapamil.** Verapamil selectively **blocks the slow inward current** carried primarily by calcium ions. The slow inward current is responsible for normal depolarization of sinus and AV nodal cells but may be pathologically induced in diseased atrial or ventricular muscle and thereby play an important role in mediating ischemic and digitalis-induced dysrhythmias. In tissues dependent on slow-channel activity, verapamil induces a concentration-dependent depression in phase 4 depolarization, resting membrane potential, and a prolongation in refractoriness, resulting in depressed automaticity and slowed conduction. Unlike group I and group II agents, verapamil has no significant effect on the action potential parameters of fast-response fibers normally located in atrial and ventricular muscle and the His-Purkinje system. The antidysrhythmic effects of verapamil thus result from its ability to depress the slow response.

In the human, the **major action** of verapamil is to slow conduction in the AV node. This effect on AV conduction is the principal mechanism by which the ventricular response in atrial fibrillation and flutter is controlled and SVTs utilizing the AV node as all or part of their reentrant circuit are abolished. Verapamil has little effect on normal sinus rate, since the drug's depressant action on sinus node automaticity is largely nullified by the reflex tachycardia that results from hypotension due to peripheral vasodilatation. Verapamil, however, may depress sinus node function in patients with sick sinus syndrome.

At therapeutic levels verapamil has mild **negative inotropic effects** that result from impairment of excitation-contraction coupling. In most patients, including those with organic heart disease, this effect is partially nullified by a reduction in afterload mediated through verapamil's direct dilating action on vascular smooth muscle. Clinically, the hypotensive effect is generally mild and transient.

A. **Absorption and excretion.** Following IV administration, the **onset of action is within 1–2 minutes,** with a peak effect occurring in 10–15 minutes. Atrioventricular nodal depression is detectable up to 6 hours following drug administration. In contrast, hemodynamic effects occur between 3–5 minutes following bolus injection but are dissipated by 10–20 minutes. Verapamil is extensively metabolized in the liver and excreted by the kidneys. Ninety percent of the drug is protein bound.

B. **Clinical utility**

   1. **Rapid conversion to sinus rhythm of paroxysmal reentrant SVTs** that incorporate the AV node as part or all of the reentrant circuit. These include AV nodal SVT and SVTs utilizing either manifest or concealed accessory pathways.

   2. **Temporary control** of rapid ventricular rate in atrial flutter or atrial fibrillation.

   3. Verapamil is **not approved** for prophylactic maintenance therapy of superventricular tachydysrhythmias.

C. **Toxicity and precautions**

   1. **Bradycardia, high-degree AV block, and asystole** have been reported. **Verapamil should not be administered** to patients with preexisting second- or third-degree AV block or to patients with sinus node dysfunction unless a temporary or permanent pacemaker is operative.

   2. **In patients with Wolff-Parkinson-White syndrome and atrial fibrillation,** verapamil may augment the ventricular response rate by enhancing antegrade conduction over the bypass tract.

   3. Transient ventricular ectopy may be seen following verapamil-induced termination of reentrant SVTs. The cause of these dysrhythmias is unknown, but they are generally self-limited and of little clinical significance.

4. Because verapamil is extensively metabolized in the liver, toxic levels may be reached quickly in patients with hepatic dysfunction who receive multiple doses.

5. Marked **hypotension** may occur following IV administration. Therapy with IV fluids and pressor agents is generally effective. Verapamil should be used cautiously in patients with mild to moderate CHF and is **contraindicated** in the presence of severe CHF or shock.

D. Drug interactions

1. Verapamil's **negative inotropic and chronotropic effects are additive** with group I agents, and combination therapy should be used with caution in patients with CHF or preexisting conduction system disease. Until further data are available, verapamil should not be used concomitantly with disopyramide.

2. **Serious adverse effects** have been reported with concomitant use of verapamil and IV beta blockers.

3. Verapamil may be used in concert with digitalis preparation. However, since both drugs impair AV conduction, patients should be monitored for AV block or profound bradycardia.

E. Preparations and dosage.
Verapamil is supplied in 2-ml vials, each containing 5 mg of drug. An **initial dose** of 5–10 mg (0.075–0.15 mg/kg) should be administered as a slow IV bolus over 2–3 minutes. This dose may be repeated after 30 minutes if the initial response is unsatisfactory.

VI. Cardioversion.
The most common cardioverter or defibrillator is the capacitor-discharge unit, which delivers an external electrical impulse and can be synchronized to avoid discharge during the vulnerable period of the ventricle. The amount of energy delivered to the heart depends on many factors, but cardioversion should be accomplished at the lowest possible energy level to reduce the incidence of complications and the degree of discomfort. The incidence of major complications with cardioversion is small. Successful reversion to sinus rhythm occurs in more than 90% of patients with atrial flutter and fibrillation, reentrant SVTs, and VT. Successful cardioversion does not obviate the need to administer antidysrhythmic drugs.

A. Indications

1. **Atrial fibrillation** is one of the most common indications for cardioversion. Cardioversion is indicated if atrial fibrillation is of short duration or if a rapid, uncontrollable ventricular rate is producing hemodynamic compromise. Atria measuring more than 4.5 cm by echocardiography rarely maintain sinus rhythm.

2. **Atrial flutter** is one of the easiest rhythms to convert to sinus rhythm. Cardioversion frequently requires less than 50 joules and often converts to atrial fibrillation with as little as 5 joules. Cardioversion should be done emergently if the patient is hemodynamically unstable or has angina.

3. **Reentrant supraventricular tachycardias.** Cardioversion is necessary if severe hypotension, CHF, or angina is present. Reentrant SVTs due to dual AV nodal pathways or manifest or concealed accessory pathways generally require 25–100 joules.

4. **Ventricular tachycardia.** Cardioversion is the treatment of choice if VT is accompanied by CHF, hypotension, or angina. Synchronized cardioversion may be accomplished with as little as 50 joules. However, the patient without blood pressure or pulse should be given 200 joules; if there is no immediate response, 360 joules should be delivered. Brief paroxysmal episodes of VT should not be treated with cardioversion.

5. **Ventricular fibrillation.** See Chap. 23.

B. Contraindications. Cardioversion is relatively contraindicated in the following circumstances:

1. **Digitalis-induced dysrhythmias.** Therapeutic levels of digitalis are not contraindications to cardioversion; however, if there is a question of digitalis intoxication, cardioversion should begin at low energy levels utilizing prophylactic lidocaine therapy. The energy delivered should be progressively increased until reversion occurs or signs of digitalis toxicity such as ventricular irritability appear.

2. **Repetitive, short-lived tachycardias**

3. Multifocal atrial tachycardia or other automatic dysrhythmias.

4. Atrial fibrillation associated with rheumatic heart disease in the immediate preoperative or postoperative period. If hemodynamic compromise is present, cardioversion may be of short-term benefit. Elective cardioversion should not be done immediately preoperatively or postoperatively, since recurrence is common.

5. Patients with supraventricular dysrhythmias and hyperthyroidism should be euthyroid prior to elective cardioversion.

6. Recurrent supraventricular dysrhythmias previously converted to sinus rhythm should not be treated by repeated cardioversion. However, if the patient has not had adequate maintenance antidysrhythmic therapy, a second cardioversion may be considered. Frequently, rapid atrial pacing is a better approach for recurrent reentrant SVT or atrial flutter, since it allows for multiple conversions over a short period while different antidysrhythmic regimens are evaluated. Rapid atrial pacing is not effective in atrial fibrillation or automatic SVTs.

7. Complete AV block.

8. Cardioversion should be done cautiously in (1) elderly patients with coronary artery disease and disease of the conducting system; (2) patients with atrial fibrillation and a slow ventricular response in the absence of digitalis; and (3) those with evidence of sick sinus syndrome.

C. Technique of cardioversion

1. The procedure is explained to the patient to decrease anxiety, and informed written consent is obtained.

2. **Digitalis should be withheld** 24–48 hours prior to the procedure unless required to prevent hemodynamic compromise.

3. The patient should take nothing by mouth for 6–8 hours prior to cardioversion.

4. **Anticoagulants** may be administered before the procedure (see sec. **IX.F.4** for details).

5. In patients with atrial fibrillation or atrial flutter, quinidine, 300 mg q6h, or procainamide, 500 mg q4h, should be started 24–48 hours before the procedure (see sec. **IX.F** and **G**).

6. The ECG should be continuously monitored.

7. The paddles should be generously coated with electrode paste or defibrillation pads applied and positioned with the posterior paddle underlying the left infrascapular region and the anterior paddle to the right of the sternum at the level of the third or fourth intercostal space. If a posterior paddle is unavailable, the second paddle should be placed just outside the cardiac apex.

8. **Amnesia** should be induced with IV diazepam or small doses of barbiturates.

Anesthesia should be available on a standby basis, since short-acting anesthetic agents may be necessary.

9. **The synchronization artifact should be checked on the defibrillator monitor.** After a stable baseline is obtained, the discharge is fired. As a result of synchronization of the energy delivered, the discharge may be delayed a short time. Do not remove the anterior paddle prematurely. Initial energy settings are **25 joules for atrial flutter, 50 joules for atrial fibrillation and SVTs, and 50 joules for VT.** Sequential increases to 100, 200, 300, and 360 joules may be necessary. If normal sinus rhythm is achieved only transiently, a higher energy setting is of no value. If ventricular dysrhythmias develop prior to cardioversion, a 50- –100-mg bolus of lidocaine should be administered if the procedure is to be continued. If bradycardia is noted, atropine, 0.6–1.0 mg IV, is generally helpful. In VF, an initial discharge of 200–300 joules is recommended.

D. **Adverse effects.** Muscle soreness, with a concomitant rise in LDH, SGOT, and CK, and irritation of the skin at the paddle site are common. Elevation of MB-CK, which generally does not occur until a total discharge greater than 425 joules has been given, is related to the total amount of energy delivered to the patient. **Dysrhythmias** may occur because of the release of catecholamines, acetylcholine, and potassium or the interaction of these substances with cardioactive drugs. Sinus pauses, as well as atrial, junctional, or ventricular ectopic beats, may occur transiently after restoration of sinus rhythm, especially in patients with long-standing atrial fibrillation and a slow ventricular response. Reports of serious dysrhythmias, such as VT, VF, or cardiac standstill, are unusual. These complications are more likely in patients with digitalis intoxication or when the defibrillator is not synchronized properly. Pulmonary edema and systemic and pulmonary embolism are rare complications.

VII. **Cardiac pacing.** Cardiac pacing may be necessary in symptomatic patients with severe bradydysrhythmias or for the therapy of tachydysrhythmias. The majority of pacemakers utilized are demand rather than fixed-rate pacemakers, although most pacemakers have a capacity to be converted to the fixed-rate mode by an external magnet. Newer programmable units allow adjustment in pacemaker rate and various pacemaker sensing and output functions. The pacemaker is generally inserted transvenously and positioned in the right ventricular apex under fluoroscopic control. In some patients with large right ventricles, adequate placement cannot be attained or maintained; in such situations, surgical placement of epicardial electrodes, either in the right or left ventricle, may be required. Atrial pacemakers and AV sequential pacemakers are also available. Newer power supplies have the potential of lasting 10–15 years.

Temporary pacemakers are invariably right ventricular endocardial electrodes placed via cutdown or percutaneously. Scrupulous aseptic techniques and a chest radiograph after the placement of the temporary pacemaker to confirm its position are mandatory. Careful attention should be paid to the pattern and axis of ventricular complexes as well as the threshold for sensing and pacing, since changes in the ECG or threshold may indicate changes in electrode position, with loss of function or perforation of the myocardial wall. An adequate threshold should be less than 1–2 mamp, and the pacemaker should be set at twice the established threshold. The pacemaker is generally set to maintain a heart rate of at least 60 beats/minute.

A. **Bradydysrhythmias: indications for temporary pacing**

1. Symptomatic second- or third-degree heart block due to transient drug intoxication or electrolyte imbalance.

2. Complete heart block, Mobitz II, or bifascicular block in the setting of acute myocardial infarction. Frequently, these conduction disturbances resolve as the acute episode evolves.

3. Symptomatic sinus bradycardia, atrial fibrillation with a slow ventricular response, or other bradycardic manifestations of conduction system disease may necessitate temporary pacing until a permanent wire can be inserted.

B. Bradydysrhythmias: indications for permanent pacing

1. Congenital complete heart block when the heart fails to accelerate with exercise or other stress

2. Symptomatic second- or third-degree AV node block

3. Second- or third-degree intra-His or infra-His block

4. Marked first-degree block in the His-Purkinje system (HV ≥100 msec; or HV 60–99 msec if symptoms present)

5. Bifascicular block that has progressed to complete heart block in the setting of acute myocardial infarctions, whether or not there is resolution of the complete heart block during the evolution of the infarction

6. Symptomatic sinus bradycardia

C. Tachydysrhythmias: indications for temporary pacing. In general, tachydysrhythmias can be adequately managed by drugs or cardioversion. In some instances, these measures are ineffective or contraindicated, and cardiac pacing may be useful in either terminating the tachycardia or preventing its recurrence.

1. **Atrial flutter** is probably the most common indication for pacing termination. Rapid atrial pacing is effective for close to 100% of patients with classic atrial flutter but is ineffective for atypical or type II flutter (rate 400, P waves upright in inferior leads). Successful conversion generally requires a critical pacing rate (125–135% of the flutter rate) and a critical duration of pacing (mean, 10 seconds).

2. **Reentrant SVTs,** especially AV nodal SVT and SVTs utilizing a manifest or concealed accessory pathway, can generally be terminated by either underdrive or overdrive pacing modalities. Sinus node and intraatrial reentrant SVTs can similarly be terminated by cardiac pacing.

3. When atrial flutter or reentrant SVTs recur frequently, a pacemaker wire may be left in the right atrium for several days, during which time repetitive conversion may be accomplished and multiple drug regimens assessed.

4. When atrial fibrillation or automatic or digitalis-induced SVTs are associated with a rapid ventricular response and hemodynamic compromise unresponsive to medical management, pacing the atrium at a rate higher than the intrinsic atrial rate generally increases the degree of AV block and thereby slows the ventricular response. Cardiac pacing is not effective in terminating these dysrhythmias.

5. Recurrent sustained VT is occasionally responsive to underdrive or overdrive ventricular pacing. Cardiac pacing during VT should be performed by experienced physicians, since **degeneration to VF** may occur.

6. In patients with bradycardia-dependent VT, or VT/VF complicating either intrinsic or drug-induced Q–T prolongation, pacing at rates faster than the intrinsic sinus rate frequently prevents spontaneous recurrences. Increasing the heart rate decreases the dispersion of refractoriness in the ventricular myocardium and abolishes the conditions necessary for reentry.

D. Tachydysrhythmias: indications for permanent pacing. Patient-activated radiofrequency underdrive and overdrive pacemakers are available for medically refractory reentrant SVTs. Similarly, underdrive patient-activated pacemakers are available for patients with refractory VT. Patients considered for pacemaker therapy should first undergo extensive electrophysiologic testing to determine the mechanism of the dysrhythmia and document a favorable response to the proposed pacing modality.

E. **Pacemaker follow-up.** The patient should take his or her pulse daily for a full minute and report variations greater than 3–5 beats/minute when the pacemaker is operational. The ECG should be repeated if symptoms occur and at reasonable intervals, to determine the discharge rate of the pacemaker, the spike amplitude, and the presence of competitive ectopic rhythms. Sophisticated monitoring techniques to evaluate the threshold, amplitude, and decay of the pacemaker spike are available and can be utilized through telephone relay mechanisms to facilitate and supplement the other observations. Pacemaker function should be checked more frequently as the projected end of battery life approaches.

F. **Complications**

1. Battery failure is the most common cause of pacemaker failure, but with the newer power supplies, this should be less frequent.

2. Electrode fracture.

3. Electrode dislodgment may occur, particularly early after placement, but can be detected by changes in both the pacing and sensing threshold and by chest x ray.

4. Infection may occur in the pacemaker site or pacemaker pocket, frequently necessitating removal of the pacemaker. However, bacteremia alone is not an indication for pacemaker removal.

5. Perforation of the myocardium can occur, with loss of pacing function.

6. Particularly with unipolar pacemakers, the muscles in proximity to the pacemaker, the power supply, or the diaphragm may be stimulated during cardiac pacing.

7. Pacemakers may irritate the ventricular cavities, resulting in mechanically induced ventricular ectopy.

8. Acceleration of the pacemaker rate is seen rarely.

9. Sensing dysfunction may occur, particularly with bipolar pacing units. It may sometimes be corrected by converting the unit to a unipolar pacemaker.

10. Rarely, a pacemaker wire may induce significant tricuspid insufficiency.

VIII. **Diagnosis and treatment of specific dysrhythmias.** Accurate diagnosis and appropriate therapy of disturbances in cardiac rhythm require a careful analysis of the patient's history (especially relating to the use of cardioactive drugs), a physical examination, and ECG findings, as well as an understanding of the nature of these rhythm disturbances and of the available therapeutic modalities. When possible, one should adhere to the approach described in **A–E** in evaluating patients with rhythm disturbances.

A. **Careful history.** The frequency, duration, mode of onset, and mode of cessation of the dysrhythmia should be determined. Symptoms and history of any disease that may directly or indirectly influence the cardiovascular system should be elicited. A careful drug history is mandatory.

B. **Physical examination.** The blood pressure, and both apical and peripheral pulses should be taken. Jugular venous pulsations should be observed for the pattern of atrial activity. The heart should be auscultated carefully for murmurs, gallops, or variations in the first heart sound. Evidence of cardiomegaly, CHF, thyroid dysfunction, or respiratory embarrassment should be specifically sought.

C. **Laboratory studies.** Electrolytes (including calcium and magnesium), arterial blood gases, drug levels, and thyroid function should be determined. A chest radiograph should be obtained.

Table 6-2. Dosages of commonly used antidysrhythmic agents[a]

Drug	Oral	Intravenous
Group I		
Disopyramide	100–300 mg q6–8h	
Quinidine[b]	Sulfate, 200–400 mg q6h, and polygalacturonate and gluconate, q8–12h	Dilute 800 mg in 50 ml, give 200-mg test dose IM, then 1 ml/min to 300–500 mg (gluconate only)
Procainamide[b]	250–1000 mg q3h; sustained release, q6h	100 mg q5min, or 50-mg/min IV infusion, up to 1 gm; maintenance IV infusion at 2–6 mg/min
Group II		
Lidocaine[b]		1.0-mg/kg bolus; repeat with a 0.5-mg/kg bolus in 5 min; maintenance IV infusion 1–4 mg/min, beginning with initial bolus
Phenytoin[b]	1 gm first 24 hr, 500 mg days 2 and 3, then 200–500 mg/day	250 mg over 10 min, then 100 mg q5min as needed, with careful monitoring
Group III		
Propranolol	10–40 mg q6h	1–3 mg diluted in normal saline; maximum dose 0.15 mg/kg, but less is generally effective
Group IV		
Bretylium[b]		VF: 5- –10-mg/kg bolus VT: 5–10 mg/kg diluted 1 : 4 over 8 min, then 1- –2-mg/min infusion, or repeat same dose IM or IV q6–8h
Group V		
Verapamil		5- –10-mg bolus (0.075–0.15 mg/kg); may be repeated in 30 min if first dose ineffective

[a]General guidelines for patients with normal pharmacokinetics. Reductions in dosages may be necessary with hepatic or renal dysfunction, CHF, shock, or electrolyte imbalance (see text).
[b]Quinidine, procainamide, lidocaine, phenytoin, and bretylium are also available for IM use (see text for details).

D. Thorough review of the ECG. It is important to define atrial activity. The following are often of help:

1. A long rhythm strip with evaluation of multiple leads. Leads aVF and V1 are generally the most valuable in identifying atrial activity. Recording the rhythm strip at 50 mm/second is often helpful.

2. **Bipolar leads** utilizing lead I with the left arm lead placed posteriorly or over the left ventricular apex and the right arm lead used as an exploring electrode are frequently of value.

Table 6-3. Emergency treatment for cardiac dysrhythmias

Type	Treatment*
Supraventricular	
Atrial premature depolarizations	(1) None; (2) quinidine, procainamide; (3) digitalis
Paroxysmal supraventricular tachycardia	
Sinus node reentry	(1) Vagal maneuvers; (2) verapamil; (3) propranolol
Intraatrial reentry	(1) Procainamide with digitalis; (2) quinidine with digitalis
AV nodal reentry	(1) Vagal maneuvers; (2) verapamil; (3) propranolol; (4) digitalis
AV reentry utilizing a concealed by-pass tract	(1) Vagal maneuvers; (2) verapamil; (3) propranolol; (4) digitalis; (5) procainamide; (6) quinidine
Automatic atrial tachycardia	
Control ventricular response	(1) Digitalis; (2) propranolol; (3) verapamil
Suppress ectopic focus	(1) Propranolol; (2) procainamide, quinidine
Paroxysmal supraventricular tachycardia with hemodynamic compromise	(1) Vagal maneuvers; (2) DC cardioversion
Atrial fibrillation	
Control ventricular response	(1) Digitalis; (2) verapamil; (3) propranolol
Terminate	(1) DC cardioversion; (2) IV procainamide, PO quinidine with digitalis
Atrial flutter	
Control ventricular response	(1) Digitalis; (2) propranolol; (3) verapamil
Terminate	(1) DC cardioversion; (2) rapid atrial pacing; (3) IV procainamide, oral quinidine with digitalis
Wolff-Parkinson-White syndrome and	
Atrial fibrillation	(1) Lidocaine; (2) procainamide; (3) DC cardioversion
Paroxysmal supraventricular tachycardia	(1) Verapamil; (2) digoxin; (3) propranolol; (4) procainamide, quinidine
Ventricular	
Ventricular premature depolarizations	(1) Lidocaine; (2) procainamide; quinidine; disopyramide
Ventricular tachycardia with critical hemodynamic compromise	(1) DC cardioversion; (2) lidocaine; (3) bretylium; (4) procainamide
Ventricular tachycardia without critical hemodynamic compromise	(1) Lidocaine; (2) procainamide; (3) cardioversion; (4) bretylium
Ventricular fibrillation	(1) Defibrillation; defibrillation with: (2) bretylium; (3) lidocaine; (4) procainamide
Torsade de pointes due to drug-induced prolonged Q–Tc	(1) Stop drug; (2) lidocaine, phenytoin; (3) isoproterenol; (4) pacemaker
Atrioventricular block or bradydysrhythmias	(1) Atropine; (2) isoproterenol; (3) pacemaker

*Numbers indicate suggested treatment sequences but may vary as the clinical situation varies. For precautions, dosage adjustments, and contraindications, see the text.

Table 6-4. Chronic treatment of cardiac dysrhythmias

Type	Treatment[a]
Supraventricular	
Atrial premature complexes	(1) Quinidine; (2) procainamide; (3) propranolol
Paroxysmal supraventricular tachycardia[b]	(1) Digitalis; (2) propranolol; (3) quinidine, procainamide
Atrial fibrillation	(1) Digitalis; (2) propranolol; (3) quinidine, procainamide
Atrial flutter	(1) Cardioversion; (2) digitalis; (3) propranolol; (4) quinidine, procainamide
Ventricular	
Ventricular premature complexes[c]	(1) Quinidine, procainamide, disopyramide; (2) digitalis; (3) propranolol
Recurrent nonsustained and sustained ventricular tachycardia	(1) Procainamide, quinidine, disopyramide; (2) digitalis (if CHF is present); (3) propranolol (if catecholamine related)
Atrioventricular block	(1) Pacemaker

[a]Numbers indicate the suggested treatment sequence, which may vary as the clinical situation varies. Precautions, dosage, adjustments, and contraindications should be read in the appropriate *Manual* sections.
[b]Therapy will vary, depending on the type.
[c]The efficacy of empirical long-term antidysrhythmic drug therapy in preventing sudden death in patients with chronic PVCs or nonsustained VT has not been established.

3. **Carotid sinus massage.** The use of vagotonic maneuvers may be helpful in slowing the ventricular response and defining atrial activity. The patient should be supine with an IV line in place and the ECG monitored. Prior to massage, the carotid vessels should be ausculated for bruits; carotid massage is rarely so essential that it need be done if bruits are heard. The right carotid sinus should be massaged first, for no more than 10 seconds. If this is ineffective, the left carotid should be massaged as well. **The left and right carotids should never be massaged simultaneously.** A simultaneous Valsalva maneuver (expiration against a closed glottis) or Müller's maneuver (sudden inspiration against a closed glottis) may further augment vagal tone. Pressure on the eyes, traction of the tongue, or testicular pressure are rarely effective and may be harmful. Adjuncts to carotid sinus massage may be found in sec. **IX.E.2.b.**

4. An **esophageal lead** may be necessary to identify atrial activity. If an esophageal lead is not available, one can be made by passing a pacemaker wire through a nasogastric tube. The electrode tip of the pacemaker wire should not be extended beyond the terminal part of the tube when it is passed into the esophagus. The nasogastric tube should be passed to approximately 50 cm and the proximal end of the pacing wire attached to an exploring (V lead) electrode. The pacemaker wire should then be extruded from the distal end of the nasogastric tube and a search made for electrical activity. Identification of atrial activity is much easier if multiple leads can be monitored simultaneously. P wave activity is generally of short duration and has a more rapid intrinsicoid deflection than does QRS activity. The lead should be withdrawn at 1-cm intervals, until the P wave and QRS morphologies are determined. On occasion, asking the patient to hold a midinspiration breath is important to reduce respiratory motion.

5. An **intraatrial** electrogram can be obtained if other methods are inadequate. This procedure should be done under sterile conditions with a well-grounded ECG machine or special amplifier.

Table 6-5. Drugs used for treatment of bradydysrhythmias

Agent	Treatment
Atropine	IV: 0.5–1.0 mg SQ: 0.5–1.0 mg
Isoproterenol	IV: 1–2 mg in 250–500 ml and titrate, generally 1–2 µg/min (maximum 10 µg/min) SQ: 0.2 mg q3h
Epinephrine	IV: 3 ml of 1 : 1000 in 300 ml and titrate SQ: 0.2–0.3 ml of 1 : 1000 q1–2h IM: 0.5–1.0 ml of 1 : 500 in oil q6–12h

E. Once the diagnosis has been established, additional therapy should be directed at **correction of underlying abnormalities** (e.g., hypoxia, acid-base or electrolyte imbalance, CHF, hypotension, anxiety). This alone may terminate the dysrhythmia and may be necessary if other therapeutic modalities are to be effective.

IX. Specific dysrhythmias

A. Sinus tachycardia is a physiologic response to physical or emotional stress.

    1. Electrocardiographic recognition. The rate is 100–160 beats/minute with minimal cyclical variation. In response to carotid sinus massage, the rate slows transiently, then returns to its previous level. In severe hypermetabolic states, in which heart rates may be greater than 160 beats/minute, there may be no response to carotid sinus massage.

    2. Therapy. Treatment of the tachycardia itself is rarely required, since it is frequently necessary to maintain cardiac output. Primary therapy is correction of the underlying abnormality. When antidysrhythmic therapy is necessary, propranolol, 10–40 mg PO q6h, or 1-mg IV aliquots (repeated q5–10 minutes, with a total IV dose not to exceed 0.15 mg/kg acutely), is generally effective. Digitalis is not useful unless CHF is present.

B. Sinus bradycardia is not in itself pathologic. Asymptomatic heart rates below 60 beats/minute (often in the range of 45–50 beats/minute) occur due to enhanced vagal tone and are frequently seen in normal persons, particularly the elderly, and usually require no therapy. If the sinus bradycardia is inappropriate for the clinical situation (e.g., hypotension, fever), or, if symptoms are present, the diagnosis of sick sinus syndrome (see sec. **XI**) should be considered. Sinus bradycardia may also be due to increased intracranial pressure.

    1. Electrocardiographic recognition. The sinus rate must be less than 60 beats/minute but is rarely less than 40 and may demonstrate marked sinus dysrhythmia. Patients with heart rates less than 40 beats/minute usually manifest angina, CHF, or CNS dysfunction.

    2. Therapy

        a. Asymptomatic patients require no treatment.

        b. Sinus bradycardia associated with hemodynamic compromise can be treated with atropine (0.5–1.0 mg IV), isoproterenol (1–10 µg/minute), or ventricular pacing. Sinus bradycardia occurring in the setting of acute myocardial infarction and in sick sinus syndrome is discussed in Chap. 4 and in sec. **XI** of this chapter respectively.

C. Atrial premature depolarizations (APDs) alone do not necessarily imply severe underlying cardiac disease. They are also seen in patients with drug intoxication, disturbances in acid-base or electrolyte balance, and compromised respiratory function.

1. **Electrocardiographic recognition.** APDs are preceded by a P wave, which may have an abnormal configuration, and are followed by a normal QRS complex. On occasion, QRS aberration may occur, most commonly with a right bundle branch block configuration. Atrial premature depolarizations usually reset the sinus node, resulting in an ectopic P–sinus P wave interval similar to the sinus P–P interval.

2. **Therapy.** APDs are usually benign and require therapy only if they are symptomatic or trigger sustained supraventricular tachydysrhythmias. Initial therapy should be avoidance of caffeine, nicotine, and alcohol and relief of anxiety. Quinidine sulfate, 200–400 mg q6h, procainamide, 250–1000 mg q4h, or propranolol, 10–40 mg q6h, is generally effective oral therapy.

D. **Ventricular premature depolarizations (VPDs)** can be associated with any myocardial pathology as well as electrolyte imbalance, hypoxia, acid-base imbalance, endocrine disorders such as thyroxtoxicosis, and a variety of drug-induced conditions, most commonly digitalis toxicity. They may also occur in patients without demonstrable organic heart disease.

1. **Electrocardiographic recognition.** VPDs generally have an abnormal QRS configuration, although in the setting of a preexisting intraventricular conduction defect or with fusion, the QRS duration may be normal.

2. **Indications for treatment**

   a. In the absence of serious underlying heart disease, specific treatment is not indicated unless the patient is symptomatic or shows evidence of repetitive dysrhythmias (couplets or VT). Frequently, these VPDs may be successfully treated with sedation or by avoidance of alcohol, caffeine, and nicotine.

   b. When VPDs are a manifestation of **underlying heart disease,** they are potentially more dangerous and should be treated if frequent ($>5/$ minute), multiform, repetitive (couplets or VT), or fall on the ascending limb of the T wave. However, documentation that treatment reduces morbidity or mortality is sparse at best.

3. **Therapy.** The **emergency treatment** of VPDs with IV antidysrhythmic agents is covered in **J.** When oral therapy is indicated, **quinidine sulfate,** 200–400 mg q4–6h, **procainamide,** 500–1000 mg q4h, or **disopyramide,** 100–300 mg q6–8h, is frequently effective. These agents require monitoring of the Q–Tc interval to prevent marked prolongation and potential exacerbation of ventricular ectopy. Propranolol, 10–40 mg q6h, may be beneficial, especially in catecholamine-related dysrhythmias. Phenytoin, 300 mg daily, is occasionally beneficial. As always, underlying abnormalities must be corrected (e.g., CHF, digitalis intoxication, hypokalemia).

E. **Paroxysmal supraventricular tachycardia** (PSVT) is most often due to reentry, generally within the AV node or a concealed bypass tract, although sinus node reentry, intraatrial reentry, and PSVT due to enhanced automaticity can also occur (M. E. Josephson and S. F. Seides, *Clinical Cardiac Electrophysiology: Techniques and Interpretations.* Philadelphia: Lea & Febiger, 1979, Pp. 147–190).

1. **Electrocardiographic recognition.** The rate of these dysrhythmias ranges from 150–250 beats/minute. The QRS complex is generally normal, but aberration may occur (Table 6-6).

   a. PSVT due to **AV nodal reentry** is the most common form of PSVT, accounting for approximately 60% of cases. The reentrant circuit is localized to the AV node and is due to longitudinal dissociation of the AV node into

Table 6-6. Electrocardiographic diagnosis of PSVT:
value of P wave position during PSVT

Type	ECG manifestations
AV node reentry	Retrograde P wave most frequently buried in QRS or with short R–P (R–P <50% R–R interval)
AV reentry utilizing a concealed bypass tract	Eccentric retrograde P wave with short R–P (R–P <50% R–R interval) and negative P wave lead I
Intraatrial reentry	Positive P wave in leads II, III, aVF (R–P >50% R–R interval), with P–R related to PSVT rate
Sinus node reentry	P-wave morphology identical to sinus rhythm (R–P >50% R–R interval) with P–R related to PSVT rate
Automatic atrial tachycardia	Positive or negative P wave in leads II, III, aVF (R–P >50% R–R interval) with P–R related to PSVT rate

two functionally distinct pathways. During PSVT, antegrade conduction occurs over one pathway and retrograde conduction over the other, resulting in nearly simultaneous ventricular and atrial activation respectively. As a result, **retrograde P waves are generally buried within the QRS complex or are visible at the end of the QRS complex.**

  b. PSVT due to a **concealed bypass tract** (CBT) is the second most common form. The antegrade limb of this macroreentrant circuit is the normal AV pathway, and the retrograde limb is an accessory AV bypass tract. During PSVT, **retrograde P waves are seen immediately following the QRS complex.** Since most reported CBTs are **left sided,** a negative P wave in lead I during PSVT strongly suggests a CBT. PSVT cannot continue in the presence of AV block.

  c. **Sinus node reentry** accounts for only 4% of PSVT cases. The reentrant circuit is localized to the sinus node, and, during PSVT, **P-wave morphology is identical to that during normal sinus rhythm.** The AV node is not part of the reentrant circuit, and the P–R interval or presence of AV block is dependent on the intrinsic properties of the AV node.

  d. **Intraatrial reentry** accounts for 5% of PSVT cases. The reentrant circuit is localized to the atria, and during PSVT, **P-wave morphology generally reflects an antegrade activation sequence.** The AV node is not part of the reentrant circuit.

  e. PSVT due to **enhanced automaticity** accounts for 5% of PSVT cases. During PSVT, **P-wave morphology is similar to that seen with intraatrial reentry.** The AV node is not part of the reentrant circuit, and the presence of AV block is dependent on the intrinsic properties of the AV node.

2. **Therapy**

  a. If the patient is **hemodynamically unstable** or is experiencing **angina,** prompt termination with electrical cardioversion is indicated.

  b. **Vagal stimulation** may terminate PSVT by increasing parasympathetic tone while inhibiting sympathetic outflow. Vagal stimulation is **particularly useful for reentrant PSVTs that utilize either the sinus or AV node as part or all of the reentrant circuit.** In addition to carotid sinus massage (see sec. **VIII.D.3**), vagal stimulation may be augmented by the following:

(1) **Edrophonium** should first be given as a 1-mg test dose, then as a 10-mg IV push over 30 seconds. Carotid sinus massage should be repeated. Edrophonium should not be used in hypotensive patients.

(2) **Methoxamine, phenylephrine, or metaraminol** may be given IV over 2–3 minutes in a dose of 5–10 mg for methoxamine and 0.5–1.0 mg for the others. These agents reflexively augment vagal tone by increasing blood pressure. They should not be used in hypertensive patients.

(3) The **diving reflex** produces intense vagal stimulation. Ice water must cover the forehead, cheeks, and temples, since the reflex is mediated by the ophthalmic branch of the trigeminal nerve. Generally, 15–30 seconds of immersion is all that can be tolerated. The maneuver is uncomfortable, and careful monitoring is essential, since ventricular ectopy or prolonged asystole can occur. This maneuver should not be performed in older patients or in those with recent myocardial infarction, a history of repetitive ventricular dysrhythmias, or suspected conduction system disease.

c. **Verapamil** is the drug of choice for terminating **reentrant PSVTs that utilize the AV node as all or part of the reentrant circuit** (AV nodal PSVT and PSVT utilizing a CBT) (see sec. **V** for dosage and precautions).

d. **Propranolol** is also effective in **terminating reentrant PSVTs involving the sinus node, AV node, or CBT.** Although the AV node is not critical to the initiation or maintenance of intraatrial reentrant PSVT or automatic PSVTs, propranolol slows the ventricular response rate during these dysrhythmias (see sec. **III** for dosage and precautions).

e. **Digoxin,** 0.5–0.75 mg IV or PO, is given initially, followed by aliquots of 0.25 mg q2h as needed. If oubain is employed, the usual dose is 0.2–0.3 mg IV, followed by 0.1 mg q30–60min for 2–4 doses. Carotid sinus massage should be carefully repeated after each dose of digoxin, since this drug increases carotid baroreceptor sensitivity. As with verapamil and propranolol, digoxin slows AV nodal conduction and is **effective in terminating AV nodal PSVT and PSVT utilizing a CBT.** Digoxin is likewise effective in slowing the ventricular response during other types of PSVT.

f. **Quinidine and procainamide** in conventional doses are helpful on occasion, especially in patients with CBT.

g. **Elective cardioversion** or **rapid atrial pacing** may be required if the preceding techniques prove unsuccessful.

h. **Prophylaxis against recurrence.** Digoxin or propranolol is generally effective in preventing recurrences of AV nodal or CBT reentrant PSVTs by altering AV nodal conduction. Type I agents are efficacious in intraatrial reentry by slowing atrial conduction and prolonging atrial refractoriness and, in some cases of CBT PSVT, by prolonging retrograde refractoriness of the accessory pathway. Sinus node reentry generally responds to propranolol, while automatic atrial tachycardias are generally resistant to therapy and have a variable response to available agents.

F. **Atrial fibrillation** may be either **chronic** (usually associated with organic heart disease due to coronary artery disease, mitral valve disease, or hypertension) or **paroxysmal,** which may be seen with preexcitation syndromes, pulmonary embolism, thyrotoxicosis, and, on occasion, without a demonstrable organic abnormality.

1. **Electrocardiographic recognition.** Discrete atrial activity is not present, and the ventricular response is usually an irregularly irregular rate between 160–200 beats/minute in the absence of digitalis. Carotid sinus massage slows the ventricular rate transiently but generally does not restore sinus rhythm.

a. Atrial fibrillation with a **regular ventricular response** should raise suspicion of **digitalis intoxication,** since it is indicative of a junctional pacemaker and AV dissociation.

b. A **slow ventricular response** in the untreated patient implies underlying AV node disease.

2. Therapy

a. **Emergent cardioversion** (see sec. **VI**) is necessary in patients with **hemodynamic compromise or angina.**

b. In **hemodynamically stable** patients, to slow the ventricular response, digitalis preparations (see sec. **E.2.e**) or propranolol (see sec. **III.E**) may be given IV or PO, or verapamil (see sec. **V.E**) may be given IV. In less emergent situations, the oral route is preferred. Propranolol may be useful even in the presence of CHF if a disease that inhibits ventricular filling is present (e.g., mitral stenosis, idiopathic hypertrophic subaortic stenosis). After initial therapy, a maintenance dosage of digitalis or propranolol should control the ventricular response between 70–90 beats/minute at rest. A combination of digitalis and propranolol is frequently beneficial.

Serum digoxin levels considered toxic in other circumstances may be necessary to control the ventricular response. Careful attention should be given to the serum potassium level when large doses of digitalis are used. An occasional patient who has difficulty because of the pulmonary effects of propranolol may respond to metroprolol (not approved by the FDA for this use at present) in a dosage of 50–100 mg PO q12h.

3. The decision to employ cardioversion selectively (see sec. **VI**) to convert atrial fibrillation to sinus rhythm should be made on the basis of (1) left atrial size (a left atrial size by echocardiogram >4.5 cm is generally not associated with long-term maintenance of sinus rhythm), (2) the duration of the dysrhythmia, and (3) the need to reestablish sinus rhythm.

Similarly, if **drug therapy** is desired, procainamide or quinidine is frequently effective in converting atrial fibrillation to sinus rhythm if the atrial fibrillation is of recent onset and atrial size is normal. **The ventricular response should be controlled prior to the administration of group I agents.** Intravenous procainamide is effective in up to 88% of patients with recent atrial fibrillation and normal left atrial size by echocardiogram. Conversion with quinidine rarely requires dosages greater than 200 mg PO q4–6h; however, a rapid pharmacologic conversion of atrial fibrillation may be attempted with quinidine, 300–400 mg PO q6h for 72 hours. The ECG should be monitored continuously for evidence of quinidine toxicity. **After conversion,** oral quinidine, 300–400 mg q6h, or procainamide, 250–1000 mg q4h, may be helpful in maintaining sinus rhythm.

4. Indications for anticoagulation

a. **Elective cardioversion** (electrical or drug). Ideally, the patient should receive a 3-week course of oral anticoagulation **before** conversion and for 2–3 weeks **after** conversion.

b. Patients undergoing **emergent cardioversion,** especially those with a history of embolism or evidence of mitral valve disease, should receive heparin therapy prior to cardioversion and continued anticoagulant therapy for 2–3 weeks thereafter unless there is a contraindication.

G. Atrial flutter. The spectrum of disease states associated with atrial flutter is similar to that associated with atrial fibrillation.

1. Electrocardiographic recognition. The rhythm is characterized by a generally constant atrial rate of 240–350 beats/minute. However, in certain patients, especially in those with large atria or those receiving group I antidysrhythmic agents, the atrial rate may be lower. The ventricular rate varies with the degree of AV block, which is usually 2 : 1 in untreated patients. Although 1 : 1 conduction is rare, it can occur, especially in patients with preexcitation syndromes or those receiving a group I antidysrhythmic agent in the absence of digitalis preparations. Atrial flutter with 1 : 1 conduction may be difficult to differentiate from VT because of aberrant conduction. **Vagotonic maneuvers** usually cause a reduction in the ventricular response because of an increase in the degree of AV block, and they reveal the characteristic flutter waves. This response is often abrupt, with the ventricular response subsequently returning to the original rate. Characteristic **flutter waves** are best seen in leads II, III, aVF, and V1.

2. **Therapy**

   a. If the patient is **hemodynamically compromised,** cardioversion should be performed promptly.

   b. If the patient is **hemodynamically stable,** initial therapy should be aimed at control of the ventricular response. Digitalis and/or propranolol are the drugs of choice if the ventricular response is rapid.

   c. If atrial flutter is **refractory to medical management,** cardioversion is the therapy of choice. In the vast majority of patients, **cardioversion** to sinus rhythm succeeds at low energies (50 joules or less), and atrial flutter may be converted to the more easily managed atrial fibrillation with even lower discharges (5–10 joules). If cardioversion is contraindicated because of underlying disease or prior drug therapy, or if the atrial flutter is recurrent and one wishes to try a variety of drug regimens, **rapid atrial stimulation may be useful.**

   d. Cardioversion may also be accomplished pharmacologically in patients with atrial flutter who are hemodynamically stable. **Intravenous procainamide** may be effective. On occasion, **oral** maintenance doses of quinidine or procainamide will be successful. **These agents should not be used until the ventricular response has been controlled.** Propranolol may be effective in converting atrial flutter to sinus rhythm if the ventricular response is lowered to 80 beats/minute. Otherwise, control of the ventricular response may be accomplished by increasing the degree of AV block with digitalis or propranolol. On occasion, atrial flutter will be converted to atrial fibrillation with this therapy. Intravenous verapamil is also useful in temporarily controlling the ventricular response.

H. **Multifocal atrial tachycardia** (MAT) usually occurs in patients with severe underlying chronic pulmonary disease or severe heart disease, often in the context of acute respiratory insufficiency. Exacerbating factors may include digitalis intoxication, theophylline administration, postoperative state, electrolyte or metabolic imbalance, pulmonary edema, septicemia, hypoxia, and hypercarbia.

1. **Electrocardiographic recognition.** Three or more different ectopic P-wave morphologies characterize MAT; frequently, there are varying P–R intervals with an atrial rate of 100–200 beats/minute. Nonconducted P waves and an isoelectric baseline are common. Chaotic atrial mechanism has the same morphologic characteristics and differs only in that the atrial rate is less than 100 beats/minute.

2. **Therapy should be directed at the underlying causes,** with particular attention to the patient's pulmonary status. **Digitalis is rarely beneficial** and may be harmful. Quinidine in maintenance dosages may be effective but should never be primary therapy until the underlying causes have been corrected. Propranolol may reduce the ventricular response but is usually contraindicated by the underlying cardiopulmonary disease.

I. Digitalis-induced dysrhythmias can take the form of essentially every known rhythm disturbance. These dysrhythmias generally reflect **enhanced automaticity** or **conduction block.** Common dysrhythmias include His escape rhythms; uniform or multiform VPDs, frequently in bigeminal or trigeminal patterns; VT; automatic atrial tachycardia with AV block; sinus arrest; and Mobitz type I AV block. There are no specific ECG features that distinguish digitalis dysrhythmias from dysrhythmias due to underlying heart disease. As a result, the diagnosis requires clinical suspicion and evidence of improvement following discontinuance of the digitalis preparation. (For specific therapy, see Chap. 5.)

J. Ventricular tachycardia may be either nonsustained or sustained. It is most commonly seen in the setting of ischemic heart disease (e.g., acute myocaridal infarction, ventricular aneurysm resulting from a myocardial infarction, variant angina). Ventricular tachycardia may also be seen in patients with prolonged Q–Tc intervals, mitral valve prolapse, metabolic disorders, drug toxicity, and occasionally in patients with no demonstrable heart disease.

   1. **Electrocardiographic recognition.** The rate is 170–220 beats/minute (accelerated idioventricular rhythms are discussed in Chap. 4), and the rhythm is generally regular. The QRS complex is greater than 0.12 seconds and is frequently of an unusual configuration. Atrioventricular dissociation is often present, and fusion beats can be seen. At times, it may be difficult to distinguish VT from SVT with aberrancy. **Additional ECG features useful in differentiating VT from SVT because they are more common in VT include the following:**

      a. The QRS width is ≥0.14 seconds.

      b. Left axis deviation is present.

      c. Atrioventricular dissociation is present.

      d. Monophasic or biphasic right bundle branch block QRS complexes are present, with left axis deviation and an R/S ratio of less than 1 in V6. This does not hold when left axis deviation is present during sinus rhythm.

   2. **Therapy.** Correction of CHF, hypoxemia, acidosis, hypokalemia, hypotension, and prolongation of the Q–Tc interval is mandatory.

      a. Acute therapy

         (1) If the patient is **without pulse,** defibrillate with 200 joules. If VT is not abolished, defibrillate with 360 joules. Lidocaine therapy (or other agents as appropriate) should be started concomitantly.

         (2) If the rate is rapid and is associated with marked **hypotension,** CHF, or angina, cardioversion may be done with a synchronized discharge of 50 joules, using higher settings as needed. Lidocaine therapy should be started concomitantly.

         (3) If VT is not accompanied by hemodynamic compromise, the following antidysrhythmic agents are generally effective in terminating an episode (but if the VT does not respond promptly, cardioversion should be performed):

            (a) Lidocaine should be given with an initial bolus of 100 mg IV (or 1.0 mg/kg), followed in 5 minutes by a second bolus of 0.5 mg/kg. Concurrent with bolus therapy, a maintenance infusion of 1–4 mg/minute should be started. (See sec. **II.A** for further information.)

            (b) Procainamide, 100 mg IV q5min or a 50 mg/minute IV infusion, up to 1 gm for both, is the second drug of choice. After loading, a constant infusion of 2–6 mg/minute should be given. Blood pressure monitoring is imperative. (See sec. **I.C.** for further information.)

(c) **Bretylium** may be of benefit when the rhythm is refractory to the preceding measures. An initial dose of 5–10 mg/kg should be given in a 1 : 4 dilution with 5% D/W by infusion over 8–10 minutes. (See sec. **IV** for further information.)

(4) In refractory cases, pacemaker therapy utilizing either underdrive or overdrive pacing modalities may be useful in terminating VT (see sec. **VII.C.5**).

b. **Chronic therapy**

(1) **Group I agents,** especially procainamide, are the most efficacious in preventing recurrences of sustained VT. Although these agents have similar electrophysiologic properties, **they are not necessarily interchangeable.** Recently, **programmed ventricular stimulation** has proved to be a reliable and safe method for studying patients with recurrent VT and objectively assessing drug efficacy. The results of these studies indicate that **high doses** of group I agents are frequently required to prevent VT recurrence. Administration of these agents should be done cautiously and under continuous ECG monitoring. (For further information on dosage and precautions, see sec. **I**.)

(2) Phenytoin is generally ineffective in preventing recurrent VT.

(3) Propranolol is likewise generally ineffective except in documented catecholamine-induced VT.

(4) In some patients with medically refractory VT not associated with immediate hemodynamic collapse, underdrive ventricular pacing is effective in terminating recurrent episodes.

(5) Recently, several new surgical approaches have been shown to be effective in treating patients with ventricular aneurysms and medically refractory VT.

3. **Torsade de pointes.** Patients with **group I–induced Q–Tc prolongation** may manifest an unusual type of recurrent VT with a corkscrew appearance (*torsade de pointes*). This type of VT is generally refractory to therapy unless the offending agent is discontinued. In many instances, active measures are required to shorten the Q–T interval while the group I drug is being withdrawn. Group II agents, sinus overdrive pacing, and isoproterenol are generally effective in shortening the Q–T interval.

K. **Ventricular fibrillation.** See Cardiac Arrest in Chap. 23.

X. **Stokes-Adams attacks.** These attacks result from transient acute cerebral ischemia that follows a sudden decrease in cardiac output due to a change in cardiac rate or rhythm. These attacks may occur during episodes of VT, VF, complete heart block with inadequate ventricular response, or prolonged asystole. Symptoms of impaired consciousness begin 3–10 seconds after transient circulatory arrest. The attacks often begin suddenly, seldom last longer than 1–2 minutes, and are not generally followed by neurologic sequelae or postictal confusion. Acute myocardial infarction or a cerebrovascular accident may be the cause or the result of such an attack. When observed, the patient suddenly becomes pale and collapses and, on regaining consciousness, often has a flushed facies. Stokes-Adams attacks may be seen with sick sinus syndrome (see sec. **XI**), carotid sinus hypersensitivity (see sec. **XIII**), and the subclavian steal syndrome. Holter monitoring may document the cause of these attacks. If the attacks are due to tachydysrhythmias, antidysrhythmic drugs should be given. If they are due to bradydysrhythmias, most commonly complete heart block, a pacemaker is indicated. Frequently, both approaches are necessary.

The **emergency treatment** of Stokes-Adams attacks due to complete heart block with slow ventricular response may include (1) a precordial thump at the midsternal level, which may initiate cardiac activity, and (2) isoproterenol or epinephrine. Isoproterenol is the drug of choice because it has a substantial chronotropic effect, is less likely to provoke ventricular dysrhythmias, and will not cause excessive blood pressure elevation.

XI. Sick sinus syndrome (SSS). This term encompasses a spectrum of disorders of impulse initiation and conduction that may include marked sinus bradycardia, sinus arrest, sinoatrial block, AV node dysfunction, and recurrent supraventricular tachydysrhythmias. It is associated with ischemic, rheumatic, hypertensive, or idiopathic heart disease. It should be distinguished from sinus bradycardia due to increased vagal tone, which is commonly recognized in older patients at rest and in physically well-conditioned individuals. In the early stages of SSS, no symptoms are apparent. Manifestations may include atrial fibrillation with a slow ventricular response, an inappropriately slow heart rate, or prolonged sinus recovery following APDs or paroxysmal supraventricular dysrhythmias. Evidence of SSS can be elicited with provocative tests such as (1) failure of appropriate acceleration of the heart rate after atropine, 1–2 mg IV, or isoproterenol, 1–2 µg/min IV infusion; (2) a prolonged sinus node recovery time following overdrive atrial stimulation; or (3) an accentuated cardioinhibitory response to carotid sinus massage (see sec. **XIII**). However, in the absence of correlated symptoms, therapy is not necessary.

SSS is frequently symptomatic. Symptoms (fatigue, light-headedness, syncope, convulsions, angina, CHF, or pulmonary edema) occur either from long pauses caused by sinus node arrest, inappropriate bradydysrhythmias, or periods of AV block. In symptomatic patients, the diagnosis can often be made from a Holter monitor. In most circumstances, **pacemaker therapy should be utilized only when the dysrhythmias diagnosed by Holter monitoring correlate with the symptom complex of the patient** and cannot be adequately treated with antidysrhythmic agents. Pacing should generally not be done in patients in whom symptoms cannot be correlated with dysrhythmias. If a patient has SSS, symptoms will persist, and the diagnosis will be made subsequently. These patients do not have a markedly increased incidence of sudden death. **Digitalis** may exacerbate the syndrome when symptoms due to bradydysrhythmias predominate. However, it may be beneficial if it suppresses APDs or improves sinus node recovery times. **Quinidine and procainamide** may also be efficacious in suppressing APDs by enhancing AV conduction and because of their vagolytic effects.

In patients with the **tachycardia-bradycardia syndrome,** there is alternation of rapid and slow heart rates. Bursts of supraventricular dysrhythmias, most frequently atrial fibrillation, may alternate with long periods of sinus node or AV node dysfunction, or both. Therapy aimed at preventing or controlling the rapid atrial dysrhythmias may enhance the bradycardic aspects. In this circumstance, a pacemaker should be employed prior to therapy of the tachydysrhythmias.

The incidence of embolism is increased in patients with SSS, but it is unclear whether or not this increased incidence justifies anticoagulant therapy.

XII. Wolff-Parkinson-White (WPW) syndrome. WPW syndrome is the most common of the preexcitation syndromes and is usually seen in young, otherwise healthy persons. During sinus rhythm, ventricular pre-excitation via an accessory bypass tract results in a **short P–R interval** (≤110 milliseconds) and a wide QRS complex due to slurring at the onset of the complex by a **delta wave.** These patterns may mimic ventricular hypertrophy, bundle branch block, or acute myocardial infarction. Patients with this syndrome are susceptible to two types of supraventricular dysrhythmias: (1) AV reentrant SVT with antegrade conduction over the normal AV pathway and retrograde conduction over the accessory pathway and (2) atrial fibrillation with a rapid ventricular response resulting from antegrade conduction over the bypass tract. The latter pattern may mimic VT because of the aberrantly conducted, bizarre QRS pattern. Although WPW syndrome is usually benign, **sudden death** may occur in patients with atrial fibrillation and antegrade conduction over the bypass tract.

In the case of reentrant SVT, therapy can be aimed at **altering antegrade conduction** in the AV node or **altering retrograde conduction** in the bypass tract. **Digoxin, propranolol,** and **verapamil are AV nodal depressants** and generally are the most effective agents. **Quinidine, disopyramide, procainamide,** and **lidocaine prolong refractoriness in the accessory pathway** and may control the dysrhythmia. In patients with WPW and **atrial fibrillation, digitalis, verapamil,** and **propranolol,** by preferentially blocking AV nodal conduction, **may favor impulse conduction over the abnormal pathway and enhance the ventricular response.** In this situation, these drugs are **contraindicated.** If a sustained tachydysrhythmia is refractory to antidysrhythmic drugs or the patient is hemodynamically compromised, cardioversion should be employed. Medically refractory SVT may be successfully managed with underdrive or overdrive pacing modalities. Surgical interruption of the accessory pathway has also been accomplished successfully but is performed only in a few clinical centers.

XIII. Carotid sinus hypersensitivity. Elderly persons frequently have an exaggerated response to stimuli affecting the carotid sinuses, as do patients with sick sinus syndrome (see sec. **XI**). Marked bradycardia or prolonged episodes of asystole may be produced by carotid sinus pressure, either due to positioning of the head or during carotid sinus massage, and may produce light-headedness or syncope. Patients may also have symptoms as a result of hypotension occurring from the withdrawal of sympathetic tone without bradycardia. **Cardioinhibitory** (reducing heart rate) and **vasodepressor** (decreasing blood pressure) components of the carotid sinus reflex must be evaluated. The technique of carotid sinus massage (see sec. **VIII.D.3**) should be used with caution.

To evaluate the patient for vasodepressor carotid sinus hypersensitivity, atropine, 1 mg IV, should be given prior to carotid sinus massage to block the bradycardic response, and changes in blood pressure evaluated. A drop in pressure of more than 50 mm Hg is thought to be significant. Because of the high incidence of carotid sinus hypersensitivity in the elderly, it is crucial that the symptoms of a particular syncopal episode be duplicated by carotid sinus massage to establish the diagnosis firmly. Patients with infrequent and mild symptoms are often successfully managed by reassurance, precautions to avoid rapid neck movements, and avoidance of tight collars. In patients with frequent symptoms accompanying periods of severe bradycardia, permanent pacemaker therapy is generally effective.

XIV. Electrophysiologic studies. Intracardiac recordings and programmed atrial and ventricular stimulation have proved to be safe and reliable methods to diagnose complex dysrhythmias accurately, reproducibly provoke paroxysmal dysrhythmias, and assess therapeutic efficacy. At present, these studies are done in only a few clinical centers.

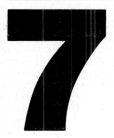

Hypertension

Hypertension, arbitrarily defined as blood pressure (BP) ≥140/90 mm Hg, affects about 20% of adult Americans. Of hypertensive persons, less than 10% have an identifiable cause of high BP (secondary hypertension) that may be amenable to operative intervention. The remaining 90% have essential (primary) hypertension, which requires long-term medical therapy. Hypertension is often detected during routine screening. Adults with a diastolic BP ≥90 mm Hg on the initial visit or outside screening should be rechecked within 3 months (within 1 month if >95 mm Hg). The diagnosis of hypertension is confirmed when the mean of diastolic measurements made on at least two "recheck" visits is ≥90 mm Hg (*Arch. Intern. Med.* 140:280, 1980).

In view of the high incidence of essential hypertension, excluding secondary causes in all hypertensive persons is currently impractical. **Initial evaluation** should include a thorough history and physical examination, emphasizing BP level, end-organ damage, and clues suggestive of secondary causes. Baseline **laboratory data** should be confined to urinalysis, blood glucose, potassium (**prior** to diuretics), creatinine, hematocrit, and ECG. Serum cholesterol, triglycerides, uric acid, calcium, fasting glucose, and a chest radiograph are desirable but not essential. **More complex diagnostic tests** should be reserved for patients (1) in whom the preceding initial evaluation suggests a secondary, potentially correctable cause; (2) whose age at onset of high BP is <30 years or >60 years; (3) with severe hypertension (>180/120 mm Hg), particularly if end-organ damage is present; and (4) whose response to medical therapy is unsatisfactory. Additional tests should be done only if the results will influence patient management.

The value of assessing the level of plasma renin activity in essential hypertension is controversial. Currently, no drugs are available that act solely as renin antagonists. High renin levels may not be pathogenically related to the hypertensive state (*J. Clin. Invest.* 64:1270, 1979). The usefulness of saralasin (an angiotensin II analogue) for demonstrating that hypertension is angiotensin dependent is hampered by its agonist properties. Angiotensin-converting enzyme inhibitors (captopril and teprotide) may produce a hypotensive response by mechanisms other than blockade of angiotensin II formation (e.g., bradykinin potentiation and prostaglandin formation). Studies employing these agents to screen and identify patients with renovascular hypertension have been reported (*Ann. Intern. Med.* 91:153, 1979), but wider experience is needed to confirm their diagnostic utility.

I. **General therapeutic considerations.** Hypertension of all degrees is associated with increased morbidity and mortality. No "cutoff" exists between safe and unsafe BP levels; the correlation between BP and longevity is inverse, even into the "normal" range. Once begun, medical therapy for hypertension tends to be lifelong, and attempts to discontinue therapy generally result in return of hypertension.

A. **Diastolic hypertension.** Effective therapy reduces the incidence of stroke, heart failure, renal impairment, and perhaps myocardial infarction. The beneficial effects of therapy in patients with mild hypertension (diastolic BP 90–104 mm Hg) are reduced morbidity from certain cardiovascular events (*Am. J. Med.* 69:725, 1980) and reduced overall mortality (*J.A.M.A.* 242:2562, 2572, 1979).

All patients with diastolic BP ≥90 mm Hg should be considered for drug therapy (see sec. III). However, a short trial of nondrug modalities (e.g. attainment and maintenance of ideal body weight, reduction in salt intake, isotonic exercise) may be effective in mild hypertension. The following factors, however, should hasten the decision to add drug(s) to nondrug therapy: (1) failure of nondrug modalities to normalize blood pressure in 3–6 months; (2) elevated systolic BP (>165 mm Hg); (3) presence of target-organ damage; (4) family history of cardiovascular disease; (5) male sex; (6) elevated blood cholesterol; (7) cigarette smoking; and (8) diabetes.

B. Systolic hypertension, independent of diastolic BP, is an established risk factor for cerebrovascular disease and ischemic heart disease. However, no data demonstrate a beneficial effect of treatment of isolated systolic hypertension (BP >160/<90 mm Hg). Reduction of systolic BP to <160 mm Hg is a reasonable goal, but hypoperfusion of vital organs may limit efforts to normalize systolic BP.

Isolated systolic hypertension occurs primarily in the **elderly,** in whom drug therapy should be instituted cautiously, beginning at smaller-than-usual doses. Drugs causing orthostatic hypotension (guanethidine) and depression (reserpine) should be avoided in the elderly. Careful monitoring for side effects, drug interactions, and patient comprehension of the regimen is essential. Sphygmomanometric measurements may overestimate BP in persons with stiff, atherosclerotic vessels; absence of end-organ damage may be a clue to this state of "pseudohypertension" (*Arch. Intern. Med.* 140:1155, 1980).

C. Therapeutic goals

    1. General goals are to minimize the risks of hypertensive complications by maintaining the lowest BP compatible with patient safety and tolerance. Pressures <140/90 mm Hg are a reasonable goal, although a lower level is preferred in younger persons. A therapeutic benefit is gained even by partial reductions in BP.

    2. Specific goals include (1) patient education, well known to improve compliance; (2) sodium restriction to about 4 gm/day; (3) achievement and maintenance of ideal body weight; and (4) cessation of smoking to reduce further the complications of atherosclerosis and to promote general health.

D. Failure to achieve blood pressure reduction

    1. Poor patient compliance is most frequently responsible for failure to achieve adequate BP reduction. Compliance can be improved by adequate patient education, stressing the asymptomatic nature of the disease, the need for periodic remeasurement of BP, the requirement for long-term therapy, and the consequences of poor control. The physician is responsible for limiting diagnostic tests, involving the patient in the therapy, and tailoring and simplifying the regimen to minimize side effects, cost, and dose frequency.

    2. Ineffective drug therapy secondary to **inadequate daily dosage** or to the presence of an **interfering substance** (excess salt intake, sympathomimetics, vasopressor decongestants, oral contraceptives, appetite suppressants) must be identified and corrected.

II. Antihypertensive medications. See Table 7-1.

A. Diuretics

    1. Thiazide diuretics are a mainstay of antihypertensive therapy because they are inexpensive, often effective as a single agent taken once or twice daily, and rarely cause serious side effects. Even in patients whose BP is not normalized with diuretics alone, long-term thiazide therapy should be continued, since it limits the fluid retention associated with the use of other antihypertensive agents, thus potentiating their effect. **Hydrocholo-**

Table 7-1. Commonly used oral antihypertensive agents

Drug (step[a])	Initial dosage (mg)	Usual daily dosage range (mg)	Ortho-stasis	Effect on RBF and GFR	Fluid reten-tion	Cardiac output	Heart rate	Effect on plasma renin	Dose change in renal or hepatic insufficiency	Available tablet or capsule sizes (mg)
Chlorthalidone (1)	50 qd	50–100	Yes	-↓	No	-	-	↑	Stop (R)	50,100
Methyldopa (2)	250 tid[b]	750–2000	Yes	-RBF ↑GFR	Yes	-→	-→	→	↓ (R,H)	125,250,500
Clonidine (2)	0.1 bid	0.2–0.8	Rare	-	Yes	-→	-→	→	↓ (R)	0.1,0.2,0.3
Reserpine (2)	0.1 qhs	0.1–0.25	No	-→	Yes	→	→	→	↓ (R)	0.1,0.25
Propranolol (2)	10–20 qid[b]	80–480	No	-	Rare	→	→	→	↓ (R,H)	10,20,40,80
Metoprolol (2)	50 bid	100–450	No		No	→	→	→	↓ (R,H)	50,100
Nadolol (2)	40 qd	80–320	No	-↓	No	-[c]	→	→	↓ (R)	40,80,120,160
Prazosin (2)	1 tid	3–20	Yes	-	Yes	↑[c]	-	-	↓ (H)	1,2,5
Hydralazine (3)	10 qid[b]	40–200[d]	Yes	↑RBF -GFR	Yes	↑[c]	↑	↑	↓ (R)	10,25,50,100
Guanethidine (4)	10 qd	10–50	Yes	→	Yes	→	→	-↓	↓ (R)	10,25
Minoxidil (4)	2.5 bid	5–40	No	↑RBF -GFR	Yes	↑	↑	↑	↓ (H)	2.5,10
Captopril (4)	25 tid, (1h ac)	75–450	No	↑RBF -GFR	No	-[c]	-	↑	↓ (R)	25,50,100

RBF = renal blood flow; GFR = glomerular filtration rate; R = renal; H = hepatic; - ↑ = unchanged or increased; - ↓ = unchanged or decreased; ↑ = increased; - = no effect.

[a] Step number (see sec. III).

[b] May be effective in moderate hypertension with the total daily dose divided into a bid regimen.

[c] Cardiac output may rise in patients with underlying CHF.

[d] Larger doses have been used effectively, but they increase the frequency of "hydralazine lupus."

rothiazide (50 mg qd or bid) and **chlorothiazide** (500 mg bid) have been the oral diuretics most widely used in antihypertensive therapy. Thiazidelike diuretics with a longer duration of effect may be given once daily: **chlorthalidone,** 50–100 mg qd, and **metolazone,** 2.5–5.0 mg qd. Common **side effects** of chronic thiazide therapy are hyperglycemia in patients with glucose intolerance, hyperuricemia, and hypokalemia. Moderate salt restriction (6 gm NaCl/day) will help minimize the development of significant hypokalemia. Hyponatremia, probably multifactorial in origin, is uncommon but may be lethal. Potentially adverse effects on lipid metabolism and the relationship between thiazides and pancreatitis require further study. Hypercalcemia may develop as a result of reduced calcium excretion and perhaps a direct effect on bone, particularly in the presence of increased bone resorption (hyperparathyroidism) or vitamin D administration. Thiazides, by reducing the renal clearance of lithium, increase the risk of lithium toxicity. Thiazides are seldom effective diuretics at glomerular filtration rates (GFRs) below 25 ml/minute and should be replaced by more potent diuretics (see **2**) in those situations. The combination of thiazide or metolazone with furosemide often produces a diuresis beyond that achieved with either agent alone, even at GFRs <25 ml/minute.

Potassium (K$^+$) supplementation should be reserved for asymptomatic patients with serum K$^+$ levels below 3.0 mEq/liter or for patients with serum K$^+$ levels less than 3.5 mEq/liter if they have symptoms or additional risk factors (e.g., concurrent usage of cardiac glycosides). The concept that increased K$^+$ intake produces antihypertensive effects remains to be substantiated by adequate clinical studies.

2. More potent diuretics, such as **furosemide (Lasix),** have not been shown to be superior to thiazides in the long-term therapy of hypertension. Furosemide may be effective in some patients resistant to thiazides. Its duration of effect is 6 hours for an oral dose, 2 hours IV. It is the diuretic of choice in patients with GFRs below 25 ml/minute. **Ethacrynic acid (Edecrin)** and furosemide may cause hearing loss, particularly in persons with renal disease.

3. Potassium-sparing diuretics may be of benefit to some patients requiring a normal serum K$^+$ level, particularly if oral K$^+$ supplements are poorly tolerated. These agents may cause serious hyperkalemia in patients with GFRs <30 ml/minute, patients taking K$^+$ supplements, and those with impaired nonrenal K$^+$ homeostatic mechanisms (e.g., those with diabetes mellitus). Because these agents have weak diuretic action, they are usually inefficacious as single agents in the treatment of essential hypertension.

   a. **Spironolactone (Aldactone),** 25–50 mg PO qid, is a mineralocorticoid antagonist that is most useful in conditions associated with hyperaldosteronism. It does not produce hyperglycemia or hyperuricemia. Large doses (especially >400 mg daily) produce gynecomastia. Amenorrhea has been reported.

   b. **Triamterene (Dyrenium),** 100 mg PO bid, blocks Na$^+$-K$^+$ exchange in the distal tubule by a mechanism independent of aldosterone. Used without a diuretic, it may produce hyperkalemia and minimal BP reduction; such use is discouraged.

   c. **Amiloride (Midamor),** 5–10 mg PO qd, blocks Na$^+$-K$^+$ exchange in the distal nephron, independent of aldosterone. The drug is excreted unchanged in the urine, making it useful for patients with liver disease but contraindicating its use in renal insufficiency.

B. **Antiadrenergic agents.** Adrenergic neural activity is involved in the maintenance of elevated BP in hypertensive patients and thus, along with the thiazide diuretics, drugs that interfere with adrenergic activity have been the mainstays of antihypertensive therapy. These drugs differ from the adrenergic-blocking drugs discussed in **C**, since they do not exert a selective blockade of either the peripheral alpha-adrenergic or beta-adrenergic receptors. The main mechanisms believed to be operative in the hypotensive effect of these drugs include (1) suppression of CNS sympathetic outflow through central alpha-adrenergic stimulation (methyldopa, clonidine); (2) depletion of norepinephrine stores (reserpine); and (3) direct inhibition of norepinephrine release (guanethidine). Despite their generally similar overall mode of action, these drugs differ in their tendency to induce orthostatic hypotension. **Tricyclic antidepressants** interfere with the hypotensive action of these drugs.

1. **Methyldopa (Aldomet)** lowers BP without compromising GFR or renal blood flow and thus is useful in patients with renal insufficiency. However, because the drug and its metabolites are excreted by the kidneys, the dose should be carefully adjusted in renal failure. Methyldopa can cause sodium retention; therefore, concomitant diuretic administration is recommended.

   Side effects include sedation (often transient), depression (less frequent than with reserpine), and orthostatic hypotension. A positive direct Coombs' test result develops in 10–20% of methyldopa-treated patients, but hemolytic anemia develops in less than 1%. In such cases the results of an indirect Coombs' test may become positive and interfere with cross matching of blood. Occasional blood counts should be performed, and the drug should be discontinued if hemolytic anemia develops. Galactorrhea (due to prolactin release), diminished libido, and impotence can occur. Hepatic damage is usually limited to mildly elevated transaminase levels, but fatal hepatic necrosis occasionally occurs. If hepatic injury develops, the drug should be stopped and never readministered. It is contraindicated in persons with underlying liver disease.

2. **Clonidine (Catapres)** is a centrally acting alpha-2–adrenoceptor agonist. Receptor activation in the medullary vasomotor center results in diminished sympathetic vasoconstrictor outflow. (This receptor is pharmacologically alpha-2, but it is anatomically postsynaptic.) Activation of peripheral alpha-2 presynaptic receptors may contribute to the antihypertensive action of clonidine by reducing norepinephrine release. Vagal tone increases during activation of the central alpha receptors and contributes to bradycardia. Sympathetic inhibition reduces resting cardiac output; however, cardiac output increases normally with upright posturing and with exercise, thus avoiding orthostatic and exercise-induced hypotension. Sedation and dry mouth occur more frequently than with methyldopa at equipotent doses (0.6 mg clonidine = 1500 mg methyldopa). Dizziness (15% of patients) and impotence (4% of males) occur as frequently as in methyldopa-treated patients.

   With sudden cessation of daily doses >1.0 mg, a rebound or **withdrawal syndrome** may occur, consisting of headache, agitation, tremor, GI symptoms, and a return of BP to pretreatment levels (occasionally higher) within 24–72 hours. This syndrome has also been reported following abrupt cessation of propranolol and methyldopa. To minimize this potential complication, planned withdrawal of clonidine should be accomplished gradually over 1 week. Discontinuance of clonidine in a patient taking a beta-adrenergic blocker allows unopposed alpha receptors to respond to circulating catecholamines; vasoconstriction and hypertension may result. Treatment of the withdrawal syndrome consists of reinstitution of clonidine or administration of IV phentolamine, diazoxide, or nitroprusside.

3. **Reserpine,** when combined with a diuretic, is useful in treating hypertension. However, the drug commonly causes **depression,** especially in doses >0.25 mg/day and in the elderly. The depression may be severe and may persist for months despite discontinuance of the drug. It is contraindicated in patients with a history of depression and should be stopped promptly if de-

pressive symptoms develop. **Other side effects** include nasal congestion, sedation, peptic ulceration, diarrhea, abdominal cramps, bronchospasm, slowed atrioventricular conduction, dysrhythmias, and edema.

4. **Guanethidine** is useful when combined with a diuretic for the treatment of moderate to severe hypertension. It may be given once daily (half-life of tissue elimination is 5 days) and rarely causes depression or sedation. **Side effects** are common and include orthostatic hypotension (exacerbated by exercise and alcohol), diarrhea, sexual dysfunction (ejaculatory impairment, reduced libido, and impotence), muscle weakness, headaches, nasal stuffiness, and reduced GFR. It is contraindicated in pheochromocytoma, because it sensitizes effector cells to catecholamines.

C. **Adrenergic-blocking agents**

1. **Alpha-adrenergic–blocking agents**

a. **Phenoxybenzamine (Dibenzyline)** and **phentolamine (Regitine)** have little place in the treatment of hypertension, except that caused by pheochromocytoma. Postural hypotension and tachycardia are the major limiting side effects. Phenoxybenzamine (20–60 mg/day) is a long-acting oral agent, useful in the preoperative management of pheochromocytoma and in chronic therapy of an unresectable tumor. Phentolamine has a short duration of effect (4–6 hours) and is more useful when given IV (5-mg doses) in the perioperative management of pheochromocytoma. Both agents are nonspecific alpha-1 and alpha-2 antagonists; the alpha-2 inhibition allows increased norepinephrine release, which probably accounts for the occasional dysrhythmias and angina. An exaggerated hypotensive response may occur when tumors produce large amounts of epinephrine.

b. **Prazosin (Minipress)** is a potent and specific alpha-1 (postsynaptic) blocker, effecting vasodilatation of both arteries and veins. The relative lack of reflex tachycardia and renin release may be due to the absence of alpha-2 (presynaptic) antagonism (*N. Engl. J. Med.* 300:232, 1979; 302:1390, 1980).

The principal **side effects** of prazosin are postural dizziness and lightheadedness. A peculiar, rare (<1%), self-limited syncopal reaction may occur after the initial dose of prazosin. Therefore, it is recommended that the initial dose not exceed 1 mg and that it be given at bedtime or with the patient in a recumbent, relaxed position. Furthermore, subsequent dosage increases should be gradual, and additional antihypertensive agents should be added cautiously. Treatment of the syncopal reaction is supportive.

Prazosin can be used cautiously in combination wih diuretics and beta-adrenergic–blocking agents to obtain an enhanced antihypertensive effect.

2. **Beta-adrenergic–blocking agents** probably exert their antihypertensive effect through a variety of mechanisms, including suppression of renin release, direct suppression of myocardial function, and suppression of central adrenergic outflow. Some data suggest that these agents are the step 2 drugs (see sec. **III**) of choice in patients who can tolerate them. Selected young patients with high renin levels and tachycardia may benefit from beta-blockers as a step 1 drug (see sec. **III**). Several beta-blockers have been developed, each with certain characteristics that may be of advantage under specific circumstances (*N. Engl. J. Med.* 301:698, 1979; 305:500, 678, 1981). **Common to these agents** are the following: (1) negative inotropic effects, which may precipitate or exacerbate congestive heart failure; (2) delay in atrioventricular conduction, which may produce atrioventricular dissociation in patients with conduction system disease or taking digitalis; (3) augmentation of insulin-induced hypoglycemia and attenuation of symptoms

thereof, thus demanding cautious use in diabetic patients, particularly those on insulin; (4) a tendency to produce bronchospasm; (5) a potential for precipitating angina or myocardial infarction with abrupt cessation. These agents are not associated with postural hypotension, and fluid retention is rare. They should not be added to one another. Agents **a–e** lack intrinsic sympathomimetic activity, a property of uncertain clinical relevance.

a. **Propranolol (Inderal),** a nonselective beta blocker, may be effective on a bid basis in some patients (qid is standard). Paradoxical hypertension may occur in patients with volume-expansion. Depression, fatigue, insomnia, and dizziness occasionally occur. Up to 5% of males taking 120 mg/day or more may become impotent.

b. **Nadolol (Corgard),** like propranolol, is nonselective. It is excreted by the kidneys and has an effective duration of 24 hours. The dosage interval should be prolonged for patients with reduced GFR. Low lipid solubility may lessen brain penetration and CNS side effects.

c. **Metoprolol (Lopressor)** preferentially antagonizes beta-1 adrenoceptors but will block beta-2 receptors at dosages of >100 mg/day. It is best avoided in patients with bronchospasm. See **a** for other side effects.

d. **Atenolol (Tenormin),** 50–100 mg PO qd, has a slight cardioselectivity at low doses. It is effective on a once-daily schedule and requires renal excretion. Drug accumulation will occur at GFRs <35 ml/minute.

e. **Timolol (Blocadren),** 10–30 mg PO bid, is a nonselective beta blocker that is minimally protein bound and metabolized in the liver. Dosage should be reduced in the presence of hepatic or renal insufficiency.

f. **Pindolol (Visken),** 10–30 mg PO bid, reduces peripheral vascular resistance while maintaining resting cardiac output. Clearance is mainly hepatic. Insomnia is a common side effect.

D. Nonadrenergic vasodilating agents

1. **Hydralazine** is a potent vasodilator, acting directly on vascular smooth muscle. Given alone, its antihypertensive effect is limited by reflex adrenergic hyperactivity (resulting in increased heart rate, stroke volume, cardiac output, and myocardial oxygen demand) and by sodium retention. In combination with a diuretic and an antiadrenergic agent (especially a beta blocker), hydralazine is a very effective antihypertensive agent. It should generally be avoided in patients with coronary artery disease (especially if symptomatic), since the reflex increase in myocardial work may precipitate myocardial ischemia or infarction.

   Hydralazine therapy can result in a clinical rheumatic syndrome resembling systemic lupus erythematosus (including the presence of serum antinuclear antibodies). This **"hydralazine lupus"** is most common (10–20%) in patients on prolonged therapy (>6 months) and with dosages exceeding 400 mg/day; it is rare with a daily dosage of 200 mg or less. Therefore, it is recommended that the daily dosage should not exceed 400 mg (200 mg in patients who have slow hepatic acetylation of the drug) and that it be discontinued (or at least reduced) if clinical or immunologic evidence of the rheumatic syndrome develops (*Am. J. Med.* 71:876, 1981).

   Impotence is not a complication of hydralazine therapy. Renal blood flow is maintained, making it a suitable agent in the treatment of hypertension complicated by renal insufficiency.

2. **Minoxidil (Loniten)** is an extremely potent oral agent whose use should be limited to the treatment of severe or refractory hypertension. It is often effective when marked hypertension is associated with renal failure. Like hydralazine, it induces fluid retention and reflex adrenergic stimulation and should be used with a potent diuretic (e.g., furosemide) and a beta blocker.

Other major **side effects** include precipitation of angina, development of hypertrichosis (which may be reduced by vitamin E or depilatory agents), reversible T wave abnormalities, and pericardial effusion. Minoxidil is not associated with orthostatic hypotension, impotence, or a lupuslike syndrome (*Ann. Intern. Med.* 94:61, 1981).

E. Angiotensin II–blocking agents are useful in the diagnostic evaluation and therapy of refractory hypertension. **Captopril (Capoten)** is an orally effective inhibitor of angiotensin-converting enzyme (also called kininase II). It is indicated in the treatment of severe or refractory hypertension, with the best responses seen in patients with inappropriately high plasma renin activity. Administration should be preceded by discontinuance of diuretics and, if possible, other antihypertensive agents. If captopril alone produces an unsatisfactory response at 150 mg/day, a diuretic should be added. The dose can then be increased to a maximum of 450 mg/day, after which other agents may be added. A triphasic response (initial sudden fall in BP, followed by gradual rise to near baseline and gradual fall to the initial low level) may occur over a week; changes in dosage are safest after this interval. **Side effects** include rash (10%), pruritis (2%), taste impairment (7%), proteinuria (1.2%), and potentially fatal neutropenia (0.3%). Excretion is primarily by the kidneys, so the dosing interval should be prolonged in patients with reduced GFR (*Hypertension* 2:567, 1980).

III. Therapeutic regimen. Empirical therapy via the **stepped-care** program is an effective and rational approach to the management of patients with mild to moderate hypertension. It obviates the need for extensive diagnostic procedures. Patients treated on the stepped-care schedule showed a clear advantage over those treated by their usual source of care ("referred-care") in overall mortality in the Hypertension Detection and Follow-up Program (*J.A.M.A.* 242:2562, 1979).

Step 1. Begin therapy with a thiazide or thiazidelike diuretic.

Step 2. If the response to thiazide alone is not satisfactory, a second drug is added (see Table 7-1 for step 2 drugs), and its dosage is gradually increased until a therapeutic result is achieved, the maximum dose is reached, or side effects become bothersome and limiting.

Step 3. If the BP is not adequately controlled with the preceding measures, an additional drug (generally hydralazine) is added.

Step 4. If the first three steps fail, guanethidine may be added. Alternatively, it may be used in lieu of the step 2 drug in the regimen that failed. To avoid the potential side effects of guanethidine, one may choose to begin minoxidil or captopril when standard triple therapy has failed.

With the failure of a **three-drug regimen,** reevaluation of the patient's hypertension and drug therapy is prudent. This may involve searching for various pressor mechanisms by additional diagnostic procedures (e.g., intravenous pyelography, digital renovascular imaging, plasma renin profiling—after discontinuing antihypertensive therapy for 2 weeks). On the basis of the additional data, more specific drug therapy or other therapeutic interventions may be instituted. Obviously, throughout the entire course of the patient's therapy, the physician should be constantly alert for factors that might prevent otherwise effective therapy (poor patient compliance, excessive fluid retention, use of interfering drugs).

For more severe hypertension (diastolic BP >115 mm Hg), initial treatment with both a diuretic and a step 2 drug is indicated. If the plasma renin profile is known and the renin-angiotensin system is felt to be a causative factor in the patient's hypertension, initial therapy with a beta-adrenergic–blocking agent may be appropriate. For renovascular hypertension captopril is the drug of choice; addition of a diuretic may be required.

In patients with mild to moderate **postoperative hypertension** who cannot take oral medications, parenteral hydralazine or methyldopa is generally effective in

Table 7-2. Drug therapy in hypertensive emergencies

Hypertensive emergency	Drug(s) of choice*	Drugs to avoid
Hypertensive encephalopathy	Nitroprusside Diazoxide	Reserpine, methyldopa
Hypertension plus renal failure	Diazoxide or nitroprusside Hydralazine	Trimethaphan
Hypertension with heart failure	Nitroprusside Diazoxide	Hydralazine
Hypertension plus intracranial bleeding	Nitroprusside	Reserpine, methyldopa, diazoxide
Malignant hypertension	Nitroprusside or diazoxide Hydralazine	
Pheochromocytoma	Phentolamine or nitroprusside	All others
Dissecting aortic aneurysm	Trimethaphan Nitroprusside plus propranolol	Hydralazine, diazoxide

*Drugs for each emergency condition are listed in order of preference.

combination with appropriate analgesic therapy. More powerful antihypertensive drugs for parenteral use are discussed in sec. **IV.**

Behavior modification techniques (biofeedback, relaxation response, and meditation) have not been shown to have prolonged BP-lowering effects or to reduce morbidity or mortality.

IV. Hypertensive emergencies. In general, patients with diastolic BP >130 mm Hg and hypertensive encephalopathy, progressive renal failure, acute pulmonary edema, a cerebrovascular accident, papilledema, or multiple fresh retinal hemorrhages should be treated aggressively with a parenteral antihypertensive agent (Table 7-2). The diastolic BP should be lowered to approximately 100 mm Hg within 30–60 minutes. Prompt lowering of BP is a key determinant of survival in these patients. In patients with advanced renal insufficiency, renal function may deteriorate further after the initiation of therapy. However, a return to pretreatment levels and even improved renal function generally occurs with continued BP control.

Many patients with diastolic BP >130 mm Hg but without the acute complications that have been mentioned do not require parenteral therapy. Vigorous oral therapy, preferably in the hospital, may suffice.

The slow onset of the antihypertensive effect of parenteral reserpine (1–3 hours) and of methyldopa (3–5 hours), as well as the side effects of these drugs, limit their value in the treatment of hypertensive emergencies.

Drug therapy in hypertensive emergencies should almost always include the administration of IV **furosemide,** which will prevent the fluid retention that accompanies the use of the antihypertensive drugs discussed in **A–D.** The role of IV propranolol in these conditions has not been established.

A. Hydralazine (parenteral) may be tried (if there are no contraindications) in relatively mild cases. A hypotensive effect is usually apparent within 10–20 minutes after IM injection of 10–20 mg of hydralazine and is usually maximal within 1 hour. If no hypotensive effect is apparent after 30 minutes, the dose can be repeated. However, failure of this second dose should prompt a change to a more potent agent. If hydralazine produces a satisfactory fall in BP, the effective dose can be repeated q2–4h as necessary while vigorous oral therapy is initiated. Generally, the agents listed in **B–D** are preferred in the treatment of hypertensive emergencies.

B. **Sodium nitroprusside (Nipride),** a direct vasodilator, is virtually 100% effective in lowering BP. It must be administered by continuous, controlled IV infusion, with the dosage adjusted as necessary to achieve BP control. The dosage range is 0.5–10 μg/kg/minute, with an average of 3 μg/kg/minute. Continuous BP monitoring is crucial, since marked changes may occur with alterations in the infusion rate. After cessation of administration, BP rises to the preinfusion level within 10 minutes.

Nitroprusside is metabolized in red blood cells to cyanide, which is then metabolized to thiocyanate by the liver prior to renal excretion. These toxic metabolites can accumulate during prolonged infusions (>3 days) with excessive doses (>10 μg/kg/minute) or in patients with renal or hepatic insufficiency. Under such circumstances, plasma thiocyanate levels should be kept under 10 mg/dl. **Nitroprusside should be used with extreme caution** in patients with hepatic or renal insufficiency (*Ann. Intern. Med.* 91:752, 1979).

A change from nitroprusside therapy to oral antihypertensive therapy should be made cautiously, since cases of sudden hypotension have been noted with simultaneous methyldopa or subsequent clonidine therapy.

C. **Diazoxide (Hyperstat)** decreases peripheral resistance and increases cardiac output. After rapid (10 seconds) IV injection (5 mg/kg, up to 300 mg) the maximal hypotensive effect is achieved within 5 minutes and is followed by a slight rise to a stable level over the next 10–30 minutes. Although the hypotensive effect may last up to 12 hours, it often lasts for a considerably shorter time. The same dose (5 mg/kg) can be repeated as needed. Although excessive hypotension is uncommon, an initial dose of 1–2 mg/kg may be appropriate, particularly if the patient is already being treated with other antihypertensive agents.

Major **sodium retention** occurs with diazoxide therapy. The concomitant administration of diuretics (e.g., furosemide, 40–80 mg IV) is recommended. Diazoxide also causes hyperglycemia through a variety of mechanisms, including suppression of insulin secretion and catecholamine-mediated acceleration of glucose production. Hyperosmolar coma and diabetic ketoacidosis have been precipitated in diabetic patients. Electrocardiographic changes and myocardial infarction have been reported following diazoxide administration. Hyperuricemia and postural hypotension may occur if plasma and extracellular fluid volume depletion results from overzealous diuretic treatment. Extravasation of diazoxide (pH 11.6) causes severe local pain and cellulitis. Diazoxide **should not be used** in patients with intracranial bleeding, dissecting aortic aneurysms, or significant coronary artery disease.

Once a therapeutic response to diazoxide has been obtained, vigorous oral antihypertensive therapy should be instituted.

D. **Trimethaphan camsylate (Arfonad)** is a potent ganglionic blocking agent with a rapid onset and short duration of action. It is the drug of choice for the treatment of hypertension associated with **aortic dissection.** Since ganglionic blockade produces primarily a postural drop in BP, the patient should be treated in the sitting position. The contents of a 500-mg ampule are diluted in 500 ml 5% D/W (final concentration, 1 mg/ml), infused IV at an initial rate of 3–4 mg/minute, and adjusted according to the BP response. The hypotensive effect is virtually immediate, and the infusion rate must be constantly monitored to maintain the desired BP.

The side effects of ganglionic blockade are largely due to parasympathetic blockade. Vigorous oral therapy with other agents should be instituted after initial control with trimethaphan, so that the drug can be discontinued as soon as possible.

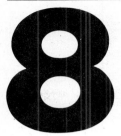

The major function of the respiratory system is to ensure an adequate exchange of oxygen and carbon dioxide. Under normal conditions, sufficient oxygen is transferred to saturate the circulating mass of hemoglobin fully, and an adequate amount of carbon dioxide is eliminated to maintain a normal arterial pH. **Respiratory failure** results when one or more components of the respiratory system fails to achieve either of these two end points of gas exchange (Table 8-1).

I. **Diagnosis.** The diagnosis of acute respiratory failure (ARF) often requires a high index of suspicion, because signs such as cyanosis, which are useful when clearly present, occur only when gas exchange is markedly impaired. The most sensitive clue may be the respiratory rate, which rarely is normal during ARF. The diagnosis of ARF, however, usually rests on an analysis of **arterial blood gases** (ABGs).

II. **Clinical setting. Acute respiratory failure** may occur in patients with a previously normal respiratory system or may be superimposed on preexisting abnormalities in alveolar gas exchange. Not only the **severity** of the alveolar gas exchange abnormality but also the **rapidity** with which it develops must be assessed. An acute rise in $PaCO_2$ to 45–50 mm Hg will drop the pH below its normal limit of 7.35, whereas a slow rise over days or weeks will produce less of an effect on pH because of compensatory bicarbonate retention. Therefore, an elevation of $PaCO_2$ indicates decreased alveolar ventilation, while a disturbance of pH indicates the **rapidity** and **severity** of the process.

Arterial oxygenation is inadequate when the hemoglobin saturation is less than 90% (PaO_2 <60 mm Hg), and most patients become symptomatic when the PaO_2 falls below 40–50 mm Hg. Thus, *acute respiratory failure* may be defined as a PaO_2 **less than 50 mm Hg or a $PaCO_2$ greater than 50 mm Hg with a pH less than 7.30 when the patient is breathing room air.**

III. **Pathophysiologic mechanisms.** Pulmonary exchange of carbon dioxide and oxygen depends on adequate alveolar ventilation and appropriate matching of ventilation to pulmonary blood flow. The types of respiratory failure may be sorted into two groups: failure to match pulmonary perfusion to alveolar ventilation (**oxygenation failure**) and failure of alveolar ventilation (**ventilation failure**).

A. **Oxygenation failure.** The transfer of oxygen from alveolar air to pulmonary capillary blood is affected by: (1) the partial pressure of oxygen in the alveolus (PaO_2), (2) diffusion of oxygen across the alveolar capillary membrane into the red cell, and (3) the matching of alveolar ventilation to capillary perfusion.

The PaO_2 can be estimated by using a simplified alveolar air equation.

$$P\bar{A}O_2 = (PB - PH_2O)(FIO_2) - \left(\frac{PaCO_2}{R}\right)$$

where PB is the barometric pressure (760 mm Hg at sea level), PH_2O the tension of water vapor (47 mm Hg), FIO_2 the fractional concentration of oxygen in inspired gas, and R the respiratory exchange ratio (usually assumed to be 0.8). Calculating $P\bar{A}O_2$ in this manner is useful primarily for assessing the factors

Table 8-1. Components of the respiratory system and common causes of malfunction

Components	Selected causes of malfunction
Central nervous system	Drug overdose, cerebrovascular accident, hypothyroidism, quadriplegia
Neuromuscular system	Guillain-Barré syndrome, myasthenia gravis, tetanus, quadriplegia
Chest wall and diaphragm	Trauma, kyphoscoliosis, upper abdominal or thoracic surgery
Airways	Laryngospasm, foreign body, asthma, chronic bronchitis
Pulmonary parenchyma	Adult respiratory distress syndrome, pneumonia, emphysema, pulmonary fibrosis
Heart and blood vessels	Pulmonary emboli, cardiac and noncardiac pulmonary edema

that affect the alveolar oxygen tension and therefore the PaO_2. Most commonly, the carbon dioxide tension changes because of changes in alveolar ventilation. However, hemodialysis may significantly decrease R, and the lowered PAO_2 may produce hypoxemia in patients with borderline oxygenation.

The difference between calculated PAO_2 and the measured PaO_2 ($P[A-a]O_2$) (normally $<10-15$ mm Hg) is also used to assess abnormalities in oxygen transfer. When hypercarbia is solely responsible for a decreased PaO_2, the $P(A-a)O_2$ remains normal. Any abnormality in diffusion or ventilation/perfusion matching, however, will widen this gradient.

Diffusion abnormalities probably do not contribute significantly to the hypoxemia of ARF, but ventilation/perfusion ($\dot{V}A/\dot{Q}$) mismatching is common. Low $\dot{V}A/\dot{Q}$ ratios seriously affect the lung's ability to oxygenate blood. When blood passes by lung units that are completely unventilated ($\dot{V}A/\dot{Q} = 0$), **intrapulmonary or right-to-left shunting** is present. The hypoxemia produced by $\dot{V}A/\dot{Q}$ mismatching generally is managed easily by supplemental oxygen, whereas the hypoxemia due to intrapulmonary shunting is relatively resistant and may require increases in airway pressure (see sec. **IV.B**).

B. The cardiopulmonary unit. A decreased mixed venous oxygen content in the presence of ventilation/perfusion inequality or shunt will lower the arterial oxygen content by an amount greater than expected from only the pulmonary abnormality. This is a result of the sigmoid shape of the hemoglobin dissociation curve. The causes of a decreased mixed venous oxygen content include (1) a decrease in the amount of hemoglobin, (2) a decreased hemoglobin saturation, (3) a rise in oxygen consumption not balanced by a rise in cardiac output, or (4) a decrease in cardiac output.

C. Hypoxia. The danger of hypoxemia (a reduced amount of oxygen in arterial blood) is that it will lead to decreased tissue oxygenation (hypoxia) and lactic acidosis. Oxygen delivery to the tissues depends on (1) an intact respiratory system to provide oxygen for hemoglobin saturation, (2) the concentration of hemoglobin for oxygen carrying capacity, (3) cardiac output, (4) an intact microvasculature, and (5) an oxyhemoglobin-unloading mechanism.

The oxyhemoglobin saturation curve relates the partial pressure of oxygen to the saturation of hemoglobin. The dissociation of oxygen from hemoglobin depends on pH, temperature, and 2,3-DPG concentration. The quantity of oxygen in the blood is proportional to the oxygen saturation and the amount of hemoglobin present. Significant points on the curve include the following:

PaO$_2$ (mm Hg)	SaO$_2$% at pH 7.4	Implications
100	97	Normal (young person)
80	95	Normal (older person)
60	90	Shoulder—beginning of steep portion
40	75	Cyanosis usually observed
27	50	Crisis
20	30	Brain death

Because a PaO$_2$ of 60 mm Hg usually ensures 90% saturation, little is usually gained by striving for a much higher PaO$_2$ especially if this requires exposing the patient to toxic concentrations of oxygen, progressive hypercapnea, or complications of positive end-expiratory pressure (PEEP). However, below a PaO$_2$ of 60 mm Hg, even small decreases in PaO$_2$ will cause large decrements in oxygen content.

D. Ventilation failure is present when the arterial PCO$_2$ is elevated and the pH is less than 7.35. The arterial carbon dioxide tension varies directly with the amount of carbon dioxide produced/unit time ($\dot{V}CO_2$) and inversely with the alveolar ventilation ($\dot{V}A$). The alveolar ventilation is the portion of total minute ventilation ($\dot{V}E$) (respiratory rate × tidal volume) that is evenly distributed to well-perfused alveoli. Ventilation in areas of the tracheobronchial tree that do not participate in gas exchange (anatomic dead space) or in areas of the pulmonary parenchyma that are relatively underperfused (alveolar dead space) is ineffective in eliminating carbon dioxide. Thus, alveolar ventilation is equal to the minute ventilation minus the dead space ventilation ($\dot{V}A = \dot{V}E - \dot{V}D$). Because PaCO$_2$ is proportional to the ratio of $\dot{V}CO_2/\dot{V}A$, PaCO$_2$ = K($\dot{V}CO_2$)/($\dot{V}E - \dot{V}D$), where K is a constant. Therefore, the tension of carbon dioxide may rise inappropriately (ventilation failure) if any of three conditions occur:

1. **A rise in carbon dioxide production not matched by a rise in alveolar ventilation.** Increases in carbon dioxide production are common in critically ill patients (fever, shivering, seizures, sepsis, parenteral alimentation with carbohydrate) but are important clinically only if unmatched by appropriate increases in minute ventilation.

2. **A decrease in total minute ventilation.** This may occur with depressed consciousness, respiratory muscle fatigue, or, rarely, intrinsic pulmonary disease.

3. **A rise in the amount of dead space not compensated by an increase in minute ventilation.** Increases in dead space occur when areas of the lung are ventilated but not perfused (e.g., pulmonary embolism) or when decreases in regional pulmonary perfusion are greater than those in ventilation (e.g., emphysema, pulmonary edema, shock). The lack of compensation is usually the result of respiratory muscle fatigue.

The consequences of ventilatory failure and the subsequent rise in PaCO$_2$ are respiratory acidosis, usually minimal hypoxemia (see **A**), and sometimes depressed ventilatory responsiveness to carbon dioxide. Whenever the PaCO$_2$ approaches 80 mm Hg in a patient breathing room air, death from acidosis and hypoxemia is imminent.

IV. Treatment. Treatment may be divided into measures directed toward correction of oxygenation failure and ventilation failure and measures appropriate to all types of acute respiratory failure.

A. Oxygen therapy. Administration of oxygen-enriched air increases arterial oxygen tension by increasing **alveolar** oxygen tension. The result is less pulmonary hypertension, less respiratory and myocardial work, and improved cellular oxygenation. Arterial blood gases are critical in evaluating and planning therapy, although clinical criteria (such as improvements in tachycardia and mental status) are also important.

1. **Patients with hypoxemia can be divided into three groups.**

   a. The first group consists of patients with mild to moderate mismatching of $\dot{V}_A/\dot{Q}$ and adequate ventilation as reflected by a normal or decreased $PaCO_2$. This is typical of pneumonia, pulmonary embolism, and moderate asthma. These patients are usually not difficult to oxygenate and may be given oxygen in any concentration necessary to achieve a satisfactory arterial PO_2 (usually 60–80 mm Hg) unless this means prolonged exposure to high concentrations of oxygen (see **3.c**).

   b. The second group consists of patients with marked $\dot{V}_A/\dot{Q}$ mismatching and right-to-left shunting but adequate ventilation (normal or low $PaCO_2$). This is typical of pulmonary edema or the adult respiratory distress syndrome (ARDS). Although these patients may initially respond to high concentrations of supplemental oxygen, they are difficult to oxygenate and often require other maneuvers to improve oxygen transfer (see **2.b**).

   c. The third group consists of patients with $\dot{V}_A/\dot{Q}$ mismatch associated with ventilation failure (elevated $PaCO_2$). This is commonly seen in patients with chronic lung disease (e.g., chronic obstructive lung disease [COPD], amyotrophic lateral sclerosis, the obesity-hypoventilation syndrome). Supplemental oxygen therapy may further elevate the $PaCO_2$ and decrease the pH, especially if respiratory acidosis is present initially. Mechanisms may include depression of hypoxic ventilatory drive or changing V_A/Q ratios in response to relief of hypoxic vasoconstriction. In most cases, the PaO_2 may be increased to acceptable levels (45–55 mm Hg) without catastrophic rises in $PaCO_2$ if oxygen is administered in controlled, low concentrations, e.g., by Ventimask with oxygen concentration of 24–28% or a nasal cannula at 1–2 liters/minute.

2. **Methods of administration.** Commonly used oxygen delivery systems provide a varying FIO_2, depending on (1) the balance between the patient's minute ventilation and inspiratory flow and (2) the gas flow of the delivery system. A high minute ventilation will result in an FIO_2 lower than expected.

   a. **Nasal cannulas** (prongs) are comfortable and effective in nontachypneic patients, including "mouth breathers." Oxygen flow rates of 1 and 2 liters/minute provide approximate oxygen concentrations of 24 and 28% respectively.

   b. **Face masks** can be used to provide a higher FIO_2 than nasal prongs. They should be replaced by nasal prongs during meals.

      (1) Light, comfortable **plastic masks** can provide 50–60% oxygen at a flow rate of 6 liters/minute.

      (2) The **Ventimask** delivers a controlled maximum oxygen concentration by entraining ambient air around a jet of oxygen. Concentrations available are 24, 28, 31, 35, 40, and 50%.

      (3) **Nonrebreathing reservoir masks** are equipped with an inflatable bag that stores 100% oxygen during expiration. On inspiration, oxygen is inhaled from the reservoir through a one-way valve. Inspired oxygen concentration may approach 90% if the mask can be properly and tightly fitted to the patient's face.

      (4) **Partial rebreathing reservoir masks,** which resemble nonrebreathing masks, permit expired air to be rebreathed. The degree of rebreathing is governed by the oxygen flow. Adequate oxygen flow (9–10 liters/minute) prevents carbon dioxide accumulation and allows the bag to deflate partially during inspiration. Inspired oxygen concentration varies from 60–80%.

c. **Face tents,** when used with a heated nebulizer, can provide heated, humidified, oxygen-enriched gas in less precise concentrations.

d. **T-tube systems** are useful for the patient breathing humidified oxygen spontaneously through an endotracheal or tracheostomy tube. The heated gas flows through the top of the T piece toward the atmosphere while the patient breathes through an endotracheal tube attached to the stem of the T. The rate of gas flow and the patient's inspiratory flow rate determine whether or not inspired gas is diluted with room air. Rebreathing of room air from the open end is reduced when the inspired gas flow is 2–3 times the patient's minute volume.

3. **Hazards.** Oxygen should be administered in a dose that provides maximal benefits with minimal risk.

   a. **Drying of secretions** may be attributed to inadequately humidified gas. Inspired gas should be humidified via bubble-jet or aerosol humidifiers.

   b. **Denitrogenation.** High concentrations of oxygen eliminate the nitrogen normally present in alveoli. This leads to instability of terminal respiratory units and promotes atelectasis.

   c. **Oxygen toxicity** is characterized by worsening oxygen transfer accompanied by diffuse pulmonary infiltrates. The occurrence of oxygen toxicity is related to the concentration of inspired oxygen and the duration of exposure. Individual susceptibility to toxicity is variable, but exposure to greater than 60% oxygen for longer than 48 hours poses a significant risk. The use of positive end-expiratory pressure (see **B.2**) usually eliminates the necessity for toxic concentrations of oxygen.

B. **Increases in airway pressure** are required when an increase in FIO_2 alone does not adequately treat oxygenation failure. Under such circumstances, the intrapulmonary $\dot{V}A/\dot{Q}$ abnormalities (especially shunts) are due to unstable terminal respiratory units that collapse at low airway pressures and decrease resting lung volume. By maintaining positive airway pressure throughout the respiratory cycle, airways remain open, resting lung volume increases, and $\dot{V}A/\dot{Q}$ matching improves. **Continuous positive airway pressure** (CPAP) may be administered through a tight-fitting face mask or an endotracheal tube.

   1. A tight-fitting **face mask** is useful when the underlying abnormality of pulmonary function is expected to be short lived. Administration of more than 10 cm H_2O of CPAP by this method is usually impractical. Complications include pressure necrosis about the face, pulmonary aspiration, gastric distention, and difficulties with eating, drinking, and expectorating. These hazards are significant but often can be avoided if the patient is alert and cooperative.

   2. **Endotracheal intubation** is necessary for the majority of patients who require CPAP. When administered during mechanical ventilation, CPAP is termed **positive end-expiratory pressure (PEEP).** The desired level of PEEP or CPAP is controversial. A conservative approach is to choose the least amount of PEEP that provides 90% saturation of blood at an FIO_2 less than 0.6. Restoration of lung compliance toward normal and maintenance of a mixed venous PO_2 ($P\bar{v}O_2$) greater than 30 mm Hg are helpful guides for balancing the effect of FIO_2 and PEEP on oxygen transport. Complications include depression of cardiac output and tension pneumothorax. The former can be partially offset by intravascular volume expansion, and the latter is uncommon when PEEP is less than 10 cm H_2O.

C. **Methods of improving alveolar ventilation**

   1. When failure to eliminate CO_2 is associated with mild acidosis (pH 7.30–7.35) and the patient is both alert and cooperative, temporizing measures such as intermittent positive pressure breathing (IPPB), deep breathing, and

airway care may prove beneficial. **Intermittent positive pressure breathing** may be useful when carbon dioxide retention is due to any of the neuromuscular diseases or chest wall deformities (e.g., amyotrophic lateral sclerosis, severe kyphoscoliosis). Intermittent positive pressure breathing is administered by tidal volume (10–12 ml/kg) with a pressure limit of 30–40 cm H_2O. Higher pressures may result in pneumothorax.

   2. More severe degrees of respiratory acidosis, especially with CNS depression, require **endotracheal intubation** and mechanical ventilation.

D. General measures

   1. Airway care. The maintenance of a patent, secretion-free airway is a critical element in the care of the patient with respiratory failure. The techniques that follow should be applied virtually to all patients in respiratory failure.

   a. Deep breathing and coughing. The patient should be taught to cough effectively following a deep breath, a short inspiratory hold, and firm contraction of the abdominal muscles.

   b. Postural drainage. The modified position, with the hips minimally elevated by pillows, will be well tolerated and provide enough elevation for gravity assistance to the mucociliary elevator.

   c. Percussion and vibration are adjuncts to postural drainage and should not be done more frequently than q4h to avoid tiring or injuring the patient. Postural drainage and coughing, however, must be done more often.

   d. Suctioning. Nasotracheal suctioning may aid the patient who is unable to raise secretions. The catheter should be of a type that minimizes mucosal trauma. Sterile technique is important, and suction should be applied for less time than one can comfortably hold one's own breath.

   e. Nasopharyngeal airway. A soft plastic airway is placed in the nasopharynx and ends above the larynx. It aids in suctioning and avoids the nasal trauma of repeated passes of the catheter.

   f. Hydration. Normal total body hydration is helpful in reducing sputum viscosity, but excessive hydration is to be avoided because it may add to cardiovascular stress.

   g. Humidification. Oxygen-enriched gases must pass through a humidification or nebulizer system.

E. Artificial airways. High-volume, low-pressure cuffs should be used to minimize the risk of tracheal necrosis.

   1. Indications. The most common uses of artificial airways are:

   a. Initiation and maintenance of mechanical ventilation or continuous positive airway pressure

   b. Facilitation of tracheal suctioning

   c. Prevention of aspiration

   d. Relief of upper airway obstruction

   2. Site of placement. Initially, either nasotracheal or orotracheal intubation is performed. Emergency bedside tracheostomy is not indicated unless the patient has an upper airway obstruction that cannot be cleared for placement of an endotracheal tube.

   a. Orotracheal placement is used for emergency intubation. Orotracheal tubes may be wider than nasotracheal tubes and therefore have a lower resistance and permit easier suctioning. However, they are harder to maintain and cause more discomfort to the patient.

  b. Nasotracheal placement is usually the choice for long-term ventilation management. They are easier to stabilize and more comfortable for the patient. The use of small-diameter (and thus high-resistance) tubes may lead to difficulty in weaning.

  c. Tracheostomy is indicated when prolonged artificial ventilation or airway care is necessary. This allows feeding of soft solids and increases patient comfort. The exact time to perform a tracheostomy is debatable, but, generally, endotracheal intubation should not exceed 2–3 weeks.

 3. Airway maintenance. See **D.1.**

 4. Cuff care

  a. Inflation. The use of high-volume, low-pressure cuffs allows for optimal sealing of the airway with the least pressure against the tracheal wall. The "minimal leak" technique allows a small (50–100 ml) amount of gas to escape from the airway during the peak of inspiration and minimizes tracheal ischemia. The cuff pressure should be monitored with a manometer and maintained below capillary filling pressure (<25 mm Hg).

  b. Deflation. Periodic deflation of the cuff is to be **discouraged,** since it does not lessen the chances of pressure necrosis and leaves the airway unprotected.

 5. Complications. See sec. **IX.**

F. Mechanical ventilation is a supportive tool that can improve alveolar ventilation, improve oxygenation, and reduce the work of breathing while other measures are applied to reverse underlying pathophysiologic processes. The decision to institute mechanical ventilation must take into account the reversibility of the process causing respiratory failure.

General guidelines for elective intubation and mechanical ventilation are provided in Table 8-2. Patients may require mechanical ventilation when the impairment in gas exchange is severe, the onset of ARF is rapid, or the response to treatment is inadequate. Therefore, the **trend** is as important as the "absolute" numbers provided in Table 8-2. The patient's overall condition, the underlying illness, and the function of other organ systems (e.g., cardiovascular) must also be considered. **Clinical judgment and individualization** for each patient is critical.

V. Guidelines for the initial management of acute respiratory failure

A. If intubation not required, then:

 1. Provide supplemental oxygen as appropriate (see sec. **IV.A**).

 2. Consider measures to improve carbon dioxide elimination if necessary (see sec. **IV.C**).

 3. Write orders for airway care (see sec. **IV.D**).

 4. Give bronchodilators, corticosteroids, and antibiotics as indicated (see Chap. 9).

 5. Seek and treat underlying and associated disease processes.

B. If intubation and mechanical ventilation are required, then:

 1. Clear the patient's airway and place an oral or nasopharyngeal airway.

 2. Provide adequate ventilation with a mask and a hand-operated resuscitation bag attached to a high-flow oxygen source.

 3. Introduce an orotracheal or nasotracheal cuffed tube, preferably >7.5 mm in internal diameter. Check cuff function prior to intubation.

 4. Inflate the cuff and ventilate with a resuscitation bag.

Table 8-2. Guidelines for elective intubation and mechanical ventilation in acute respiratory failure

Process	Usual indication	Useful parameters	Comment
Acute respiratory failure without underlying respiratory disease			
Neuromuscular illness, (e.g., Guillain-Barré syndrome, myasthenia gravis)	Imminent failure of bellows mechanism	Inspiratory force <25 cm H_2O; Vital capacity <15 ml/kg; Respiratory rate >40/min	Onset of abnormalities in gas exchange often sudden and **follows** signs of weakness
Central airway obstruction	Presence of inspiratory stridor		Emergency tracheotomy may be necessary
Lung parenchymal or airway disease (e.g., ARDS, pulmonary edema, pneumonia, asthma)	Progressive refractory hypoxemia; Progressive respiratory acidosis; Excessive work of breathing	PaO_2 <60 mm Hg, with FIO_2 ≥0.6; $PaCO_2$ >45, pH <7.3; Respiratory rate >40/min	Hypercarbia often a late manifestation
Stupor or coma (e.g., drug overdose)	Airway protection	Poor gag reflex, ineffective cough	Onset of apnea may be abrupt
Circulatory failure (e.g., myocardial infarction, cardiogenic shock)	Inadequate gas exchange; Increased O_2 consumption	As above (parenchymal lung disease)	Decreased work load for the **severely** failing or ischemic heart can be critical
Acute-on-chronic respiratory failure (e.g., acute exacerbations of COPD or chronic neuromuscular disease)	Impaired mental status; Refractory hypoxemia; Progressive respiratory acidosis	PaO_2 <35–40 mm Hg despite controlled O_2 therapy; pH <7.2–7.25; Respiratory rate >40/min	Implies hypoxia or CO_2 narcosis; O_2 therapy resulting in progressive respiratory acidosis is an indication for mechanical ventilation

5. Immediately auscultate the chest for proper tube placement, and order a chest radiograph for confirmation.

6. Stabilize the airway securely with tape.

7. Suction with sterile technique.

8. Order ventilator settings, as follows:

    a. FiO_2: 0.9–1.0

    b. Tidal volume: 10–15 ml/kg; rate 8–15/minute

    c. Mode: intermittent mandatory ventilation, control, or assist/control

9. Ensure proper function of alarms, humidifier, and pressure limit.

10. Institute airway care (see sec. **IV.D.1**).

11. Obtain ABGs in 10–20 minutes, and adjust the ventilator accordingly.

12. **Always remember:** If ventilator malfunction occurs, disconnect the patient from the ventilator and ventilate with a resuscitation bag and high-flow oxygen.

C. **After initiation of mechanical ventilation:**

1. Anticipate the need for PEEP if PaO_2 is <60 mm Hg with FiO_2 >0.5.

2. Restrict fluids in the presence of increased pulmonary capillary permeability, but maintain cardiac ouptut and urine output.

3. Use blood transfusions if volume expansion is indicated and if the hematocrit is <36.

4. Support plasma oncotic pressure if albumin is <2.0 gm/dl (e.g., with whole blood transfusion, hyperalimentation).

5. Give bronchodilators, corticosteroids, and antibiotics as indicated.

6. Consider the need for pulmonary artery catheterization if oxygenation failure is severe, or if hypotension or oliguria is present.

7. Treat underlying and associated disease processes.

VI. **Mechanical ventilation**

A. **Goals**

1. **Oxygenation.** Ensure a PaO_2 of at least 60 mm Hg (saturation of 90%) by adjustments in FiO_2 and PEEP.

2. **Ventilation.** Adjust minute ventilation and mode of ventilation, so that the $PaCO_2$ that is achieved results in a pH of 7.35–7.45.

3. Provide airway and cuff care (see **IV.D.1** and **IV.E.4**).

4. **Oxygen delivery.** Tissue oxygenation is paramount. Utilization of hemodynamic monitoring and transfusions may be necessary to maintain mixed venous PO_2 ($P\bar{v}O_2$) >30 mm Hg.

B. **Selection of ventilator.** Many types of ventilators are available. Minimal requirements include controls for providing variable oxygen concentrations, tidal volume, and respiratory rate, as well as alarms for pressure limits, exhaled volume, and disconnection.

C. **Modes of mechanical ventilation.**

1. **Controlled ventilation** (ventilator initiating every inspiration) is required if the patient is not breathing spontaneously. It may also be necessary when the ventilator is operating near its pressure limit (severe asthma) or when respiratory rates are rapid (>25/minute). Control may be accomplished by

sedation with modest doses of morphine, a barbiturate, or diazepam. Patients with noncompliant lungs are often tachypneic and restless despite sedation, and unless intermittent mandatory ventilation (see **3**) is used, the patient may have to be paralyzed. If necessary, this must be done under very strict supervision and monitoring. Pancuronium bromide, a nondepolarizing neuromuscular-blocking agent with hemodynamic advantages over curare, may be the safest paralyzing agent. The initial intravenous dose is 0.08 mg/kg body weight, followed by maintenance doses of 0.01–0.04 mg/kg IV as needed to maintain control of ventilation. The action of pancuronium can be reversed by the use of a neostigmine-atropine combination. Since paralysis can be a terrifying experience, the patient should also be sedated. The paralyzed patient must never be left unattended, because a disconnection in the ventilator circuit can be rapidly fatal.

2. **Assist/Control.** In this mode, every inspiratory effort of the patient triggers a fixed volume breath from the ventilator. The sensitivity should be set so that a 2–3 cm H_2O inspiratory effort will initiate a mechanical breath. A backup rate is also selected to ensure mechanical ventilation in case of apnea. Alkalosis and its subsequent complications may develop in the tachypneic patient. Moreover, the patient receives no graded exercise of the respiratory muscles and may eventually have difficulty in being weaned from the ventilator.

3. **Intermittent mandatory ventilation** (IMV) allows breathing at the patient's own rate and volume via an auxiliary gas flow through the ventilator circuit while the ventilator intermittently adds a breath of fixed volume at a preset rate.

   a. Intermittent mandatory ventilation is useful for the following reasons:

      (1) Patients contribute as much of the required alveolar ventilation as possible on their own, while the ventilator supplements minute ventilation. This usually prevents hypocarbia and alkalosis.

      (2) The deleterious hemodynamic effects of intermittent or continuous positive airway pressure are minimized.

      (3) Sedation, paralysis, or both are generally unnecessary.

      (4) The patient is compelled to do respiratory work, so that the respiratory muscles receive graded exercise training.

      (5) Ventilator support can be gradually removed as the patient improves.

   b. A disadvantage of IMV is that oxygen consumption may be greater than during controlled ventilation if the patient provides a significant portion of the minute ventilation. This increased work of breathing may have deleterious effects in certain clinical circumstances (e.g., shock, myocardial infarction with severe oxygenation failure).

   c. Most spontaneously breathing patients who require prolonged ventilatory management should be started immediately on IMV. An initial ventilator rate of 10–12 breaths/minute is usually sufficient to ensure appropriate alveolar ventilation. The ventilator rate is gradually reduced as clinical status and arterial blood gases improve.

   d. Not all IMV circuitry is the same, and these differences can have a major impact on how well IMV is tolerated. Older ventilators (MA-1, Emerson) were designed before IMV came into use. Consequently, special circuits are usually added to provide an auxiliary flow of gas during spontaneous breathing. The most common of these is "continuous-flow, closed circuit" IMV, in which a continuous flow of fresh gas is presented to the patient at the Y connector to the endotracheal tube. Its major advantage is that it minimizes respiratory work done by the patient during spontaneous breathing. On the other hand, the makeshift nature of the apparatus makes it susceptible to human error and ventilator failure.

Newer ventilators (MA-2, Siemens, Bear-1) have incorporated IMV circuitry into their manufacture. They use a demand valve in which a separate circuit is opened by the patient when a spontaneous breath lowers airway pressure by 1–2 cm H_2O. However, gas must still travel along several feet of tubing from the ventilator to the patient, and a significant pressure drop is thus possible, especially in tachypneic patients with high inspiratory flow rates. Since respiratory work is related to changes in airway pressure, respiratory work can therefore increase. This should be evident by a deflection greater than 2–3 cm H_2O in the negative direction on the ventilator's airway pressure manometer. A change to a different ventilator with continuous-flow IMV or a change in ventilator mode to assist-control should be considered in this setting.

4. **Additional considerations.** The peak airway pressure limit should be set approximately 10 cm H_2O above the pressure needed to deliver the tidal volume. Sighs are not necessary with the use of large tidal volumes and small amounts of PEEP. If used, sigh volume should be about 1.5 times the set tidal volume, and the frequency 6–10/hour.

D. **Initial ventilator orders.** When the patient has been intubated, the physician must select the FIO_2, $\dot{V}E$, PEEP, and mode of mechanical ventilation.

1. **FIO_2.** Hypoxemia and hypoxia are more dangerous than brief overoxygenation. An initial FIO_2 of 0.9–1.0 alleviates hypoxemia due to all but the lowest of $\dot{V}A/\dot{Q}$ ratios. After initial oxygenation, the FIO_2 may be changed to obtain a PaO_2 of approximately 60 mm Hg.

2. **Positive end-expiratory pressure** (see sec. **IV.B.2**). Many physicians use small amounts of PEEP (2–5 cm H_2O) immediately, because many causes of ARF are associated with decreased resting lung volume (functional residual capacity), and this level of PEEP is maintained until the time of extubation. Such practice is probably inappropriate when respiratory failure is the result of severe bronchospasm.

3. **$\dot{V}E$.** A minute ventilation of 100 ml/kg is an appropriate starting point. This can be accomplished at a respiratory rate of 8–15 breaths/minute, and a tidal volume of 10–15 ml/kg. Minute ventilation should be adjusted until a normal pH is achieved. Slower rates may be preferred in COPD, while faster rates may be useful when pulmonary compliance is diminished (e.g., in ARDS).

An important consideration in adjusting the tidal volume is "ventilator compliance," i.e., loss of the machine-delivered tidal volume to expand flexible tubing instead of the patient's lungs. An approximate value for this effect is 4 ml/cm H_2O of developed airway pressure. Thus, if tidal volume was set at 800 ml and peak airway pressure was 60 cm H_2O, 240 ml (or 30%) would be lost to ventilator compliance.

VII. **Monitoring during acute respiratory failure.** Although many variables may be measured to monitor the course of ARF, relatively few have proved to be of value in guiding patient management. In many cases, absolute values are less useful than changes or trends.

A. **Mechanical properties of the respiratory system**

1. Measurements of **respiratory rate, tidal volume,** and **vital capacity** provide useful data. In general, a respiratory rate >25/minute, a tidal volume of <5 ml/kg, and a vital capacity <1 liter indicates a need for continued mechanical ventilation. **Maximum inspiratory pressure** reflects the effectiveness of the "bellows." An inspiratory pressure of 25 cm H_2O usually can be expected to correlate with a vital capacity of 1 liter. However, this pressure-volume

relationship may not hold in patients with severe airway obstruction or hyperinflation.

2. Serial measurements of the **compliance** of the respiratory system are helpful in assessing clinical changes. **Lung compliance** is strictly defined as the change in lung volume divided by the change in pleural pressure measured near functional residual capacity under quasistatic, equilibrium conditions (no airflow). However, liberties are taken with this definition in the intubated and mechanically ventilated patient.

   a. **Static compliance** is assessed by plotting the relationship between the change in "static" airway pressure and tidal volume. Increasing tidal volumes (400–1000 ml) are delivered, and airway pressure is measured on the ventilator pressure gauge during a brief "inspiratory hold." The value for PEEP is subtracted from the pressure obtained during inspiratory hold. The ratio of tidal volume to the static pressure change gives information about the elastic properties of the respiratory system and will decrease as the lungs become less compliant, as seen in pulmonary edema or pneumonia (see **IV.B.2**).

   b. **Dynamic compliance** is measured similarly, except that the **peak** pressure reading (minus the PEEP) is used. Dynamic compliance is a function of both elastic and nonelastic (resistance) properties of the entire system. Increasing differences between static and dynamic measurements signify changes in airway resistance, commonly associated with bronchoconstriction or mucous plugging. Significant deterioration of oxygenation without a change in static or dynamic measurements suggests pulmonary vascular abnormalities (e.g., thromboembolism).

B. **Oxygenation.** Although the PaO_2 can be used to estimate hemoglobin saturation, it does not yield information about the efficiency of oxygen transfer or about the adequacy of tissue oxygenation. Calculation of the alveolar-arterial oxygen difference, the arterial-alveolar oxygen ratio, or the "venous admixture" may demonstrate the efficiency of oxygen transfer. The mixed venous oxygen tension ($P\bar{v}O_2$) and saturation ($S\bar{v}O_2$) demonstrate the adequacy of tissue oxygenation, but their measurement requires pulmonary artery catheterization.

1. The $P\bar{A}O_2$ is calculated by use of the alveolar air equation (see sec. **III.A**) or approximated by the "rule of sevens," i.e., $700 \times FIO_2 = P\bar{A}O_2$. The PaO_2 is obtained from ABGs. Since $PaO_2/P\bar{A}O_2$ remains relatively constant as FIO_2 is changed, it can be used to decrease FIO_2 to obtain a desired PaO_2.

$$\frac{700 \times \text{current } FIO_2}{\text{measured } PaO_2} = \frac{700 \times \text{new } FIO_2}{\text{desired } PaO_2}$$

2. Measurement of intrapulmonary **shunt** requires use of 100% oxygen to eliminate the contribution of $\dot{V}A/\dot{Q}$ abnormality, but this predisposes to absorption atelectasis. Therefore, it is recommended that the FIO_2 in use be used to calculate venous admixture ($\dot{Q}va/\dot{Q}t$) via the following equation:

$$\dot{Q}va/\dot{Q}t = (Cc'O_2 - CaO_2)/(Cc'O_2 - C\bar{v}O_2)$$

where $\dot{Q}va$ is venous admixture, $\dot{Q}t$ is total cardiac output, and $Cc'O_2$, CaO_2, and $C\bar{v}O_2$ are the content of oxygen in pulmonary capillary, arterial, and mixed venous blood respectively. Oxygen content in milliliters/deciliter is calculated by the formula

$$C\text{-}O_2 = (Hb \times 1.36)SO_2 + 0.003\ PO_2$$

where $C\text{-}O_2$, SO_2, and PO_2 are respectively content, saturation, and partial pressure of oxygen in the blood, and Hb is hemoglobin concentration.

The $Cc'O_2$ is calculated using the calculated alveolar oxygen tension as the PO_2 in end-capillary blood. The arterial oxygen content is obtained either by direct measurement or calculated using the measured arterial oxygen tension and saturation. The mixed venous oxygen content may be obtained by assuming it is 4.5 ml/dl less than the arterial content or by obtaining blood from a pulmonary artery catheter and either measuring the content or calculating it from the measured mixed venous oxygen tension and saturation.

The normal value for $\dot{Q}va/\dot{Q}t$ is less than 0.05. Values above 0.20 are usually associated with a need for mechanical ventilation and positive airway pressure. In addition, when venous admixture exceeds this level, decreases in $S\bar{v}O_2$ may have profound effects on arterial oxygenation (see sec. **III.C**).

3. **Adequacy of tissue oxygenation** is the primary goal of therapy. The amount of oxygen delivered to the tissues is the product of the cardiac output and the arterial oxygen content. Normally,

$$(5.0 \text{ l/min}) \times (200 \text{ ml O}_2/\text{liter of blood}) = 1.0 \text{ liter of delivered O}_2/\text{min}$$

The mixed venous oxygen tension ($P\bar{v}O_2$) and saturation ($S\bar{v}O_2$) obtained through a pulmonary artery catheter are good indicators of tissue oxygenation. Normal values of $P\bar{v}O_2$ range from 35–40 mm Hg. When $P\bar{v}O_2$ is below 30 mm Hg, tissue hypoxia and lactic acidosis are likely.

The measurement of $S\bar{v}O_2$ and $P\bar{v}O_2$ is especially useful in patients with severe impairment of oxygen transfer (e.g., ARDS) and in patients with compromised left ventricular function. The goal is to maintain aerobic tissue metabolism and thus a $P\bar{v}O_2$ of >30 mm Hg or a $S\bar{v}O_2$ of $>55\%$. The use of these criteria allows the clinician to select the lowest possible PEEP and FIO_2 while minimizing the risks of oxygen toxicity, barotrauma, and depressed cardiac output. Furthermore, judicious utilization of transfusions, preload regulation, and inotropic agents may improve cardiac output and support oxygen delivery.

C. **Ventilation.** The total minute ventilation is not the same as alveolar ventilation (see sec. **III.D**) and cannot be used to evaluate either the adequacy or efficiency of ventilation.

1. **Alveolar ventilation** is inversely proportional to $PaCO_2$. Maintenance of normal pH (7.35–7.45) is an accepted criterion for adequate ventilation.

2. **Efficiency of ventilation** can be judged by measuring the proportion of gas in each breath that does not participate in gas exchange, i.e., the ratio of **dead space** to **tidal volume** (VD/VT). However, since the minute ventilation required to maintain a normal $PaCO_2$ also reflects wasted ventilation, measurement of respiratory rate and total exhaled minute volume also reflects the relative efficiency of the gas exchange process.

D. **Noninvasive techniques for monitoring gas exchange**

1. The **ear oximeter** provides a quantitative assessment of arterial oxygen saturation. It is used primarily in the patient with mild oxygenation failure and adequate alveolar ventilation.

2. **Mass spectrometry** and **capnography** allow rapid analysis of carbon dioxide concentrations (and thus partial pressures) in expired gas. The end-tidal carbon dioxide ($PETCO_2$) is close to the value for arterial PCO_2 in patients with normal lungs. In patients with acute or chronic lung disease, this relationship no longer holds. Nevertheless, if an initial correlation is made between the two values, $PETCO_2$ can then be followed serially as a guide to ventilator management. Significant changes in $PETCO_2$ can be used to alert the physician to obtain ABGs and recheck arterial PCO_2. A rise in $PETCO_2$ almost always indicates a rise in $PaCO_2$ and therefore usually a decrease in alveolar ventilation. A fall in $PETCO_2$ indicates either an increase in alveolar ventilation or a rise in dead space, which must then be correlated with a new measurement of $PaCO_2$.

E. Hemodynamic monitoring. Pulmonary artery catheterization via a balloon-flotation catheter allows collection of the following data: $S\bar{v}O_2$; $P\bar{v}O_2$; cardiac output; and right atrial, right ventricular, pulmonary artery, and pulmonary artery occlusive ("wedge") pressures. The pulmonary artery occlusive pressure (PAOP) is often used to guide fluid therapy during ARF, but several factors make interpretation during mechanical ventilation problematic:

1. **Transmural pressure.** Intravascular pressures are always measured with atmospheric pressure as a zero reference, but **transmural** vascular pressure is more accurate. Since pleural pressure is normally a few centimeters H_2O negative with respect to atmospheric pressure but changes little during quiet, spontaneous breathing, no correction is necessary. However, in the dyspneic patient being mechanically ventilated with PEEP, the PAOP relative to atmospheric pressure may rise while transmural pressures fall. Such artifactual increases in the measured PAOP are rarely significant when PEEP is less than 10 cm H_2O. Above this level, the magnitude of the artifact is often significant but unpredictable.

2. **Respiratory variation.** The PAOP shows little respiratory variation during quiet, spontaneous breathing. This is not true when patients are dyspneic, when exhalation is not passive, and when mechanical ventilation is used. For this reason, measurements must be made at a given point in the respiratory cycle (usually at **end-exhalation**) directly from a written paper tracing of the wedge pressure. Reliance on digital readings from bedside monitors can seriously overestimate or underestimate the actual value, especially during marked respiratory variation.

   Similarly, measurements of cardiac output by thermodilution vary with the phase of respiration in patients on mechanical ventilation. Therefore, cardiac output should always be measured at end-exhalation.

3. **Ventricular compliance.** The use of the PAOP to estimate the left ventricular preload implies a direct relationship to both left atrial and left ventricular end-diastolic pressure. Furthermore, it is assumed that left ventricular end-diastolic pressure and left ventricular end-diastolic volume (LVEDV) maintain their normal relationship (normal ventricular diastolic compliance). This assumption may not be true during ARF or sepsis, especially when pulmonary vascular resistance or PEEP levels are high. Under such circumstances, the PAOP may be high for a given LVEDV. Since it is actually LVEDV that determines the effect of myocardial stretch on cardiac output, the use of the PAOP (as an estimate of LVEDV) can be misleading, and changes should be correlated with measured changes in cardiac output.

   In conclusion, a low PAOP (<5–8 mm Hg) measured at end-exhalation usually indicates relative hypovolemia; a high value (>18–20 mm Hg) usually indicates left ventricular failure. Intermediate values must be interpreted with the potential effects of altered ventricular compliance and high airway pressure in mind.

VIII. Supportive care of the intubated patient

A. Physiotherapy should include turning the patient at least hourly, flotation devices, heel pads, and passive motion of immobilized extremities to prevent subsequent physical impairment and skin ulcers. Early institution of graded exercise training often will facilitate withdrawal of ventilatory support. Having the patient stand, sit, or walk short distances while being mechanically ventilated by machine or anesthesia bag is an example of the level at which such a program might begin.

B. Care must be taken to **prevent eye damage** in the unconscious patient. Moisturizing eyedrops (methyl cellulose) should be used, and the eyes may be padded and taped shut.

C. **Emotional support.** Effective communication with the intubated patient, using sign language, lip reading, and written materials, is extremely important. Calendars, clocks, television, radio, and other visual and auditory stimuli can maintain a frame of reference with the outside world.

D. **Nutrition.** When oral intake is limited, alimentation is appropriate (parenteral or enteric, by nasogastric feeding tube, gastrostomy, or jejunostomy; see Chap. 11). **The formula for providing calories is particularly important in the patient with respiratory failure.** Calories provided in excess of needs and nonprotein calories provided solely in the form of carbohydrate can lead to excess carbon dioxide production and ventilatory demand. An inability to be weaned from mechanical ventilation may be partly due to such excess carbon dioxide production.

E. **Drugs**

1. The use of **antibiotics, cardiovascular agents, corticosteroids, diuretics, and bronchodilators** is described in Chap. 9.

2. The long-acting **respiratory stimulant** medroxyprogesterone acetate (100 mg IM qd) occasionally can improve alveolar ventilation in patients with underlying chronic obstructive lung disease. Some physicians have used the short-acting stimulant doxapram HCl, although its effectiveness is unproved.

3. **Acetazolamide** is used occasionally when the arterial pH exceeds 7.45, serum bicarbonate exceeds 29 mEq/dl, and the serum K^+ is in the normal range. Administration of 2 doses of acetazolamide (125–250 mg IV q6h) may promote a sufficient bicarbonate diuresis to normalize the pH, increase alveolar ventilation, and facilitate weaning from the ventilator. A few additional doses can be given, depending on the initial response.

IX. **Complications**

A. **Airway problems**

1. **Improper artificial airway placement** in the esophagus or right main stem bronchus may cause inadequate ventilation, hypoxemia, and pneumothorax (see sec. **V.B**).

2. **Cuff overinflation** regularly produces late development of tracheal stricture (see sec. **IV.E.4**).

3. **Endotracheal tube dislodgment** or cuff leak should be suspected when there is a sudden decrease in expired volume associated with a fall in airway pressure.

B. **Barotrauma.** Subcutaneous emphysema, pneumomediastinum, and pneumothorax are associated with high peak airway pressures and PEEP. Pneumothorax should be considered when lung compliance or blood pressure falls. Frequent palpation of the neck for crepitation and auscultation of the lung are necessary. Chest tube-insertion equipment should be readily available for mechanically ventilated patients.

C. **Rapid acid-base shifts.** Sudden overventilation can result in hypocarbia and respiratory alkalosis, which can lead to decreased cardiac output, cardiac dysrhythmias, and CNS disturbances. **Altered clinical states should be corrected at a rate proportional to their development.**

D. **Hemodynamic effects.** Positive pressure ventilation can result in decreased venous return, especially if associated with intravascular fluid volume depletion. This may decrease cardiac output and blood pressure. To assess extracellular fluid status, measure blood pressure during mechanical ventilation and after a few seconds of spontaneous ventilation. An increase in systolic pressure >10 mm Hg during spontaneous breathing suggests extracellular fluid depletion.

E. Positive fluid balance and hyponatremia tend to develop in patients mechanically ventilated with well-humidified gas. This effect may be accentuated by the use of PEEP.

F. Cardiac dysrhythmias are common in respiratory failure and should be treated in the usual fashion. **Multifocal atrial tachycardia** is frequently associated with acidosis, hypoxia, electrolyte imbalance, theophylline intoxication, and digitalis toxicity. Therapy should be directed at the underlying causes. Antidysrhythmic drugs are less helpful.

G. Oxygen toxicity. See sec. **IV.A.3.c.**

H. Pulmonary thromboembolism is common and should be treated in the standard fashion (see Chap. 16). Subcutaneous heparin (5000 units SQ q12h) may be prophylactic.

I. Aspiration can occur despite a cuffed tracheal tube, especially in patients receiving enteral nutrition. Aspiration may be demonstrated by testing tracheal secretions either for glucose with Dextrostix or for a blue discoloration after the enteral administration of methylene blue.

J. Upper gastrointestinal bleeding can be life-threatening. Frequent antacid titration, keeping the pH of gastric contents greater than 3.5, significantly decreases the incidence of bleeding. **Cimetidine** may achieve the same goal (pH >3.5), although proof of its clinical efficacy awaits confirmation.

K. Metabolic complications

1. The **syndrome of inappropriate antidiuretic hormone** (SIADH) often complicates respiratory failure. Fluid restriction (often difficult) or demeclocycline, 150 mg PO qid, provides effective control.

2. **Hypokalemia and hypochloremia,** when not associated with SIADH, should be treated by replacement of these electrolytes.

3. **Severe hypophosphatemia** (<1.0–1.5 mg/dl) should be treated with oral phosphosoda or IV potassium phosphate to improve respiratory muscle and red cell function.

L. Nosocomial infections can largely be prevented with strict adherence to sterile technique during intratracheal suctioning, avoidance of cross-contamination, and frequent changes of ventilator tubing and equipment. **Careful handwashing techniques by all personnel are essential.**

M. Long-term airway complications

1. Postintubation tracheal **stricture** is caused by high cuff pressures. A significant number of patients will have asymptomatic tracheal narrowing after extubation. Stricture is prevented by using a highly compliant cuff inflated to allow a minimal leak (see sec. **IV.E.4**).

2. **Tracheoesophageal fistula,** a rare but serious complication, requires immediate attention. The use of large-bore nasogastric tubes in intubated patients predisposes to this complication.

3. Erosion of the **innominate artery with hemorrhage** is a rare catastrophic event and is associated with a low-lying tracheostomy (fifth tracheal ring or below) and poor stabilization of the airway.

N. Muscle wasting occurs after prolonged inactivity and inanition. A comprehensive rehabilitation and feeding program should be initiated in the ICU as early as possible.

O. Drug toxicity

1. **Theophylline** preparations are the bronchodilators most often used. Serum levels should be monitored (see Chap. 9).

2. The potential for **digitalis toxicity** may increase with hypoxemia and respiratory failure. Nevertheless, digitalis preparations should be administered when left ventricular failure is present.

P. **Psychiatric complications,** including "intensive care unit psychosis," depression, and agitation, can often be avoided by effective communication among patient, staff, and family, as well as by maintaining the patient's awareness of the outside world. Organic causes of behavioral disturbance, such as carbon dioxide narcosis, hyponatremia, or drug toxicity, must be evaluated before implicating psychiatric dysfunction.

X. **Weaning** is the **gradual** withdrawal of mechanical ventilatory support. In general, patients requiring mechanical ventilation for less than 3 days do not require weaning. Furthermore, patients generally will no longer require mechanical ventilation when the underlying process that originally caused the need for mechanical ventilation is markedly improved. Successful withdrawal of ventilatory support depends on the general condition of the patient and the status of the cardiovascular and respiratory systems. All weaning methods require close monitoring of the patient's overall condition, the respiratory rate, and arterial blood gases. **Common problems** that prolong the weaning process include (1) incompletely treated pulmonary infection or bronchospasm, (2) excessive airway secretions, (3) poor nutrition, and (4) narrow endotracheal tubes. The last can be especially important in patients with increased airways resistance as part of their chronic lung disease.

Although complete cessation of mechanical support is necessary prior to extubation, the final decision to extubate must include a determination of the need for continued airway control. Patients who cannot protect their airway adequately (severe obtundation, repeated aspiration) may require prolonged tracheostomy even after mechanical ventilation is no longer required. Some patients, especially those with chronic abnormalities in alveolar gas exchange, can be weaned despite failure to meet the guidelines presented in Table 8-3.

A. When **oxygenation failure** is the major clinical problem, the focus must be on a gradual withdrawal of positive airway pressure (primarily PEEP) and FiO_2 until the patient can sustain a PaO_2 >60 mm Hg on an FiO_2 of <0.5 and ≤5 cm H_2O PEEP. Until this point is reached, the ventilator should be adjusted to provide a minute ventilation sufficient to maintain a normal arterial pH; intermittent mandatory ventilation (IMV) frequently is useful in achieving this goal in the tachypneic patient. The overall respiratory rate of the patient plus machine should be less than 25/minute. It is usually possible to lower PEEP and the IMV rate in tandem, but this must be checked against blood gas values and the patient's respiratory effort. Once 5 cm H_2O PEEP is required for oxygenation (with an FiO_2 of <0.5), reductions in IMV rate usually can be rapid. Extubation may be considered after a trial of 2–6 hours of CPAP.

Table 8-3. Guidelines for assessing withdrawal of mechanical ventilation

1. An awake and alert mental state
2. PaO_2 >60 mm Hg with an FiO_2 <0.5
3. PEEP ≤5 cm H_2O
4. $PaCO_2$ acceptable, with pH in the normal range
5. Vital capacity >10–15 ml/kg
6. Minute ventilation <10 L/min; respiratory rate <25/min
7. Maximum voluntary ventilation double that of minute ventilation
8. Peak inspiratory pressure more negative than −25 cm H_2O
9. Spontaneous ventilation via T-tube (with or without CPAP) for 2–6 hr with acceptable blood gases and without marked increases in respiratory rate, heart rate, or change in general status

B. When **ventilation failure** is the primary clinical problem, the focus must be on tidal volume and rate. Two weaning methods are available:

   1. The **intermittent mandatory ventilation technique** allows a gradual transition from mechanical ventilation to spontaneous breathing. This is accomplished by gradually decreasing the fixed ventilator rate until the patient is totally self-supporting. A combination of IMV and T-tube weaning is often successful in selected patients.

   2. **T-tube technique.** Weaning should be initiated during the day when the full staff is readily available. Humidified oxygen-enriched gas is given via a T tube during spontaneous ventilation for short periods (5–15 minutes/hour). The use of end-tidal PCO_2 in the expired gas that is continuously monitored by either mass spectrometry or capnography can be particularly useful at this time. The duration of spontaneous ventilation is increased progressively as tolerated. During the period of spontaneous ventilation, intermittent hyperinflation via an anesthesia bag, or small amounts (3–5 cm H_2O) of positive airway pressure, may prevent early airway closure and microatelectasis. Patients with **chronic ventilation failure** often need mechanical ventilation at night to prevent hypoventilation and fatigue. After 2–6 hours without mechanical ventilation, extubation may be appropriate. A FiO_2 higher than that used during mechanical ventilation usually is necessary immediately after extubation.

XI. Extubation

A. Procedure. When indications for an artificial airway are no longer present, proceed with extubation as follows:

   1. Begin early in the day.

   2. Educate the patient about the procedure.

   3. Elevate head and trunk 20–40 degrees.

   4. Check the clinical baseline (vital signs and arterial blood gases).

   5. Have a high-humidity, oxygen-enriched gas source with a higher FiO_2 available at bedside.

   6. Have equipment available should reintubation become necessary.

   7. Carefully suction through the airway and in the oropharynx above cuff.

   8. Deflate the cuff completely, extubate, and administer high-humidity oxygen.

   9. Encourage vigorous coughing; suction as necessary.

   10. Check vital signs and arterial blood gases; watch for evidence of laryngospasm (e.g., listen with the stethoscope for inspiratory stridor).

   11. Reintubate for progressive hypoxemia, hypercarbia, acidosis, or laryngospasm not responsive to therapy.

B. Postextubation complications

   1. Hoarseness and sore throat are common. Additional humidity may help.

   2. Glottic edema is manifested by inspiratory stridor. It usually takes several hours for the edema to reach its maximum. Treatment is racemic epinephrine (0.5 ml) in 3 ml of saline administered via an intermittent positive pressure breathing apparatus. If postextubation edema does not respond rapidly, subglottic edema or stenosis must be presumed and an artificial airway reintroduced.

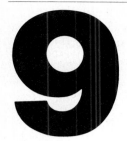

Pulmonary Disease

Asthma

Ddx: lrg. airway obstruction, cardiogenic pulm edema, anaphylaxis, chronic bronchitis

Asthma is a chronic, episodic disease characterized by increased reactivity of the airways. The consequent bronchial smooth muscle contraction, mucosal edema, and increased mucous secretion result in reversible obstruction of airflow. Coughing, wheezing, or dyspnea characterize an acute attack. Factors that precipitate episodes of asthma include allergens, chemical irritants, exercise, drugs, and infections. Large airway obstruction (by tumor or foreign body), cardiogenic pulmonary edema, anaphylaxis, and exacerbations of chronic bronchitis can mimic asthma.

I. Assessment of severity of an asthmatic attack

A. A relevant **history** includes the number of previous hospitalizations, the prior need for corticosteroids or intubation, the relative severity of the current attack, precipitating factors, recent emergency room visits, and compliance with current medications.

B. **Sternocleidomastoid muscle contractions** and an inspiratory fall in systolic blood pressure greater than 12 mm Hg (**increased pulsus paradoxus**) indicate severe airway obstruction but are insensitive and may disappear after only minor improvements in airflow. The intensity of **wheezing** can be misleading, since it may decrease with worsening obstruction. Somnolence or agitation are ominous signs representing severe respiratory decompensation.

C. Laboratory studies

1. Arterial blood gases (ABGs) are used to assess the severity of an attack.

   a. Between attacks, ABGs usually are normal.

   b. Early in an attack, mild hypoxemia and respiratory alkalosis are noted. The PO_2 is below 80 mm Hg, the PCO_2 is less than 35 mm Hg, and the pH is greater than 7.4.

   c. Over the next several hours, metabolic compensation for the respiratory alkalosis begins. The serum bicarbonate falls below 24 mEq/liter and the pH normalizes. The PCO_2 may decrease to less than 20 mm Hg; the PO_2 may also decrease.

   d. With a severe, prolonged attack, muscle fatigue may decrease ventilation. As a result, the PCO_2 begins to rise and the pH falls. **Intubation and mechanical ventilation** should be considered if the PCO_2 is greater than 35 mm Hg and the pH is less than 7.4. Any further clinical deterioration will rapidly lead to respiratory failure. The resultant respiratory acidosis will be especially severe, because there is less bicarbonate available to buffer the carbon dioxide (see **c**).

   e. The ABGs of an **improving patient** will also demonstrate a rise in PCO_2, but the pH will be greater than 7.4.

2. **Measurement of airflow** is the best method to assess both the severity of an attack and the response to therapy. Bedside spirometry is used to measure the volume of air expired in the first second of a forced expiration (FEV$_1$). **Hospitalization** is recommended if the initial FEV$_1$ is less than 800 ml or if the increase in FEV$_1$ is less than 400 ml after 3–4 hours of vigorous outpatient therapy.

[handwritten: Hospitalize]
[handwritten: FEV$_1$ < 800 ml]
[handwritten: ↑ in FEV$_1$ < 400ml after 3-4 hrs therapy]

3. **Sputum** should be examined for eosinophils and neutrophils with a wet mount preparation. Bacteria should be sought with a Gram stain.

4. The **complete blood count** with differential should be obtained to determine the presence or absence of eosinophilia.

5. **Chest radiography** can exclude conditions that mimic asthma and can reveal complications such as pneumomediastinum.

II. **Acute therapy.** The goals of therapy are rapid reversal of bronchospasm and prevention of respiratory failure.

A. **Oxygen** (2–3 liters/minute via nasal prongs) should be administered immediately to all patients. Bronchodilator-induced increases in pulmonary blood flow precede bronchodilatation and worsen ventilation/perfusion mismatch. The resultant transient fall in PO$_2$ may be prevented by adequate oxygen therapy. Further adjustments in flow rate are made according to the ABGs.

[handwritten: O$_2$]
[handwritten: 2-3 L/min]

B. **Dehydration** may result from poor oral intake, the increased work of breathing, fluid loss from the respiratory tree, and the diuretic effect of theophylline. Oral intake should be encouraged. Intravenous fluids at 100–200 ml/hour are usually necessary during severe attacks. Serum electrolytes should be monitored daily during the acute attack, since hyponatremia may occur secondary to excessive hydration or inappropriate secretion of antidiuretic hormone.

C. Parenteral or inhaled **bronchodilators** provide the most rapid reversal of obstruction.

1. **Parenteral sympathomimetics**

   a. Aqueous **epinephrine** (0.3–0.5 ml of a 1 : 1000 dilution) is given SQ and may be repeated 2–3 times at 20-minute intervals. Relative contraindications include severe hypertension, a pulse rate over 140/minute, and cardiac dysrhythmias. The drug should be used cautiously in patients over 40 years old.

   b. **Terbutaline,** a beta-2 agonist, should not be used to initiate treatment because of its delayed onset of action (30–60 minutes). However, it has a longer serum half-life than epinephrine and may be used after improvement is noted. Parenteral administration is relatively contraindicated in patients with cardiac disease, because the drug causes systemic vasodilatation with compensatory tachycardia.

2. **Inhalation therapy** is as effective as parenteral sympathomimetics except in very severe cases in which adequate inspiration is impossible. Its systemic effects are few. Nonspecific airway irritation by the aerosol may exacerbate bronchospasm in some patients.

[handwritten: Ventolin by mask]
[handwritten: 0.03 cc/kg q 1-2 hr in children]
[handwritten: 0.5 - 1 cc in 2cc NS for adults]

   a. **Metaproterenol** is administered via a hand-held nebulizer (0.2–0.3 ml in 2.5 ml of saline q4–6h) or via a metered-dose inhaler (two inhalations q4–6h).

   b. **Albuterol** is available only as a metered-dose inhaler. The dosage is two inhalations q4–6h.

   c. **Isoetharine** has more systemic effects (e.g., tachycardia) and must be given more frequently than the previous agents. The dosage is 0.5 ml in 2.5 ml of saline q2–4h via a hand-held nebulizer.

3. **Theophylline,** a xanthine derivative, relaxes bronchial smooth muscle by increasing intracellular cAMP. Aminophylline (a soluble ethylene diamine salt containing 85% theophylline by weight) is a frequently used parenteral form. Intravenous aminophylline alone is less effective in the initial therapy of an acute attack than either inhaled or parenteral sympathomimetics. However, the combination of sympathomimetics and aminophylline is more effective and no more toxic than epinephrine alone.

   a. The **loading dose** is 5–6 mg/kg IV over 20 minutes. Maintenance therapy is given by constant infusion at a rate of 0.2–0.5 mg/kg/hour.

   b. The loading dose should be reduced or omitted if the patient is currently taking a theophylline preparation. Congestive heart failure, liver disease, advanced age, and the concurrent administration of cimetidine, propranolol, or erythromycin slow aminophylline metabolism and require the lower infusion rate. Smokers and adolescents may rapidly metabolize aminophylline and may require higher rates (e.g., 0.8 mg/kg/hour).

   c. **Serum theophylline concentrations** must be monitored. The maintenance dose is adjusted to maintain serum levels between 10–20 μg/ml.

   d. Nausea, vomiting, and cardiac dysrhythmias occur more frequently when levels exceed 20 μg/ml. Seizures may occur when the serum level exceeds 30 μg/ml and can present without any preceding signs of toxicity.

D. **Corticosteroids** reduce airway obstruction by decreasing bronchial inflammation. They are indicated for patients not responding significantly to bronchodilator therapy within 1 hour. The onset of therapeutic effect takes at least 12 hours. Recommended starting doses are 250–1000 mg IV of hydrocortisone (or its equivalent). The maintenance dosage is 100–300 mg IV q4–6h. Oral prednisone is administered after airflow improves. The dosage is 25–50 mg PO bid. This dosage is rapidly tapered over the following week as long as improvement continues.

E. **Antibiotics** are administered when purulent sputum, fever, or a pulmonary infiltrate is present. Sputum eosinophilia may make sputum appear grossly purulent.

F. **Percussion and postural drainage** may exacerbate bronchospasm and are used only in patients with copious secretions or mucous plugs.

G. **Sedatives are contraindicated** during an acute attack unless the patient is intubated.

H. **Intermittent positive pressure breathing** is used to deliver inhaled bronchodilators when the patient is unable to take an adequate inspiration. For therapy to be effective, the volume delivered must exceed the patient's tidal volume. Bronchospasm may be worsened by intermittent positive pressure breathing.

III. **Chronic therapy.** Once the acute attack has subsided, further therapy is aimed at relieving residual bronchospasm and preventing recurrence. Pulmonary function tests may not return to normal for weeks after an acute attack.

A. Known **precipitating factors** should be avoided. These may include animal danders, dust, aspirin, nonsteroidal anti-inflammatory agents, exercise in the cold, and agents containing tartrazine.

B. **Bronchodilators**

   1. **Inhaled agents** (metaproterenol or albuterol) are used as needed in patients with infrequent or mild attacks. They have few systemic effects and provide rapid relief.

   2. A **theophylline preparation or sympathomimetic** should be added when inhaled agents fail to control attacks. Long-acting theophylline preparations

encourage compliance; their usual dosage is 200–400 mg PO bid. Serum concentrations must be measured to ensure therapeutic levels (10–20 µg/ml).

The beta-2 agonists **terbutaline** (2.5–5.0 mg PO tid) and **metaproterenol** (20 mg PO tid or qid) have minimal cardiac side effects. Drug-induced tremors may limit the dosage in some patients.

   3. Formulations containing multiple drugs at fixed dosages should be avoided.

C. Corticosteroids are used in patients with frequent, severe attacks despite optimal bronchodilator therapy. The lowest effective corticosteroid dosage is administered, and, if tolerated, alternate-day therapy is preferred. **Beclomethasone,** a corticosteroid administered by inhalation, may reduce or obviate the need for orally administered corticosteroids. The usual dosage is two puffs (100 µg) qid.

D. Cromolyn sodium is useful as a prophylactic agent in patients with exercise- or cold-induced asthma. The usual dosage is 1 capsule (20 mg) qid by inhalation with the turboinhaler.

Chronic Obstructive Pulmonary Disease

Chronic obstructive pulmonary disease (COPD) is characterized by the limitation of airflow secondary to airway disease (chronic bronchitis) or destruction of pulmonary parenchyma (emphysema). Most patients have a combination of both. In chronic bronchitis, expiratory airflow is limited by mucous gland hypertrophy, mucous plugging, and obliteration of airways. In emphysema, enlargement of the air passages distal to the terminal bronchioles and destruction of alveolar walls lead to loss of elastic recoil and reduced expiratory airflow.

I. Diagnosis. Typically, the disease is silent for years or minimally symptomatic, with cough and sputum production. Patients seldom seek attention until they are short of breath.

A. Spirometry shows an obstructive pattern characterized by a reduction of the volume of air expired in the first second of a forced expiration (FEV_1), and an FEV_1–forced vital capacity ratio less than 75%.

B. Arterial blood gases reveal a widened alveolar-arterial (A-a) oxygen gradient. Patients with chronic bronchitis are more hypoxemic and more prone to carbon dioxide retention than patients with emphysema of comparable obstructive severity.

C. Chest radiographs often show flattened diaphragms and increased anteroposterior diameter. In emphysema, vascular markings may be decreased, and bullae may be evident.

II. Management. Adequate oxygenation must be maintained and reversible causes of airway obstruction, such as increased secretions, airway inflammation, and bronchospasm, corrected.

A. Acute exacerbations are manifested by worsening dyspnea and signs of fatigue. Sputum may be increased or decreased in amount but usually is thicker than normal. In severe cases, confusion, cyanosis, and right-sided heart failure may supervene.

   1. Oxygen is administered at rates sufficient to maintain arterial PO_2 between 45 and 60 mm Hg. Intubation and mechanical ventilation are necessary if supplemental oxygen and optimal medical management cannot maintain the PO_2 above 40 mm Hg with a pH greater than 7.25.

   2. Bronchodilators are given to reverse bronchospasm (see Asthma, sec. **II.C**).

Acute respiratory failure may slow aminophylline metabolism and increase the risk of toxicity.

3. **Antibiotics**

   a. **Empirical treatment** with ampicillin (500 mg PO q6h) or tetracycline (500 mg PO q6h) is given when sputum is purulent and radiographic evidence of pneumonia is absent. Sputum cultures in COPD may reflect bacterial colonization and are rarely helpful.

   b. **Intravenous antibiotics** are administered if pneumonia is present. Potential pathogens include *Streptococcus pneumoniae, Haemophilus influenzae,* and, less commonly, *Klebsiella pneumoniae, Staphylococcus aureus,* and *Legionella pneumophila.* Initial therapy is guided by the radiographic and clinical presentation and the predominant organism seen on sputum Gram stain (see Chap. 10). Therapy is modified to cover specific organisms recovered from initial sputum or blood cultures. Infiltrates may resolve slowly, and it is unwise to change antibiotics if the patient's clinical status is improving.

4. **Percussion and postural drainage** are recommended for patients with coexisting bronchiectasis.

5. **Corticosteroids** (e.g., methylprednisolone, 0.5 mg/kg IV q6h for 3 days) significantly improve airflow in patients with acute respiratory insufficiency due to COPD.

B. **Long-term management**

1. The patient and family should be taught about the disease and its management. Exacerbations should be recognized and reported before they become serious.

2. Daily administration of **bronchodilators** may increase airflow even in patients who fail to show immediate improvement after inhalation of isoproterenol. These agents should be used only in patients with a corresponding symptomatic improvement.

3. **Corticosteroids** (e.g., prednisone, 20–40 mg PO qd) are started in patients with bronchospasm refractory to optimal bronchodilator therapy. Therapy is continued (at the lowest effective dosage) only if pulmonary function tests improve after 3–4 weeks of treatment.

4. **Continuous low-flow oxygen therapy** is the only form of therapy documented to improve survival in patients with chronic hypoxemia or cor pulmonale. Oxygen therapy should be used only when optimal inpatient management has failed to correct hypoxemia. The flow rate of oxygen is adjusted to maintain the resting PO_2 close to 60 mm Hg. Increases in the flow rate may be required if hypoxemia worsens during exercise or sleep. Most patients tolerate the oxygen-induced increases in PCO_2.

5. **Nocturnal oxygen therapy** reduces cardiac dysrhythmias and may retard the development of cor pulmonale in patients with sleep-induced hypoxemia.

6. Correction of **exercise-induced** hypoxemia with supplemental oxygen may improve exercise tolerance.

7. **Digitalis and diuretics** should be used only when left ventricular dysfunction is present. Digitalis increases the risk of dysrhythmias, and diuretics may further depress respiration by causing a metabolic alkalosis.

8. **Antibiotic therapy** should be initiated by the patient when there is a change in the color or consistency of the sputum. Ampicillin, tetracycline, and trimethoprim-sulfamethoxazole are the drugs of choice.

9. **Influenza and pneumococcal vaccines** are recommended for patients with COPD.

10. **Sedatives and tranquilizers** are avoided because they suppress respiratory drive and cough. Nervousness or irritability in a patient with COPD can be the first sign of respiratory decompensation.

11. **A general rehabilitation program,** including exercise training, helps improve the patient's sense of well-being and exercise tolerance.

12. **Percussion and postural drainage** are especially useful in patients with significant sputum production and may be performed by a trained family member.

Pulmonary Embolism

The diagnosis of pulmonary embolism requires a high index of clinical suspicion. Risk factors include cardiomegaly, congestive heart failure, venous disease of the lower extremities, carcinoma, oral contraceptive use, recent pelvic or lower extremity surgery, and prolonged immobilization. Signs and symptoms often are subtle and nonspecific, but the sudden onset of dyspnea, wheezing, chest pain, hemoptysis, unexplained hypoxemia, or tachycardia suggests the possibility of pulmonary embolism.

I. Diagnosis

A. **Arterial blood gases** show a widened A-a gradient. Hypocarbia usually is present, and the PO_2 is below 80 mm Hg in 90% of cases.

B. The **ECG** is usually normal, but it may show an S1Q3 pattern, signs of right heart strain, or P pulmonale.

C. **Chest radiographs** are most often unremarkable, but occasionally show strip atelectasis, hemidiaphragm elevation, or, rarely, an area of hypolucency reflecting decreased blood flow to the area. The classic radiographic findings of a pleural effusion and a pleural-based infiltrate (Hampton's hump) are uncommon.

D. **Ventilation-perfusion lung scans** can confirm or exclude pulmonary emboli with high degrees of specificity and sensitivity if strict criteria are used in their interpretation. Perfusion scans alone are less specific, especially if there is underlying lung disease. An equivocal or nondiagnostic scan may direct the attention of the angiographer to the most suspicious areas of the lung.

E. **Selective pulmonary angiography** is indicated whenever clinical data and lung scans are equivocal. In expert hands it carries less mortality and morbidity than long-term anticoagulation.

II. Treatment

A. **Supportive treatment** includes oxygen administration and maintenance of cardiac output and blood pressure.

B. **Prophylaxis** against further emboli is the primary goal in the majority of cases.

1. **Anticoagulation** is instituted with heparin and then switched to oral therapy (see Chap. 16). Although anticoagulation prevents further clot formation, the patient remains at risk of further emboli for 3–7 days, until normal physiologic mechanisms dissolve existing thrombi. Therapy is discontinued after 2–3 months if the risk factors for embolism are no longer present. Patients at continued risk may require lifelong therapy.

2. **Inferior vena cava interruption** is required in a minority of patients to prevent further emboli. It is accomplished either with a transvenous umbrella filter or with a surgically placed clip on the vessel. **Indications** include:

a. **A critically ill patient** in whom a recurrent embolus would likely prove fatal

b. **Recurrent emboli** despite 7 days of adequate anticoagulation

c. **A contraindication** to or **complications** of heparin therapy

d. **Septic emboli** arising from below the renal veins that recur after 24–48 hours of conservative therapy with antibiotics, anticoagulation, and control of the local infection

C. Definitive therapy

1. **Embolectomy** is used only in patients who have documented massive emboli that prevent adequate perfusion of the lungs and left ventricle.

2. **Systemic thrombolytic therapy** with streptokinase or urokinase hastens the resolution of emboli but has not been shown to improve survival.

Adult Respiratory Distress Syndrome

The adult respiratory distress syndrome (ARDS) is a nonspecific pulmonary reaction to a wide variety of insults. Disorders leading to ARDS include sepsis, shock of any cause, lung trauma, head injury, aspiration of gastric juices, near-drowning, smoke inhalation, and overdoses of heroin, methadone, and barbiturates, among other drugs. Adult respiratory distress syndrome is characterized by progressive accumulation of extravascular fluid within the lung due to a derangement of alveolar-capillary permeability. The excess fluid leads to decreased pulmonary compliance and to increased dead space ventilation and intrapulmonary shunt fraction.

I. Diagnosis. The diagnosis requires the appropriate clinical setting and exclusion of other causes of respiratory failure (e.g., COPD, left ventricular failure, acute pneumonia). Clinical signs include tachypnea, intercostal retractions, and use of accessory muscles of respiration. The arterial PO_2 is less than 50 mm Hg despite inspired oxygen tensions (FIO_2) of 60% or greater. Chest radiographs demonstrate a diffuse parenchymal infiltration that is initially interstitial but rapidly progresses to an alveolar pattern.

II. Management. Management is directed at maintaining adequate tissue oxygen delivery at the lowest possible FIO_2 while treating the underlying cause. Hemodynamic monitoring via a balloon-flotation (Swan-Ganz) catheter is essential. (See Chap. 8 for a more extensive discussion of hemodynamic monitoring in patients with pulmonary disease.)

A. **Mechanical ventilation with positive end-expiratory pressure** (PEEP) is currently the most effective means of respiratory support for the patient with ARDS. This technique decreases the fraction of cardiac output distributed to the intrapulmonary shunt compartment. The resulting increase in arterial PO_2 allows reduction of the FIO_2. Positive end-expiratory pressure can also reduce cardiac output, and thus tissue oxygen delivery may decrease despite the increased arterial PO_2. Calculation of the tissue oxygen delivery or measurement of the mixed venous oxygen tension (see Chap. 8, sec. **VII.B**) is essential to document that PEEP-induced increases in arterial PO_2 are not negated by decreased cardiac output.

B. **The pulmonary artery occlusive pressure** (PAOP) is kept at the lowest level compatible with adequate tissue perfusion in order to minimize pulmonary interstitial fluid accumulation. Inotropic agents should be used if cardiac output is inadequate despite a PAOP of 10 mm Hg or greater.

C. Intravenous volume is maintained with **crystalloid** rather than colloid solutions, since the latter may increase extravascular lung water. The hematocrit should be kept within the normal range with packed red blood cells to maintain adequate tissue oxygen delivery.

D. The use of **high-dose corticosteroids** is controversial. Despite a theoretical basis for their efficacy in some patients, there is no conclusive evidence that corticosteroids are of any benefit.

Pleural Effusions

Pleural effusion is the accumulation of fluid within the pleural space. Although visualization on posteroanterior radiographs requires the presence of 300–500 ml of fluid, lateral decubitus views may demonstrate as little as 50 ml. Ultrasonography facilitates the localization of loculated effusions. Thoracentesis is indicated to establish a cause unless the pleural effusion is judged to be secondary to a known underlying condition such as congestive heart failure.

I. **Diagnosis.** Pleural effusions are divided into those caused by altered Starling forces (transudates) and those caused by inflammation or malignancy (exudates).

  A. Transudates are defined by the following criteria:

    1. Pleural fluid lactic dehydrogenase less than 200 international units/dl

    2. A ratio of pleural fluid to serum lactic dehydrogenase of less than 0.6

    3. A ratio of pleural fluid to serum protein of less than 0.5

  B. Pleural effusions lacking any one of these characteristics are **exudates.**

  C. Common causes of **transudates** include congestive heart failure, cirrhosis, and the nephrotic syndrome.

  D. Exudates may result from infection, tumor, pulmonary infarction, and collagen vascular disease. Laboratory tests useful in determining the etiology of exudates include:

    1. Cytology. Several hundred milliliters should be submitted if possible.

    2. Stains and cultures for bacteria (aerobic and anaerobic), mycobacteria, and fungi.

    3. Cell count and differential. Gross blood is associated with pulmonary infarct, tumor, or trauma.

    4. Glucose may be less than 40 mg/dl in empyema, rheumatoid arthritis, and tuberculosis.

    5. Amylase exceeds the serum level in pancreatitis and esophageal rupture.

    6. Triglycerides are increased in chylous effusions.

    7. pH is less than 7.3 in empyema, malignancy, collagen vascular disease, and esophageal rupture.

  E. A **needle biopsy** of the pleura should be considered when the preceding laboratory tests fail to establish a cause.

II. **Treatment**

  A. Symptomatic pleural effusions may require the removal of large amounts of pleural fluid. The sudden aspiration of more than 1 liter of pleural fluid may result in ipsilateral pulmonary edema. If a chest tube is placed, the fluid should be removed in stages by clamping the tube for an hour after each liter is drained.

  B. Parapneumonic effusions occur in approximately 40% of bacterial pneumonias. Thoracentesis is mandatory for appropriate treatment.

1. **Prompt drainage** via tube or open thoracostomy is required if pleural fluid cultures are positive or if thoracentesis demonstrates purulence, a positive pleural fluid Gram stain, a pleural fluid glucose less than 40 mg/dl, or a pH less than 7.2.

2. Effusions that do not meet the preceding criteria should resolve with therapy directed at the underlying pneumonia. **Repeat thoracentesis** should be performed if the effusion reaccumulates or clinical improvement is delayed.

C. **Chronic empyema** results from the incomplete resolution of a parapneumonic effusion. A thick pleural peel may develop and compress the underlying lung. Surgical obliteration of the empyema space is necessary in these cases.

D. **Malignant pleural effusions** may be due to obstruction of venous or lymphatic drainage, pleural implants, or malignant cells growing freely in the pleural space.

1. Effusions should be drained completely by thoracentesis or tube thoracostomy.

2. **Systemic chemotherapy** may control some effusions due to lymphoma or to breast, ovarian, testicular, or small-cell lung carcinoma.

3. Recurrent symptomatic malignant effusions require closed-tube thoracostomy and sclerosis of the pleural space. **Tetracycline** (500 mg in 50 ml of saline) or nitrogen mustard (10 mg in 50 ml of sterile water) should be instilled as soon as drainage is complete. The patient should be repositioned frequently over the next several hours to maximize dispersal of the sclerosing agent.

Aspiration

Aspiration may be divided into three categories: massive aspiration of gastric contents, aspiration of infected secretions, and aspiration of foreign bodies.

I. **Massive aspiration of gastric contents.** Aspiration of gastric contents usually occurs in patients with altered consciousness or impaired cough and swallowing mechanisms. It may also occur during cardiopulmonary resuscitation or during induction of anesthesia in patients with full stomachs. The severity of the subsequent pulmonary dysfunction is determined by the pH of the gastric contents, the volume of aspirated fluid, and the presence of food particles. Corticosteroids and prophylactic antibiotics are of no proved benefit. The adult respiratory distress syndrome develops in only a small subset of patients. The remainder experience rapid clinical and radiographic improvement. A subsequent deterioration should suggest a secondary pneumonia.

II. **Aspiration of infected material.** Aspiration of infected material may be acute (e.g., the unconscious patient), or recurrent (e.g., the debilitated or alcoholic patient). A pneumonia or abscess develops in a dependent segment. If aspiration occurs when the patient is supine, the superior segment of the upper lobe is usually involved. Treatment is directed toward the eradication of pulmonary infection (see Lung Abscess).

III. **Foreign bodies**

A. **Large foreign bodies** obstructing the airway above the glottic opening present with sudden onset of marked respiratory distress with vigorous but ineffective respiratory efforts. The victim, though highly agitated, is unable to talk and may quickly asphyxiate unless the material is removed by the first reflex cough. The **Heimlich maneuver** has been lifesaving in these instances. If this is unsuccessful, an emergency tracheostomy is required.

B. **Small foreign bodies** may lodge more distally in the tracheobronchial tree, producing atelectasis or pneumonia. These may be removed by rigid bronchoscopy.

Lung Abscess

Lung abscess most often develops following aspiration. Extensive gingival and dental disease is common. The clinical course may be insidious in onset, with constitutional symptoms of fever and weight loss. Copious amounts of foul-smelling sputum may be produced. Anaerobic bacteria are the most frequent pathogens.

I. **Diagnostic procedures.** The diagnosis of lung abscess should be made only when other causes of cavitary lung disease (tuberculosis, fungal disease, acute necrotizing pneumonia, carcinoma, vasculitis, septic embolism, and bland pulmonary embolism with infarction) have been excluded. Sputum should be cultured for aerobic bacteria, fungi, and mycobacteria. An intermediate-strength PPD should be placed. Bronchoscopy is indicated to exclude the presence of an obstructing tumor or foreign body. If transthoracic needle aspiration is indicated (see sec. II), specimens should be cultured for aerobic and anaerobic bacteria, mycobacteria, and fungi. Complications of this procedure include empyema, hemorrhage, and bronchopleural fistula.

II. **Therapy.** Postural drainage of the involved segment is mandatory. Seriously ill patients require aqueous penicillin G at a dosage of 1–2 million units IV q4h. Patients with minimal symptoms and no underlying medical problems may be treated with procaine penicillin at a dosage of 600,000 units IM q6h. Therapy may be switched to oral penicillin (500 mg PO q6h) when there is a definite clinical response and should be continued until the cavity closes. Even with adequate treatment, fever may persist for up to 3 weeks, the cavity for 10–12 weeks, and an infiltrate for 18–20 weeks. Progression of the disease despite adequate therapy warrants repeat bronchoscopy or a transthoracic needle aspiration in an effort to secure an exact diagnosis.

Hemoptysis

The causes of hemoptysis include the following: (1) infection (bronchitis, bronchiectasis, lung abscess, tuberculosis, and pneumonia); (2) neoplasm (carcinoma and bronchial adenoma); (3) cardiovascular disease (mitral stenosis, pulmonary embolus, or pulmonary vascular malformations); or (4) inflammation (Wegener's granulomatosis or Goodpasture's syndrome). In a significant number of patients, the cause of hemoptysis is never determined. The severity of any episode of hemoptysis is determined by the rate of blood loss and the patient's underlying pulmonary status. **Asphyxiation** by aspirated blood is the major cause of immediate mortality. Quantifying the amount of bleeding is often difficult because it may be mixed with varying amounts of saliva, and the blood may be swallowed or aspirated.

I. **Diagnosis**

   A. The **history** should include questions regarding smoking habits, past pneumonias, bronchiectasis, exposure to tuberculosis, recent seizures or loss of consciousness, and recent weight loss.

   B. **Physical examination** should include careful inspection of the upper airway to rule out a nonpulmonary source of bleeding. Signs of systemic disease (e.g., telangiectasias, hepatomegaly, congestive heart failure) should be sought.

   C. **Laboratory studies** include a chest radiograph; sputum cytologies; sputum stains and cultures for bacteria, fungi, and mycobacteria; tests of hemostasis; and ABGs. A urinalysis may demonstrate the red cell casts seen in Goodpasture's syndrome or Wegener's granulomatosis.

   D. **Bronchoscopy** may localize the source of bleeding. Rigid bronchoscopy is required when bleeding is brisk. Fiberoptic bronchoscopy allows evaluation of a greater portion of the bronchial tree and is preferred when bleeding is mild. Appropriate washings, brushings, and biopsies are taken at the time of bronchoscopy.

II. **Therapy.** Therapy is tailored to the severity of the episode and the findings at bronchoscopy.

    A. Therapy in patients with **minor hemoptysis** (e.g., blood-streaked sputum) is directed at treating the underlying cause.

    B. Prevention of asphyxiation, support of vital signs, and control of bleeding are the aims of treatment in patients with **gross hemoptysis.**

        1. Patients in **clinically stable condition** should be positioned with the bleeding side down to prevent aspiration of blood into the contralateral lung. Sedatives aid patient cooperation, but excessive sedation may totally suppress coughing and mask signs of respiratory decompensation.

        2. **Blood loss greater than 600 ml in 48 hours or respiratory or hemodynamic compromise** is a medical emergency. Rigid bronchoscopy localizes the site of bleeding and can isolate and ventilate the uninvolved lung. Fiberoptic bronchoscopy has no role in these patients. Prompt surgical resection of the bleeding site is the therapy of choice. Surgical contraindications include inoperable lung cancer and previous pulmonary function studies precluding pulmonary resection (e.g., a predicted postoperative FEV_1 less than 800 ml). Potential therapeutic maneuvers in inoperable patients include tamponade of the bleeding bronchial segment with a Fogarty catheter or embolization of the arterial supply to the bleeding segment.

Carbon Monoxide Poisoning

Carbon monoxide avidly binds to hemoglobin and shifts the oxyhemoglobin saturation curve to the left. The resulting impairment in oxygen release causes acute tissue hypoxia.

I. **Symptoms.** Symptoms are related to the **carboxyhemoglobin level,** the rapidity with which this level is attained, preexisting cardiac and neurologic status, and factors influencing oxygen demand and delivery.

    A. Levels of **20–40%** are associated with headache, dizziness, weakness, nausea, vomiting, and diminished visual acuity.

    B. Levels of **40–60%** are associated with ataxia, syncope, and convulsions.

    C. **Levels greater than 60%** are associated with coma and death.

II. **Diagnosis.** The presence of symptoms or the history of probable exposure to carbon monoxide justifies hospitalization and immediate institution of therapy. "Cherry-red" lips are not invariably present, and cerebral hypoxia may prevent the expected increase in pulse rate and ventilation. Arterial PO_2 is usually normal, and the ABGs may be misleading unless the carboxyhemoglobin level or oxygen content is measured. The pH is usually markedly decreased secondary to hypoxia-induced metabolic acidosis.

III. **Treatment.** Treatment requires the displacement of carbon monoxide from hemoglobin. High concentrations of **oxygen** are administered as soon as possible (e.g., at the scene of a fire); 100% oxygen improves tissue oxygen delivery and decreases the biologic half-life of carboxyhemoglobin from 250 to 40–50 minutes. Hyperbaric oxygen further diminishes the half-life and, when available, is used to treat life-threatening cerebral or coronary hypoxia. Adequate tissue oxygen delivery should be assured by maintenance of cardiac output and the correction of anemia. Factors that increase tissue oxygen demand should be controlled.

Smoke Inhalation

Smoke is a suspension of small particles in heated gases. Patients who are exposed to a large quantity of smoke in a closed space, or who experience facial burns or singed vibrissae, are at high risk of respiratory complications and require hospitalization for close observation. Respiratory distress may develop immediately after exposure or may be delayed for as long as 2 days.

I. **Complications**

A. **Early complications** (0–24 hours) may arise from thermal injuries, exposure to toxic fumes, or carbon monoxide poisoning.

1. **Thermal injuries** are largely confined to the upper airways because of the rapid cooling of inhaled gases that occurs in the larynx. Massive edema of the upper airway may progress rapidly, especially after fluid therapy is instituted. Careful endotracheal intubation or, less preferably, tracheostomy is required.

2. **Toxic fumes** released by pyrolysis include hydrochloric acid, sulfur dioxide, ammonia, cyanide, phosgenes, oxides of nitrogen, and low molecular weight alcohols and aldehydes. They produce epithelial injury and result in increased mucosal permeability, airway edema, and mechanical obstruction by desquamated tissue and secretions.

3. **Carbon monoxide.** See Carbon Monoxide Poisoning.

B. The most frequent **intermediate complication** (24 hours–5 days) is **pulmonary edema.** This may result from decreased oncotic pressure due to protein loss, increased hydrostatic pressure due to fluid resuscitation, or increased capillary permeability due to toxic fumes.

C. **Late complications** (after more than 5 days) include pneumonia and pulmonary emboli.

II. **Management.** See Chap. 8 for general measures. An outline of specific therapy follows.

A. **Intubation** with a large-bore endotracheal tube is required at the first sign of upper airway obstruction or progressive hypoxia.

B. Scrupulous **airway care** with frequent suctioning is required. Bronchoscopy may be necessary for adequate toilet.

C. **Corticosteroids** increase the already high risk of infection and are of no proved benefit.

D. **Antibiotics** are used only when a pulmonary infection is strongly suspected. They should not be used prophylactically.

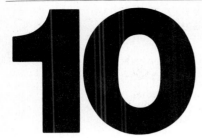

Antimicrobials and Infectious Diseases

The Use of Antimicrobial Agents

Antimicrobials should be chosen only after considering the most likely infecting organism(s) and the clinical status of the patient.

I. **Infecting organism.** Because the infecting organism is usually unknown at the time therapy is begun, the initial empirical treatment must be directed at the most likely pathogens (Table 10-1).

A. **Gram stain.** During the initial evaluation, all potentially infected material should be examined with the Gram stain. Careful examination of this material may permit both a more rapid diagnosis and more reliable interpretation of subsequent culture results.

B. **Culture.** Because the morphology of an organism with Gram stain provides only a general indication of its likely identity, cultures should be done whenever possible. Specimens obtained for culture should be delivered promptly to the laboratory, because delays may allow fastidious organisms to die or contaminating flora to overgrow. Whenever organisms with special growth requirements are suspected, the microbiology laboratory should be consulted to ensure appropriate specimen transport and processing. Specimens from potential anaerobic infections must be kept free of air (e.g., in a syringe or anaerobic transport system) and cultured anaerobically as soon as possible. A candle jar is not anaerobic.

C. **Antimicrobial susceptibility testing.** Susceptibility testing permits a more rational choice of chemotherapeutic agents, although clinical and in vitro correlations are not always precise. Disk-diffusion susceptibility testing provides qualitative data about the inhibitory activity of commonly used antimicrobials against the isolated pathogen and is usually sufficient. In serious infections, such as infective endocarditis, quantitation of the drug concentrations necessary to inhibit and to kill the pathogen is often helpful. The lowest drug concentration that prevents the growth of a defined inoculum of the isolated pathogen is the **minimal inhibitory concentration** (MIC); the lowest concentration that kills 99.9% of the inoculum is the **minimal lethal concentration** (MLC). Knowledge of the pathogen's MLC can aid in planning dosing schedules, since peak serum drug levels should exceed the MLC (Table 10-2). For bactericidal drugs, the MIC and MLC are usually similar. When the MLC is substantially greater than the MIC with the cell wall–active antibiotics, the organism is considered to be tolerant to those drugs. However, the clinical significance of tolerance is controversial, particularly for staphylococci (*Ann. Intern. Med.* 93:924, 1980). Finally, the antimicrobial activity of the treated patient's serum can be quantitated by measuring **serum bactericidal titers.** Clinical experience suggests that intravascular infections usually are controlled when the peak serum bactericidal titers are 1:8 or greater.

Table 10-1. Primary pathogens associated with specific infections

Burns

Streptococcus pyogenes (early)
Pseudomonas aeruginosa
Klebsiella-Enterobacter-Serratia group
Staphylococcus aureus

Skin Infections

Staphylococcus aureus
Streptococcus pyogenes
Haemophilus influenzae (in children)
Dermatophytes
Candida albicans
Herpes simplex virus (whitlow)

Surgical wounds and decubiti

Staphylococcus aureus
Gram-negative enteric bacilli
Pseudomonas aeruginosa
Bacteroides
Anaerobic streptococci
Enterococci
Clostridium spp.

Meningitis

Viruses (enteroviruses, mumps, and
  others)
Neisseria meningitidis
Streptococcus pneumoniae
Haemophilus influenzae (in children)
Cryptococcus neoformans and other
  fungi
Escherichia coli (or other
  gram-negative bacilli)
Staphylococcus aureus (after
  neurosurgery)
Listeria monocytogenes
Leptospira

Paranasal and middle ear infection

Streptococcus pneumoniae
Streptococcus pyogenes
Haemophilus influenzae
Gram-negative enteric bacilli and
  Pseudomonas aeruginosa (chronic
  otitis media)
Bacteroides and anaerobic streptococci
  (chronic sinusitis and otitis)
Mucor, Aspergillus (especially in
  diabetics)

Pharyngitis

Streptococcus pyogenes
Neisseria gonorrhoeae
Respiratory viruses
Epstein-Barr virus
Coxsackieviruses group A
Herpes simplex virus
Bacteroides, Fusobacterium, spirochetes
  (Vincent's angina)

Candida albicans
Corynebacterium diphtheriae

Pneumonia

Streptococcus pneumoniae
Respiratory viruses
Haemophilus influenzae
Mycoplasma pneumoniae
Legionella pneumophila
Klebsiella, Pseudomonas aeruginosa
  (and other gram-negative bacilli)
Staphylococcus aureus
Fungi (*C. neoformans, H. capsulatum,*
  C. immitis, B. dermatitidis)
Mycobacterium tuberculosis
Cytomegalovirus
Herpes simplex virus

Encephalitis

Herpes simplex virus
Arboviruses
Toxoplasma gondii (in
  immunosuppressed patients)
Rabies virus

Brain abscess

Streptococci (aerobic and anaerobic)
Bacteroides
Staphylococcus aureus
Nocardia (e.g., in immunosuppressed
  patients)

Lung abscess

Bacteroides, Fusobacterium
Anaerobic streptococci
Staphylococcus aureus
Klebsiella (and other gram-negative
  bacilli)
Actinomyces

Empyema

Staphylococcus aureus
Streptococcus pneumoniae
Gram-negative bacilli
Anaerobic streptococci
Bacteroides, Fusobacterium
Streptococcus pyogenes
Mycobacterium tuberculosis
Actinomyces

Endocarditis

Viridans group of streptococci
Staphylococcus aureus
Enterococci
Staphylococcus epidermidis
Gram-negative bacilli
Candida albicans and other
  fungi

Table 10-1 (Continued)

Peritonitis

Escherichia coli (and other enteric bacilli)
Bacteroides fragilis
Anaerobic streptococci
Enterococci
Streptococcus pneumoniae (e.g., spontaneous bacterial peritonitis)
Staphylococcus aureus (in presence of a peritoneal shunt)
Neisseria gonorrhoeae
Mycobacterium tuberculosis

Biliary tract infections

Escherichia coli and other enteric bacilli
Enterococcus
Clostridium spp.

Pyelonephritis and cystitis

Gram-negative bacilli (e.g., *E. coli*)
Enterococcus
Candida albicans
Mycobacterium tuberculosis
Staphylococcus aureus (perinephric abscesses)

Urethritis

Neisseria gonorrhoeae
Chlamydia trachomatis
Trichomonas vaginalis
Ureaplasma urealyticum

Epididymitis and orchitis

Gram-negative enteric bacilli
Neisseria gonorrhoeae
Chlamydia trachomatis
Mumps and other viruses
Mycobacterium tuberculosis

Prostatitis

Gram-negative enteric bacilli
Staphylococcus aureus
Neisseria gonorrhoeae

Osteomyelitis

Staphylococcus aureus
Salmonella spp. (and other enteric bacilli)
Pseudomonas aeruginosa
Bacteroides and anaerobic streptococci
Mycobacterium tuberculosis

Septic arthritis

Staphylococcus aureus
Neisseria gonorrhoeae
Streptococcus pyogenes
Gram-negative bacilli
Streptococcus pneumoniae
Neisseria meningitidis
Haemophilus influenzae (in children)
Mycobacterium tuberculosis
Fungi

D. **Local susceptibility patterns.** Because culture and susceptibility testing require 2–3 days, treatment usually is begun with a regimen effective against the suspected pathogen. This choice must be based on local data, because susceptibility patterns vary widely among communities and hospitals. Therapy should then be altered in accordance with the patient's clinical course and the laboratory results, as those data become available.

II. **Status of the host.** The clinical status of the patient determines the speed with which therapy must be instituted, the route of administration, and the choice of therapy.

A. **Timing for the initiation of antimicrobial therapy.** If the clinical situation is acute, empirical therapy is usually begun after appropriate cultures have been taken. However, if the patient's condition is stable, a delay of several days may permit specific chemotherapy based on the results of cultures and susceptibility testing and may avoid toxicity from the use of unnecessary drugs.

B. **Route of administration.** Patients with either serious infections or hypotension should be given antimicrobial agents IV. In less demanding circumstances, IM or oral therapy is sufficient, although IM injections are contraindicated in patients with bleeding disorders. Oral therapy is acceptable if GI absorption is normal and if the serum antimicrobial levels achieved are sufficient to ensure adequate drug concentrations at the site of infection.

C. **Choice of therapy.** Bactericidal therapy is usually the treatment of choice for

Table 10-2. Relationship of antimicrobial dose to serum and urine concentrations in adults with normal renal and hepatic function[a]

Antimicrobial	Dose	Peak serum concentration or serum concentration 30–60 minutes after IV infusion (μg/ml)	Peak urine concentration (μg/ml)[b]
Penicillins			
Aqueous PCN G	3 million units IV	18–80	>1000
Procaine PCN G	300,000 units IM	1.5	
PCN VK	500 mg PO	3–5	400–600
Oxacillin	500 mg IV	25	
Nafcillin	1 gm IV	20–40	500–1000
Dicloxacillin	500 mg PO	10–18	300–700
Ampicillin	500 mg PO	2–6	250–500
	500 mg IV	7–25	250–500
Amoxicillin	500 mg PO	6–8	>1000
Carbenicillin	5 gm IV	200–300	>1000
Ticarcillin	3 gm IV	119–217	>1000
Mezlocillin, piperacillin	3–4 gm IV	60–130	>1000
Cephalosporins			
Cephalothin, cephapirin	1 gm IV	25–100	>1000
Cefazolin	500 mg IM	30–42	>1000
Cephalexin	500 mg PO	13–18	500–1000
Cefaclor	500 mg PO	13	900
Cefamandole	2 gm IV	70–100	>1000
Cefoxitin	2 gm IV	24–85	>1000
Cefuroxime	1 gm IV	27–43	>1000
Cefoperazone	2 gm IV	80–120	>1000
Cefotaxime	1 gm IV	100	>1000
Moxalactam	1 gm IV	100	

Aminoglycosides			
Gentamicin, tobramycin	1.5 mg/kg IV, IM	4–6	100–500
amikacin, kanamycin	7.5 mg/kg IV, IM	20–30	500–1000
Erythromycin	500 mg PO	0.3–1.9	Low
	1000 mg IV	9.9	Low
Clindamycin	300 mg PO	3–5	Low
	600 mg IV	8.4–17.1	Low
Vancomycin	1 gm IV	20–35	100–300
Tetracycline	500 mg PO	2.88–3.25	200–300
Chloramphenicol	15 mg/kg PO	10–20	Low
Metronidazole	500 mg PO	11.5–13	88
	500 mg IV	26	88
Trimethoprim-sulfamethoxazole	160 mg TMP and 800 mg SMZ PO	1.2–2.0 TMP, 26–63 SMZ	11–206 TMP, 27–125 SMZ
	160 mg TMP and 800 mg SMZ IV	6–8 TMP, 45–100 SMZ (1.5 hr after infusion)	38–45 TMP, 137–237 SMZ
Rifampin	600 mg PO	4–32 (mean 7)	450
Amphotericin B	50 mg IV	0.5–2.0	
Flucytosine	2 gm PO	30–40	200–500
Amantadine	200 mg PO	0.3	
Acyclovir	5.0–7.5 mg/kg IV	10–22	
Vidarabine	10 mg/kg IV	3 (hypoxanthine arabinoside)[c]	

[a]These values are general guidelines; individual patients can demonstrate a wide variation.
[b]The actual urinary concentration depends on the urine volume and the amount of drug excreted by the kidneys and varies significantly among patients.
[c]Vidarabine is rapidly metabolized in vivo to hypoxanthine arabinoside.

patients with immunologic compromise or life-threatening infection. Other patients may be treated effectively with either bacteriostatic or bactericidal drugs. Although synergistic combinations are useful in certain clinical situations (enterococcal endocarditis, gram-negative septicemia in cancer patients), combinations of antimicrobial agents should be used judiciously because they also may produce significant antagonism in vivo and enhanced toxicity.

D. Effects of renal and hepatic disease on the choice and dosage of antimicrobials. Renal and hepatic excretion are the major pathways of antibiotic elimination. The dosage of antibiotics excreted by the kidney, such as the aminoglycosides, must be reduced in patients with renal failure (Table 10-3). Thus, drugs excreted by the liver often are useful in patients with renal failure, and drugs excreted by the kidney similarly may be helpful in patients with significant liver disease. Furthermore, drugs excreted by the liver may be valuable particularly for treating hepatobiliary infection, analogous to the use of drugs excreted by the kidney for the treatment of lower urinary tract infection. The measurement of serum drug levels is helpful particularly in the treatment of patients with hepatic or renal failure.

E. Pregnancy and the puerperium. Although no antibiotics are known to be completely safe in pregnancy, the penicillins and cephalosporins are often used. Tetracycline is specifically contraindicated, and the sulfonamides and aminoglycosides should not be used if alternatives are available. The dosage of most antimicrobials must be increased to compensate for the increased maternal volume of distribution in pregnancy. In addition, all antibiotics are present in mother's milk and thus are administered inadvertently to the nursing child.

III. Drug interactions. In current practice the patient who is taking more than one drug is the rule rather than the exception. The possibility of either incompatibilities in solution or in vivo drug interaction should be considered each time a new drug is prescribed (P.D. Hansten, *Drug Interactions* [4th ed.]. Philadelphia: Lea & Febiger, 1979).

IV. Failure to respond to therapy. When a patient does not respond to treatment, the current therapy must be reconsidered. If no obvious problems are apparent, the following questions should be asked: (1) Is the isolated organism really the etiologic agent? (2) Is a previously unsuspected infection present? (3) Is adequate antimicrobial therapy being given, i.e., the correct dosage by the appropriate route? (4) Is the antimicrobial penetrating to the site of the infection? (5) Is drainage necessary? (6) Have resistant organisms or superinfection developed? (7) Is the fever due to an underlying disease, an iatrogenic complication such as phlebitis, or a drug reaction?

Antimicrobials

Physicians have a bewildering array of antimicrobials at their disposal. The number of these agents available and the differences in their action, side effects, and dosage make it difficult to consider them individually. Accordingly, they will be discussed as chemically and clinically related groups of drugs.

I. The penicillins. The penicillins (PCNs) remain among the most effective and least toxic antimicrobials available. Whenever a choice exists between penicillins and other drugs, PCNs are usually preferred. Because the penicillins are usually rapidly excreted by the kidneys, **probenecid** (0.5 gm PO q6h) may be used to increase their short serum half-lives. Similarly, the dosage of most PCNs should be reduced in renal insufficiency.

Hypersensitivity is the most common side effect of the PCNs and may vary from fever or eosinophilia to serum sickness, interstitial nephritis, and anaphylaxis. Persons who are known to be allergic to one *penicillin* PCN preparation should not

Table 10-3. Modification of antimicrobial regimens for systemic infections in the presence of renal insufficiency[a]

Antimicrobial[b]	Primary excretion route[c]	Serum half-life (hr)		Maintenance dosage[d] based on creatinine clearance (ml/min)				Modifications for dialysis	
		Normal	Renal failure	100	80–50	50–10	<10	Hemodialysis	Acute peritoneal dialysis
Penicillins									
PCN G	R	0.5	7–10	100% q4–6h	100% q4–6h	100–75% q6–12h	50–25% q12h	Supplemental maintenance dose after dialysis	Add to dialysis fluid at desired serum levels
Ampicillin	R (H)	1.0–1.5	10–20	q6h	q6h	q6–12h	q12h	Supplemental maintenance dose after dialysis	Add to dialysis fluid at 50 mg/L
Amoxicillin	R (H)	1	10–15	q8h	q8h	q8–12h	q12–16h	Supplemental maintenance dose after dialysis	None
Carbenicillin, ticarcillin	R (H)	1.0–1.5	10–20	100% q4h	100–75% q4h	75–50% q4–12h	25% q12h	Give 2 gm after dialysis	Add to dialysis fluid at desired serum levels
Mezlocillin, piperacillin	R (H)	1	3–8	100% q4h	100% q4h	100–50% q4–8h	33–25% q8–12h	Give 3 gm mezlocillin or 1 gm piperacillin after dialysis	No data available
Cephalosporins									
Cephalothin	R (H)	0.5–1.0	3–18	100% q6h	100% q6h	75–50% q6h	25% q8–12h	Give 1 gm after dialysis	Add to dialysis fluid at desired serum levels
Cefazolin	R	1.5–2.0	15–40	100% q6–8h	100% q8h	75–50% q12h	25% q24–48h	Give 250 mg after dialysis	Add to dialysis fluid to desired serum levels

Table 10-3. (Continued)

Antimicrobial[b]	Primary excretion route[c]	Serum half-life (hr)		Maintenance dosage[d] based on creatinine clearance (ml/min)				Modifications for dialysis	
		Normal	Renal failure	100	80–50	50–10	<10	Hemodialysis	Acute peritoneal dialysis
Cephalosporins									
Cephalexin	R	1.0–1.5	5–30	q6h	q6h	q6–8h	q12h	Give 500 mg after dialysis	No data available
Cefamandole	R	1	5–18	100% q4–6h	75–50% q4–6h	50–25% q6–12h	25% q12–24h	None	None
Cefoxitin	R	0.75–1.0	13–22	100% q4–6h	100% q4–6h	75–50% q8–24h	33% q24–36h	Give 1–2 gm after dialysis	Add to dialysis fluid at desired serum levels
Cefuroxime	R	1–2	15–22	100% q8h	100% q8h	67% q8h	50% q8h	Supplemental maintenance dose after dialysis	No data available
Cefotaxime	R (H)	1.0–1.5	2–6	100% q4–6h	100% q4–6h	100% q4–6h	50% q8–12h	No data available	No data available
Moxalactam	R	2.0–2.5	5–20	100% q8h	75% q8h	50% q8–12h	25% q12–24h	Give 1 gm after dialysis	None
Aminoglycosides									
Gentamicin, tobramycin	R	2.0–2.5	24–60	100% q8h	75–50% q8–12h	50–25% q12–24h	25% >q48h	Give ½–¾ loading dose after dialysis	Add to dialysis fluid at 5 mg/L
Amikacin, kanamycin	R	2–3	30–96	100% q12h	75–50% q12–18h	50–25% q24–36h	25% >q48h	Give ½–¾ loading dose after dialysis	Add to dialysis fluid at 20–25 mg/L
Vancomycin	R	6–8	120–216	q12h	q24h	q48–96h	>q144h	None	None

Drug	Excretion[c]	Half-life Normal	Half-life ESRD	Normal	>50	10–50	<10	Supplement for dialysis	
Trimethoprim-sulfamethoxazole	R	10–15 (TMP) 9–11 (SMZ)	24 (TMP) 20–50 (SMZ)	100%	100%	100–50%	e	Dosage supplement after dialysis based on serum levels[e]	No data available
Sulfisoxazole	R	3–7	6–12	q6h	q6h	q8–12h	q18–24h	Dosage supplement after dialysis based on serum levels	No data available
Doxycycline	H (R)	14–25	15–36	q12h	q12h	q12h	q12–18h	None	None
Flucytosine	R	3–6	70	q6h	q6h	q12–24h	q24–48h	Give 20 mg/kg after dialysis	No data available
Ethambutol	R (H)	4	8	100%	100%	100%	60%	Give the daily dose after dialysis on dialysis days	No data available
Isoniazid	H (R)	0.5–4.0	4	100%	100%	100%	100–67%	Give the daily dose after dialysis on dialysis days	No data available
Acyclovir	R	2.5	19.5	100% q8h	100% q8h	100% q12–24h	50% q24h	Supplemental maintenance dose after dialysis	No data available

aThese are general recommendations, intended to guide initial therapy. Because individual patients may have varying pharmacokinetics, the measurement of serum drug levels is necessary for appropriate dosing in the presence of renal insufficiency.

bThe following antimicrobials do not require a reduction in dosage in the present of renal failure, and dialysis does not alter their dosing schedules: amphotericin B, cefaclor, cefoperazone, chloramphenicol, clindamycin, dicloxacillin, erythromycin, ketoconazole, metronidazole, miconazole, nafcillin, oxacillin, and rifampin. However, dosage reductions may be required in hepatic disease. The following agents should not be used in renal insufficiency: chlortetracycline, methenamine mandelate, and tetracycline.

cPrimary modes of excretion are abbreviated as R (renal) or H (hepatic); significant secondary excretion routes are noted in parentheses.

dThe percentage (%) of the recommended daily dosage to be administered and the usual dosing interval. Dosage may be adjusted by changing the length of the dosing interval or the total amount of drug administered per day. These recommendations presume normal hepatobiliary function.

eTrimethoprim-sulfamethoxazole is not recommended when the creatinine clearance is <15 ml/min. However, several investigators have used it in this setting when serum levels could be closely monitored.

be given other PCNs if possible. In questionable cases, skin testing with both major and minor PCN determinants may be carried out. A negative reaction makes anaphylaxis unlikely but does not exclude the possibility of other allergic reactions.

Coombs'-positive hemolytic anemia, bone marrow suppression and CNS irritation with grand mal seizures have all been described, but are uncommon. The CNS complications usually occur in patients with renal insufficiency who have excessively high blood levels (and presumably cerebrospinal fluid [CSF]) levels of PCN.

The various PCN preparations are produced by modification of the 6-aminopenicillanic acid nucleus. Only the most widely used will be discussed here.

A. **Acid-labile PCNs** are destroyed by β-lactamase. Because they are hydrolyzed by gastric acid, they should not be taken PO, except by patients with achlorhydria. All are modifications of benzyl penicillin (PCN G).

   1. **Aqueous PCN G** is given IM or IV. It is usually supplied as the potassium salt (1.7 mEq K/million units), although sodium salts may be useful, particularly for hyperkalemic patients with renal failure. Because of rapid renal excretion, IV infusions do not provide sustained blood levels although simultaneous probenecid treatment reduces the excretion rate. The dosage of PCN should be reduced in renal insufficiency. An upper limit of 4–6 million units/day is suggested in severe renal failure (glomerular filtration rate [GFR] < 10 ml/minute).

   2. **Procaine PCN G,** for IM administration, gives detectable blood levels for 8–12 hours. Procaine hypersensitivity is a contraindication to its use.

   3. **Benzathine PCN** is for IM injection only; 1.2 million units provides detectable blood levels for 4 weeks. Meningeal penetration is unreliable, because only low serum levels are obtained (≤0.1 μg/ml). The only indications for benzathine PCN are rheumatic fever prophylaxis and the treatment of syphilis.

   4. Methicillin is discussed in **D.**

   5. Carbenicillin, ticarcillin, mezlocillin, and piperacillin are discussed in **C.**

B. **Acid-stable PCNs** are relatively resistant to hydrolysis by gastric acid and thus may be given PO. In general, food diminishes their absorption.

   1. **β-Lactamase–susceptible PCNs**

      a. **Phenoxymethyl PCN (PCN VK)** is the oral drug of choice for infections caused by gram-positive cocci that do not produce β-lactamase. Each 125 mg is equivalent to 200,000 units of PCN G. The usual dosage is 250–500 mg PO q6h.

      b. **Ampicillin, amoxicillin, and indanyl carbenicillin** are discussed in **C.**

   2. **β-Lactamase–resistant PCNs** that are acid-stable are discussed in **D.**

C. **Extended-spectrum PCNs** provide expanded coverage against many gram-negative bacilli. They usually are not recommended for the treatment of infections caused by gram-positive cocci, because PCN G and PCN VK are more active against these organisms in vitro and are also less expensive.

   1. **Ampicillin** is an excellent agent for the treatment of urinary tract infection (UTI), because of its excretion into the urinary tract and its activity against the gram-negative bacilli responsible for most community-acquired UTIs. It also is useful for the treatment of biliary tract infections without obstruction and for respiratory infection due to *Haemophilus influenzae*. Ampicillin is hydrolyzed by β-lactamase and is therefore ineffective against organisms that produce that enzyme, i.e., *Staphylococcus aureus, Pseudomonas, Enterobacter,* and the β-lactamase–producing strains of both *H. influenzae* and *Neisseria gonorrhoeae*. In addition, *Klebsiella pneumoniae* usually is resis-

tant to ampicillin. The usual ampicillin dosage is 0.5–1.0 gm PO q6h for mild infections and 1.0–2.0 gm IM or IV q4–6h for moderate to severe infections. **Bacampicillin,** a carbonate ester of ampicillin, is metabolized to ampicillin in vivo when taken PO. Although the ampicillin serum levels achieved with this drug are twice those achieved with similar doses of ampicillin, its current expense precludes its routine use.

2. **Amoxicillin** is an analogue of ampicillin with a nearly identical spectrum, although it is less effective in the treatment of shigellosis. Because the gastrointestinal absorption of amoxicillin and bacampicillin is more rapid and complete than that of ampicillin, these drugs may be less likely to produce antibiotic-associated diarrhea. The recommended adult dosage of amoxicillin is 250–500 mg PO q8h.

3. **Carbenicillin and ticarcillin** have antibacterial spectra similar to that of ampicillin. They are also active against *Pseudomonas aeruginosa* and some strains of *Proteus* and *Enterobacter* that are resistant to ampicillin. When administered IV, these drugs are effective (in combination with an aminoglycoside) against systemic *P. aeruginosa* infections and may also be effective alone (in high doses) for *Bacteroides fragilis* infections. However, *K. pneumoniae* usually is resistant to carbenicillin and ticarcillin.

   The CSF penetration of carbenicillin and ticarcillin is modest (10% of serum levels) and is not sufficient for the treatment of gram-negative bacillary meningitis. Because these drugs are cleaved by staphylococcal β-lactamase, they are ineffective for infections caused by *S. aureus*.

   The **dosage** for severe systemic infections is 400–500 mg/kg/day IV in 6 divided doses for carbenicillin and 200–300 mg/kg/day IV in 6 divided doses for ticarcillin. Parenteral dosages for uncomplicated UTI are 1–2 gm q6h for carbenicillin and 1 gm q6h for ticarcillin. Dosages should be reduced in renal insufficiency.

   Indanyl carbenicillin, an acid-stable oral preparation of carbenicillin, is effective for UTI due to *Pseudomonas* and other ampicillin-resistant organisms. Because it produces low serum levels, it should not be used for the treatment of systemic infections. The dosage is 0.5–1.0 gm PO qid.

   The **adverse effects** of carbenicillin and ticarcillin include phlebitis, platelet dysfunction, hypokalemia, and congestive heart failure. Both drugs contain substantial amounts of sodium (4.7 mEq/gm carbenicillin and 5.2 mEq/gm ticarcillin). Because ticarcillin is 2–4 times more active than carbenicillin in vitro, and because hypokalemia, congestive heart failure, and the inhibition of platelet aggregation are dose-related side effects, many physicians prefer to use ticarcillin rather than carbenicillin when treating patients with thrombocytopenia or cardiac disease.

4. **Piperacillin and mezlocillin** have antibacterial spectra similar to those of carbenicillin and ticarcillin, although they usually are more active in vitro against susceptible strains of Enterobacteriaceae. *K. pneumoniae* often is susceptible to piperacillin and mezlocillin. Carbenicillin-ticarcillin–resistant strains of *P. aeruginosa* may be susceptible to mezlocillin and particularly to piperacillin. However, both piperacillin and mezlocillin are inactivated by staphylococcal β-lactamase. The **indications** for their use are serious infections caused by susceptible gram-negative bacilli. They should be used in **combination with an aminoglycoside** to prevent the emergence of resistance, e.g., parenchymal infections with *P. aeruginosa*.

   The **potential advantages** of mezlocillin and piperacillin include their lower sodium content (1.7 mEq/gm mezlocillin and 1.98 mEq/gm piperacillin). Although piperacillin inhibits platelet aggregation, it prolongs the bleeding time less than carbenicillin and ticarcillin. Significant platelet dysfunction has not been reported with mezlocillin in vivo.

Recommended **dosages** are 3–4 gm IV q4h for mezlocillin and piperacillin. Dosages should be reduced in patients with renal insufficiency.

D. **β-Lactamase–resistant (semisynthetic) PCNs** should be used for the treatment of infections caused by β-lactamase–producing staphylococci. Staphylococci resistant to one of these agents (e.g., methicillin) in vitro are also resistant to the other semisynthetic penicillins and to the cephalosporins. The drug of choice for infections due to these methicillin-resistant staphylococci is vancomycin.

1. **Oxacillin** is given IV (1–2 gm q4h). Serum transaminase elevations and cholestatic jaundice have occasionally been reported with its use.

2. **Dicloxacillin** is very similar to oxacillin. Because its absorption is better than that of oxacillin or cloxacillin, it generally has replaced those agents for oral use. The dosage is 500 mg PO q6h.

3. **Nafcillin** should be given parenterally because of its erratic oral absorption. Because it is excreted by the liver, it is useful when treating patients with renal failure. The dosage is 1.5–3.0 gm IV q6h.

4. **Methicillin** may produce a greater incidence of interstitial nephritis, cholestatic hepatitis, and agranulocytosis than oxacillin and nafcillin. Therefore, many physicians prefer to avoid its use.

II. **Cephalosporins, cephamycins, and oxa-β-Lactams.** These agents continue to proliferate in such great numbers that it is now useful to consider generations of cephalosporins that share similar antibacterial activity and pharmacokinetics. Succeeding generations of cephalosporins tend to have increased activity against gram-negative bacilli, usually at the expense of staphylococcal coverage. **These agents are never indicated for the treatment of enterococcal infections.**

Properties common to most of the cephalosporins include renal excretion by both glomerular filtration and tubular secretion and the enhancement of their serum levels by probenecid. Thus, their dosage usually should be reduced in renal failure. In addition, all cephalosporins may produce **hypersensitivity reactions** similar to those observed with the penicillins, and some PCN-allergic patients are also allergic to the cephalosporins. **Toxic reactions** to the cephalosporins, other than hypersensitivity, include phlebitis (with IV administration), sterile abscesses (when given IM), antibiotic-associated diarrhea, and serum sickness (cefaclor). The use of cephalosporins should always be considered carefully, since they are rarely the drugs of choice, and they often are significantly more expensive than the alternatives.

A. **The first-generation** cephalosporins include cephalothin, cephapirin, cefadroxil, cefazolin, cephalexin, cefaclor, cephaloridine, and cephradine. Their in vitro antibacterial spectrum encompasses the gram-negative bacilli that cause most community-acquired infections, including *Klebsiella,* and gram-positive cocci. However, *B. fragilis, P. aeruginosa,* and *Enterobacter* are typically resistant to the first generation cephalosporins. **None of the first generation cephalosporins crosses the meninges** in concentrations sufficient for the treatment of meningitis.

1. **Cephalothin and cephapirin** are usually given IV q4–6h. The dosage of 4–6 gm/day is adequate for mild infections; a larger dosage (8–12 gm/day) is used for serious infections. Cephalothin and cephapirin are the cephalosporins most resistant to staphylococcal β-lactamase.

2. **Cefazolin** is the only cephalosporin often given IM. Not only is it less painful IM than the other cephalosporins, but it also produces a higher serum level with a longer half-life. The dosage is 0.5–1.0 gm IM q6–8h.

3. **Cephalexin** is well absorbed orally. The usual dosage is 250–500 mg PO q6h. Its major use is in the treatment of UTI. Although cephalexin should not

generally be used for systemic infections, larger doses (combined with probenecid) have occasionally been used for the prolonged oral treatment of osteomyelitis and other systemic infections (after an initial response to 2–4 weeks of IV treatment with cephalothin or cephapirin).

4. **Cefaclor** is an oral agent with a spectrum similar to that of cefoxitin (see **B.2**), which is also active against β-lactamase–producing *H. influenzae.* The usual adult dosage is 250–500 mg PO q8h.

5. **Cephaloridine** should not be used because of its nephrotoxicity.

B. **The second-generation** agents include cefamandole, cefoxitin, and cefuroxime. They offer expanded coverage against gram-negative bacilli when compared with the first-generation cephalosporins. It is important to note that their antibacterial spectra are sufficiently different to require individual susceptibility testing. Their **CSF penetration is unreliable,** and they should not be used for the treatment of meningitis. Their major role is in the treatment of infections caused by cephalothin-resistant gram-negative bacilli. They may also be used against pathogens of known susceptibility to avoid the risk of aminoglycoside toxicity. The dosages of cefamandole and cefoxitin (1–2 gm IV or IM q4–6h) and cefuroxime (1–2 gm IV or IM q8h) should be reduced in renal insufficiency.

1. **Cefamandole** is active in vitro against most Enterobacteriaceae, including indole-positive *Proteus,* and against β-lactamase–producing *H. influenzae.* It is not active against *P. aeruginosa, B. fragilis,* or *Serratia* and may induce resistance mediated by β-lactamase in *Enterobacter.*

2. **Cefoxitin** (a cephamycin) and **cefuroxime** are particularly resistant to β-lactamase. They are more active against *Serratia, B. fragilis,* and β-lactamase–producing *N. gonorrhoeae* than cefamandole.

C. **The third-generation cephalosporins** now available include cefotaxime, moxalactam (an oxa-β-lactam), and cefoperazone. In general, these agents are more active in vitro against most gram-negative bacilli than the first- and second-generation cephalosporins, i.e., the MICs are lower. The value of these drugs will be determined by their activity against organisms resistant to the older cephalosporins and aminoglycosides, which varies among hospitals. The third-generation drugs now available have not been shown to be effective alone against *P. aeruginosa* infections, and none is effective (even when combined with an aminoglycoside) for the treatment of enterococcal infections. Due to their expense, we recommend restricting their use to the treatment of infections by pathogens susceptible to them and resistant to other antimicrobials. They should not be used for surgical prophylaxis, because their activity against gram-positive cocci, including *S. aureus,* is less than that of first- and second-generation cephalosporins. Until controlled trials have determined whether or not the third-generation cephalosporins alone can replace the β-lactam antibiotic plus aminoglycoside combinations currently used for the empirical treatment of possible sepsis, we recommend that these drugs not be used alone for that purpose.

1. **Cefotaxime and moxalactam** produce significant CSF levels with the usual therapeutic doses and have been shown to be effective in the treatment of **gram-negative bacillary meningitis.** Both drugs are excreted primarily by the kidneys. However, cefotaxime is rapidly desacetylated in vivo and produces serum levels only half of those observed after similar doses of moxalactam or cefoperazone. Moxalactam serum levels are not enhanced by probenecid. In addition to hypersensitivity, moxalactam may produce a prolonged prothrombin time (depression of the vitamin K–dependent clotting factors) by its action on the bowel flora and a disulfiramlike effect with alcohol. The usual recommended dosages for serious infections are 1–2 gm IV q4–6h for cefotaxime and 1–2 gm IV q8h (with a maximum dosage of 3–4 gm q8h) for moxalactam. These dosages should be reduced in renal insufficiency.

2. **Cefoperazone** is more active in vitro against *P. aeruginosa* than cefotaxime or moxalactam, although it is less active against most other gram-negative pathogens. However, clinical experience with this drug is limited, particularly in the treatment of *Pseudomonas* sepsis in compromised hosts. Despite its hepatic excretion, it may have only a modest role in the treatment of biliary sepsis because of its limited anaerobic coverage. Cefoperazone may also produce a prolonged prothrombin time and a disulfiram effect.

III. **Erythromycin and clindamycin.** These agents produce bacteriostasis by inhibiting ribosomal protein synthesis. They are distributed widely in the body and produce high tissue concentrations, although their **CSF penetration is unreliable.** Both drugs are excreted primarily by the liver into the bile, with about 20% excreted into the urine. Consequently, dosage reductions are not necessary in renal insufficiency but should be employed with severe hepatic dysfunction. Gastric irritation and diarrhea are frequent, but hypersensitivity is rare.

  A. **Erythromycin** is used most frequently as an alternative to PCN for PCN-allergic patients with infections due to *Listeria, Staphylococcus,* or *Streptococcus.* Erythromycin is the drug of choice for infections due to *Legionella* and *Mycoplasma,* and may be used for the treatment of chancroid. The usual adult dosage is 0.25–1.0 gm PO q6h and 0.5–1.0 gm IV q6h. The erythromycin estolate formulation is hepatotoxic and should not be used.

  B. **Clindamycin** has a gram-positive spectrum similar to that of erythromycin and is also active against most anaerobes, including *B. fragilis.* Except for anaerobes, it is rarely the drug of choice. Clindamycin is well absorbed orally, and parenteral formulations are available. The recommended adult dosages are 150–450 mg PO q6h and 250–750 mg IV q6h.

  Clindamycin often produces diarrhea, which may progress to pseudomembranous colitis in a fraction of patients (1–3%). This colitis is due to a toxin produced by *Clostridium difficile,* an anaerobe that may proliferate when antibiotics alter the normal bowel flora. Vancomycin, 125–500 mg PO qid in water or juice, has been effective in the treatment of this disorder. Other adverse effects of clindamycin include nausea, vomiting, and skin rashes.

IV. **Vancomycin.** Vancomycin is a bactericidal agent active only against gram-positive cocci. Its major clinical uses are in the treatment of severe infections due to methicillin-resistant staphylococci and for patients allergic to both PCNs and cephalosporins. Vancomycin in combination with an aminoglycoside is also effective in treating enterococcal endocarditis. Oral vancomycin is indicated for the treatment of pseudomembranous colitis caused by toxin-producing *C. difficile* (see sec. III.B). Systemic vancomycin should be given IV over 30 and 60 minutes for doses of 500 and 1000 mg respectively; shorter administration times have been associated with histaminelike reactions (the "red-neck syndrome"). The recommended adult dosage is 500 mg IV q6h or 1 gm IV q12h. Vancomycin is excreted by the kidneys, and its dosage must be reduced in patients with decreased renal function.

  Vancomycin is particularly well suited for the treatment of gram-positive infections in anephric patients, since 1 gm IV will provide adequate blood levels for 7–10 days. Because its CSF penetration is unreliable, CSF levels must be measured if vancomycin is used for the treatment of meningitis. **Toxic effects** include deafness, skin rash, phlebitis, chills, and the "red neck syndrome." Serum levels (30 minutes after the IV infusion) should not exceed 50 μg/ml, to minimize the risk of ototoxicity.

V. **Tetracyclines.** Tetracyclines reversibly inhibit ribosomal protein synthesis and produce bacteriostasis against a wide variety of pathogens, including *Rickettsiae, Chlamydia, Nocardia, Actinomyces,* and *Borrelia.* The most important clinical uses of the tetracyclines are for nongonococcal urethritis, chronic bronchitis, and Rocky Mountain spotted fever. Because the antimicrobial activity of the various tetracyclines is very similar, the significant differences among the available preparations relate to their absorption and excretion.

A. Pharmacokinetics. Although all tetracyclines are well absorbed when taken PO on an empty stomach, the absorption of the tetracyclines, except doxycycline, is decreased substantially if they are taken with milk, antacids, calcium salts, or iron. The tetracyclines are distributed throughout the body, although their penetration into the CSF is unreliable, and levels in breast milk are approximately half of those in serum. The serum levels of the tetracyclines are relatively stable because of their enterohepatic circulation.

B. Preparations and dosage

1. **Tetracycline and oxytetracycline** are excreted primarily by the kidneys. The usual dosage is 250–500 mg PO or IV q6h.

2. **Chlortetracycline** is given in similar doses and has a similar serum half-life (6–9 hours) but is excreted primarily by the liver.

3. **Doxycycline** is almost completely absorbed PO, even in the presence of food or milk, and has a prolonged serum half-life (17–20 hours). It has been used for 1–3 weeks for the short-term prevention of traveler's diarrhea (100 mg PO qd) and for patients with renal failure because of its hepatobiliary excretion. The usual oral dosage is 200 mg on the first day of treatment, then 100 mg qd or 50 mg bid. More severe infections may require 100 mg bid.

4. **Minocycline** is another long-acting preparation (serum half-life is 17–20 hours). Although it is used for *Nocardia* infection in patients allergic to sulfonamides, minocycline is no longer recommended for general use because of its vestibular toxicity, which may be dose related. The frequency of vestibular toxicity is controversial and has varied from 4–96% among different studies.

C. Toxicities. With prolonged use, the tetracyclines may alter the normal flora markedly and produce oral or vaginal candidiasis. Other side effects include diarrhea; vomiting; phlebitis (when given IV); discoloration of the teeth in children; photosensitivity (especially with doxycycline); and elevation of the BUN, presumably from the inhibition of human protein synthesis (all preparations except doxycycline are contraindicated in uremia). Dosages greater than 2 gm/day should not be given IV, especially in pregnancy, because they may produce fatal fatty degeneration of the liver.

VI. Chloramphenicol. Chloramphenicol reversibly inhibits ribosomal protein synthesis and produces bacteriostasis against a wide variety of gram-negative and gram-positive pathogens, including anaerobes.

A. Pharmacokinetics. Because chloramphenicol is metabolized by the liver to the biologically inactive glucuronide, liver disease may permit the accumulation of excessively high levels of the unconjugated (biologically active) drug. It usually is unnecessary to modify the dosage in patients with renal failure.

Chloramphenicol penetrates into all body compartments, including the eye, saliva (where it may produce a bitter taste), fetal circulation, and CSF; CSF penetration is excellent (30–50% of serum levels) and is one of the major reasons for the use of the drug.

B. Indications. Chloramphenicol is rarely used to treat gram-positive infections because of the low toxicity of the PCNs and cephalosporins. Despite its toxicity, chloramphenicol is useful for infections due to *Salmonella* (especially typhoid fever), ampicillin-resistant *H. influenzae, Rickettsiae,* and anaerobes such as *B. fragilis.*

C. Dosage and administration. Chloramphenicol is given IV or PO; IM administration is not used because absorption is unreliable. Chloramphenicol palmitate is administered PO (500–750 mg PO q6h). Chloramphenicol succinate is administered IV in the same dosage, although some physicians use a larger dosage in the initial treatment of meningitis (1.0–1.5 gm q6h for 1–3 days).

D. Toxicity. Although the major concern with chloramphenicol is often fatal aplastic anemia, the frequency of this idiosyncratic complication (1:25,000) is roughly similar to the risk of anaphylactic death from penicillin (1:50,000–60,000). Therefore, the risk of this complication should not prevent the use of the drug for potentially life-threatening infections. However, oral, parenteral, or ophthalmic formulations of chloramphenicol should not be used indiscriminately or for infections that will respond equally well to other antimicrobials.

In addition to aplastic anemia, chloramphenicol may produce dose-related suppression of erythropoiesis, as well as leukopenia and thrombocytopenia. Suppression of erythropoiesis is preceded by a falling reticulocyte count or by an increased saturation of transferrin; bone marrow suppression is usually reversible within 7–10 days after stopping the drug. Dose-related hematologic toxicity can usually be avoided by maintaining peak serum levels <25 µg/ml. Other side effects include hemolysis (in glucose 6-phosphate dehydrogenase–deficient patients), allergy, peripheral and optic neuritis, and superinfection.

VII. Aminoglycosides. Aminoglycosides irreversibly inhibit protein synthesis by binding to the bacterial ribosome. Gentamicin, tobramycin, amikacin, kanamycin, and streptomycin can be considered as a group because of their similar activity, pharmacology, and toxicity.

A. Pharmacokinetics. Aminoglycosides are polycationic, water-soluble agents that are distributed throughout the extracellular space (excluding the CSF) and are rapidly excreted by normal, functioning kidneys (serum half-life ≤ 2 hours). Parenteral administration is necessary to produce therapeutic levels, because gastrointestinal absorption is poor. However, significant amounts of aminoglycosides may be absorbed PO if the mucosal surface is inflamed or disrupted.

Factors that increase the volume of distribution (e.g., burns, peritonitis, retroperitoneal infection) also increase the amount of aminoglycoside necessary to achieve a given peak serum level. Critically ill patients with an increased cardiac output (and thus an increased GFR) also require more frequent doses due to the shortened serum half-life of these drugs. Conversely, renal failure prolongs the serum half-life of these drugs and necessitates an increase in the dosing interval. Although nomograms are available to estimate the appropriate initial dosage, the measurement of serum drug levels is invaluable in most unstable patients. The measurement of serum aminoglycoside levels is usually not necessary in young patients with normal renal function receiving short courses of therapy.

B. Indications. Aminoglycosides are bactericidal for a wide range of gram-negative and gram-positive organisms and mycobacteria. However, they are not active in an anaerobic environment or at a low pH. Therefore, they are ineffective against anaerobes and in the treatment of abscesses and may require urinary alkalinization for maximum efficacy in the treatment of UTI.

Although the aminoglycosides have similar in vitro activity against most pathogens, tobramycin is more active than gentamicin against *P. aeruginosa,* and gentamicin is more active than tobramycin against *Serratia.* Widespread resistance has limited the routine use of kanamycin in adult populations. Plasmid-mediated aminoglycoside resistance results from the enzymatic modification of specific amino or hydroxyl groups; organisms that are resistant to one aminoglycoside are often susceptible to others. Therefore, the clinician must utilize **local susceptibility patterns** when selecting an aminoglycoside for therapeutic use.

Aminoglycosides are used for the treatment of serious infections caused by gram-negative bacilli, including bacteremia in immunocompromised hosts, hospital-acquired aspiration pneumonia, and peritonitis. The limited indications for **streptomycin** include plague, tularemia, and tuberculosis. Aminoglycosides are not systemically effective for meningitis, because **they do not cross the blood-brain barrier.** They are not used for most gram-positive infections, because the PCNs and cephalosporins are less toxic.

C. **Dosage.** The aminoglycosides are administered IM or IV in doses adjusted to body weight. The loading doses are 2 mg/kg for gentamicin and tobramycin and 7.5 mg/kg for amikacin and kanamycin. The usual maintenance dosages in patients with normal renal function are 3–5 mg/kg/day in 3 divided doses for gentamicin and tobramycin and 15 mg/kg/day in 2 or 3 divided doses for amikacin and kanamycin. These dosages must be reduced in patients with renal insufficiency (Table 10-3).

D. **Nephrotoxicity** and **ototoxicity** are the greatest disadvantages of the aminoglycosides. Nephrotoxicity is usually reversible, but may range from mild renal tubular dysfunction to acute tubular necrosis with azotemia. Although tobramycin has been reported to cause less nephrotoxicity than gentamicin (*N. Engl. J. Med.* 302:1106, 1980), other investigators have found a much lower incidence of nephrotoxicity (<1%) for gentamicin when serum levels were carefully monitored (*Antimicrob. Agents Chemother.* 21:407, 1982).

Otoxicity is particularly difficult to assess because cochlear and vestibular testing often are not feasible for the patients who receive these drugs. If possible, serial audiometry should be conducted on patients treated for extended periods. Loop-active diuretics, especially ethacrynic acid, may enhance the risk of ototoxicity when administered concurrently.

In an effort to minimize the risks of these dose-related toxicities, many physicians keep trough levels < 2 μg/ml for gentamicin and tobramycin and < 8–10 μg/ml for amikacin and kanamycin. Renal function should be monitored closely during treatment.

VIII. **Sulfonamides.** The sulfonamides are bacteriostatic drugs that interfere with the synthesis of folic acid by bacteria. Mammalian cells usually are not affected because of their ability to use preformed folic acid. There are few indications for the use of sulfonamides alone, because many organisms are resistant to them and because the same therapeutic effect often can be achieved more rapidly with a bactericidal drug. Sulfonamides are excreted by the kidneys, and their dosage should be reduced in renal insufficiency.

A. **Indications.** The antimicrobial spectrum of sulfonamides includes *Escherichia coli, Nocardia,* and susceptible strains of *Haemophilus ducreyi* (the cause of chancroid). Important uses include the treatment of UTI, prophylaxis against meningococcal disease due to susceptible organisms, topical therapy of burns, and the treatment of nocardiosis and chancroid.

B. **Selected preparations. Sulfadiazine** is often used for nocardiosis. Gastrointestinal absorption is rapid, and therapeutic CSF levels are achieved. Because urine solubility is relatively low, adequate urine flow and alkalinization are required to prevent crystalluria. **Sulfisoxazole** is recommended for treatment of UTI because its gastrointestinal absorption is excellent, and it is rapidly excreted into the urine where it is very soluble. **Topical sulfonamides** for burns include mafenide acetate and silver sulfadiazine creams.

C. **Toxicity** occurs in 5–10% of patients. The most common adverse reactions are nausea, diarrhea, a variety of skin manifestations (photosensitivity, urticaria, and other types of skin rash), the Stevens-Johnson syndrome, drug fever, and a serum sickness–like syndrome. Sulfonamides are oxidants and may induce hemolytic anemia in persons with glucose 6-phosphate dehydrogenase deficiency; agranulocytosis, aplastic anemia, and thrombocytopenia also have been reported. Crystallization of the free drug or its acetyl conjugate (both acidic), may occur in an acid urine and may result in tubular obstruction, particularly with sulfadiazine. Urinary alkalinization and adequate hydration minimize the risk of this complication.

IX. Trimethoprim. Trimethoprim, a pyrimidine analogue, inhibits bacterial dihydrofolate reductase. It is bacteriostatic in vitro against most gram-negative bacilli except *P. aeruginosa*. At present, the only approved use of trimethoprim alone is the treatment of UTI (100 mg PO bid for 10 days), although it has no known advantages over the other standard therapeutic regimens. Its long-term use is discouraged because bacterial resistance develops. Side effects include megaloblastic anemia, thrombocytopenia, neutropenia, and skin rash.

X. Trimethoprim-sulfamethoxazole. Trimethoprim-sulfamethoxazole (TMP-SMZ) is a fixed-dose combination of trimethoprim and sulfamethoxazole in a ratio of 1:5. These agents act at sequential steps in the folic acid pathway and may be bactericidal in combination. The dose ratio and the sulfonamide component were chosen to provide steady-state serum levels that approximate the optimal synergistic ratio of 1:20 for most bacteria. The antibacterial spectrum of this combination encompasses most gram-positive and gram-negative pathogens except *P. aeruginosa* and enterococci.

A. Preparations are available for PO and IV use. Tablets are available in two sizes: 80 mg TMP/400 mg SMZ (single strength) and 160 mg TMP/800 mg SMZ (double strength). The oral suspension contains 40 mg TMP and 200 mg SMZ/5 ml. The IV preparation is a 5-ml ampule containing 80 mg TMP and 400 mg SMZ that is dissolved in 125 ml 5% D/W and is stable for 6 hours. If fluid restriction is necessary, 75 ml 5% D/W can be used; however, this higher concentration of TMP-SMZ is stable only for 2 hours. Dosage recommendations are outlined under Treatment of Specific Infections. Dosage should be halved when the GFR is 15–30 ml/minute, and TMP-SMZ is not recommended if the GFR is less than 15 ml/minute.

B. Indications

1. Treatment and prophylaxis of UTI.

2. *Pneumocystis carinii* infection.

3. *Shigella* gastroenteritis.

4. Serious infections caused by susceptible gram-negative bacilli resistant to other antimicrobials, e.g., typhoid fever, meningitis, osteomyelitis.

5. Acute otitis media in children, particularly in the PCN-allergic patient.

6. Other uses include gonorrhea, chancroid, prostatitis, acute and chronic bronchitis, and nocardiosis.

C. Toxicity. Megaloblastosis, leukopenia, or thrombocytopenia may develop in patients who are folate deficient. Folinic acid prevents this complication without interfering with the antibacterial activity of TMP-SMZ. Many adverse reactions, including skin eruptions, are similar to those produced by the sulfonamides alone (see sec. **VIII.C** above). The large volumes of free water required for parenteral TMP-SMZ may be hazardous in patients with cardiac or renal disease.

XI. Metronidazole. Metronidazole is a nitroimidazole active against most gram-negative anaerobic bacteria, several protozoa (*Trichomonas vaginalis, Giardia lamblia, Entamoeba histolytica*), and *Dracunculus medinensis*. Its bacterial spectrum is primarily anaerobic and includes *B. fragilis*.

A. Indications. Metronidazole is useful in the treatment of anaerobic bacterial infections. These include brain abscess, intraabdominal infections, pelvic infections, osteomyelitis, and the rare patient with *B. fragilis* endocarditis. Metronidazole must be combined with other antimicrobials when treating mixed aerobic-anaerobic infections.

B. Dosage and administration. The GI absorption of metronidazole is excellent, and its distribution is widespread, including the CSF, where therapeutic levels are obtained. The recommended IV dosage for serious infections is an initial loading dose of 15 mg/kg infused over 1 hour, followed by 7.5 mg/kg q6h infused over 1 hour. The oral dosage for serious infections is 7.5 mg/kg q6h. The dosage should be decreased in patients with severe hepatic disease, because the drug is metabolized by the liver prior to excretion by the kidneys.

C. Adverse effects include nausea, dry mouth and metallic taste, disulfiramlike effects with alcohol, and neurologic reactions, including peripheral neuropathy, ataxia, and seizures. Because metronidazole is mutagenic in bacteria and carcinogenic in rodents, it should not be used in pregnant women.

Systemic Antiviral Agents

Viruses are obligate intracellular parasites that principally utilize host biosynthetic mechanisms for replication. Consequently, there are few virus-specific processes suitable for attack by antiviral agents. The presently available antiviral agents suppress viral replication, but viral containment or elimination requires a relatively intact host immune response. The **latency** of the herpes-viruses is unaffected by these antiviral agents.

I. **Amantadine.** Amantadine, a tricyclic amine, blocks an early replication step of the influenza A virus.

    A. Indications. Uncomplicated influenza A infection usually resolves within 3 days, and most patients do not need prophylaxis or treatment with amantadine. However, patients at high risk of complications (e.g., the elderly, patients with pulmonary or cardiovascular disease) may benefit from treatment or prophylaxis. Amantadine has no effect against infections due to influenza B or C.

    B. Administration. Orally administered amantadine is well absorbed. The **dosage** for treatment or prophylaxis is 200 mg PO qd in 1 or 2 divided doses. Because amantadine is excreted by the kidneys, its use should be restricted to patients with adequate renal function. **Treatment** should begin as soon after exposure as possible or within 48 hours after the onset of symptoms. Treatment can be discontinued 48 hours after symptoms have disappeared. **Prophylaxis** should begin whenever influenza A is documented in the community. Because amantadine does not interfere with the immunogenicity of inactivated influenza vaccine, it may be started concurrently with vaccination, then discontinued 14 days later when protective antibodies have developed.

    C. Adverse effects. Central nervous system symptoms are the most common toxicities and include confusion, slurring of speech, blurred vision, and sleep disturbances. Amantadine is teratogenic and should not be administered to pregnant women.

II. **Vidarabine.** Vidarabine (adenine arabinoside) is an adenosine analogue that inhibits DNA synthesis. It is active in vitro against many DNA viruses, especially herpes simplex viruses types 1 and 2, and varicella-zoster virus.

    A. Indications. Vidarabine currently is indicated for the treatments of **herpes simplex encephalitis** and neonatal herpes simplex infections.

    Herpes simplex virus is the most common cause of nonepidemic infectious encephalitis. Early vidarabine treatment of patients with biopsy-proven herpes simplex encephalitis significantly reduces the morbidity and mortality of this disease. **Disseminated varicella-zoster infections,** which rarely are fatal, usually occur in immunocompromised patients. Early treatment of these patients with vidarabine may accelerate the healing process, although the incidence of postherpetic neuralgia is unchanged. Vidarabine has no proven role in the treatment of other viral infections, e.g., cytomegalovirus, Epstein-Barr virus, or adenovirus.

B. Administration. Treatment for herpes simplex encephalitis is 15 mg/kg/day IV infused over 12–24 hours for 10 days. Because the drug is excreted by the kidneys, its dosage should be reduced in renal failure. Each 1 milligram of drug requires 2.22 ml of IV infusion fluid; this large fluid load may prove hazardous for patients with underlying cardiac or renal disease.

C. Adverse effects include nausea, diarrhea, and bone marrow suppression. Serious CNS complications, including coma and death, have been observed in patients with renal failure.

III. Acyclovir. Acyclovir (acycloguanosine) is phosphorylated to acyclovir monophosphate by a virus-coded thymidine kinase found in some herpesviruses. Acyclovir monophosphate is further phosphorylated and eventually inhibits viral DNA polymerase and halts DNA synthesis. Acyclovir is most active against herpes simplex types 1 and 2 and varicella-zoster virus.

A. Indications. Preliminary studies indicate that acyclovir is effective for the suppression of mucocutaneous and disseminated herpes simplex infections in immunocompromised patients. Infection usually recurs after treatment, however, if the underlying immunodeficiency persists. Treatment with acyclovir may also shorten the infectivity periods of herpes simplex types 1 and 2 infections in normal hosts. Although acyclovir reduces the infectivity of varicella-zoster infections, its benefits for the treatment of the normal host have not been defined.

B. Dosages and administration. Although bioavailability of an **oral** dose is only 15–30%, adequate serum levels may be achieved for effective therapy. The **intravenous** dosage is 5.0 mg/kg infused over 1 hour q8h. Parenteral dosages should be reduced in renal failure, because the kidneys excrete acyclovir by glomerular filtration and tubular secretion (Table 10-3). The recommended dosage for a 5% **topical** ointment is the application of amounts sufficient to cover the lesions every 3 hours 6 times/day for 7 days. The patient should use a finger cot or glove to avoid autoinoculation or transmission to others.

C. Adverse effects have been minimal and include cutaneous irritation if extravasated, elevations in serum creatinine, and transient elevations in serum transaminases.

Treatment of Infectious Diseases

I. General principles

A. The choice of an antimicrobial is not the only important therapeutic measure in treating infectious diseases. Several other measures that should be considered follow.

1. **A direct attack on protected sites of infection** requires the removal of foreign bodies, drainage of abscesses and empyema, and relief of obstruction.

2. **Treatment of predisposing conditions.** Conditions such as diabetes, uremia, cardiac failure, hepatic coma, and adrenal insufficiency must be treated. Iatrogenic immunosuppression should be decreased or stopped whenever possible.

3. **Optimal supportive care** includes the maintenance of adequate hydration and oxygenation, electrolyte balance, and hemodynamics.

4. **Passive immunization** is indicated in the treatment of rabies, tetanus, and diphtheria and is useful in persons with immunoglobulin deficiencies.

B. Fever does not require therapy unless the patient manifests complications. Antipyretics are indicated if there is a probability of cardiac or respiratory insufficiency, or a possibility of CNS damage. Care must be exercised not to obscure fever due to inadequate therapy or emerging complications. **Antipyretics should never be administered routinely.**

C. Isolation techniques (contact, respiratory, intestinal, general) should be specified and **rigidly enforced.** Experience has shown that the persons least likely to practice good isolation techniques are physicians.

D. An acute-phase serum is often valuable when uncertainty exists about the admitting diagnosis. Serum should be collected and frozen until a convalescent sample can be obtained. Demonstration of a high serologic titer or changing titers may establish a diagnosis, particularly in atypical pneumonias, systemic mycoses such as histoplasmosis and coccidioidomycosis, infectious vasculitides, viral diseases, and certain parasitic diseases.

E. Antimicrobial combinations. The use of multiple antimicrobials is generally justified in critically ill patients when (1) the identity of the infecting organism is not apparent, (2) the suspected pathogen has a variable antimicrobial susceptibility, and (3) high morbidity or mortality may be associated with failure to initiate correct antimicrobial therapy promptly. Antimicrobial combinations specifically are indicated to (1) produce synergism (enterococcal endocarditis and gram-negative sepsis in cancer patients), (2) treat infections probably due to multiple organisms (e.g., peritonitis following a ruptured viscus), and (3) prevent the emergence of antimicrobial resistance (e.g., tuberculosis). The indiscriminate use of multiple antimicrobials should be avoided because of their toxicity and potential pharmacologic antagonism.

F. Duration of therapy. Treatment of acute, uncomplicated infections should be continued until the patient has been afebrile and clinically well for a minimum of 72 hours. Chronic infections (e.g., bacterial endocarditis) require longer treatment (Table 10-4), and follow-up cultures should be obtained to assess the effectiveness of therapy. Changes in the normal flora are to be expected but do not require treatment unless there is evidence of infection.

II. Pneumonia. Pneumonia accounts for about 10% of all admissions to medical wards and remains an important cause of death during the productive years of life. Although the pneumococcus is the most common etiologic agent, many bacteria, viruses, and fungi can cause pneumonia.

A. Diagnosis

   1. Sputum examination. An adequate sputum specimen must be obtained for gross and microscopic examination. If the patient can cough, other measures should not be necessary. If the patient cannot produce a sputum specimen, aerosolization of warmed saline may be helpful. Specimens containing more than 10 epithelial cells/low-power field on Gram's stain represent oral rather than pulmonary secretions and are inadequate for microscopic examination and culture.

   2. Nasotracheal suction, when properly performed, can be helpful in inducing cough as well as in obtaining diagnostic sputum.

   3. Transtracheal aspiration may be valuable when: (1) adequate sputum cannot be obtained by more conventional methods; (2) anaerobic infection is a possibility; and (3) the pneumonitis is not resolving despite therapy. The complications of this procedure are inversely related to expertise and include death in hypoxic patients, hemorrhage, and pneumomediastinum.

   4. Direct needle aspiration, bronchial brushings, transbronchial biopsy, and **open lung biopsy** are often helpful in diagnosing severe pneumonias caused by organisms not normally recoverable from sputum (e.g., *Pneumocystis carinii, Nocardia,* or fungi).

Table 10-4. Suggested duration of antimicrobial therapy.[a]

Site	Clinical diagnosis	Therapy (days)
Bone	Acute osteomyelitis	42
Endocardium	Acute bacterial endocarditis	28–42
	Subacute bacterial endocarditis:	
	Viridans streptococci	28
	Enterococci	42
Genital Tract	Acute salpingitis	10
Joints	Septic arthritis	14
	Gonococcal arthritis (nonpurulent)	7
Kidneys	Upper UTI (pyelonephritis)	14
Lungs	Staphylococcal pneumonia	21–28
	Tuberculosis	180–270
	Legionnaire's disease	21
Meninges	Bacterial meningitis	14
	Cryptococcal meningitis	42
Pharynx	Group A streptococcal pharyngitis	10[b]
	Gonococcal pharyngitis	1 or 5

[a]The recommended duration is a minimum or average time and should not be construed as absolute.
[b]Drug and dosage: PCN VK, 250 mg PO qid. A more efficient treatment that assures compliance is a single dose of benzathine PCN, 1.2 million units IM.

5. **Cultures.** An adequate specimen of sputum should always be cultured (see **II.A.1**). Approximately 30% of persons with pneumococcal pneumonia will have a transient bacteremia, and thus blood cultures are often positive. Sputum should not be cultured anaerobically, because contaminating pharyngeal organisms may produce false-positive results.

6. **Leukocyte count.** Neutrophilia suggests bacterial infection. However, the leukocyte count may be low or normal in patients with overwhelming infections, in immunocompromised patients, and in the elderly or debilitated.

7. **A chest roentgenogram** is helpful in confirming the diagnosis of pneumonia, although it is not specific. It is valuable particularly in detecting small effusions, abscesses, and cavities. Small effusions are best demonstrated by placing the patient in the lateral decubitus position with the involved side dependent.

B. **General therapeutic measures.** Adequate hydration is essential. **Antitussives** are unnecessary unless continued coughing is exhausting the patient. Control of **pleuritic pain** may be accomplished with anti-inflammatory agents, analgesics, or intercostal nerve block. Nerve block is especially useful when the pain is well localized or is due to fractured or bruised ribs. **Oxygen** should be administered when indicated (see Chap. 8); nasal administration is preferred, because a mask interferes with coughing. Continuous gastric suction may be necessary when **gastric dilatation** or **paralytic ileus** complicates pneumonia.

C. **Antibiotic therapy**

1. **Pneumonias caused by gram-positive organisms**

a. *Streptococcus pneumoniae* **(pneumococcus).** In uncomplicated cases, the drug of choice is procaine PCN G, 600,000 units IM q12h. After clinical improvement, oral agents may be used, e.g., PCN VK, 250 mg q6h. Seriously ill patients are treated with PCN G, 5–10 million units/day IV in 4–6 divided doses. In patients allergic to PCN, erythromycin may be substituted. Although outbreaks of disease due to multiply resistant *S. pneumoniae* have occurred, these organisms have not been endemic in the United States and have uniformly been susceptible to vancomycin.

b. **Staphylococcus aureus.** Because the majority of staphylococcal infections are caused by organisms resistant to PCN, a β-lactamase–resistant PCN (e.g., oxacillin, 6–12 gm/day IV) should be used to initiate therapy. If the organism is susceptible to PCN G (by MIC), it is reasonable to substitute this less expensive drug in a dose of 4–6 million units/day. Treatment of staphylococcal pneumonia usually should be continued for a minimum of 3–4 weeks.

2. **Gram-negative bacillary pneumonias** usually result from aspiration in elderly, immunosuppressed, or otherwise debilitated patients, particularly those with an impaired gag reflex. When the infecting species is unknown, it is advisable to begin with two drugs (e.g., a cephalosporin plus an aminoglycoside) and then adjust the regimen according to the results of culture and susceptibility testing.

   a. **Klebsiella** pneumonia is a virulent, necrotizing infection generally seen in alcoholic or otherwise debilitated patients. Abscess formation is frequent. This is one of the few situations in which **cephalothin** is the drug of choice; the dosage is 2 gm IV q4h. Aminoglycosides may be used in combination with cephalothin in severe infections or as alternative drugs in patients allergic to the cephalosporins. Treatment should be continued until recovery is complete.

   b. **Haemophilus influenzae** pneumonia often follows severe viral respiratory infection. The drug of choice is ampicillin, 1–2 gm IV or PO q6h if the pathogen is β-lactamase negative. Alternatives acceptable for β-lactamase–positive organisms include cefamandole, TMP-SMZ, cefaclor, and chloramphenicol.

   c. **Pseudomonas** pneumonia is a severe necrotizing infection that requires intensive parenteral therapy with a **combination** of tobramycin or gentamicin (5 mg/kg/day) plus carbenicillin (30–40 gm/day) or ticarcillin (15–24 gm/day). The combination is preferred, because it produces synergism in vitro and because resistance to carbenicillin or ticarcillin alone develops rapidly in vivo. Amikacin may be substituted for tobramycin or gentamicin. Piperacillin or mezlocillin may be substituted for carbenicillin or ticarcillin. Empyema is common in this disease.

3. **Atypical pneumonias**

   a. **Mycoplasma pneumoniae pneumonia.** The drug of choice is erythromycin (500 mg PO q6h). Tetracycline is an effective alternative, given in the same dosage.

   b. **Chlamydia psittaci pneumonia (psittacosis).** The drug of choice is tetracycline, 500 mg PO qid. Treatment should be continued for 2–3 weeks to minimize the danger of relapse. In severe infections, tetracycline should be given IV until the patient is afebrile and then continued orally.

   c. **Legionnaire's disease (Legionella pneumophila** and other **Legionellaceae).** The drug of choice is erythromycin, 0.5–1.0 gm q6h for 21 days. Critically ill patients should be given IV therapy initially.

   d. **Pneumocystis carinii pneumonia.** The treatment of choice is TMP-SMZ for at least 14 days. The therapeutic dose is 5 mg/kg TMP and 25 mg/kg SMZ PO or IV q6h. Peak serum levels of 5–8 μg/ml for TMP and 100–150 μg/ml for SMZ may be necessary for therapeutic efficacy. If the drug is given PO, serum levels of SMZ alone or of both SMZ and TMP should be measured to document adequate GI absorption. Alternative therapy with pentamidine isethionate is obtainable from the Centers for Disease Control (telephone: 404-329-3670). The dosage for **prophylaxis** is 2 mg/kg TMP and 10 mg/kg SMZ PO bid.

e. Q fever *(Coxiella burnetii)* is a systemic disease with occasional pulmonary involvement. Although the response to antibiotics is often disappointing, most clinicians administer tetracycline (500 mg PO q6h). Chloramphenicol is an alternative.

D. Complications of pneumonia include empyema, abscess formation, and purulent pericarditis. Empyema requires drainage by either repeated thoracenteses or by chest tube if the effusion is thick and cannot be adequately drained by thoracentesis.

III. Lung abscess. Lung abscess is discussed in Chap. 9.

IV. Urinary tract infections. Urinary tract infections clinically present as lower UTI (urethritis or cystitis) or upper UTI (pyelonephritis). **Lower UTI** is characterized by pyuria, often with dysuria, urgency, or frequency. A properly collected and promptly cultured clean-voided, midstream urine specimen from a patient with significant bacteriuria should yield $>10^4-10^5$ bacteria/ml on quantitative culture. A rapid, suggestive diagnosis is afforded by Gram stain of an unspun, clean-voided urine specimen; more than one organism/oil-immersion field correlates with at least 10^5 organisms/ml urine. Quantitative routine urine cultures in patients with urethritis are negative ($<10^4$ bacteria/ml), whereas significant bacteriuria is usually present in cystitis.

Upper UTI is an infection of the renal parenchyma. Presenting symptoms vary but may include fever and flank pain, as well as lower tract symptoms. Urine specimens characteristically demonstrate significant bacteriuria, pyuria, and occasional leukocyte casts.

Other sites of infection in the genitourinary tract (epididymis, prostate gland, perinephric areas) often are associated with $<10^3$ bacteria/ml urine and have different clinical manifestations.

A. Acute urethritis syndrome is usually a sexually transmitted disease due to *Chlamydia trachomatis* or *N. gonorrhoeae.* The urethral exudate should be cultured for *N. gonorrhoeae.* **Treatment** is with tetracycline (500 mg PO qid for at least 7 days) or doxycycline (100 mg PO bid for at least 7 days). Erythromycin is an alternative for the pregnant patient with nongonococcal urethritis.

B. Lower UTI in adults usually occurs in women, the incidence increasing linearly with age. Recurrent symptomatic UTI may be associated with sexual activity. The significance of asymptomatic bacteriuria in the nonobstructed adult urinary tract is controversial; it should be documented by at least two cultures. Infections in men under 50 are uncommon and suggest anatomic or functional abnormalities of the GU tract. **Men should have a complete GU evaluation after the first infection; women should have a similar evaluation only after three or more recurrences.** Chronic UTI is usually associated with significant urine residual, as with obstruction or neurogenic bladder dysfunction, or with frequent instrumentation or catheterization.

The most common urinary pathogen in community-acquired UTI is *E. coli* susceptible to most antimicrobials. Gram-positive organisms, including the enterococci, account for less than 10% of all UTI. Chronic complicated infections may be due to *E. coli* but are also frequently due to *Klebsiella-Enterobacter* species, *Proteus, Pseudomonas,* and enterococci.

1. Therapy. Single-dose oral regimens are sufficient for nonpregnant females with no known anatomic or functional abnormalities. Standard oral regimens (7–10 days) are administered to all other patients, including males, pregnant females, patients with symptoms of upper UTI, and patients with underlying renal disease or renal obstruction. Children and pregnant women with asymptomatic bacteriuria should be treated according to standard regimens.

    a. Single-dose oral regimens: amoxicillin 3 gm; sulfisoxazole 2 gm; or 160 mg TMP/800 mg SMZ.

    b. Standard oral regimens

        (1) Sulfisoxazole, 2-gm initial dose, then 1–2 gm qid for 10 days.

        (2) Ampicillin, 500 mg qid for 10 days.

        (3) Cephalexin 500 mg qid for 7–10 days.

        (4) Indanyl carbenicillin, 500–1000 mg qid for 7–10 days, may be used for organisms resistant to other antimicrobials.

  2. Failure of therapy for an infection due to a susceptible organism suggests an anatomic or functional urinary tract abnormality or persistent renal infection.

  3. Prophylaxis may be helpful for patients with frequent lower UTIs. Sterilization of the urine with a standard regimen is necessary before initiating prophylaxis. Then 40 mg TMP and 200 mg SMZ every night or every other night usually is sufficient. For female patients with relapses that correlate with sexual intercourse, ampicillin, 250 mg, or 80 mg TMP with 400 mg SMZ after coitus may provide adequate prophylaxis.

  4. Catheters. Although a urinary catheter may be indispensable for patient care, the indications for its use always should be clear. Catheters are placed with aseptic technique and removed as soon as possible. Follow-up urine cultures should then be obtained. When an indwelling catheter must be inserted, a closed urinary drainage system should be used. The catheter should not be irrigated unless it is obstructed. The care of patients with chronic indwelling catheters is controversial. The development of bacteriuria is inevitable, and long-term antimicrobial suppression simply selects for multiply resistant bacteria. We recommend that patients with indwelling catheters and bacteriuria be treated with systemic antimicrobials only if they become symptomatic.

C. Upper UTI is usually associated with the same pathogens responsible for lower UTI. **Acute nonobstructive pyelonephritis** should respond to antimicrobials and hydration without sequelae. Ampicillin, 1 gm IV q4–6h for 10–14 days, is the drug of choice for susceptible organisms in nonallergic patients. Alternative agents include gentamicin, tobramycin, and TMP-SMZ. **Acute obstructive pyelonephritis** may require more prolonged treatment, and relief of the underlying obstruction is critical for long-term cure.

D. Chronic pyelonephritis (chronic interstitial nephritis) is a pathologic diagnosis. There may be multiple causes, including vesicoureteral reflux and infection, obstruction, and analgesic nephropathy. Appropriate treatment of these patients requires an etiologic diagnosis.

E. Infected calculi, particularly struvite, often are associated with *Proteus* species and other urea-splitting organisms. Pyelolithotomy may be helpful in conjunction with prolonged therapy with an appropriate antibiotic, usually penicillin or ampicillin (*J. Urol.* 122:592, 1979). Struvite stones may dissolve with prolonged antimicrobial therapy alone.

F. Prostatitis may not produce bacterial counts $> 10^3$ organisms/ml urine. Therefore, special techniques, such as quantitative urine culture before and after prostatic massage, may be necessary to demonstrate this infection (*Invest. Urol.* 5:492, 1968). Prostatitis is usually caused by enteric gram-negative bacilli. **Acute prostatitis** should be treated for 14 days with any of the drugs to which the pathogen is susceptible (e.g., ampicillin, TMP-SMZ, cephalexin). Patients with **chronic bacterial prostatitis** should receive prolonged treatment (for at least 3 months) with drugs to which the pathogen is susceptible that also presumably enter the prostatic fluid, such as TMP-SMZ or erythromycin.

V. Meningitis. Meningitis is a medical emergency. The prognosis in bacterial meningitis depends more on the interval between the onset of the disease and the institution of therapy than on any other single factor. Therefore, when bacterial meningitis is suspected, diagnostic procedures and the initiation of therapy should be completed within an hour after the patient is first seen. Adjunctive radiographic studies, such as sinus x rays and computed tomography of the brain, may be performed electively **after** the initiation of antimicrobial therapy.

Meningitis should be considered in any patient with a fever and mental or neurologic symptoms, especially if there is a history of head trauma or previous infection (e.g., pneumonia). Cerebrospinal fluid pleocytosis with negative cerebrospinal fluid cultures may be associated with viral meningoencephalitis, parameningeal foci of infection, neoplastic disease, subarachnoid hemorrhage, trauma, and prior antimicrobial therapy. **S. pneumoniae and N. meningitidis are responsible for most adult bacterial meningitides;** *H. influenzae,* other gramnegative bacilli, streptococci, staphylococci, and *Listeria monocytogenes* should be considered but are less frequent in adults. *H. influenzae* is responsible for the majority of cases in children below the age of 4.

A. Diagnostic measures. Lumbar puncture should be performed prior to antibiotic therapy.

1. **Cultures.** Because of the fastidiousness of meningococci, CSF specimens should be taken immediately to the microbiology laboratory. Alternatively, **warmed** culture media may be inoculated directly at the bedside and placed in a candle jar. Blood, nasal swabs, and aspirates of skin lesions should be handled similarly. If **viral meningitis** is a possibility, CSF specimens should be cultured promptly. If this is not possible, specimens of CSF and serum may be frozen (preferably at $-70°C$) for subsequent viral culture and serologic investigation. Viral cultures of the throat and stool may provide additional evidence for viral infection.

2. **Cerebrospinal fluid examination** should include cell counts with differential and Gram-stained smears of the centrifuged sediment. Neutrophilic pleocytosis is usually seen in bacterial meningitis. Acid-fast stains and India ink preparations should be examined if the Gram stain is negative. Similarly, a wet-mount examination of the sediment may reveal motile amebas in patients with amebic meningoencephalitis. If no organisms are seen, repeat smears can be made aseptically from the CSF after 6–8 hours of incubation at 37°C in a candle jar.

3. **Cerebrospinal fluid protein and cerebrospinal fluid and blood sugar concentrations.** The CSF protein is commonly elevated (>100 mg/dl) and glucose decreased (< 40% of blood glucose) in bacterial meningitis.

4. **Detection of capsular polysaccharide antigens** may provide a rapid diagnosis of bacterial or fungal meningitis. Antigen detection is often helpful when the CSF Gram stain or India ink preparation is negative or when antibiotics have been administered previously. **Counterimmunoelectrophoresis** can detect the antigens of *S. pneumoniae, H. influenzae* type b, and *N. meningitidis* (groups A and C) in CSF, urine, or serum. **Latexagglutination** assay for the capsular antigen of *Cryptococcus neoformans* in CSF or urine may provide a rapid diagnosis for this systemic mycosis. Newer techniques for CSF antigen determination (principally used in pediatric infections) include **latex-agglutination** for *H. influenzae* type b and group B streptococcus and **coagglutination** for *H. influenzae* type b, group B streptococcus, and *S. pneumoniae.*

B. Antimicrobial therapy. When bacterial meningitis is a reasonable possibility, high-dose parenteral therapy should be administered until bacterial infection can be excluded. Antimicrobial combinations generally should be avoided, although they may be reasonable if the pathogen is unknown or if polymicrobial infection (e.g., brain abscess) is suspected. Most investigators recommend that the antimicrobial CSF concentration exceed the MLC of the pathogen.

Because *S. pneumoniae* and *N. meningitidis* cause most cases of adult bacterial meningitis, large doses of **aqueous PCN G** will usually provide effective therapy. However, if the cause of the meningitis is in doubt, additional antimicrobials should be chosen on the basis of the clinical setting and CSF Gram stain.

Intrathecal antimicrobials generally need not be administered. Exceptions to this rule occur in meningitis due to some gram-negative bacilli, fungi, and amebas.

C. Supportive measures are important, especially maintenance of electrolyte balance and patency of the airways. Fluid intake should be restricted to two-thirds maintenance to minimize cerebral edema and to lessen the consequences of inappropriate secretion of antidiuretic hormone. Deeply comatose patients may require tracheal intubation. Phenytoin or barbiturates should be given parenterally for seizures, although barbiturates may be more likely to suppress respiration. Diazepam, 5 mg IV, may be used initially in patients who are convulsing.

D. Therapy for specific infections

1. *S. pneumoniae.* Penicillin G, 2 million units IV q2h for 10–14 days. Patients allergic to PCN may be treated with chloramphenicol (sec. **3**).

2. *N. meningitidis.* Penicillin G is given as in **1** for at least 5 days after the patient has become afebrile. Patients allergic to PCN may be treated with chloramphenicol. Corticosteroids probably do not reduce the mortality associated with fulminant meningococcemia, except as replacement therapy for hemorrhagic destruction of the adrenal glands (Waterhouse-Friderichsen syndrome).

   Patients with meningococcal meningitis should be placed in a private room on respiratory isolation for at least the first 24 hours of treatment. **Close contacts** and **family members** should receive prophylaxis with sulfadiazine (1 gm PO bid for adults for 2 days) if the pathogen is susceptible. If the pathogen's susceptibility to sulfadiazine is unknown, prophylaxis with rifampin, 600 mg PO bid for 2 days (adult dosage) is indicated.

3. *H. influenzae.* Ampicillin is the drug of choice for β-lactamase–negative strains. Dosage is 300 mg/kg/day in 6 divided doses in infants and children and at least 2 gm IV q4h in adults. For strains that may be β-lactamase positive, current recommendations include the addition of **chloramphenicol,** 100 mg/kg/day IV in 4 divided doses in children and 1.0–1.5 gm IV q6h in adults, until susceptibility results are available. Serum levels of chloramphenicol should be monitored. Treatment should be continued for a minimum of 10 days. Alternative treatment regimens include TMP-SMZ, moxalactam, or chloramphenicol alone. *H. influenzae* is a rare cause of meningitis in adults. When it occurs, one should consider the possibility of a parameningeal focus of infection associated with head injury, mastoiditis, sinusitis, pneumonitis, or an immunoglobulin deficiency.

4. *S. aureus.* This rare cause of meningitis is often fatal regardless of the treatment employed. Meningitis is usually the result of a high-grade staphylococcal bacteremia, direct extension from a parameningeal focus (e.g., mastoiditis, otitis), a neurosurgical procedure, or skull trauma. Initially, **nafcil-**

lin or **oxacillin** (16–20 gm/day) should be administered IV q4h. Cephalothin should not be used because it does not penetrate into the CSF. If vancomycin is used, CSF drug levels should be measured to ensure adequate penetration.

5. ***Staphylococcus epidermidis*** meningitis usually is secondary to an infected ventricular shunt. Vancomycin is employed initially, because *S. epidermidis* frequently is resistant to the β-lactam antibiotics. Although combinations of vancomycin with rifampin frequently are used if they enhance serum antibacterial activity, removal of the infected shunt often is necessary for cure.

6. **Gram-negative bacillary meningitis** usually occurs in the setting of head trauma and neurosurgical procedures or, rarely, in debilitated patients (e.g., alcoholism). Because the pathogen is often unidentified at the time treatment is begun, the initial therapy should be chosen to provide wide-spectrum coverage. Clinical trials suggest that moxalactam (2–4 gm IV q8h) or cefotaxime (2 gm IV q4h) may be effective (*Am. J. Med.* 71:693, 1981), although one group of investigators reports that moxalactam has a variable CNS penetration (*J. Pediatr.* 99:975, 1981). Alternatives for susceptible organisms are TMP-SMZ, ampicillin, and chloramphenicol. If the infecting organism is *P. aeruginosa* or *Acinetobacter,* ticarcillin should be used with an aminoglycoside for a potential synergistic effect. Effective therapy may require both IV and intrathecal (or intraventricular) administration of the aminoglycoside. The adult intrathecal dosage for gentamicin is 4–8 mg/day, which produces CSF levels of approximately 20 μg/ml.

7. ***Listeria monocytogenes*** is an important cause of meningitis in immunosuppressed adults. The drugs of choice are ampicillin, 2 gm IV q4h (or PCN G, 2 million units IV q2h), in combination with a systemically administered aminoglycoside. Treatment should be continued for at least 4 weeks.

VI. Infective endocarditis. Infective endocarditis (IE) is usually caused by grampositive cocci, although gram-negative bacilli and fungi may also produce the disease. Viridans streptococci typically produce the clinical picture of subacute bacterial endocarditis (SBE); whereas *S. aureus* endocarditis more frequently presents as an acute bacterial endocarditis (ABE). However, SBE can be produced by *S. aureus* and ABE by viridans streptococci. Patients with ABE are sick generally for a short time (3–10 days) and present critically ill. In contrast, patients with SBE often are chronically ill, with symptoms of fatigue, weight loss, low-grade fever, immune complex disease (nephritis, arthalgias), and emboli (petechiae and renal, cerebral, and splenic infarcts).

A deformed or damaged valve is the usual focus of infection in SBE. Left-sided disease, involving the aortic or mitral valves, occurs most commonly in middle-aged to older patients with preexisting valvular disease (e.g., rheumatic, calcific). Dental procedures, instrumentation of the GU tract, and other distant foci of infection are frequent seeding events. Right-sided endocarditis, involving the tricuspid or pulmonic valves, is seen most frequently in parenteral drug abusers and in hospitalized patients with septic phlebitis from IV catheters. Despite the frequency of bacteremia in immunosuppressed and neutropenic patients, the incidence of infective endocarditis is not increased in these patients.

Streptococci and staphylococci are the most common causes of SBE and ABE respectively. However, the **microbiology** of IE also reflects the epidemiology of specific high-risk patients. Parenteral drug abusers and patients with catheter-associated sepsis have an increased risk of staphylococcal disease. Gram-negative and fungal IE, although infrequent, usually occur in drug addicts or in patients with prosthetic valves.

A. Diagnosis. The most reliable criterion is persistent septicemia in a compatible clinical setting.

1. **Blood cultures** are positive in > 90% of patients. Three or four blood cultures taken over a 24-hour period usually are adequate in patients presenting with

Treatment of Infectious Diseases **193**

SBE. However, the yield may be reduced significantly if the patient has received prior antibiotic therapy within 1–2 weeks. Cultures should be incubated for 4 weeks if fastidious pathogens (e.g., *Cardiobacterium hominis*) are suspected. Because ABE is a medical emergency, three or four cultures should be taken over 1-hour period prior to beginning empirical therapy.

2. M-mode and two-dimensional **echocardiography** are complementary techniques that provide noninvasive means for assessing valvular and myocardial function. Echocardiography may detect valvular vegetations as small as 2 mm in diameter, although false-positive findings are possible and can result from myxomatous valvular degeneration, ruptured chordae tendineae, and atrial myxomas. The visualization of vegetations identifies a population of patients at higher risk of embolism, congestive heart failure, and valvular disruption (*N. Engl. J. Med.* 295:135, 1976; *Circulation* 61:374, 1980). However, vegetations visualized by echocardiography may persist unchanged for at least 3 years after clinical cure.

B. **Treatment** requires high doses of antibiotics for extended periods, because organisms in endocardial lesions may be protected from antimicrobials in serum and from immune defense mechanisms. Although the adequacy of therapy must be assessed clinically, helpful ancillary studies include quantitative susceptibility testing (MICs and MLCs) and the measurement of serum drug levels and serum bactericidal activity (see sec. **I.C**).

1. **Viridans group and nonenterococcal group D streptococci** cause most cases of subacute IE. These organisms are susceptible to PCN, which produces a recovery rate of > 95%.

   a. **Penicillin G,** 2 million units q2–4h for 4 weeks, is effective. The addition of streptomycin is controversial, although some investigators use it for the first 2 weeks of therapy if the PCN MIC is > 0.1 μg/ml. A recent report suggests that 2 weeks of treatment with procaine PCN G, 1.2 million units IM q6h, plus streptomycin sulfate, 500 mg IM q12h, may be effective (*J.A.M.A.* 245:360, 1981), although the pathogen must be susceptible to both antimicrobials (PCN MIC ≤ 0.1 μg/ml; streptomycin MIC < 2000 μg/ml). If possible, streptomycin should be avoided in the elderly and in patients who could not tolerate its renal toxicity and ototoxicity (e.g., renal disease, blindness).

   b. **Cephalothin** or **vancomycin** are alternative antimicrobials for patients allergic to PCN. Penicillin skin testing and desensitization also should be considered.

2. *Streptococcus faecalis* **and other group D enterococci** cause 10–20% of cases of subacute IE. These bacteria are resistant to PCN alone. The **combination of penicillin plus an aminoglycoside** produces synergism against these bacteria and is the **treatment of choice for enterococcal endocarditis.**

   Patients with endocarditis due to other streptococci with PCN MICs > 1.0 μg/ml may require combination therapy. Recommended dosages are 20 million units of PCN/day plus 3–5 mg/kg/day of gentamicin. In patients who do not respond to this regimen, serum bactericidal activity should be examined. Inadequate bactericidal activity suggests either inappropriate dosing or high-level aminoglycoside resistance. Pathogens with high-level aminoglycoside resistance (MIC >2000 μg/ml) are resistant to synergism with PCN plus that specific aminoglycoside.

   Vancomycin in combination with an aminoglycoside is effective against the enterococcus and is used for the treatment of PCN-allergic patients. The usual dosage (500 mg IV q6h) should be reduced in patients with renal insufficiency. Serum levels of both vancomycin and the aminoglycoside should be monitored.

3. **S. aureus.** Older patients with aortic valve infection have a high mortality and often require surgical intervention. They are treated with oxacillin or nafcillin (2 gm IV q4h) for 6 weeks. An aminoglycoside often is added to achieve serum bactericidal titers exceeding 1:8 against tolerant strains, although the clinical significance of tolerance is controversial. The prognosis is better in parenteral drug abusers with right-sided endocarditis, and treatment with oxacillin or nafcillin alone for 4 weeks is usually sufficient for these patients; they rarely require surgery. Alternative agents include cephalothin or vancomycin for PCN-allergic patients.

4. **S. epidermidis** is an increasingly frequent cause of IE, particularly after cardiac surgery. These organisms often are resistant to PCN, semisynthetic penicillins, and the cephalosporins. Pending the results of susceptibility studies, the treatment of choice is vancomycin, 500 mg IV q6h, in combination with rifampin, 300 mg PO q12h, or gentamicin, or both. Treatment should be continued for at least 6 weeks.

5. **Streptococcus pyogenes (group A) and S. pneumoniae.** Penicillin G, 12 million units/day IV, should be administered for 4 weeks.

6. **Empirical therapy.** When the diagnosis of IE seems well established on clinical grounds, or when the illness is progressing rapidly, it is essential to initiate therapy before culture results become available.

   a. **Subacute bacterial endocarditis. Penicillin G,** 24 million units/day in divided doses q2–4h, **plus an aminoglycoside.** In culture-negative SBE, this regimen should be continued for 4–6 weeks.

   b. **Acute bacterial endocarditis,** or when staphylococcal or gram-negative infections are suspected: **oxacillin or nafcillin,** 2.0–2.5 gm IV q4h, **plus gentamicin or tobramycin,** 5 mg/kg/day IV in 3 divided doses.

C. **Prosthetic valve endocarditis** occurs in 1–4% of patients after valve replacement. **Early** cases (within 2 months of surgery) are commonly caused by *S. aureus, S. epidermidis,* gram-negative rods, *Candida* species, and other opportunistic organisms. The diagnosis is difficult, because fever and transient bacteremia often occur after cardiac surgery. However, endocarditis must be considered in any patient with sustained bacteremia after valve surgery. Treatment should continue for at least 6 weeks and should be guided by the results of MLC and serum bactericidal studies.

   Late prosthetic valve endocarditis usually is caused by organisms similar to those seen in SBE on natural valves. Treatment should be continued for at least 6 weeks.

D. **Role of surgery.** Surgical intervention may be necessary when natural valve endocarditis is complicated by refractory congestive heart failure, major systemic emboli, mycotic aneurysm, or persistent septicemia. Natural valve or prosthetic valve endocarditis due to fungi or gram-negative bacilli usually is refractory to medical therapy and requires surgery. Although 10 days of preoperative antibiotics are desirable, surgery must not be delayed in patients whose condition is rapidly deteriorating.

E. **Response to therapy.** The institution of appropriate antibiotic therapy in IE frequently leads to defervescence and an increased sense of well-being within 3–10 days. However, low-grade fever may persist throughout the entire period of therapy in up to 12% of patients. Drug fever or rash occasionally may supervene and complicate the febrile course but usually is not an indication for changing therapy.

F. **Prophylaxis.** The population at risk of the development of IE includes patients with prosthetic valves, rheumatic heart disease, calcific aortic stenosis, most forms of congenital heart disease, mitral valve prolapse with mitral insufficiency murmur, idiopathic hypertrophic subaortic stenosis, and other intravascular prostheses. Parenteral prophylaxis generally is preferred for high-risk patients, e.g., those with prosthetic valves or rheumatic valvular disease.

The recommendations for the prevention of bacterial endocarditis in adults that follow are adapted from the American Heart Association (*Circulation* 56:139A, 1977) and the *Medical Letter on Drugs and Therapeutics* consultants (*Med. Lett. Drugs Ther.* 23:91, 1982).

1. **Dental and upper respiratory tract procedures.** Parenteral therapy is preferred.

   a. **Aqueous PCN G** (1 million units) mixed with **procaine PCN G** (600,000 units), is given IM 30–60 minutes before the procedure. The addition of **streptomycin** (1 gm IM) is recommended for high-risk patients with prosthetic valves and for those receiving PCN prophylaxis for rheumatic heart disease. **Penicillin V** (500 mg PO q6h) is then given for 8 doses.

   b. **Oral therapy** is PCN V, 2 gm, given 30–60 minutes before the procedure, followed by 500 mg q6h for 8 doses.

   c. **Penicillin-allergic** patients may be given either:

      (1) **Vancomycin** (1 gm IV infused over 60 minutes) begun 60–90 minutes prior to the procedure and followed by erythromycin, 500 mg PO q6h for 8 doses.
      or

      (2) Erythromycin, 1.0 gm PO 30–120 minutes prior to the procedure, followed by 500 mg PO q6h for 8 doses.

2. **Gastrointestinal and genitourinary procedures**

   a. **Aqueous PCN** (2 million units IV or IM) or **ampicillin** (1.0–2.0 gm IV or IM), **plus gentamicin** (1.5 mg/kg IM) 30–60 minutes prior to the procedure. This regimen is repeated q8h for 2 additional doses.

   b. **Penicillin-allergic patients** should receive **vancomycin** (1 gm IV infused over 60 minutes) as a substitute for the penicillin or ampicillin in **a.** The vancomycin and gentamicin combination is then repeated once 12 hours later.

   c. The American Heart Association recommends that antibiotics be given before urethral catheterization in patients with valvular heart disease, but they are not required in most patients with heart disease for upper GI endoscopy without biopsy or for percutaneous liver biopsy, proctoscopy, sigmoidoscopy, barium enema, pelvic examination, dilatation and curettage of the uterus, uncomplicated vaginal delivery, or the insertion or removal of intrauterine devices. (**Note:** Since patients with prosthetic valves are at especially high risk, it is recommended that such patients be treated with antibiotics for these procedures.)

VII. Enteric infections

A. *Salmonella* **infections** may present as enteric fever, septicemia, or enterocolitis. The usual sources of nontyphoidal salmonellae are contaminated meat and poultry products.

   1. **Enteric fever** usually is caused by *S. typhi,* although other species may produce a similar picture. Laboratory confirmation is made by isolation of the organism from the blood (first week), feces (second through sixth weeks), or urine (second and third weeks). Bone marrow culture is a very sensitive diagnostic tool.

   Chloramphenicol (50 mg/kg/day IV or PO) should be given in 6 divided doses until the temperature is normal and then reduced to 30 mg/kg/day in 4 divided doses for the balance of a 2-week course. Therapy for chloramaphenicol-resistant strains is amoxicillin (1 gm PO qid) or ampicillin (1–2 gm IV qid) for 2 weeks, although ampicillin has a higher failure rate. Multiple drug resistance, especially for strains with R factors, has been a problem in Mexico and other nations but has not been significant to date in the United States. Organisms resistant to ampicillin and chloramphenicol should be treated with 160 mg TMP and 800 mg SMZ q12h for 14 days. **Salicylates should be avoided, since they may cause hypothermia and cardiovascular collapse.**

   a. **Complications** include intestinal hemorrhage in the second or third week and intestinal perforation. Relapse occurs within 2 weeks after the cessation of antibiotic therapy in 5–15% of patients.

   b. **Carriers.** Approximately 3% of patients recovering from typhoid fever intermittently or continuously excrete organisms in the stools for more than 3 months and are a reservoir of the disease. These patients should be instructed to avoid occupations (especially food handling) in which there is danger of spreading infection; public health authorities should be notified. Cholecystectomy usually is necessary to terminate the chronic carrier state in patients with cholelithiasis. **Ampicillin** (2 gm PO qid) plus **probenicid** (0.5 gm PO qid) for 6 weeks or **amoxicillin** (2 gm PO tid) for 4 weeks may terminate the carrier state in patients with normal gallbladder function. Therapy with 160 mg TMP and 800 mg SMZ PO bid for at least 4 weeks may also be effective.

2. **Septicemia** frequently presents as fever without GI symptoms. *Salmonella choleraesuis* is the most common agent, but all *Salmonella* serotypes are capable of producing this form of disease. Focal manifestations that may develop subsequent to bacteremia include osteomyelitis, endocarditis, and infections at other sites in the vascular system. The choice and duration of antibiotic therapy depend on the location of the infection; intravascular infections require antimicrobials for at least 6 weeks, often combined with surgery. If no focal manifestations are present, the choice and dosage of antibiotics are identical with the treatment of enteric fever discussed in **1.** Therapy should be continued until the patient has been afebrile for at least 1 week, with a minimum of 14 days of antibiotic treatment.

3. **Enterocolitis** is the most common form of salmonellosis. Blood cultures are usually not positive, although the causative organism can be cultured from the feces. Supportive therapy is adequate in the normal host, although antibiotics may be useful in compromised hosts, the very young, and the very old.

B. ***Shigella* infections.** Bacillary dysentery is primarily a disease of children in whom transmission is by the fecal-oral route. However, the infection also is prevalent among the homosexual population, in whom transmission is primarily by oral-genital contact. The diagnosis is generally made by isolation of the organism from stool cultures. The majority of patients with shigellosis will undergo a spontaneous cure after about a week and do not require treatment other than supportive therapy. However, antibiotics may hasten clinical recovery in severely ill patients. If treatment is necessary, the drug of choice is **ampicillin**, 500 mg q6h PO or IV for 5–6 days. One uncontrolled study suggests that nonpregnant adults may be treated successfully with a single dose of tetracycline hydrochloride, 2.5 gm PO (*J.A.M.A.* 239:853, 1978). Infection with **ampicillin-resistant strains,** which are prevalent in Mexico and the southwestern United States, may be treated with 160 mg TMP and 800 mg SMZ PO or IV q12h for 5 days. Nonabsorbable antibiotics and sulfonamides should not be used, and antidiarrheal agents should be avoided if possible, since they may increase the duration of symptoms and the risk of toxic megacolon.

C. ***Campylobacter jejuni*** gastroenteritis usually presents as an acute illness, with fever, chills, abdominal pain, and bile-stained inflammatory diarrhea. Less frequent symptoms include headache, myalgias, and vomiting. The disease is often mild and self-limiting within 4–5 days, although serious life-threatening disease has been described, and prolonged infection may be confused with inflammatory bowel disease. The diagnosis is established by positive stool culture. The microbiology laboratory should be notified when the diagnosis is considered, since the enriched media and elevated temperature required for isolation may not be included in routine stool culturing. When treatment is necessary, the drug of choice is erythromycin, 0.5–1.0 gm PO qid. Alternative therapy includes oral tetracycline or parenteral gentamicin. Serious infections require 3–4 weeks of therapy to prevent relapse.

D. **_Yersinia_ species** may produce enterocolitis, mesenteric adenitis, or septicemia. Childhood infection with _Y. enterocolitica_ may present as an inflammatory enterocolitis. However, infection with _Y. entercolitica_ or _Y. pseudotuberculosis_ in older children and adults may present as an acute mesenteric lymphadenitis and terminal ileitis that are clinically indistinguishable from acute appendicitis. Subsequent extraintestinal complications that may occur include polyarthritis, erythema nodosum, and Reiter's syndrome. Isolation of the pathogen from stool requires special techniques (e.g., alkali treatment or cold enrichment) and should be discussed with the microbiology laboratory. Septicemia is rare and usually occurs in the setting of an underlying disease, such as cirrhosis.

Enterocolitis and mesenteric adenitis usually are self-limiting and require only supportive care. Sepsis requires treatment. _Y. entercolitica_ usually is susceptible to aminoglycosides, TMP-SMZ, chloramphenicol, and tetracycline. _Y. pseudotuberculosis_ is susceptible in vitro to ampicillin, aminoglycosides, and tetracycline.

VIII. **Osteomyelitis.** Osteomyelitis is an important but uncommon disease in the adult population. The diagnosis must be considered in patients with localized bone pain who are febrile or septic. The diagnosis is made by **culturing the pathogen from bone at biopsy.** The radiographic changes of soft tissue swelling, periosteal elevation, and lysis and sclerosis of bone may be absent when the patient is first seen and may lag 1–2 weeks or more behind the clinical presentation of osteomyelitis. In contrast, a bone scan is often helpful early in the course of the disease, because it may be positive before x-ray changes are apparent. Persons especially prone to osteomyelitis are those with (1) vascular insufficiency (e.g., diabetic patients), (2) soft tissue foci of infection contiguous to bone, (3) bacteremia, (4) hemoglobinopathy (_Salmonella_ osteomyelitis), or (5) recurrent UTI (vertebral osteomyelitis).

A. **Acute osteomyelitis.** In the absence of either vascular insufficiency or a foreign body, in most patients acute osteomyelitis may be treated successfully with antimicrobial therapy alone. The selection of antimicrobial therapy depends on the results of culture and susceptibility testing. If a causative organism cannot be identified, the choice of antimicrobial therapy should be based on the most likely pathogen.

Hematogenous osteomyelitis is most frequently due to _S. aureus_. Osteomyelitis associated with contiguous foci of infection (e.g., vertebral osteomyelitis and UTI infections) may be due to _S. aureus,_ as well as gram-negative bacilli (_E. coli, Pseudomonas, Klebsiella, Enterobacter,_ and _Proteus_). Cure requires high-dose parenteral therapy with appropriate antibiotics for at least 6 weeks. Most physicians measure the serum bactericidal activity of the parenteral regimen to assure peak killing titers > 1:8. This may be helpful, particularly when considering a switch to oral therapy (after an initial clinical response to parenteral therapy) to ensure that the oral regimen has similar serum bactericidal activity.

Osteomyelitis in the presence of internal fixation devices usually cannot be eradicated by antimicrobials alone. Cure typically requires removal of the foreign material. Similarly, osteomyelitis associated with vascular insufficiency (e.g., diabetic patients) is seldom cured by drug therapy alone; amputation is often required.

B. Chronic osteomyelitis is usually associated with the presence of dead and sclerotic bone (sequestrum) that serves as a chronic nidus of infection. Eradication requires a combined medical and surgical approach, with excision of the sequestrum, although suppressive antibiotics may be used if an operation is not feasible. Inadequately treated osteomyelitis, without obvious sequestra, occasionally may be treated successfully by an additional 6-week course of an appropriate antimicrobial.

IX. Sexually transmitted diseases. Sexually transmitted diseases (STDs) are a diverse collection of diseases caused by a variety of bacterial, fungal, protozoal, and viral pathogens. Nevertheless, certain common principles should be applied when caring for any patient with a presumed STD. The **history** should include the patient's sexual practices to identify risk factors for particular infections. For example, male homosexuals have high incidences of infection with *Treponema pallidum, Shigella,* cytomegalovirus, hepatitis B virus, and *Entamoeba histolytica,* among other pathogens. The **physical examination** and **microbiologic studies** should be directed toward the oral, pharyngeal, rectal, and urogenital areas. Because multiple infections are common, studies for several pathogens (at least gonorrhea and syphilis) should be included when evaluating a patient. When possible, cultures should be done in **sexual contacts,** who should be treated to reduce the spread of infection, because asymptomatic carriers are often important in the transmission of these infections. **Follow-up** cultures or serologic studies should be obtained after completion of therapy to document cure. An STD refractory to therapy may represent reinfection, a concomitant, previously undiagnosed STD, or antimicrobial resistance.

A. Gonorrhea usually presents as a purulent urethritis in males and as a urethritis or cervicitis in females after an incubation period of 2–8 days. Humans are the only reservoir. Both sexes, particularly females, may be asymptomatic carriers.

   1. Diagnosis. Gram stain of the urethral discharge that demonstrates gram-negative intracellular diplococci is the best single diagnostic aid in males. It is not reliable in females, because cervical and urethral saprophytic *Neisseria* may cause false-positive smears. Cultures should be obtained with noninhibitory swabs (e.g., calcium alginate) of the urethral discharge in men and from the rectum and cervix of women, plated **immediately** on **warm** chocolate agar or Thayer-Martin medium, and incubated in a candle jar or a carbon dioxide incubator.

   2. Treatment. The recommendations of the U.S. Public Health Service (1982) are:

      a. Uncomplicated gonorrhea. Recommended regimens include tetracycline, 0.5 gm PO qid for 7 days; doxycycline, 100 mg PO bid for 7 days; amoxicillin (3.0 gm PO) or ampicillin (3.5 gm PO) plus probenecid (1.0 gm PO); and procaine PCN G (4.8 million units IM at two injection sites) plus probenecid (1.0 gm PO). The advantage of the tetracycline and doxycycline regimens is the treatment of possible coexisting chlamydial infections. Their disadvantages include the requirement for patient compliance for a minimum of 7 days and their ineffectiveness against anorectal gonococcal infections in men.

      b. Penicillinase-producing N. gonorrhoeae (PPNG) is increasingly frequent in many parts of the nation. The physician should be aware of the prevalence of PPNG strains in the area where the patient contracted the disease. The treatment of choice for uncomplicated anogenital disease is a single injection of spectinomycin (2 gm IM).

c. **Spectinomycin-resistant PPNG** is rare. Treatment for uncomplicated anogenital disease is cefoxitin (2 gm IM) plus probenecid (1.0 gm PO); or cefotaxime (1 gm IM).

d. **Pregnant patients** usually are treated with amoxicillin or ampicillin, each with probenecid as described in **a**. Women allergic to PCN or probenecid should be treated with spectinomycin (2.0 gm IM). **Tetracycline and TMP/SMZ should not be used for pregnant women or nursing mothers.**

e. **Pharyngitis.** Patients with pharyngitis should be treated with tetracycline, doxycycline, or procaine PCN G as described in **a**. Pharyngitis due to PPNG and spectinomycin-resistant PPNG should be treated with TMP/SMZ, 9 single-strength tablets daily (in a single dose) for 5 days (45 tablets total dosage). Ampicillin, amoxicillin, spectinomycin, and cefoxitin are ineffective for pharyngeal infection.

f. **Acute salpingitis.** Gonococcal and nongonococcal salpingitis are clinically indistinguishable. Although first episodes usually are due to *N. gonorrhoeae* or *Chlamydia trachomatis,* subsequent infection may also involve secondary invaders, including facultative gram-negative bacilli and anaerobes. The treatment of choice is not established. Because no single antimicrobial provides adequate coverage against all of these potential pathogens, the U.S. Public Health Service currently recommends several antimicrobial combinations. However, comparative clinical studies to assess their relative efficacy are not presently available.

   (1) **Outpatient** treatment may be attempted if there is no evidence of septicemia or abscess formation, and if the patient is able to take oral medication. Single-dose therapy should not be used because of the high-failure rate. The following combinations are recommended: cefoxitin (2.0 gm IM), amoxicillin (3.0 gm PO), ampicillin (3.5 gm PO), or procaine PCN G (4.8 million units IM at two injection sites), each with probenecid (1.0 gm PO). Each of these regimens is followed by doxycycline, 100 mg PO bid, for 10–14 days.

   (2) **Inpatient** treatment is given IV for at least 4 days and at least 48 hours after defervescence, and then is followed by oral treatment for a total of 10–14 days of therapy. Suggested regimens include doxycycline (100 mg IV q12h) plus cefoxitin (2 gm IV q6h) followed by doxycycline (100 mg PO bid); or clindamycin (600 mg IV q6h) plus gentamicin or tobramycin (1.7 mg IV q8h), followed by clindamycin (450 mg PO qid); or doxycycline (100 mg IV q12h) plus metronidazole (1.0 gm IV q12h) followed by both drugs orally at the same dosage.

g. **Disseminated gonococcal infection (arthritis-dermatitis syndrome).** Several regimens are available for infection due to PCN-susceptible strains: aqueous PCN G (10 million units IV/day) until improvement occurs, followed by ampicillin (0.5 gm PO qid) or amoxicillin (0.5 gm PO qid), to complete at least 7 days of treatment; amoxicillin (3.0 gm PO) or ampicillin (3.5 gm PO) plus probenecid (1.0 gm PO) followed by amoxicillin (500 mg PO qid) or ampicillin (500 mg PO qid) for at least 7 days; tetracycline (500 mg PO qid) for at least 7 days; or erythromycin (500 mg PO qid) for at least 7 days. The treatment of choice for infection by a PPNG is cefoxitin (1.0 gm IV q6h) or cefotaxime (500 mg IV q6h) for at least 7 days. Patients who are unreliable, toxic, or have septic arthritis should be hospitalized. Patients with a purulent joint may require aspiration and more intensive antibiotic therapy.

B. **Nongonococcal urethritis** (NGU), cannot be differentiated reliably from gonorrhea on the basis of symptoms. *C. trachomatis* is responsible for approximately 40% of NGU in the United States and Britain. The cause in the remaining cases is still unclear, although *Ureaplasma urealyticum* may have a pathogenic role. Neither organism is susceptible to PCN. Postgonococcal urethritis may represent coinfection with both gonococci and an agent causing NGU and may present as persistent urethritis in a patient treated for gonorrhea with PCN.

1. The **diagnosis** is based on a negative culture and Gram stain for *N. gonorrhoeae* in a patient with urethritis. Culture of *Chlamydia* requires special techniques that generally are not available. Therapy usually is initiated on the basis of a negative Gram stain and a compatible history without waiting for a negative culture report.

2. **Treatment** of nongonococcal and postgonococcal urethritis is doxycycline (100 mg PO bid) or tetracycline (500 mg PO qid) for at least 7 days; erythromycin is a less effective alternative (500 mg PO qid for at least 7 days). Patients with cultures positive for *N. gonorrhoeae* should receive an additional antibiotic if they have been treated for NGU with erythromycin alone.

C. **Syphilis.** The incubation period for the primary lesion (hard chancre) is usually 2–6 weeks. Manifestations of secondary lues usually appear 2–12 weeks later and may occur several times during subsequent years. Both primary and secondary syphilitic lesions are infectious; the diagnosis may be made by dark-field examination of the primary or secondary lesions or by serologic testing.

1. **Serologic tests** are of major importance in diagnosis but present difficulties in interpretation, because false-positive nontreponemal tests occur in many nonsyphilitic patients.

   a. **Nontreponemal tests** for serum syphilitic reagin (VDRL, RPR) are useful for screening because they are easy to perform. They require a minimum of 1–3 weeks from the onset of infection to turn positive and are invariably positive in secondary syphilis. However, they are not specific for syphilis; biologic false-positive tests occur in pregnancy, in many acute nonsyphilitic infections (e.g., infectious mononucleosis and *Mycoplasma* pneumonia), and in a variety of chronic disorders, particularly the collagen-vascular diseases.

   In addition, the VDRL is used in the **diagnosis of neurosyphilis.** This test should be performed on the CSF of all patients with suspected neurosyphilis or latent syphilis.

   b. **Treponemal tests** (FTA, TPHA) are specific. Their greatest value is in distinguishing between biologic false-positives and true positive reagin tests for syphilis and in diagnosing late syphilis when blood and CSF reagin tests may be nonreactive.

   c. **Serologic response to therapy.** The VDRL titer generally decreases by at least two dilutions within several months of adequate therapy for primary or secondary disease. The CSF titers should also diminish with successful therapy for neurosyphilis. However, the VDRL titer may not change in patients with late or latent syphilis, although it should not rise. The FTA-ABS test is not useful in monitoring the serologic response to therapy, because titers remain positive for life.

2. **Treatment.** The following recommendations are established by the U.S. Public Health Service (1982).

   a. **Early syphilis. Benzathine PCN G** (2.4 million units as a single IM dose) is the treatment of choice for primary and secondary syphilis, latent syphilis of less than 1 year's duration, and case contacts. PCN allergic patients should be treated with tetracycline, 500 mg PO qid, for 15 days.

   b. **Syphilis exceeding 1 year's duration.** For latent syphilis (exceeding 1 year's duration) and for cardiovascular syphilis, the treatment is benzathine PCN G, 2.4 million units IM weekly for 3 successive weeks (a total of 7.2 million units). In patients allergic to PCN, tetracycline (500 mg PO qid for 30 days) or erythromycin (500 mg PO qid for 30 days) may be given.

The treatment of **neurosyphilis** has not been adequately studied. Potentially effective regimens include aqueous PCN G (2–4 million units IV q4h) for 10 days followed by benzathine PCN G, 2.4 million units IM, weekly for 3 doses; procaine PCN G (2.4 million units IM daily) plus probenecid (500 mg PO qid) for 10 days, followed by benzathine PCN G, 2.4 million units IM, weekly for 3 doses; and benzathine PCN G, 2.4 million units IM, weekly for 3 doses. This last regimen achieves a satisfactory clinical response in approximately 90% of patients.

    c. Syphilis during pregnancy should be treated with one of the preceding regimens but not with either erythromycin estolate or tetracycline because of their potential adverse effects on the mother and fetus.

D. Herpes simplex infection (primarily type II) usually presents as painful vesicles or shallow ulcerations (unroofed vesicles) involving the vulva, labia, or cervix in women or the penis in men. Primary infection may be associated with fever and inguinal adenopathy, whereas recurrent disease usually does not produce constitutional symptoms. Preliminary studies suggest that **acyclovir** effectively suppresses disease activity in primary and recurrent infection (see Systemic Antiviral Agents, sec. III). Dyes plus light, ether, and other topical antiviral chemotherapeutic agents (iododeoxyuridine, adenine arabinoside) have not been proven useful in controlled studies. Pain may be treated with analgesics and topical anesthetics (e.g., benzocaine spray), and sitting in a warm bath to urinate may relieve the severe dysuria frequently seen in women. Pregnant women with active genital lesions at the time of delivery should be delivered by cesarean section to reduce the likelihood of transmission to the neonate during vaginal delivery.

E. Vaginitis presents as a vaginal discharge, often associated with dysuria, burning, pruritus, and malodor. The most common etiologic agents are *Trichomonas vaginalis, C. albicans,* and *Gardnerella (Haemophilus) vaginalis,* possibly in combination with anaerobic bacteria.

    1. Diagnosis. Although the gross appearance of the discharge may be characteristic, the clinical diagnosis requires microscopic verification. Wet mount examination under high-dry magnification of a drop of discharge in 1 ml of normal saline will demonstrate the pear-shaped, motile organisms of *T. vaginalis.* One drop of 10% potassium hydroxide may be added to lyse the epithelial cells. *Candida* organisms appear as budding yeast forms, with or without pseudohyphae. Because *G. vaginalis* and anaerobes require culturing for identification, a diagnosis of **nonspecific vaginitis** usually is based on a malodorous discharge, a wet mount examination remarkable for coccobacilli possibly with "clue cells," and the absence of other known pathogens.

    2. Therapy

        a. *T. vaginalis* infection in nonpregnant women and in men is treated with single-dose metronidazole, 2 gm PO.

        b. *C. albicans* vaginitis responds to miconazole vaginal cream applied at bedtime for 7 days. Alternatives include nystatin vaginal tablets and clotrimazole vaginal tablets or cream. Refractory or recurrent infection is often associated with pregnancy, birth control pills, diabetes, or broad-spectrum antibiotic therapy. Wearing cotton underwear and avoiding tight clothing may be helpful.

        c. Nonspecific vaginitis is treated with metronidazole, 500 mg PO bid for 7 days. Ampicillin is a less effective alternative (500 mg PO qid for 7–10 days).

F. The **acquired immune deficiency syndrome** occurs primarily among homosexual men, although it also has been observed among drug addicts, hemophiliacs, and Haitian refugees. Associated with a profound immunosuppression (manifested by lymphopenia, anergy, and a lack of blastogenic responsiveness to multiple antigens), affected patients have an increased incidence of several infections (e.g., *P. carinii* pneumonia, cytomegalovirus disease, and anogenital herpes simplex ulcerations) and a neoplasm (Kaposi's sarcoma). Such severely ill patients are uncommon, but they represent a major problem in therapeutics because appropriate dosages of antimicrobials have often failed to prevent their deaths from potentially treatable infections such as *Pneumocystis* pneumonia.

X. Antibiotic therapy in sepsis of unknown cause.

A. Early bactericidal treatment is essential in the therapy of septicemia. The broadest coverage with the least potential toxicity is provided by a **β-lactam antibiotic plus an aminoglycoside.** The actual drugs used should be determined by the clinical situation. If staphylococcal sepsis is likely, a β-lactamase–resistant PCN should be used. For enterococcal infection, PCN G or ampicillin plus an aminoglycoside is the best choice. In immunosuppressed patients, particularly neutropenic patients, when *P. aeruginosa* sepsis is possible, a combination of an aminoglycoside plus an effective extended spectrum penicillin (piperacillin, ticarcillin, carbenicillin, or mezlocillin) is indicated. Gentamicin or tobramycin are usually the aminoglycosides of choice, except when resistance is suspected, in which case amikacin should be used. A first-generation cephalosporin is often added to cover for staphylococci, but it may enhance aminoglycoside nephrotoxicity.

B. Septic shock may complicate fungemia or viremia, although the most common cause is bacteremia. Early recognition of bacteremic shock is critical, since any delay in instituting appropriate therapy will increase mortality. Cardiovascular collapse occurs in approximately 30% of gram-negative bacillary bacteremias and has an overall mortality of 40%. The GI and GU tracts are the most common sources of infection, but any infection can be the source, including pneumonia, meningitis, abscesses, and wounds. Clinically, there may be two stages of bacteremic shock. In the early hyperdynamic phase ("warm shock"), the cardiac output is elevated, peripheral vascular resistance is decreased, and the patient is warm, diaphoretic, and peripherally vasodilated. This may progress to a second hypodynamic phase ("cold shock") that is manifested by normal or increased peripheral vascular resistance, cool vasoconstricted skin, and finally decreased cardiac output.

Initial evaluation should include a careful physical examination, chest radiographs, urinalysis, evaluation of clinically indicated body fluids (e.g., CSF, pleural effusions), and several sets of blood cultures from separate venipuncture sites. **Treatment of bacteremic shock** should proceed in the following manner:

1. Stabilize the cardiovascular system. These patients frequently have a decreased effective blood volume secondary to decreased systemic resistance and increased venous capacitance. Crystalloid fluids should be administered initially to achieve normal blood pressure; if this is unsuccessful, vasopressor drugs should be utilized. The placement of a central venous catheter or a Swan-Ganz catheter may be necessary for hemodynamic monitoring and fluid management. In addition, electrolyte and acid-base disorders must be corrected and adequate ventilation ensured.

2. Treat the underlying infection with a β-lactam antibiotic plus an aminoglycoside as previously discussed.

3. Corticosteroid use is controversial, although in one study it was found that either methylprednisolone (30 mg/kg) or dexamethasone (3 mg/kg) given IV over 20 minutes significantly reduced mortality in gram-negative septicemia (*Ann. Surg.* 184:333, 1976). However, the beneficial effect was observed only if the corticosteroids were given within 24 hours of clinical presentation.

4. Laboratory evidence of **disseminated intravascular coagulation** may occur, but restoration of blood pressure and appropriate antimicrobials usually are adequate to reverse this problem. Other modes of treatment (e.g., heparin, fresh-frozen plasma) rarely are necessary.

5. Although β-**endorphins** may be important in the pathogenesis of shock, the use of the opiate and β-endorphin antagonist naloxone (*Lancet* 1:529, 1981) for the treatment of bacteremic shock is investigational.

Tuberculosis

I. **General comments.** The diagnosis of tuberculosis is established by culturing the organism. Positive fluorochrome or acid-fast (Kinyoun or Ziehl-Neelsen) smears are presumptive evidence of active tuberculosis, although nontuberculous (atypical) mycobacteria are also positive with these techniques, and *Nocardia* are usually positive with modified acid-fast staining. Pulmonary disease is the most frequent clinical presentation of tuberculosis. Less common clinical manifestations include meningitis, renal disease, vertebral osteomyelitis (Pott's disease), skin involvement (lupus vulgaris), and miliary dissemination.

The **initial treatment** of tuberculosis may include a period of hospitalization to initiate therapy and patient education. Respiratory isolation precautions should be instituted for patients with pulmonary disease. These should include covering the mouth and nose when coughing and the use of a mask if the patient must be moved from his or her room. During this time, the physician must instruct the patient about the disease and the need to take antituberculosis drugs for an extended period. If the patient does not understand the chronicity of the disease and the need for prolonged therapy, it is unlikely that he or she will do so for the many months required for adequate treatment.

Members of the patient's immediate family and other close contacts, especially children, should have an intermediate-strength tuberculin skin test (PPD) at the time of diagnosis and again 3 months later. The local health department should be notified of all cases of tuberculosis, so that studies of other contacts can be made.

II. **Antituberculous drugs**

A. **Primary drugs** have excellent bactericidal activity for both intracellular and extracellular mycobacteria.

1. **Isoniazid (INH)** inhibits the synthesis of mycolic acid and is bactericidal for *Mycobacterium tuberculosis, M. kansasii,* and *M. bovis.*

a. **Pharmacokinetics.** Oral INH is well absorbed and widely distributed, including the CSF. The drug is acetylated and hydroxylated by the liver; these metabolites are then excreted into the urine. Because isoniazid potentiates levels of phenytoin, dosage adjustments of phenytoin may be necessary to avoid toxicity.

b. **Dosage.** The most commonly employed adult dosage is 300 mg/day PO. Larger doses (10 mg/kg/day) are used occasionally for the initial treatment of widespread disease, although the incidence of toxicity is increased. The IM preparation is rarely employed.

c. **Toxicities.** Drug-induced **hepatitis** is an unpredictable complication. Whether or not patients with rapid hepatic acetylation have an increased risk of hepatitis is unclear. The incidence of INH-induced hepatitis increases with age, i.e., 0.3% for patients 20–34 years old, 1.2% for those 35–49, and approximately 2.3% for patients 50 years of age or older. A prior history of unrelated nonalcoholic liver disease does not increase the risk of INH-induced hepatitis. However, daily alcohol consumption and alcoholic liver disease do increase the risk of this complication. Hepatitis induced by INH usually resolves after the drug is discontinued. Although asymptomatic serum transaminase elevations may occur during the first few months of therapy in up to 20% of patients receiving INH, serum levels usually return to the normal ranges as drug therapy continues. Therefore, most investigators do not routinely monitor serum transaminase levels during treatment with INH.

Peripheral neuritis and other nervous system disorders are dose-related complications of INH therapy. They are more common in marginally nourished patients (e.g., diabetic and alcoholic patients), because INH increases the excretion of pyridoxine. The administration of pyridoxine (50 mg PO qd) prevents these complications. Other **untoward effects** include skin rashes, arthritis symptoms, and lowering of seizure thresholds in patients with a seizure disorder.

2. **Rifampin,** an inhibitor of DNA-dependent RNA polymerase, is bactericidal for gram-positive cocci, many gram-negative bacilli, and most species of *Mycobacterium*. Its GI absorption and distribution, including CNS penetration, are excellent. Rifampin participates in an enterohepatic circulation while being progressively metabolized by the liver. Because it induces hepatic microsomal enzymes, rifampin may reduce the therapeutic effects of drugs metabolized by these enzymes, including anticoagulants, corticosteroids, oral contraceptives, quinidine, digitoxin, and barbiturates. The **dosage** for tuberculosis is 600 mg PO qd. Patients should be warned about the harmless, orange-red discoloration of tears, saliva, urine, feces, and sweat that occurs with rifampin. **Toxicities** include hepatitis that may be potentiated by other types of liver disease or confused with INH hepatitis, mild GI disturbances, and a rare influenzalike syndrome characterized by dyspnea and thrombocytopenia.

B. **Secondary drugs** usually are reserved for patients with extensive extrapulmonic disease, in whom the infecting organisms have known or suspected resistance to the primary drugs or who are infected with atypical mycobacteria. Selection of a secondary drug should be aided by the in vitro susceptibility studies of the isolated organism.

1. **Ethambutol,** a bacteriostatic agent, is well absorbed after oral administration. The recommended dosage is 15 mg/kg/day. The drug is excreted primarily by the kidneys; the dosage should be reduced in patients with renal failure. The only significant dose-related toxicity is **optic neuritis,** which occurs in less than 1% of patients at a dosage of 15 mg/kg/day. The earliest manifestations may include decreased color perception, impaired visual fields, or reduced visual acuity. Eye examinations should be included in the follow-up of these patients, because the ophthalmic complications are often reversible with early drug withdrawal.

2. **Streptomycin** is bactericidal for extracellular mycobacteria. The dosage is 0.5–1.0 gm IM daily or 20 mg/kg twice weekly. Except for occasional hypersensitivity (skin rash, fever, or malaise), the major toxicities of streptomycin are ototoxicity and nephrotoxicity.

3. **Pyrazinamide** is bactericidal for intracellular mycobacteria. The drug is well absorbed from the GI tract and is excreted by the kidneys. It is usually given as a single daily dose: 1.5 gm qd for patients weighing under 50 kg, 2.0 gm qd for patients weighing 50–74 kg, and 2.5 gm qd for patients weighing over 75 kg. If administered 3 times/week, these dosages should be increased to 2.0, 2.5, and 3.0 gm for patients weighing less than 50, 50–74, and over 75 kg respectively. Hepatotoxicity is the most common untoward effect.

4. **Para-aminosalicylic acid,** an antagonist of folate synthesis, is a bacteriostatic agent. The usual adult dosage of 10–12 gm/day PO in 3 or 4 divided doses is often limited by the GI side effects, especially diarrhea. Hypersensitivity reactions are also frequent; rarely, they may be fatal. Ethambutol is preferred because it is more active and less toxic.

C. **Tertiary drugs** have the lowest therapeutic ratio for treatment of mycobacterial disease and should not be used without consultation and susceptibility testing.

1. **Ethionamide** is absorbed rapidly from the GI tract and widely distributed, including the CSF. The drug is acetylated by the liver and excreted in the urine. The usual dosage is 0.5–1.0 gm/day PO in 3 divided doses. Untoward effects include gastric irritation, hepatotoxicity, and ganglionic blockade.

2. **Cycloserine** is absorbed rapidly from the GI tract and widely distributed with good CSF penetration. Excretion is primarily by the kidneys. The usual dose is 0.5–1.0 gm/day PO in 3 divided doses. Untoward effects include seizures, somnolence, muscle twitching, and hepatic damage. Large doses of pyridoxine, 100 mg PO tid, may prevent the CNS toxicity.

3. **Kanamycin**, 500 mg IM bid; toxicity is manifested by eighth nerve or renal dysfunction.

4. **Viomycin**, 1 gm IM daily; toxicity is the same as for kanamycin.

III. **Corticosteroid therapy.** Corticosteroid therapy in tuberculosis remains controversial but has been used with the primary antituberculosis drugs in patients with tuberculous pneumonitis, pericarditis, or meningitis. Patients with these life-threatening complications may benefit from glucocorticoid therapy (1 mg/kg prednisone initially, with gradual withdrawal and discontinuance within 4–8 weeks), although it should not be used for less severely ill patients.

IV. **Antituberculosis therapy.** Antituberculous therapy is based on three principles: (1) the incidence of primary drug resistance to a single drug is 1 in 10^6 tubercle bacilli; (2) extended therapy is necessary because of the prolonged generation time of mycobacteria (>20 hours); and (3) successful regimens must include at least two drugs to which the organism is susceptible.

Uncomplicated pulmonary tuberculosis (including cavitary disease) is treated with INH, 300 mg qd, and rifampin, 600 mg qd, for a minimum of 9 months with self-administered drugs. When directly supervised, treatment may be given twice weekly (15 mg/kg INH and 600 mg rifampin per dose) after an initial clinical response to daily therapy for 2–8 weeks as described above. **Treatment must be continued for at least 6 months after the conversion of the sputum culture from positive to negative.** Patients should be observed for at least 12 months after the completion of treatment for the possibility of relapse. Ethambutol (15 mg/kg/day) should be added to the preceding regimens until susceptibility results are available if the patient is from an area with known drug resistance, e.g., Asian refugees.

Complicated tuberculosis includes patients with compromised immunity, silicosis, renal failure, diabetes, and extrapulmonic disease such as meningitis. These patients should be treated with three drugs for 18–24 months. If possible, the drug combination employed should include INH and rifampin. The selection of the third drug is individualized.

V. **Chemoprophylaxis.** The decision to initiate chemoprophylaxis balances the risk of the development of active disease against the risks of drug toxicity. In up to 5% of persons whose skin tests (intermediate-strength PPD) convert from negative to positive, disease will develop within the first year of exposure if left untreated. Adequate prophylaxis has reduced this risk in several studies. The groups of patients in **A–E** should be considered for prophylactic INH, 300 mg qd (adult dosage) for 12 months, as recommended by the American Thoracic Society (1974).

A. Although children have the greatest risk of the development of active disease, all **household contacts** and other close associates of patients with active tuberculosis should begin treatment at the time of diagnosis, even if their initial PPD is negative. Treatment can be stopped if the repeat PPD is negative 3 months later.

B. Positive PPD reactors over 35 years of age with radiographic evidence of previous infection, e.g. apical scars.

C. Patients of any age whose PPD skin tests have converted within the past 2 years (defined as an increase of at least 6 mm from less than 10 mm induration to greater than 10 mm, excluding a booster phenomenon).

D. Other high-risk patients with positive tuberculin skin tests who may benefit from chemoprophylaxis include patients receiving immunosuppressive drugs; patients with immunocompromising diseases, such as lymphoreticular malignancies, diabetes mellitus, and silicosis; and patients who have had a gastrectomy. The duration of chemoprophylaxis should be individualized for these patients, although there is no evidence that more than 1 year of chemoprophylaxis provides additional protection.

E. Positive PPD reactors under 35 years of age. **Note:** Chemoprophylaxis for patients 21–35 years old is controversial, particularly in the absence of the risk factors that have been described (*Ann. Intern. Med.* 94:808, 817, 1981).

Actinomycotic Infections

I. **Actinomycosis.** Penicillin is the drug of choice for actinomycosis and 10–20 million units/day IV should be given for at least 6 weeks, followed by 6–12 months of oral PCN V, 2–4 gm/day, to prevent relapse. Tetracycline is an alternative in the PCN-allergic patient. Surgical drainage of localized lesions may be helpful.

II. **Nocardiosis.** Most infections require a prolonged course of therapy. Sulfonamides are the drugs of choice, given in amounts sufficient to produce peak serum levels of 120–150 μg/ml. This usually can be accomplished by the administration of 6–8 gm/day of sulfisoxazole or sulfadiazine IV or PO. Minocycline is an alternative in patients with sulfonamide sensitivity. Therapy should be given for a minimum of 6 weeks.

Systemic Mycoses

I. **General comments.** The major primary fungal pathogens of North America are *Histoplasma capsulatum, Coccidioides immitis, Blastomyces dermatitidis,* and *Sporothrix schenckii.* The most common opportunistic (or secondary) fungal pathogens are *C. neoformans, Torulopsis glabrata, Candida, Aspergillus, Mucor,* and *Rhizopus.* However, the primary pathogens (e.g., *H. capsulatum*) also cause disease in immunoincompetent patients, and the opportunistic pathogens (e.g., *C. neoformans*) can afflict normal hosts.

The **diagnosis** of a systemic mycosis depends on culturing the organism from appropriate specimens or on the histologic demonstration of tissue invasion. Antibody determinations are helpful in the diagnosis of histoplasmosis and coccidioidomycosis. (**Caution:** Histoplasmin skin tests may elevate agglutinin and complement-fixation titers in the absence of systemic disease.)

II. **Antifungal drugs**

A. **Amphotericin B** is a polyene antibiotic that disrupts the fungal cell by binding to ergosterol in the membrane. It is fungicidal and is the treatment of choice for most systemic mycoses.

1. **Pharmacokinetics.** Amphotericin B is formulated in a bile salt and buffer complex that forms a colloidal suspension. Administration is IV, because the drug is not absorbed from the GI tract. Only low drug concentrations are obtained in the CSF. Although the metabolism and excretion of amphotericin B are poorly defined, its dosage should not be reduced in renal failure, because it is not excreted by the kidneys.

2. **Dosage and administration.** The drug must be suspended in 5% D/W in a concentration less than 0.1 mg/ml. Each dose should be infused over 4–6 hours. A common empirical regimen is to begin with a 1-mg test dose, followed by 0.2 mg/kg the first day, and to increase the dosage by 0.1–0.2 mg/kg/day until a daily dosage of 0.5–1.0 mg/kg is reached (1.0–1.5 mg/kg in children). Daily dosages greater than 0.5 mg/kg usually increase toxicity without affecting efficacy. This protocol may be accelerated in patients with fulminant disease by following the 1-mg test dose with 0.25 mg/kg on the first day and beginning full therapeutic doses (0.5–1.0 mg/kg) 24 hours later. The dosage may be doubled and given on alternate days but should not exceed 1.5 mg/kg/dose. The alternate-day regimen often reduces patient discomfort and may decrease renal toxicity. Intrathecal and intraventricular therapy are occasionally used in the treatment of fungal meningitis but often produce significant toxicity.

3. **Toxicity.** Fever, chills, headache, nausea, and vomiting usually occur but may be reduced by premedicating the patient with acetaminophen or aspirin (0..6–1.2 gm PO) and diphenhydramine (25–50 mg PO or IV) and by adding 25–50 mg of hydrocortisone to the infusion. Thrombophlebitis may be reduced by the addition of heparin, 1000 units/infusion. Patients often become tolerant to these effects of amphotericin B and may not require premedication after the first few weeks of therapy.

   Nephrotoxicity develops in all patients treated with amphotericin B. However, the amount of permanent renal damage is not usually significant unless underlying renal disease is present or the total dosage has exceeded 4 gm. Only serious renal dysfunction (i.e., > 75% decrease in GFR) generally requires a reduction in dosage or temporary discontinuance of therapy. If treatment is interrupted for more than 7 days, dosage should begin at 0.25 mg/kg and be increased gradually. If possible, other nephrotoxic drugs should be avoided during therapy with amphotericin B.

   Other **adverse effects** include distal renal tubular acidosis, isosthenuria, hypokalemia, and possibly serious pneumonitis when combined with leukocyte transfusions (*N. Engl. J. Med.*, 304:1185, 1981). Neuritis and arachnoiditis may occur with intrathecal administration.

B. **Flucytosine,** an inhibitor of nucleic acid synthesis, is effective orally against some isolates of *Candida* and *C. neoformans*. Susceptible organisms are inhibited in vitro by concentrations < 5 μg/ml, which are achieved easily in serum. The usual dose (37.5 mg/kg PO q6h) produces therapeutic peak serum levels of 50–75 μg/ml. Oral doses are well absorbed and achieve therapeutic CSF levels. Because flucytosine is excreted in the urine, the dosage should be reduced in patients with renal insufficiency as follows: 37.5 mg/kg q12h if the GFR is 20–40 ml/minute; 37.5 mg/kg q24h if the GFR is 10–20 ml/minute. Flucytosine is hemodialyzed; patients should receive an additional 20 mg/kg after each dialysis. The major disadvantage of the drug is that resistance develops during treatment in a significant proportion of *Candida* and cryptococcal isolates. Flucytosine is used with amphotericin B in the treatment of cryptococcal meningitis and alone for *Candida* UTI that persists after removal of a catheter.

   Hematologic toxicity is dose related. Serum levels > 100 μg/ml are associated with bone marrow suppression. Other **adverse effects** include elevations in serum hepatic enzymes, nausea, diarrhea, and, rarely, intestinal perforation.

C. **Imidazoles** are static agents for various fungi. Because they are metabolized by the liver, their dosage need not be adjusted in azotemic patients.

   1. **Miconazole** is a second-line antifungal agent and should be used only if amphotericin B either cannot be tolerated or is not effective. Some clinical efficacy has been demonstrated against coccidioidomycosis, paracoc-

cidioidomycosis, and systemic candidiasis. Miconazole is not indicated for aspergillosis or histoplasmosis. Intravenous miconazole always is infused in at least 200 ml of 5% D/W or saline over 30–60 minutes. A 200-mg test dose should be administered initially. The recommended dosage is 400–1200 mg IV q8h. Because miconazole does not cross the blood-brain barrier, direct intrathecal or intraventricular instillation is necessary to produce significant CSF concentrations.

Adverse reactions include pruritus, rash, vomiting, diarrhea, flushes, thrombocytopenia, leukopenia, hyperlipidemia, and artifactual hyponatremia (due to the PEG-40 castor oil vehicle). Rare but serious toxicities include anaphylaxis and dysrhythmias. Phlebitis may be minimized by administration through a central venous catheter.

2. **Ketoconazole** is an orally administered agent active against *Candida* species, *C. immitis, H. capsulatum,* and *B. dermatitidis.* Although clinical studies are limited, it may be the long-term suppressive therapy of choice in chronic mucocutaneous candidiasis. Systemic disease due to *C. immitis* and *H. capsulatum* also may be suppressed for prolonged periods. Penetration of *CSF* is unreliable.

   Ketoconazole is supplied as a 200-mg tablet. Absorption after an oral dose on an empty stomach is nearly complete within 4 hours. Absorption can be enhanced by dissolving the tablet in orange juice or in 4 ml of 0.2N HCl (drinking it through a plastic straw to protect the teeth and then drinking a glass of water). Any measures that decrease gastric acidity also decrease absorption. **Adverse reactions** are minimal and include nausea, gynecomastia, fever, and diarrhea. Transient serum transaminase elevations and hepatitis have been reported. Toxicities with prolonged use may include the inhibition of sterol synthesis by the adrenals.

III. **Treatment of selected systemic mycoses.** The treatment schedules for most mycoses are based on clinical experience. The successful treatment of opportunistic pathogens often reflects the prognosis of the underlying host disease more than the specific antifungal regimen employed. Therefore, the recommendations that follow are general guidelines.

   A. **Cryptococcosis.** Pulmonary cryptococcosis in a normal host is typically a self-limited disease that requires only observation. However, treatment is necessary when the patient is immunocompromised (e.g., lymphoreticular malignancy, immunosuppressive therapy). **Disseminated disease,** including **meningitis,** always requires treatment. The treatment of choice for meningitis is amphotericin B (0.3 mg/kg/day IV) plus flucytosine (37.5 mg/kg PO q6h) for a total duration of 6 weeks. Pulmonary disease may be treated with the same regimen for 4–6 weeks. Ketoconazole may have a role as alternative therapy.

   B. **Blastomycosis** rarely demonstrates spontaneous remission; therefore, treatment usually is indicated. Amphotericin B (2 gm total dosage) is most effective. Ketoconazole may be an alternative in certain cases. Some physicians have used hydroxystilbamidine isethionate (225 mg/day IV to a total dosage of 8 gm) for limited, noncavitary lung disease.

   C. **Histoplasmosis.** Treatment is indicated for chronic fibronodular and cavitary pulmonary disease, disseminated disease, and disease in immunocompromised patients. The treatment of choice is amphotericin B, usually 1.5–2.5 gm total dosage. Limited studies suggest a possible role for ketoconazole as alternative therapy.

   D. **Invasive aspergillosis** usually presents as a pulmonary infiltrate or sinusitis in severely immunocompromised patients. Treatment of this life-threatening infection requires amphotericin B, total dosage 2.0–2.5 gm. The synergistic addition of rifampin is investigational.

E. Sporotrichosis. Cutaneous and subcutaneous disease is best treated with local heat and **oral iodides** (saturated solution of potassium iodide [SSKI]). The dose of SSKI is begun at 1 ml tid in milk or juice and increased slowly until a maximum of 8 ml tid is attained or drug intolerance develops. Treatment should be continued for 1–2 months after all lesions have healed. **Toxicities** include increased lacrimation and salivation, an unpleasant brassy taste, gastric irritation, and diarrhea. Amphotericin B (1.5–2.5 gm total dosage) should be used for patients with disseminated disease and those unable to tolerate iodine.

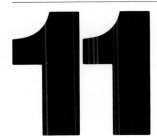

Nutritional Therapy

I. Basic concepts in nutrition. Food energy values are usually given in kilocalories (kcal). There is an average of 4.0 kcal/gm of carbohydrate, 4.0 kcal/gm of protein, and 9 kcal/gm of fat. A caloric intake in excess of daily needs results in weight gain, while an insufficient caloric intake results in weight loss. A negative balance of approximately 3500 kcal is required to lose 1 lb.

A. The total daily energy expenditure is the sum of the **basal metabolic rate (BMR),** the energy expenditure of activity, and the specific dynamic action of food. The energy requirements for a normal subject can be easily calculated, so that the proper caloric needs can be supplied (D. W. Wilmore, *The Metabolic Management of the Critically Ill.* New York: Plenum, 1977).

1. The BMR can be determined as follows:

$$\text{BMR (kcal/M}^2\text{/hr)} = 37 - \left(\frac{\text{age} - 20}{10}\right)$$

The BMR increases in the presence of fever (13% for each degree centigrade elevation), cardiac failure (15–25%), simple postoperative states (0–5%), peritonitis (5–25%), severe infection or multiple trauma (30–50%), multiple trauma with a patient on a ventilator (50–75%), and burns over 50% of the body (100%). These increases must be added to the calculation of the BMR.

2. The energy expenditure of activity must be estimated. The level of daily activity in the healthy person is the major variable determining energy needs. Sedentary activity may expend 400–800 kcal/day; light work may expend 800–1200 kcal/day; moderate mechanical work may expend 1200–1800 kcal/day; and prolonged heavy labor or exercise may expend 1800–4500 kcal/day. The average adult male who does not do heavy labor needs about 2500 kcal/day to maintain energy balance.

3. The **specific dynamic action of food** is the heat production above basal levels that occurs with food ingestion. The specific dynamic action of food = 0.10 × (BMR + energy expenditure of activity).

4. The total daily energy expenditure (kcal) = BMR + energy expenditure of activity + specific dynamic action of food.

5. **Example:** What is the total daily energy requirement of a 30-year-old man (height 5 feet 11 inches, weight 175 lb) one day after surgery for an inguinal hernia?

   a. BMR (in kcal/M^2/hr) = $37 - \left(\dfrac{30 - 20}{10}\right)$

   BMR = 36 kcal/M^2/hr

   b. Daily energy expenditure due to BMR:

   = 36 × 2 (M^2) × 24 (hr)

   = 1728 kcal

Add about a 5% increase to the BMR for the simple postoperative state. The daily energy expenditure due to BMR = 1814 kcal.

    c. Energy expenditure of activity: Since the patient is sedentary, add about 500 kcal = 2314 kcal.

    d. Specific dynamic action of food = 0.10 × (1814 + 500) = 231 kcal.

    e. Total daily energy expenditure = 1814 + 500 + 231 = 2545 kcal.

B. Metabolic adaptations take place in response to stresses, such as short-term starvation, long-term starvation, and catabolic states.

    1. Short-term starvation. During short-term starvation, there is a continuous utilization of body protein for gluconeogenesis because (1) there is no net glucose synthesis from fatty acids in humans, (2) certain tissues (brain) have obligate glucose requirements, and (3) carbohydrate reserves (liver glycogen) are depleted after approximately 12–24 hours of starvation. After carbohydrate depletion, the rate of protein breakdown (catabolism) is 60–75 gm/day, resulting in 10–12 gm of urinary nitrogen excretion (gm protein ÷ 6.25 = gm nitrogen) and a loss of about 0.5 lb/day of lean body mass. A more rapid weight loss indicates either a loss of body fluids or an increased catabolic state (fever, burns, or the postoperative state). Urinary nitrogen losses are decreased to as little as 2–3 gm/day by the provision of 100 gm/day of carbohydrate (approximately 400 kcal). The protein-sparing effect of small amounts of carbohydrate is important to remember when deciding the composition of fluids to be administered to patients who cannot eat for short periods. Increasing the carbohydrate content above 100 gm does not increase the protein-sparing effect. A positive nitrogen balance (anabolism) cannot be attained unless an exogenous source of protein also is provided.

    2. Long-term starvation. If fasting persists for several days, a series of adaptations occurs to limit the rate of protein breakdown. The brain begins to consume ketone bodies as an alternative oxidative fuel. Since less glucose is required, gluconeogenic processes are decreased, and the flow of amino acids from muscle is reduced. Urinary nitrogen decreases to about 3 gm/day (the result of the catabolism of about 20 gm protein/day).

    3. Catabolic states. Patients with major burns, fever, or traumatic injuries have increased demands for energy, resulting in increased protein catabolism. Positive nitrogen balance in these states requires an exogenous source of amino acids plus sufficient calories in the form of carbohydrate or fat to meet the increased energy demands.

C. Essential nutrients

    1. Protein constitutes 15% of the typical American diet. Of the 22 amino acids, 8 are essential for endogenous protein synthesis: phenylalanine, methionine, lysine, threonine, tryptophan, valine, leucine, and isoleucine. The minimal dietary allowance for the mixed proteins is 0.8 gm/kg/day. This requirement increases to 1.25 gm/kg/day with catabolic stress, such as major trauma or the complicated postoperative state. The requirement is 1.5 gm/kg/day with sepsis and it may be even greater with major burns. If caloric intake is insufficient, a large proportion of dietary amino acids will be diverted to the provision of energy rather than being used for anabolic purposes.

    2. Carbohydrate constitutes 50% of the typical American diet and is an essential energy source for the brain. A minimal daily consumption of 400 kcal of digestible carbohydrates is recommended.

    3. Fats constitute 35% of the typical American diet. Two polyunsaturated fatty acids, linoleic acid and arachidonic acid, are essential. Linoleic acid must be supplied by the diet, but arachidonic acid can be formed in vivo from linoleic acid. Food fat also serves as a vehicle for the absorption of the fat-soluble vitamins. In contrast to long-chain triglycerides, medium-chain triglycerides (MCTs) (fatty acids with 8 to 10 carbon atoms) enter the circulation via the portal system and are rapidly hydrolyzed by pancreatic lipase and absorbed by the small intestine.

4. **Vitamins** act as critical metabolic cofactors and must be obtained by dietary means. Sufficient quantities of both fat-soluble and water-soluble vitamins must be provided to avoid deficiency.

5. **Trace elements** are provided in the ordinary American diet, and the risk of deficiency is small. Special provisions must be made for patients receiving chronic IV nutritional support. Essential trace elements include zinc, copper, cobalt, iodine, magnanese, iron, and chromium.

D. **Assessment of nutritional status.** The clinical assessment of nutritional status by a history and physical examination is both a simple and a valid technique. Anthropometric measurements and laboratory data may provide supportive information (*N. Engl. J. Med.* 306:969, 987, 1982).

1. **Nutritional history.** The history should stress the presence or absence of weight loss, anorexia, vomiting, diarrhea, bizarre food habits, chronic illness, edema, heavy alcohol intake, and drug usage. A daily calorie count, including protein as well as caloric intake, is helpful in determining an inadequate intake.

2. **Physical signs.** Signs of nutritional and vitamin deficiency are most often seen in the visible organs, such as the hair, eyes, skin, and teeth. Attention should be specifically directed to the presence of cheilosis, glossitis, loss of subcutaneous fat, muscle wasting, edema, jaundice, and changes in hair color and texture.

3. **Anthropometric measurements.** The height and weight should be measured and compared with ideal weight. A weight of less than 85% of ideal weight usually signifies nutritional deficiency. A decrease of greater than 10% of normal weight over a 6-month period is a significant weight loss. Supplemental data may include evaluation of fat stores by measuring triceps skinfold thickness. Skeletal mass can be evaluated by measuring the upper midarm circumference. Both of these measurements are subject to error in obese or edematous patients and are best made by an experienced observer.

4. **Laboratory tests.** The serum albumin, serum transferrin, total iron-binding capacity, total lymphocyte count, and serum levels of vitamins A and C are useful in assessing nutritional status. Cellular immunity may be depressed in protein-calorie malnutrition and can be assessed by appropriate skin tests.

II. **Types of nutritional therapy.** The type of nutritional therapy is dependent on caloric requirements and function of the gastrointestinal tract. In many instances, some combination of the following modes of caloric supplementation will be necessary:

A. **The standard hospital diet** will be appropriate for many patients. A soft diet should be considered if poor dentition is noted. A low-residue diet may be necessary prior to GI procedures. Particular nutritional adjustments will be required with known diseases (e.g., diabetes, gluten enteropathy).

B. **Nutritional supplements.** See Table 11-1.

1. **Indications.** Supplements should be used to supply extra dietary calories, protein, and fat. They are not to be used as a complete diet.

2. **Available products.** Citrotein is a low-fat, low-residue, gluten-free caloric supplement supplied in a 1.2-oz packet. Casec is a high-protein supplement. Medium-chain triglycerides alone or in a complete nutrition such as **Travasorb MCT** (containing 80% of the fat calories as MCTs) or **Portagen Powder** supply extra calories as fat and can be administered to patients with

Table 11-1. Oral supplemental feedings

Product	Amount (oz)	Osmolality (mOsm/kg H_2O)	Kcal	Protein (gm)	Fat (gm)	Carbohydrate (gm)
Citrotein	1.2	496	127	7.67	0.33	23.3
Casec powder	1	12	34	8.0		
MCT Oil	0.5	0	115		14.0	
Polycose (liquid)	2	850	120			30.0
Portagen powder	8	236	640	22.4	30.5	73.6
Forta Pudding	5		250	6.8	9.7	34.0

Table 11-2. Oral complete feedings in ready-to-use form[a]

Product	Protein Source	Osmolality (mOsm/kg H_2O)	Kcal	Protein (gm)	Fat (gm)	Carbohydrate (gm)
Meritene[b]	IP	560	240	14.4	7.2	27.6
Sustacal[b] (vanilla)	IP	640	240	14.6	5.5	33.6
Travasorb MCT	IP	375	400	19.7	13.2	49.1
Ensure	PI	450	254	8.8	8.8	34.8
Isocal	PI	350	254	8.1	10.5	31.6
Precision Isotonic	PI	300	230	6.8	3.7	34.8
Precision LR	PI	520	266	6.2	0.2	59.7
Flexical	PH	550	240	5.3	8.1	36.6
Vivonex HN	CAA	810	240	11.04	0.2	50.4
Amin-Aid	CAA	1050	700	6.3	22.0	118.0
Hepatic-Aid	CAA	900	560	14.5	12.3	98.1

IP = intact protein; PI = protein isolates; PH = protein hydrolysates; CAA = crystalline amino acids.
[a]Values based on 8-oz feeding.
[b]Contains lactose.

malabsorption due to either intestinal or pancreatic disease. **Polycose** can provide extra calories as carbohydrate. Oral complete feedings may also be used as nutritional supplements. **Forta Pudding** is available in many flavors. Each 5-oz serving supplies 250 calories and 6.8 gm of protein.

3. **Complications.** Palatability may be a major problem with any of the supplements. Polycose is usually diluted by mixing it into foods or beverages. Even diluted polycose may be hyperosmolar and can cause diarrhea and cramps if given too rapidly.

C. **Liquid diets.** See Table 11-2.

1. **Indications.** Liquid diets may replace a soft, solid diet in patients with normal GI tracts. They are particularly useful in patients who have difficulty with mastication, and are also useful in patients with anorexia, food prejudice, and severe depression. Liquid diets can also supplement caloric intake in patients recovering from surgery, burns, or other injuries.

2. **Selection criteria.** A liquid diet should be selected on the basis of palatability, osmolality, and composition. Several liquid diets have an acceptable

taste, and a variety of flavors is available. Palatability can be further enhanced by chilling and drinking these diets through a straw. These supplements may be used in the preparation of puddings, flavored shakes, gelatin desserts, and toppings. The osmolality of these liquid diets is high (500–700 mOsm/kg H_2O), with the exception of Ensure (450 mOsm/kg H_2O) and Travasorb MCT (375 mOsm/kg H_2O). Lactose and gluten content, protein source, residue, and cost should be considered when selecting a nutritional supplement.

3. **Available products.** The caloric content per volume of most liquid diets is approximately the same. Lactose-free liquid diets are available as **Ensure, Travasorb MCT,** and **Precision LR.** The latter may be helpful to patients requiring low-residue diets. **Hepatic-Aid** has an amino acid composition that is high in branched-chain amino acids and low in aromatic amino acids. Since patients with hepatic encephalopathy have abnormal amino acid patterns with increased concentrations of aromatic amino acids (phenylalanine, tryosine, tryptophan) and decreased concentrations of branched-chain amino acids (valine, leucine, and isoleucine), Hepatic-Aid may be useful in their treatment. **Amin-Aid** may be a suitable liquid diet for patients with acute renal failure not undergoing regular dialysis therapy. Each package contains the minimum daily requirements of the eight essential amino acids (6.35 gm) plus histidine (0.25 gm).

4. **Complications.** Patients generally are unwilling to ingest more than 3 cans (8-oz servings) daily by mouth, but larger amounts can be delivered by tube feedings. Diarrhea, cramps, and dehydration can result from the hyperosmolality of the diets, especially if they are administered too rapidly. If diarrhea occurs, liquid diets should be diluted with water to half-strength and then slowly increased in concentration as tolerated. Obviously, this means more volume will be required to achieve the same caloric intake. Lactose intolerance can result in similar symptoms.

D. **Low-residue diets** are more completely absorbed in the proximal small intestine, so that little residue is presented to the distal small intestine.

1. **Indications.** Low-residue diets are **expensive** and often require a period of patient adaptation because of their high osmolality. For these reasons, they should be used only when necessary. Indications include: (1) short bowel syndrome, (2) GI fistulas, (3) inflammatory bowel disease, (4) acute diarrhea, (5) postoperative management of patients with colonic or rectal surgery, and (6) preoperative bowel preparations.

2. **Selection criteria.** Amino acids and oligopeptides have a disagreeable flavor and odor. **Flexical** and **Vivonex HN** use crystalline amino acids or protein hydrolysate for part or all of their protein source and are often referred to as *elemental diets.* Flexical supplies the majority of its protein as hydrolyzed casein, but it also contains three essential crystalline amino acids and MCTs. The entire protein source in Vivonex is crystalline amino acids. **Precision LR** uses egg albumin as its protein source and is more palatable and less expensive than most elemental diets.

3. **Therapy.** The low-residue diets can be given orally or via a feeding tube. **Vivonex HN** is available in an 80-gm packet, which must be mixed with water to a total volume of 300 ml. Each milliliter of the liquid mixture contains 1 kcal; 10 packets will provide 3000 kcal. **Flexical** contains about 250 kcal in a 2-oz portion mixed with 8 oz of water. A 1-lb can provides a daily intake of 2000 kcal. **Precision LR** is supplied in 3-oz packets to be mixed with 8 oz of water and supplies approximately 320 kcal.

4. **Complications.** The high osmotic and/or carbohydrate load of some products (see Table 11-2) can lead to nausea, vomiting, diarrhea, hyperglycemia, nonketotic hyperosmolar coma, and disturbances of water and electrolyte bal-

ance. These problems can be reduced by slow administration and frequent monitoring of blood glucose and electrolytes. These diets may be contraindicated in diabetic patients and should be used cautiously in patients with glucose intolerance. Hypoprothrombinemia has been attributed to a decreased population of intestinal bacteria that make vitamin K. Vitamin K (10 mg IM) should be administered twice weekly, and prothrombin times should be checked regularly. Elemental diets significantly reduce the amount of residue, and their prolonged use may cause constipation.

E. Tube feedings are liquid diets administered through a nasogastric feeding tube.

1. **Indications.** They are useful in patients who cannot swallow because of an esophageal motility problem, tumor, coma, neurologic disorder (leading to incoordination of the swallowing mechanism), or confusion. Other indications include resistance to feeding, inability to tolerate an elemental diet, apathy, nausea, anorexia, or debility. Use of the intact GI tract averts the major problems of sepsis and metabolic derangements that occur with total parenteral nutrition.

2. **Technique.** Large-bore feeding tubes have been replaced by a variety of narrow-diameter (8F), flexible feeding tubes that are long enough to reach the duodenum. Available products include the Dobbhoff and Entriflex tubes. The latter is supplied with a stylet for easy fluoroscopic placement. **It is essential** that the tube tip be placed into the duodenum to decrease the risk of aspiration. Extra and larger holes can be made in the tubes to prevent clogging by viscous liquid diets.

3. **Selection criteria. Isocal** and **Precision Isotonic** can be used as a sole source of nourishment. Both contain adequate vitamins and minerals, and neither contains lactose. Both are low residue. Isocal also contains MCTs.

4. **Administration.** To minimize the risk of gastroesophageal reflux, the patient should not be placed in the supine position during feeding. The feeding solution should be administered by a volumetric infusion pump but also can be dripped in by gravity from IV bags. These feedings should be instituted slowly regardless of the method used. The volume can be increased to 2 liters over the first 48 hours. As much as 4000 kcal daily can be given via the tube. The patient should be encouraged to ambulate and, depending on the underlying problem, may take food orally in addition to the tube feedings.

5. **Complications.** The infusion rate should be decreased if diarrhea occurs. Constipation may occur with long-term usage.

F. Short-term intravenous nutrition. The major goals of short-term IV nutrition are protein sparing and fluid and electrolyte balance. Administration of 100 gm of carbohydrate over 24 hours achieves protein sparing in most patients but may not be effective in severe catabolic states. The carbohydrate, fluid, and electrolyte requirements of short-term IV therapy may be provided by 1000 ml 5% D/W with 20 mEq KCl over 12 hours and 1000 ml of D5½NS with 20 mEq KCl over 12 hours. This provides approximately 350 kcal (there are 3.4 kcal/gm dextrose) (see also Chap. 2, sec. II).

G. Peripheral alimentation should be considered only when enteral feeding is undesirable. Peripheral alimentation systems provide fewer calories than either the enteral or total peripheral nutrition (TPN) systems and are useful only in a limited number of situations. Examples of such situations are (1) patients on TPN whose central venous catheter is removed because of infection; (2) patients who require caloric supplementation while enteral nutrition rates are gradually increased until full needs are met; and (3) patients in whom maintenance nutrition is desired for a short period following an uncomplicated recovery from surgery. Amino acids and dextrose solutions can be used either alone or in combination with a lipid emulsion.

Table 11-3. Comparison of different parenteral regimens

Regimen (3 L/day)	Protein (gm)	Nonprotein calories (kcal)	Osmolarity* (mOsm/L)
Dextrose infusion (5% dextrose)	0	510	253
Protein sparing (4.25% amino acids in 5% dextrose)	128	510	680
Lipid system (4.25% amino acids [2 L] plus 10% lipid [1 L])	85	340 1100	480
Total parenteral nutrition (4.25% amino acids in 25% dextrose)	128	3000	1700

*Does not include added electrolytes or vitamins.

1. **Types of parenteral regimens.** See Table 11-3.

   a. **Intralipid** is the most commonly used fat emulsion and is composed of 10% soybean oil, 1.2% egg yolk phospholipids, and 2.25% glycerin. The osmolarity is approximately 280 mOsm/liter, and the caloric content is 1 kcal/ml. The caloric content of Intralipid containing 20% soybean oil is 2.0 cal/ml. The use of 20% Intralipid should only be considered when volume restriction is necessary. The size of fat particles in these emulsions is approximately the same as chylomicrons. These fat particles release triglycerides in vivo that are hydrolyzed by lipoprotein lipase to yield glycerol and free fatty acids. Temporary hyperlipemia occurs initially after an infusion. Maximal serum triglyceride levels are reached 4 hours after the end of an infusion and return to the preinfusion levels about 2 hours later. The patient's ability to clear the infused fat from the circulation should be monitored by checking serum triglyceride levels and the appearance of the serum approximately 6 hours after the end of the lipid infusion.

   Fever, chills, and chest or back pain are rarely reported acute reactions. Adverse reactions to long-term administration may include an impairment of biliary function associated with jaundice, elevated SGOT, increased Bromosulphalein retention, and a mild drop in hemoglobin and hematocrit. Thrombocytopenia has been reported as a rare complication. Intralipid is **contraindicated** in patients with abnormalities in lipid metabolism or severe liver disease.

   b. **Amino acid solutions.** Peripheral amino acid infusions initially were suggested as a form of short-term protein sparing therapy for surgical patients. However, because of their expense, the sole use of peripheral amino acid infusions is not justified in the great majority of postoperative surgical patients. However, protein-sparing therapy may be useful in the postoperative diabetic patient who needs short-term maintenance support. A 3.0–3.5% solution of amino acids containing maintenance electrolytes is used (see Table 11-4).

   When peripheral alimentation is the sole source of calories and protein, **Aminosyn** 7%, **FreAmine** 8.5%, or **Travasol** 8.5% is used. Since each will be diluted to one-half strength by the addition of 10% D/W or 20% D/W, the final concentration of the amino acid–dextrose solution will be 3.5% or 4.25% amino acids in 5% D/W or 10% D/W. To avoid phlebitis, the final

Table 11-4. Composition of several commercially available amino acid solutions for parenteral nutrition

Solution	Amino acid content (gm/L)	Protein equivalent (gm/L)	Osmolarity (mOsm/L)	Na$^+$ (mEq/L)	K$^+$ (mEq/L)	C$^+$ (mEq/L)	Mg (mEq/L)	P (mmol/L)
FreAmine III 8.5%	85	81	810	10	0	2	0	10
Aminosyn 7.0%	70	62	700	0	5.4	0	0	0
Nephramine II 5.4%	54	40	440	6	0	0	0	0
Travasol 3.5%	35	36	450	25	15	25	5	7.5

Source: Modified from the *Barnes Hospital TPN Manual*, 1981.

concentration of dextrose in the peripheral line should not exceed 10% D/W. The concentration of potassium and other electrolytes present in each of the baseline amino acid solutions (Table 11-4) must be taken into account when ordering additional electrolytes. Monitoring of electrolytes and serum phosphorus must be done during the duration of peripheral alimentation.

2. **Administration of peripheral alimentation**

   a. The initial infusion rate of Intralipid should be 1 ml/minute. If no adverse reactions have occurred after the first 15–30 minutes of infusion, the rate can be increased. The infusion rate should not exceed 500 ml/4 hours. No more than 60% of the total caloric intake should come from **Intralipid** (normally about 35–45% of daily caloric intake comes from fat).

   b. The simultaneous administration of 1 liter of lipid along with 2 liters of amino acid solution in a 5% dextrose solution over a 24-hour period provides 3 liters of water, 85 gm of protein (12 gm of nitrogen), and approximately 1800 calories.

   c. Intralipid is a delicate emulsion, and a Y connector must be used so that minimal mixing of the amino acid–dextrose solution occurs with the Intralipid during simultaneous infusion. All electrolytes and supplements should be mixed into the amino acid solution after consultation with the pharmacist to ensure that no incompatibilities exist. The lipid emulsion has a low specific gravity and should be hung higher than the amino acid solution to prevent backflow of the amino acid mixture into the Intralipid line. The flow rates of each solution should be controlled separately by infusion pumps.

   d. Intralipid is minimally irritating to peripheral veins, but the amino acid solution is hypertonic and causes thrombophlebitis. Simultaneous infusion helps to reduce the incidence of this complication. Hydrocortisone (5 mg) and/or heparin (500–1000 units) may be added to each liter of amino acid solution to reduce the incidence of thrombophlebitis.

   e. Steel scalp vein needles, which do not irritate veins, are impractical because of their easy dislodgment. Silicone Elastomer catheters are the preferred catheters. They should be changed q24–36h.

   f. Antibiotic ointment and Opsite (Acme United Corporation, Bridgeport, Conn.), a clear dressing material applied over the catheter to allow inspection and minimize catheter disturbances, will help decrease the incidence of local infection.

H. **Total parenteral nutrition**

   1. **Indications.** Because the use of TPN may result in a number of potentially life-threatening complications, its use should be restricted to the following two groups of patients:

      a. Those with poorly functioning GI tracts who cannot tolerate other means of nutritional support.

      b. Those with high caloric requirements that cannot otherwise be met.

   2. **Catheter placement.** The TPN solution cannot be given through a peripheral vein, because administration of a high-osmolality solution causes sclerosis. The catheter should be electively placed in the subclavian or internal jugular vein by physicians experienced in this procedure. Elastic catheters, which are tunneled subcutaneously (e.g., Broviac, Hickman), are desirable for long-term therapy. Sterile technique must be employed during catheter placement and maintenance. **No fluid other than the TPN solution should be given through the TPN line.**

Complications of subclavian vein catheter insertion include pneumothorax, hemothorax, subclavian artery puncture, brachial plexus damage, lymphatic leak, catheter embolism, myocardial perforation, great vein thrombosis, and air embolism. A chest radiograph should be obtained immediately following placement to rule out pneumothorax. The risk of air embolism is minimized by placing ointment and a small air-occlusive dressing over the puncture site when the catheter is removed.

3. **Rationale for formulation of TPN solutions**

   a. **Protein and nitrogen requirement.** Protein requirements change, depending on the type of catabolic stress (see sec. **I.C.1**). Gravely ill patients may require as much as 2.25 gm of protein/kg/day. The variance in amino acids solutions permits individualized therapy. FreAmine III 8.5%, 500 ml, provides 41 gm of amino acids. This is equivalent to 41 gm of protein or 6.5 gm of nitrogen and approximately 180 kcal.

   b. **Calories.** Most calories should come from the carbohydrate source to achieve a maximal protein-sparing effect. The stressed patient should receive 150–200 kcal of carbohydrate/gm of utilizable nitrogen.

   c. **Electrolytes.** Commercially available amino acid solutions contain widely varying amounts of electrolytes. This must be taken into consideration when totalling electrolytes (see Table 11-4). Since TPN orders specify final electrolyte concentration, the pharmacist should include the electrolyte content of the commercial amino acid solution in the final calculations.

      (1) **Sodium.** The daily amount of sodium can range from 15–200 mEq, and wide ranges are compatible with a liter of TPN solution. The sodium content will depend on nutritional requirements and cardiovascular function.

      (2) **Potassium.** Daily potassium needs range from 12–240 mEq and tend to increase as the patient becomes anabolic. No more than 80 mEq should be added to any liter of TPN solution.

      (3) **Chloride.** The daily supplements range from 40–220 mEq and wide ranges are compatible with mixed amino acid solutions.

      (4) **Magnesium.** The median daily requirement is approximately 25 mEq. Regulation depends on renal function and serum concentrations of calcium and phosphorus. No more than 12 mEq of magnesium should be added to any liter of mixed amino acids.

      (5) **Calcium.** The usual daily requirement can be based on serum levels. No more than 10 mEq of calcium should be added to any liter of mixed amino acids.

      (6) **Phosphate.** Since tissue synthesis requires 4 mEq of phosphate/gm of nitrogen, hypophosphatemia should be anticipated during effective TPN. Daily supplements of phosphate range from 20–80 mEq (10–40 mmol phosphorus). Phosphate is supplied as a sodium or potassium salt. No more than 20 mEq of phosphate (10 mmol phosphorus) should be added to any liter of mixed amino acid solution.

      (7) **Sodium bicarbonate.** Sodium bicarbonate should not be added to TPN solutions. The TPN solution is acidic (pH 6.5 for 500 ml FreAmine III 8.5% in any equal volume of hypertonic dextrose), and bicarbonate may be lost through the effervescence of carbon dioxide. In addition, if magnesium or calcium is present in sufficient quantity, insoluble carbonate salts may be produced. It is preferable to balance pH with acetate supplied as the sodium or potassium salt. This provides a readily metabolizable bicarbonate precursor for the prevention or

Table 11-5. Daily multivitamin infusion for addition to total parenteral nutrition solution*

Vitamin	Amount
Vial 1 (5 ml)	
Ascorbic acid (C)	100 mg
Vitamin A (retinol)	3300 IU
Vitamin D (ergocalciferol)	200 IU
Thiamine (B_1)	3.0 mg
Riboflavin (B_2)	3.6 mg
Pyridoxine HCl (B_6)	4.0 mg
Niacinamide	40.0 mg
Pantothenic acid	15.0 mg
Vitamin E	10 IU
Vial 2 (5 ml)	
Biotin	60 μg
Folic acid	400 μg
Vitamin B_{12}	5 μg

*This product (MVI-12, USV Laboratories, Tuckahoe, N.Y.) contains two vials labeled Vial 1 and Vial 2. Both are used on a daily basis.

treatment of metabolic acidosis. The acetate ion is also used by the pharmacist to balance the sodium and potassium ions.

   d. Vitamins. Deficiencies of water-soluble vitamins occur rapidly in the debilitated state. Vitamin K should be administered once a week, and vitamin B_{12} should be given once monthly. Commercially available multivitamin supplements may be helpful. A multivitamin infusion (MVI-12, USV Laboratories, Tuckahoe, N.Y.) contains biotin, folic acid, vitamin B_{12}, and the fat-soluble vitamins in dosages that are compatible with daily administration for prolonged periods (Table 11-5).

   e. Trace minerals. Trace mineral deficiency may become evident during long-term treatment with TPN. A commercially available trace mineral solution is available (Travenol Laboratories, Deerfield, Ill.). Each milliliter of this solution contains 1 mg of zinc, 0.4 mg of copper, 0.1 mg of manganese, and 4 μg of chromium, and 3 ml of this solution is added daily to the hyperalimentation solution. Prolonged TPN therapy will eventually result in depletion of the existing iron stores. Iron can be replaced orally or IV on a monthly schedule.

4. Specific formulations. The basic formulations that follow (**a–d**)* are based on the use of **FreAmine III 8.5%** as the protein source and 50% dextrose as a carbohydrate source. Five hundred milliliters of each solution are mixed together to provide 1 liter of TPN solution with a final dextrose concentration of 25% and a final amino acid concentration of 4.25%. One liter of this solution provides 39 gm of protein and 1030 kcal. Other combinations of amino acids (see Table 11-4) and dextrose solutions may be desirable in certain clinical settings. Critically ill patients may benefit from a mixture of **Travasol 10%** or **Aminosyn 10%** and 70% dextrose. One liter of this type of solution provides 50 gm of protein and 1190 calories.

Commercially available amino acid solutions contain electrolytes in mark-

*Modified from *Procedures for Nutritional Support,* developed by the Hyperalimentation Team of The New York Hospital–Cornell Medical Center and approved by the Medical Board of The New York Hospital, 1978.

edly varying amounts (see Table 11-4). When TPN orders are written, the final concentration of electrolytes desired is ordered. Although the pharmacist preparing the TPN amino acid solution is responsible for including the electrolyte content of the base amino acid solutions in the final solution, the physician ordering these solutions should be aware of these calculations. It is preferable for the physician to order electrolytes in their individual form (e.g., potassium) rather than as a salt (e.g., potassium chloride), because the pharmacist is then able to use acetate to balance the cations. Individualizing electrolyte requirements is essential. The serum electrolyte concentrations are the major determinants of the amount of a particular electrolyte to be ordered each day.

a. **Standard amino acid solution.** This can be used for the great majority of patients who do not have renal or cardiac failure and who do not require additional supplementation or potassium restriction.

FreAmine III 8.5% (180 kcal)	41 gm (500 ml)
50% D/W (850 kcal)	250 gm (500 ml)
Calcium	4.7 mEq
Magnesium	8.0 mEq
Potassium	54.0 mEq
Sodium	30.0 mEq
Acetate	41.0 mEq
Chloride	34.0 mEq
Gluconate	4.8 mEq
Phosphorus	14.0 mmol
Sulfate	8.0 mEq
Approximate volume	1050 ml
Approximate osmolarity	1900 mOsm/L
Total caloric value (approximately 1 kcal/ml)	1030 kcal
Nitrogen content	6.5 gm

b. **Cardiac failure formula.** Patients with cardiac failure require fluid and sodium restriction. To reduce the volume, 70% dextrose is added to a smaller volume of FreAmine III 8.5%.

FreAmine III 8.5% (120 kcal)	30 gm (360 ml)
70% D/W (1190 kcal)	350 gm (500 gm)
Magnesium	8.0 mEq
Potassium	49.0 mEq
Sodium	3.6 mEq
Acetate	40.0 mEq
Sulfate	8.0 mEq
Phosphorus	10.0 mmol
Approximate volume	890 ml
Approximate osmolarity	2280 mOsm/L
Total caloric value (approximately 1.6 kcal/ml)	1390 kcal
Nitrogen content	4.8 gm

c. **Renal failure solution.** There is a significant mortality when acute renal failure occurs in the postoperative state. Some studies have indicated a diminished mortality when a parenteral nutrition solution of essential amino acids and hypertonic dextrose is used, as compared with mortality with hypertonic dextrose alone. The amino acid solution most commonly used is **Nephramine,** which contains the eight essential amino acids as the only source of nitrogen and sodium, 6 mEq/liter; 250 ml of this solution is combined with 500 ml of 70% dextrose for a final volume of 750 ml. Generally, 1500 ml/day is given. **Electrolyes are not routinely added to this solution.** Rather, daily serum electrolytes should be measured to determine what additives, if any, are needed.

Nephramine (54 kcal)	12.8 gm (250 ml)
70% D/W (1190 kcal)	350 gm (500 ml)
Sodium	2 mEq
Approximate volume	750 mg
Osmolarity	2125 mOsm/L
Total caloric value	1245 kcal
(approximately 1.7 kcal/ml)	
Nitrogen content	1.46 gm

d. **Hepatic failure.** These patients often have underlying malnutrition. An abnormal plasma amino acid pattern with high concentrations of aromatic acids (phenylalanine, tyrosine, tryptophan) and reduced concentrations of branched-chain amino acids (leucine, isoleucine, valine) are often found. A solution with reduced aromatic amino acids and increased branched-chain amino acids **(HepatAmine)** is available for intravenous use.

Patients with hepatic failure should not be given Intralipid, since the liver is required to metabolize the triglycerides. Every attempt should be made to provide nutrition to these patients via the intestinal tract. Complete liquid feedings **(Hepatic-Aid** or **Travasorb-Hepatic)** should be administered by mouth or through a small-bore tube. If this is not possible, TPN should include only a small amount of amino acids, because hepatic encephalopathy may be precipitated or worsened. Requirements for sodium will generally be low, while those for potassium, phosphorus, and magnesium may be high.

5. **Administration of TPN.** The initial TPN solution should be infused only after the position of the catheter tip has been confirmed by a radiograph. A volumetric infusion pump is essential for maintaining a constant infusion rate. The initial rate of administration should not exceed 50 ml/hour and can be increased by daily increments of 5 ml/hour until the rate is 125–150 ml/hour. This slow increase in infusion rate allows time for the patient's pancreas to respond to the high glucose load. No attempt should be made to speed up the infusion if the patient has not received the desired volume during a specific time period, because rapid changes in the infusion rate may lead to undesirable glucose intolerance. Urines should be checked q6h for glucose and acetone. A blood glucose should be obtained daily until the rate of infusion is stable and then routinely twice a week. In renal and cardiac patients who are given TPN formulas with higher glucose loads, the blood glucose should be checked q6h until the infusion is stable. **No fluid other than the TPN solution is to be given through the TPN line.**

6. **Routine orders for TPN.** Institution of TPN requires careful patient monitoring and catheter care. Daily laboratory monitoring of electrolytes and glucose may be necessary in the first week of TPN, but, after stabilization, venipuncture may be limited to approximately 3 times/week. A major attempt should be made to have blood drawn no more than once daily. The patient whose condition is unstable will require more frequent monitoring, and orders must be individualized. If a lipid solution has been given within the 6 hours prior to blood drawing, lipemia may interfere with accurate blood testing.

a. **Routine nursing orders**

(1) Vital signs q4h.

(2) Daily weights.

(3) Intake and output (charted on TPN flowsheet).

(4) Urine spot checks qid for glucose.

(5) Change TPN tubing daily.

(6) Change the sterile dressing 3 times weekly or according to the established TPN protocol (specific protocols vary among institutions).

(7) Flush the catheter twice daily with 50 units of heparin solution when the catheter is not in use.

(8) Provide additional catheter care as per the TPN protocol.

(9) The catheter is to be used for TPN only.

b. Laboratory tests

(1) Urine glucose spot check q6h

(2) Serum electrolytes and glucose qd or, when the patient is stable, every Monday, Wednesday, and Friday

(3) Blood urea nitrogen or creatinine every Monday and Friday

(4) Complete blood count and platelet count every Monday and Friday

(5) SMA-12 (liver function tests, Ca, P) every week

(6) Serum magnesium every week

(7) Prothrombin time every week

7. Metabolic complications

a. Hyperglycemia. In the normal patient, hyperglycemia at the start of TPN will be followed by a relatively hyperinsulinemic state, and the blood glucose concentration will return to normal. However, this may not occur in patients with liver disease, pancreatitis, pancreatic resection, and diabetes. When significant hyperglycemia (> 250 mg/dl) and glycosuria persist beyond the initial day of TPN, the infusion rate should be slowed or exogenous regular insulin should be added to the TPN solution. An initial concentration of 15 units of regular insulin/liter can be increased as necessary. If hyperosmolar nonketotic coma occurs, the TPN infusion should be stopped and IV insulin and hydration begun.

b. Hypoglycemia. Abrupt cessation of hyperalimentation results in hypoglycemia. If TPN is discontinued, 10% D/W should be given peripherally and tapered over 24 hours.

c. Reactions to amino acids. The infusion of crystalline amino acids may lead to hyperchloremic metabolic acidosis, but the introduction of the newer amino acid formulations containing acetate salts has lessened the risk of this complication. Hyperammonemia, however, can develop in pediatric patients or patients with liver disease.

d. Other metabolic complications. Abnormalities in serum concentration of potassium, calcium, magnesium, and phosphate can lead to severe metabolic disturbances. Levels of these electrolytes should be monitored and the TPN solution composition adjusted appropriately.

e. Infectious complications. Septicemia related to TPN therapy is a frequent and serious problem. Its incidence is clearly related to catheter insertion technique and the quality of catheter care practiced. To minimize infections due to skin bacteria, the IV tubing should be changed daily, and dressings over the insertion site should be changed only by trained personnel. **The catheter should be used solely for TPN** and not for blood products, drugs, or other fluids. No stopcocks or manometers for central venous pressure measurements should be permitted. If sepsis is suspected, blood cultures should be drawn simultaneously from the peripheral blood and from the catheter itself. This is the only time that blood is drawn through the line. In addition, the hyperalimentation fluid should be cultured and the bottle and tubing changed. If no other source of sepsis is found, the catheter should be removed and the tip cultured.

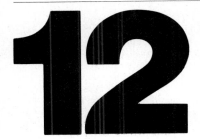

Liver Disease

Viral hepatitis

Viral hepatitis may be caused by the virus of hepatitis A, hepatitis B, or at least two other viruses, called non-A, non-B. **Hepatitis A:** Several sensitive immunoassays are now available for testing IgM antibody to hepatitis A virus. This antibody appears early during infection and is short lived (6 months or less). Thus, its detection is virtually diagnostic of acute hepatitis A. Infection is usually transmitted via the fecal-oral route, and large-scale outbreaks are occasionally described that are traced to contamination of food or drinking water.

Hepatitis B: The presence of hepatitis B surface antigen (HBsAg) in serum is associated with hepatitis B virus infection and indicates a potential for infectivity. Spread via percutaneous inoculation (e.g., needle stick) is a common mode of in-hospital transmission. Although blood is the most consistently effective vehicle for transmission, the presence of HBsAg in other body fluids (e.g., saliva, sneeze specimens, semen) supports a role for these fluids as well. Hepatitis B surface antigen is not normally found in feces. Hepatitis B is a common problem among drug addicts, male homosexuals, and sexual partners of persons with this infection. A high risk of acquiring hepatitis B has been reported for patients and staff in hemodialysis units and hematology-oncology wards and for workers in clinical pathology laboratories and plasma fractionation facilities.

Non-A, non-B hepatitis: Infection with these agents cannot be diagnosed by specific serologic tests and remains a diagnosis of exclusion. Non-A, non-B hepatitis occurs most notably following transfusion and has been associated with epidemiologic features similar to those of hepatitis B, i.e., illicit drug use, hemodialysis, nosocomial spread. However, as many as 50% of patients hospitalized with sporadic HBs-Ag–negative hepatitis may have non-A, non-B infection (*Ann. Intern. Med.* 87:1, 1977).

I. Measures to prevent spread of infection

A. Reduction of exposure

1. **Hepatitis A.** Careful attention to hand washing by the patient and close contacts is an essential part of the preventive regimen. Although the period of greatest infectivity is during the 2 weeks prior to the onset of clinical illness, stool isolation precautions are indicated during the first 2–3 weeks of clinical illness in all patients. This corresponds to the time during which virus may be excreted in the feces. Isolation beyond this interval is not warranted. Separate toilet facilities are probably not indicated unless the patient is fecally incontinent. Viremia is very brief, accounting for the observation that infection is not blood borne.

2. **Hepatitis B.** Good personal hygiene, including hand washing after examination of patients and contact with potentially infected surfaces, should be consistently practiced. Gloves should be worn when handling body fluids from infected patients. Disposable needles and syringes should be discarded

with care. Blood tubes sent to the laboratory should be clearly labeled as coming from a hepatitis patient, and all nondisposable instruments in contact with the blood or other tissue fluids must be carefully autoclaved. During procedures that could result in splattering or splashing of infective material, a surgical face mask to protect the nose and mouth may have value. The U. S. Public Health Service currently indicates that HBsAg-positive patients need not be placed in isolation; they can be cared for in semiprivate or ward accommodations, provided blood and instruments are handled appropriately. The hepatitis B patient must be warned never to become a blood donor.

3. **Non-A, non-B hepatitis.** Sensitive and cost-effective screening measures for non-A, non-B hepatitis are not available. The risk is highest in commercial blood or donor blood that is positive for high titers of antibody to hepatitis B core antigen or elevated SGPT. Due to similar epidemiologies, it is probably wise to employ isolation measures as for hepatitis B.

B. **Prophylaxis: gamma globulin (immune globulin, hepatitis B immune globulin) and hepatitis B vaccine**

1. **Hepatitis A.** Numerous field studies during the past two decades have documented that protection against hepatitis A is conferred by immune globulin (IG) administered before exposure and during the early incubation period. When administered in the appropriate dose, before or within 1–2 weeks after exposure, IG prevents illness in more than 90% of those exposed. Also, since IG may permit subclinical infection (passive-active immunity), long-lasting natural immunity may result. Specific recommendations for prophylaxis of hepatitis A depend on the nature of the exposure (Table 12-1).

2. **Hepatitis B. Hepatitis B immune globulin (HBIG)** is produced from selected donors who have high titers of neutralizing antibody to HBsAg. To be dispensed as HBIG, the Bureau of Biologics of the Food and Drug Administration requires that each lot be tested for antibody potency to ensure that a titer of 1 : 100,000 or greater is detectable. Each 5-ml vial (HBIG or Hep-B-Gammagee) costs $135–150. Clear-cut indications exist for two forms of exposure:

   a. Postexposure prophylaxis is recommended following either needle stick or direct mucous membrane inoculation (e.g., accidental splash) or oral ingestion (e.g., accident with a pipette) involving HBsAg-positive materials, such as blood, plasma, or serum. The **recommended dose** is 0.06 ml/kg body weight. The globulin should be administered as soon as possible following exposure (preferably within 24–48 hours). An identical dose is recommended 1 month later. **Confirmation of HBsAg in the donor is essential, and anti-HBs screening of the potential recipient is desirable prior to receipt of this material.** An algorithm to reduce the likelihood of improper use of HBIG when these serologic tests are not readily available is suggested in Figure 12-1.

   b. Hepatis B immune globulin is also indicated for neonatal exposure to HBsAg-positive mothers. Infants should be given 0.5 ml of globulin as soon as possible, preferably within 24 hours of delivery. Identical doses are recommended at 3 and 6 months.

   The use of HBIG as opposed to IG for sexual contacts of patients with acute type B hepatitis is controversial, but recent data suggest that many **currently produced lots of IG** may provide passive-active immunity (*Hepatology* 1:536, 1981). If IG is employed, it is recommended that 0.12 ml/kg body weight be administered as soon as possible after identification. If HBIG is utilized, a dose of 0.06 ml/kg is sufficient.

3. **Non-A, non-B hepatitis.** Studies of the prophylactic efficacy of IG for posttransfusion hepatitis are difficult to evaluate, but no clear-cut advantages

Table 12-1. Immune globulin for protection against viral hepatitis type A

Circumstance	Dose (ml/kg)	Frequency of administration
Preexposure		
Travelers to endemic areas:		
Residence for <3 months	0.02	Once
Residence for >3 months	0.06	Once every 5 months
Postexposure		
Close personal contacts (e.g., household members, sexual partners)		
Outbreaks in day care centers: staff, attendees, and households of diaper-age children		
Outbreaks in custodial care facilities (e.g., prisons, institutions for the mentally retarded):	0.02	Once
Residents and staff having close contact with patients		
Casual school, hospital, office, and factory contacts	Not recommended	
Common source exposure	Not recommended once cases have begun to occur	

Source: Based on recommendations of the Immunization Practices Advisory Committee of the Public Health Service, as published in *Morbid. Mortal. Weekly Rep.* 30:423, 1981.

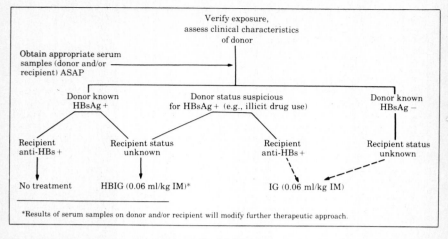

Fig. 12-1. Algorithm for managing needle stick hepatitis exposures if rapid serologic confirmation is not available.

have been demonstrated. Whether current lots of IG would prove effective against other forms of non-A, non-B exposure (e.g., needle stick) is not known. However, due to its low cost and relative lack of side effects, a single dose of 0.06 ml/kg is recommended by the authors for sexual partners and individuals exposed by needle stick to patients suspected of having non-A, non-B infection. It is also recommended that a single dose of 0.5 ml of IG be given to infants born to mothers with acute or chronic non-A, non-B hepatitis.

4. **Hepatitis B vaccine.** Clinical trials employing a pepsin-formalin–treated vaccine made from the blood of HBsAg carriers have been conducted among certain high risk groups. A randomized, controlled study among a large group of male homosexuals has indicated that this vaccine is more than 95 percent effective in preventing infection (*Hepatology* 1:377, 1981). The same vaccine was only slightly less effective among dialysis patients and dialysis staff. The vaccine has now been licensed by the Federal Drug Administration under the trade name of Heptavax-B. Three 20-μg doses are recommended, the first two spaced 1 month apart and the third at 6 months.

   a. The following populations should be strongly considered for vaccination:

   (1) Medical and laboratory personnel who have frequent contact with hepatitis B–positive blood or blood products (e.g., hepatitis researchers, dialysis workers, blood bank and chemistry lab technicians)

   (2) Hemodialysis patients

   (3) Male homosexuals

   (4) Neonates of infected mothers

   (5) Spouses of chronic HBsAg carriers

   b. **It has been recommended that anti-HBs or anti-HBc screening tests should be done on all potential recipients of the vaccine who are at high risk prior to administration.** Since the cost of the vaccine is approximately $100 for three doses, this may be particularly important for certain populations, such as male homosexuals, users of illicit drugs, and spouses of HBsAg carriers, in whom antibody detection rates may be as high as 50%.

II. General measures in acute viral hepatitis

A. Diet. No specific benefit accrues from the use of high-calorie, high-protein diets. Initially, the patient should be allowed to eat an ad lib diet. Hard candy, carbonated drinks, and fruit juices may cause less aggravation of the nausea that is frequently present than do other foods. Fats should not be arbitrarily restricted, since they make the diet more palatable as recovery ensues. If anorexia is severe, 10% glucose IV or supplemental tube feedings may be required. The use of alcohol should be discouraged until liver chemistries have normalized (usually 8–12 weeks after the onset of symptoms).

Vitamins are recommended for malnourished or seriously anorectic patients. In hypoprothrombinemic patients, parenteral vitamin K (10 mg IM) should be given. Those with severe hepatocellular disease are unlikely to respond.

B. Rest. In general, early ambulation can be allowed if the patient feels well and biochemical test are improving. Modified activity should be recommended only if clinical and laboratory data do not improve or if a relapse occurs with full ambulation.

C. Glucocorticoids. There is no indication for the use of glucocorticoids in acute viral hepatitis no matter how severe the illness. Although they may increase appetite and the sense of well-being and decrease serum bilirubin and transaminase levels, controlled studies have not shown that routine use of these agents prevents necrosis of liver cells, reduces the incidence of fulminant hepatic failure, accelerates healing, or improves survival. Methylprednisolone is no more effective than placebo in enhancing the survival of patients with severe hepatitis, including those in whom extensive necrosis was noted on liver biopsy (*N. Engl. J. Med.* 294:681, 1976). The risk of relapse and the chronic HBsAg carrier state may increase when corticosteroids are used during the acute episode.

III. Complications of viral hepatitis

A. Fulminant hepatic failure (massive hepatic necrosis). Less than 1% of adult patients with icteric acute viral hepatitis will progress within 4 weeks to fulminant hepatic failure manifested by increasing jaundice, shrinkage of the liver, and hepatic encephalopathy. Severe clotting abnormalities will be present. Once coma ensues, reported mortality is 80–90%. Advanced age, coexistence of other disease, and prolonged duration of coma worsen the prognosis. Death usually ensues from bleeding, coma, or infection. Other causes of fulminant hepatic failure include halothane exposure, acetaminophen overdose, carbon tetrachloride poisoning, isoniazid hepatitis, surgical shock, fatty liver of pregnancy, and Reye's syndrome. All except the last two are associated with massive hepatic necrosis.

Treatment is supportive (see Chronic Hepatic Insufficiency). The use of glucocorticoids in high doses (200 mg/day or more of hydrocortisone) cannot be recommended on the basis of available data. Clotting abnormalities should be corrected by administration of fresh-frozen plasma. Various heroic measures have been reported, including exchange transfusion, plasmapheresis, saline washout, charcoal hemoperfusion, and extracorporeal pig liver perfusion. Of these, only exchange transfusion has been subjected to a controlled therapeutic trial and was found to offer no advantage over conservative management. **None of these measures can be recommended.**

B. Chronic hepatitis, defined as hepatitis present for at least 6 months, may develop insidiously or follow an episode of acute viral hepatitis. Chronic hepatitis may develop following infection with hepatitis B or non-A, non-B viruses or as an idiopathic form. **Liver biopsy** is essential to determine the necessity for

Table 12-2. Drugs reported to be associated
with chronic active hepatitis and/or cirrhosis

Acetaminophen	
Aspirin	Sulfonamides
Alpha methyldopa	Nitrofurantoin
Chlorpromazine	Oxyphenisatin
Dantrolene	Danthron, dioctyl sodium sulfosuccinate
Halothane	
Isoniazid	Propylthiouracil

therapy, since prognosis correlates best with the hepatic histologic picture.
Regardless of the cause, there are two major histologic variants.

1. **Chronic persistent hepatitis** has a good prognosis with little evidence to
   date of progression to chronic active hepatitis or cirrhosis. Restriction of
   activity and the use of glucocorticoids are not warranted.

2. **Chronic active hepatitis** (CAH) is characterized by chronic progressive inflammation in the portal tracts and periportal parenchyma that may progress to cirrhosis. The viral form is frequently associated with HBsAg and
   male predominance. Idiopathic or autoimmune CAH is characterized by a
   major elevation of globulin, a positive ANA, and female predominance.
   Chronic active hepatitis may also follow drug ingestion (Table 12-2), and it
   may be a component of metabolic diseases, such as Wilson's disease and
   alpha$_1$ antitrypsin deficiency.

   a. **Idiopathic ("Autoimmune") CAH.** Three controlled trials have shown
      definite improvement in life expectancy when patients with CAH are
      treated with glucocorticoids, and one study has demonstrated im-
      provement in histologic abnormalities (*Gastroenterology* 73:1422, 1977).
      **The majority of the patients studied in these trials presented with
      jaundice or symptoms and major elevations (at least 5–10 times nor-
      mal) in serum glutamic oxaloacetic transaminase (SGOT).**

      For severe idiopathic CAH, regimens employing corticosteroids alone or
      in combination with azathioprine yield equally good results. However,
      combination therapy is associated with the fewest side effects. Prednisone
      may be given initially at 60 mg/day and then tapered to a maintenance
      dosage of 20 mg/day. Alternatively, a fixed dosage of azathioprine, 50 mg/
      day, may be given with lower doses of prednisone (30 mg/day initially,
      with a maintenance dose of 10 mg/day). Azathioprine alone has not been
      effective. Once histologic remission is obtained, slow discontinuance of
      therapy over a 6-week or longer period may be tried. The patient should
      then be maintained on the smallest dose possible that will control his-
      tologic and biochemical evidence of disease.

      Although corticosteroid therapy of severe CAH induces histologic remis-
      sion and enhances the immediate life expectancy in as many as 80% of
      patients with idiopathic disease, not everyone who responds continues to
      do well after withdrawal of medication. Within 6 months after cessation
      of therapy, relapse occurs in 50% of patients. When therapy is recom-
      menced, the probability of achieving remission is the same as initially, but
      the likelihood of subsequent relapse increases. **Although the majority of
      patients who enter remission do so within 3 years, approximately 15%
      fail to improve during this period.** Continuance of therapy for an addi-
      tional period is not recommended, since it is associated with a less than
      10% likelihood of achieving remission and a similar or greater risk of
      drug-related complications (*Mayo Clin. Proc.* 56:311, 1981).

The natural history of subclinical CAH and CAH associated with minor abnormalities in SGOT (e.g., less than a threefold elevation) is not known. Whether or not therapy is indicated in such patients has not been determined.

b. **Patients with HBsAg-positive CAH** often present without specific symptoms and with substantially lower transaminase values than those with the idiopathic form. Although the natural history of this disorder is not completely defined, many instances are reported of histologic progression to cirrhosis, with complications of bleeding esophageal varices and hepatocellular carcinoma.

The findings of one study suggest that the presence of HBsAg does not preclude a satisfactory response to corticosteroids (*Gut* 17:781, 1976); a more recent investigation has demonstrated that the long-term use of these agents may actually prove harmful in this setting (*N. Engl. J. Med.* 303:380, 1981). The condition of many patients with HBsAg-positive CAH is stable for prolonged periods. **In the relatively few instances in which frank clinical and histologic deterioration are progressive, however, the authors consider it reasonable to employ a therapeutic trial (3–6 months) of corticosteroids.** In such instances, prednisone, 30 mg qd, and azathioprine, 50 mg qd, should be prescribed initially. If a response occurs, the patient should be maintained on the smallest dosage of prednisone that improves symptoms and histologic appearance. **If these agents fail to induce improvement, they should be discontinued.** Histologic documentation of improvement is essential prior to decisions about long-term use (i.e., >6 months) of these agents.

Other treatment options are greatly needed in this disease. Conventional doses of corticosteroid enhance hepatitis B virus proliferation. Antivirals such as adenine arabinoside and interferon and immunostimulants such as levamisole and transfer factor are currently under study.

c. **Non-A, non-B infection** appears less likely to evolve into cirrhosis and hepatic failure than does HBsAg-positive CAH. Corticosteroids cannot be recommended for the majority of cases. However, when clinical and histologic deterioration occurs, consideration may be given to a therapeutic trial of steroids and azathioprine as has been described.

Toxic and Drug-Related Liver Disease

According to the presumed mechanism of injury, hepatotoxins may be classified as either intrinsic (predictable) toxins or dependent on the host (idiosyncratic, unpredictable). According to the morphologic pattern of injury, hepatotoxins may be classified as cytotoxic, cholestatic, or mixed. The cytotoxic injury pattern potentially is more serious, with a likelihood of hepatic failure and significant mortality. The cholestatic injury pattern is less likely to result in hepatic failure. Table 12-2 lists agents that have been implicated in the development of chronic hepatocellular injury. The reader is referred to *Semin. Liver Dis.* 1:91, 1981, for a complete discussion of drug-induced liver disease.

I. **Mechanisms of hepatic injury**

A. **Intrinsic hepatotoxins**

1. **Direct hepatotoxins** (e.g., carbon tetrachloride, arsenicals, phosphorus, and *Amanita phalloides* [mushroom toxin]) disrupt all elements of the liver cell. There are no known therapeutic agents for such hepatotoxins. Zonal necrosis or steatosis, or both, are noted on liver biopsy. Other life-threatening side effects such as renal failure must be sought. **Treatment** is supportive (see

Viral Hepatatis, sec. II). If the patient is seen soon after ingestion of the hepatotoxin, it should be removed from the GI tract by lavage or cathartics.

2. **Indirect hepatotoxins** (e.g., tetracycline, L-asparaginase, methotrexate, 6-mercaptopurine, mithramycin) include antimetabolites and related compounds that interfere with metabolic and secretory processes of the liver cell. Cholestatic indirect hepatotoxins include C-17 alkylated anabolic and contraceptive steroids. **Treatment** is supportive after withdrawal of the offending agent.

Oral contraceptives have been associated with abnormalities in sulfobromphthalein retention and liver enzymes, hepatic venous thrombosis (Budd-Chiari syndrome), cholestatic jaundice, and hepatic adenoma. The association with hepatic adenoma has become increasingly recognized, and in one series the relative risk of the development of this complication was noted to increase dramatically with duration of use, particularly after 5 years or longer.

B. Idiosyncratic hepatotoxins

1. **Hypersensitivity** is presumed to be the mechanism when the hepatic injury is characterized by the following: (1) a relatively fixed "sensitization" period of 1–4 weeks; (2) a prompt recurrence of injury on readministration of small doses of the agent; (3) an association with fever, rash, or eosinophilia; and (4) the presence of eosinophils on liver biopsy.

   Hypersensitivity may be responsible for injury caused by sulfonamides, para-aminosalicylic acid, chlorpromazine, organic arsenicals, methyldopa, and halothane. Glucocorticoids have been given to patients with apparent hypersensitivity reactions, but their efficacy has not been proved.

2. **Metabolic idiosyncrasy** permits either slow clearance or accelerated production of hepatotoxic metabolites of drugs. Reactions mediated through this mechanism are characterized by (1) a variable latent period of days to weeks; (2) no accompanying rash, fever, or eosinophilia; (3) no eosinophilic infiltration on liver biopsy; and (4) failure to reproduce the reaction by a single challenge dose of the agent. Drug toxicities in this category include isoniazid (see Ch. 10), acetaminophen, pyrazinamide, and possibly some cases of halothane and methoxyflurane toxicity. **Therapy** consists of supportive management after withdrawal of the offending agent. After the patient recovers, structurally similar drugs should be given cautiously, if at all.

II. Alcohol and the liver

A. Toxic effect and interaction with other drugs.
Alcohol exerts a direct toxic effect on the liver, although the role of malnutrition in promoting or modifying hepatic damage is not clearly defined. Acutely intoxicated patients may be especially sensitive to the CNS-depressive effects of barbiturates and sedatives (e.g., diazepam, chlordiazepoxide) that are metabolized by the smooth endoplasmic reticular enzyme system. However, after alcohol withdrawal, patients may require relatively larger dosages of these drugs because of the induction of detoxifying enzymes by ethanol.

Alcohol may potentiate liver damage induced by therapeutic doses (3–5 gm/day) of acetaminophen (*Ann. Intern. Med.* 92:511, 1980), probably as a result of accelerated acetaminophen conversion to a toxic intermediate in the presence of ethanol. For this reason, attempts should be made to restrict the use of acetaminophen in heavy alcohol users, particularly those with concomitant alcoholic liver disease.

B. Alcoholic liver disease
presents in three clinical forms that may occur singly or in combination:

1. **Alcoholic fatty liver** generally has a good prognosis. This disorder is self-limited, provided alcohol intake is stopped and an adequate, nutritionally

balanced diet is ingested. Multivitamins (initially administered parenterally to avoid malabsorption) should be given to correct vitamin deficiencies. Special diets and bed rest are not of therapeutic value. In most instances, conservative treatment substantially reduces hepatic triglyceride within 6 weeks.

2. **Alcoholic hepatitis** may be clinically silent or so severe as to lead to the rapid development of hepatic encephalopathy and death. A prolonged prothrombin time, not corrected by parenteral vitamin K, is associated with a poor prognosis during the acute illness. Treatment during the acute phase is supportive. Sodium restriction is necessary in the treatment of ascites and edema, and treatment of portosystemic encephalopathy must be started early (see Chronic Hepatic Insufficiency, sec. **II.B**). Glucocorticoids probably are not beneficial in the treatment of alcoholic hepatitis, and their routine use in this disorder is not advised.

3. **Alcoholic or Laennec's cirrhosis.** In the United States, alcohol is the most common cause of cirrhosis, accounting for over 50% of cases. The treatment of cirrhosis is supportive, as discussed under Chronic Hepatic Insufficiency.

Chronic Hepatic Insufficiency

I. **General measures.** The following principles of management apply to all types of chronic liver failure:

A. **Diet.** Improved nutritional status is an important part of the therapeutic regimen.

1. High-protein diets (100–125 gm) have been recommended, but in patients with severe hepatic insufficiency or portacaval shunts, signs of portasystemic encephalopathy may develop after a protein load. This risk can be reduced by limiting initial protein intake to 40 gm/day in such patients and increasing this by 10-gm increments every 2–3 days. Larger amounts of dietary protein may be tolerated by patients with milder degrees of hepatic insufficiency.

2. About one-half of total calories should be supplied as carbohydrates.

3. Salt restriction (see sec. **III.A**) is indicated if fluid retention develops.

4. Multivitamin preparations should be given to all patients; absorption of the fat-soluble vitamins A, D, and K may be particularly impaired. Parenteral administration of vitamins is preferred initially, because intestinal absorption may be impaired in cirrhosis. Macrocytic anemia is commonly associated with folic acid deficiency. Vitamin K should be given parenterally if the prothrombin time is depressed.

B. **Rest.** Bed rest is indicated when fever, infection, or marked constitutional symptoms occur or when hepatic function tests deteriorate. Bed rest may also be useful in the treatment of refractory ascites.

C. **Alcohol.** Complete abstinence is mandatory. Ingestion of even small amounts of alcohol by the cirrhotic patient may worsen liver function. In cases of mild and moderately advanced cirrhosis, abstinence from alcohol significantly improves 5-year survival.

D. **Sedation.** Narcotic and sedative drugs metabolized by the liver (e.g., secobarbital, amobarbital) and drugs associated with liver toxicity should be **withheld**. The effect of liver disease on the metabolism of sedatives, such as chlordiazepoxide, diazepam, phenobarbital, and diphenhydramine, has not been extensively studied in humans, and such drugs should be used cautiously, particularly when long-term usage is contemplated. Pulmonary elimination of paraldehyde is relatively inefficient and not reliable in the presence of liver disease. **Oxazepam**, a tranquilizer-sedative of the benzodiazepine group, is eliminated normally in patients with cirrhosis and acute viral hepatitis;

however, only an oral preparation of this agent is available presently. Small doses of IV diazepam may be preferable if sedation of patients with chronic hepatic insufficiency is absolutely indicated.

II. Portasystemic encephalopathy. Portasystemic encephalopathy represents a state of altered cerebral metabolism produced by the accumulation of various metabolic products originating from protein breakdown in the gut. These products normally are cleared from the portal blood by the intact liver. However, in the presence of hepatocellular failure or portasystemic shunting, large amounts of these toxic metabolites may accumulate. The exact cerebral toxin or group of toxins involved is uncertain. Ammonia has been most extensively studied and is formed in the GI tract from ingested ammonium salts, the action of bacterial deaminases on amino acids, and the action of bacterial ureases on urea. Normally, ammonia is rapidly removed from the portal venous system and converted to urea by the liver. In some instances (alkalosis, hypokalemia, or diuretic therapy complicated by hypovolemia), the kidney contributes to the production of significant amounts of ammonia. In addition, in renal failure, the quantity of urea available for bacterial breakdown increases.

A. Precipitating factors are detailed in Table 12-3.

B. Treatment of portasystemic encephalopathy **should be started as early as possible.** It is directed for the most part at reducing nitrogenous substrates in the GI tract and eliminating precipitating causes.

1. Established therapy

a. Gastrointestinal bleeding should be sought and, if documented, arrested as quickly as possible (see Chap. 13). Blood should be removed from the intestinal tract by constant gastric aspiration if upper GI bleeding is active or by administration of a cathartic (50 gm sorbitol in 200 ml water or 200 ml of magnesium citrate solution) if bleeding has ceased. Cleansing enemas are of value.

b. Administration of narcotics, sedatives, tranquilizers, diuretics, and drugs containing ammonium or amino compounds should be stopped.

c. Dietary protein should be reduced to zero initially and adequate calories (1600–2000 daily) provided. This may necessitate the placement of a central venous line to deliver 20% D/W (1000 ml provides 800 calories). If clinical improvement occurs after several days of treatment, 20–40 gm/day of protein may be allowed in the diet, with increments of 10–20 gm every 3–5 days as tolerated.

d. Removal of fecal material from the colon through laxatives or enemas effectively reduces nitrogenous substrate loads and should be instituted early. Cleansing enemas or oral magnesium citrate may be used for this purpose.

e. Lactulose, a nonsoluble synthetic disaccharide, is effective in the treatment of hepatic encephalopathy. Its mechanism of action has not been completely determined. Lactulose is not entirely metabolized in the small intestine but is hydrolyzed by bacterial action in the colon, producing an acidic diarrhea. Lactulose is supplied as a syrup, and it may be effective either orally or in an enema consisting of 300 ml of 50% lactulose added to 700 ml of tap water. The clinically effective oral dosage ranges from 60–160 gm/day, but is usually 2–3 tblsp (20–30 gm) tid–qid. Hourly doses of 30–45 ml may be used to induce the rapid laxation indicated in the initial phase of therapy of severe encephalopathy. The dosage should be adjusted to produce two to three soft stools daily. Excessive dosage may cause diarrhea with severe dehydration and hypernatremia. Continuous long-term therapy with lactulose may be indicated to improve protein tolerance, lessen the severity of encephalopathy, or prevent its recurrence.

Table 12-3. Factors precipitating portosystemic encephalopathy

Factor	Mechanism
Azotemia, associated with renal failure or diuretics	Increases urea available for bacterial breakdown in the GI tract
Tranquilizers, narcotics, or sedatives	Decreased metabolic clearance and increased cerebral sensitivity; production of hypoxia
Gastrointestinal hemorrhage	Provides substrate for increased ammonia production (100 ml of blood = 15–20 gm of protein); also, contribution from ammonia in stored blood; production of shock, hypoxia, and hypovolemia
Hypokalemia and alkalosis	Increased renal venous ammonia; increased resorption of ammonia from GI tract and renal tubule; enhanced transfer of ammonia across blood-brain barrier
High-protein diet	Increased availability of urea and toxicogenic amino acids
Constipation	Increased production and absorption of ammonia and other nitrogenous products
Infection	Increased endogenous nitrogen load from tissue catabolism; hypovolemia and renal failure; hypoxia
Progressive hepatocellular disease	Failure to detoxify nitrogenous products from GI tract; nitrogenous products bypass liver via portosystemic collaterals
Portacaval shunt	Same as above
Surgery	Cerebral sensitivity to anesthetics and sedatives; increased endogenous nitrogenous substrate; hypovolemia and hypoxia

Controlled studies have demonstrated that lactulose is as effective as either neomycin plus sorbitol or neomycin plus magnesium sulfate in the treatment of portasystemic encephalopathy. Lactulose is less expensive than neomycin and potentially beneficial in patients with renal failure or when prolonged therapy is likely. The combined use of both drugs should be considered when single-agent therapy fails. The suggestion that neomycin inhibits the effectiveness of lactulose by suppressing the activity of bacteria responsible for lactulose degradation has not been confirmed.

f. Neomycin (1 gm q4–6h) may be given PO or through a nasogastric tube. Oral administration of this poorly absorbed antibiotic will decrease urease-producing intestinal flora. Neomycin can also be given by enema: 1–2 gm is added to 100–200 ml of isotonic saline and administered bid–tid as a retention enema. Approximately 1% of oral or rectal neomycin is absorbed, with some risk of nephrotoxicity and ototoxicity. The risk of toxicity increases in patients with renal impairment. The prolonged administration of neomycin may be complicated by bacterial overgrowth or a malabsorption syndrome caused by direct mucosal damage or precipitation of luminal bile salts.

g. Infection can precipitate portasystemic encephalopathy and requires prompt treatment. All infections should be vigorously sought, including hypostatic pneumonia, pyelonephritis, and IV catheter sepsis. **Spontaneous bacterial peritonitis** occurs in 5–8% of cirrhotic patients with ascites and is associated with a high mortality (50–90%). Characteristically, the patient has fever, abdominal pain or rebound tenderness, reduced or absent bowel sounds, and encephalopathy. However, bacterial peritonitis may be present **without** specific clinical signs and **must be excluded** by diagnostic paracentesis in all cirrhotic patients with ascites and deterioration. A Gram stain of ascitic fluid reveals the causative organism in 25–50% of cases, but culture of the ascitic fluid is positive in greater than 90% of instances. Gram-negative bacilli, particularly *Escherichia coli,* constitute the most common pathogens found, although gram-positive cocci and anaerobes may also be present. Successful control of infection has not been associated with increased survival in many instances, since such patients often die from other complications of advanced liver disease.

h. Electrolyte abnormalities, especially hypokalemia and alkalosis, should be corrected. Hypokalemic alkalosis is best treated by infusion of KCl, and when contraction of extracellular fluid volume occurs, cautious expansion should be tried, preferably with central venous pressure monitoring. Human serum albumin, 25–50 gm IV, may be given over 4–6 hours, but it should be anticipated that this will provide temporary, if any, benefit. Blood loss should be replaced. Pulmonary congestion or edema must be avoided during volume expansion. Hyponatremia is usually dilutional and best treated by water restriction.

2. Unestablished therapy

a. Vegetable-protein diets contain lower amounts of certain amino acids, such as methionine and other putative materials that may be important in the pathogenesis of hepatic encephalopathy. Preliminary experience with these diets (*Am. J. Dig. Dis.* 22:845, 1977) has demonstrated decreased encephalopathy, decreased arterial ammonia levels, and improved intellectual performance. Such diets offer the advantages of being inexpensive and readily available in most hospitals.

b. Supplemental feedings enriched with branched-chain amino acids (Hepatic-Aid) may be better tolerated by patients with portasystemic encephalopathy than other sources of protein. Each packet provides approximately 560 cal and 14 gm of protein. **However, minimal data are available to justify the expense of their routine use.**

Intravenous amino acid solutions designed to normalize plasma amino acid levels have had mixed results. A parenteral solution enriched with branched-chain amino acids (HepatAmine) is available.

  c. **Ketoanalogues** of essential amino acids offer the theoretic advantage of combining with urea precursors to yield essential amino acids. At present, ketoanalogues are restricted to investigational use only.

  d. The place of **L-dopa** and **bromocriptine** in the therapy of hepatic coma is uncertain. L-Dopa is a precursor of the neurotransmitters norepinephrine and dopamine, while bromocriptine is a dopamine-receptor agonist. In theory, both agents reduce the effect of false neurotransmitters produced in the gut. A prospective, controlled study, however, demonstrated L-dopa to be no more effective than placebo in the management of chronic hepatic encephalopathy; absorption may be erratic, and GI intolerance is a frequent side effect. Controlled trials employing bromocriptine have demonstrated conflicting results, and thus this agent cannot be recommended at this time.

III. Ascites and edema. The development of ascites and edema results from increased portal hydrostatic pressure, decreased plasma oncotic pressure, direct movement of newly synthesized albumin into the free peritoneal space, and an avid sodium-retaining state, probably mediated by decreased effective plasma volume. Treatment of ascites **should be undertaken cautiously and gradually,** since it is seldom life-threatening, whereas electolyte imbalance, hypokalemia, or intravascular volume depletion caused by overly aggressive therapy may lead to hepatic encephalopathy, compromised renal function, and death.

  A. **Salt restriction** is the most important measure; no more than 500 mg sodium/day should be allowed at first. Occasionally, rigid restriction of sodium to 250 mg/day will be necessary, but such diets are unpalatable and restricted in protein; to supply adequate protein, powdered protein supplements of low-sodium milk may be given. When diuresis has occurred, more sodium (e.g., 750–1000 mg/day) may be allowed.

  B. **Water restriction** should not be imposed on all patients, but restriction to 1500 ml/day or less will help prevent development of dilutional hyponatremia in patients with impaired free water clearance. Reduction of fluid intake to less than 1000 ml/day is indicated for patients with dilutional hyponatremia and may be required when progression to renal circulatory failure with severe oliguria occurs.

  C. **Diuretics.** Numerous complications may follow diuretic administration; electrolyte abnormalities are the most frequent and serious. Because the capacity to absorb ascitic fluid appears to be limited to 700–900 ml/day under optimal conditions, overvigorous use of diuretics may result in marked contraction of the intravascular fluid volume and azotemia, with worsening of the hepatic encephalopathy. Patients undergoing sustained diuresis should not lose more than 10–12 lb/week.

    1. **Spironolactone** is the preferred agent to add when more conservative measures fail to mobilize gross fluid overload. It must be given for 2–7 days before effective aldosterone blockage in the distal tubule occurs. It may potentiate ethacrynic acid, furosemide, and the thiazides. The usual initial dosage is 100–200 mg/day; a total dosage of 200–400 mg/day may prove necessary to effect an optimal diuresis.

    2. **Ethacrynic acid** and **furosemide** are often effective treatment for ascites in

cirrhotic patients unresponsive to other measures. **Both drugs are potent and may precipitate encephalopathy.** Hypokalemia, hypochloremic alkalosis, and extracellular fluid contraction are common. The usual initial daily dosages are 50 mg for ethacrynic acid and 40 mg for furosemide.

3. **Thiazide diuretics** are effective, but hypokalemia and increased blood ammonia concentrations following administration may precipitate encephalopathy. Thiazides must be given cautiously, usually with potassium supplements. The usual initial dosage is 500 mg of chlorthiazide or 50 mg of hydrochlorthiazide daily. **Concurrent administration** with spironolactone is often more effective in producing sustained diuresis than the administration of either of the drugs individually. An additional benefit of combined therapy is protection against hypokalemia, and potassium supplements may not be necessary.

4. **Triamterene and amiloride** are alternative potassium-sparing diuretics that exert their effect at the site of sodium-potassium exchange. Both are weak diuretics when used alone. Potassium supplements **should not be used concomitantly** unless the serum levels of potassium are monitored frequently.

D. **Bed rest** may prove useful in inducing a diuresis in the patient with refractory ascites. After diuresis has begun, a gradual increase in activity may be permitted.

E. **Paracentesis** should be performed **only** for diagnostic purposes (e.g., suspicion of malignant ascites or spontaneous peritonitis) or when pressure symptoms caused by abdominal distention are severe. Aspirated ascitic fluid rapidly reaccumulates; rarely, shock, hypotension, and encephalopathy may follow withdrawal of as little as 1000–1500 ml. Other complications include hemorrhage, infection, and protein depletion.

F. **Salt-free albumin.** The administration of 50–100 gm/day of salt-free albumin for 3–4 days is occasionally beneficial, even when hypoalbuminemia is not a problem. The effects are seldom long lasting, but a protracted diuresis is occasionally initiated. This is most safely given with a central venous pressure line in place.

G. **Prostaglandins** may provide a natriuretic effect in patients with cirrhosis and ascites. The use of indomethacin or other prostaglandin inhibitors should be avoided whenever possible in such patients, for they may appreciably worsen fluid overload.

H. **Peritoneovenous (Le Veen or Denver) shunt** can be a rapidly effective surgical treatment for resistant, noninfected ascites. Patient selection criteria are incompletely defined at present; subjects with active liver disease, e.g., alcoholic hepatitis, appear to do most poorly. A high incidence of disseminated intravascular coagulation has been reported as a complication. Such shunts should not be employed in patients with recent esophageal variceal bleeding that has not been treated surgically. With current forms of medical therapy, insertion of a shunt should prove necessary in a very small percentage of patients.

Primary Biliary Cirrhosis and Other Cholestatic Disorders

Primary biliary cirrhosis, a progressive disorder of unknown cause that primarily effects middle-aged women, is characterized by cholestasis, elevation of serum cholesterol, and the presence of antimitochondrial antibody in the serum. Pruritus is often the most troublesome symptom. **Glucocorticoids are contraindicated,** since they do not affect the course of the disease and hasten osteoporosis. A controlled, prospective trial to assess treatment with azathioprine has demonstrated no apparent long-term advantage with this agent.

Pruritus in this and other cholestatic diseases (e.g., viral hepatitis, granulomatous liver disease, mechanical biliary obstruction) may be treated with cholestyramine, a bile-acid sequestrant resin. This drug will have its maximal benefit when bile salt concentration in the small bowel is greatest, i.e., at breakfast time. Therefore, cholestyramine should be given as 1 packet (4 gm) before and 1 packet after the first meal of the day. Further doses should be given before lunch and dinner. Cholestyramine may be mixed with fruit juice or applesauce. Nausea and constipation may occur, and hyperchloremic acidosis has been reported. Patients with prolonged cholestasis will require supplemental parenteral doses of vitamins A, D, and K.

Biliary tract obstruction by either inflammatory or neoplastic lesions may be treated in some cases by percutaneous placement of externally or internally draining catheters or stents.

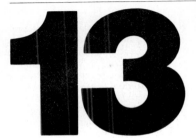

Gastrointestinal Bleeding

Acute gastrointestinal bleeding may vary in severity from hemorrhoidal bleeding without associated change in vital signs or hematocrit to ongoing exsanguinating hemorrhage. Thus, the therapeutic-diagnostic approach cannot be "cookbook" but rather must be based on the assessment of blood loss (actual severity) and assessment of risk factors (potential severity). The overall mortality in upper GI bleeding is 8–10% but varies in the individual patient as governed by the following **risk factors:** (1) As one would expect, severe or continuing blood loss correlates with high mortality. The death rate increases 6–25 times when more than 10 units of blood are required preoperatively. This may reflect the severity of the hemorrhage, but the same result can occur if the clinician fails to appreciate the amount of blood lost, resulting in undertransfusion or delayed transfusion. (2) Recurrent hemorrhage during the same hospitalization has been associated with a mortality 4–7 times greater than in patients who do not have recurrent bleeding. The propensity to rebleed may be predicted in patients with gastric or duodenal ulcers shown to have a "visible vessel" at endoscopy (*N. Engl. J. Med.* 305:915, 1981). (3) Age directly affects mortality. The relatively young, healthy patient rarely dies from ulcer hemorrhage, while mortality is greater than 35% in patients over age 80. (4) The cause of the bleeding has significant consequences. Mortality in unrecognized or unoperated-on aortoenteric fistulas is 100%. Bleeding from esophageal varices is associated with at least a 50% mortality (independent of the therapeutic approach) while a Mallory-Weiss tear usually has a benign course, with cessation of bleeding in 90%.

I. Initial measures

A. Assessment of blood loss. An estimate of the severity of bleeding is determined by combining the following signs and symptoms into an overall assessment of blood loss. Shock is evidenced by hypotension, tachycardia, decreased urine output, diaphoresis, and metabolic acidosis (see Shock, Chap. 23). Postural hypotension represents a postural (supine to upright) drop in systolic blood pressure of more than 10 mm Hg or a postural increase in pulse greater than 20/minute and may indicate a 20–25% decrease in circulating blood volume. An estimate of continuing blood loss may be established by determining the volume of hematemesis and bloody bowel movements. Since blood acts as a laxative, frequent tarry bowel movements associated with unstable vital signs indicate continued bleeding. Inadequate urine output is evidenced by an output of less than 20–30 ml/hour in the absence of renal disease. Skin appearance can be a reflection of inadequate circulatory volume (e.g., pallor, diaphoresis). A fall in hematocrit is the least sensitive indicator of acute blood loss, because fluid shifts from the extravascular space, so that hemodilution is only one-third complete in 2 hours and one-half complete in 8 hours. Thus, the hematocrit can be normal in the acutely bleeding patient.

B. Replacement and maintenance of blood volume must assume top priority in the overall management. A large-bore IV line (14–18 gauge) should be inserted for administration of volume expanders and blood. A separate central venous pressure (CVP) catheter is recommended, particularly in patients with uncertain cardiovascular status. The blood bank should be notified of the impending demand on its services, and 3 units of whole blood should be available at all times. Acute GI bleeding with shock is an indication for the use of whole blood. Packed red blood cells are appropriate in patients in stable condition with subacute or chronic blood loss or in those with congestive heart failure. With moderate to severe hypotension, transfusion should begin at a rate of 500 ml of whole blood q15–30min and continue until the indicators of diminished circulatory volume are stabilized. The hematocrit should be maintained at 30–35%; the CVP should be maintained at 8–15 cm H_2O. Each unit of whole blood (500 ml) should raise the hematocrit 3–4%. Once the initial volume deficit has been replaced, estimates of continuing blood loss can be based on the amount of blood and fluid required to maintain a stable circulatory state.

II. Diagnosis: upper gastrointestinal bleeding

A. History. A number of patients with a history of a potential bleeding site in the GI tract will actually be found hemorrhaging from a different lesion on endoscopic examination. About one-sixth of the patients who bleed from a duodenal ulcer have had no prior symptoms of ulcer disease. A patient with alcoholic cirrhosis and varices may be bleeding from varices (40%) but is as likely to have nonvariceal bleeding from a duodenal ulcer (20%) or gastric sites (30%), such as in gastritis or gastric ulcer. In patients with nonalcoholic cirrhosis, bleeding from varices is about 4 times as likely as from peptic ulcer, and gastritis is rare. Recent excessive ingestion of alcohol or salicylates suggests erosive gastritis, but endoscopy can sometimes prove this history misleading. Hematemesis following prolonged or forceful vomiting suggests a mucosal tear (Mallory-Weiss) at the gastroesophageal junction. In a patient with a history of an abdominal aortic graft placement, aortoenteric fistula should be strongly suspected as the cause of the bleeding. Gastrointestinal bleeding associated with abdominal pain should raise the consideration of bleeding into the biliary tract (hematobilia).

B. Nasogastric tube. Hematemesis or bloody nasogastric return indicates upper GI bleeding proximal to the jejunum.

1. In patients without hematemesis, a nasogastric tube should be inserted into the stomach as a means of detecting fresh or old blood.

2. A gastric aspirate should be considered positive for blood only if there is evidence of significant fresh blood (not tube trauma) or very dark aspirate that is strongly positive for occult blood. Guaiac card tests may be unreliable in the determination of occult blood in gastric juice (*Ann. Intern. Med.* 94:774, 1981).

3. A negative gastric aspirate does not rule out the upper GI tract as the bleeding source. The tube may be placed incorrectly, or there may not be any reflux of blood from a duodenal ulcer through the pylorus. Conversely, bright red blood per rectum may have its source in the upper GI tract if the bleeding is profound and intestinal transit rapid. Nevertheless, a positive gastric aspirate will be associated with an identified upper bleeding site 93% of the time, while a negative aspirate will have an upper source in only 1% of patients (*J.A.M.A.* 241:576, 1979).

4. In the presence of hematemesis or massive bleeding, a large-bore (at least 1 cm in diameter) tube can be passed through the mouth into the stomach and used for iced normal saline lavage. Gentle lavage with 1–2 liters of iced saline should be done with the patient in the left lateral or prone position with the head lowered. (**Note:** The therapeutic value of iced saline lavage is unproved.) It is usually not necessary to leave a nasogastric tube in place to monitor bleeding, since the recurrence of bleeding may be judged by other means (e.g., a change in vital signs and the passage of bloody stools). An indwelling tube can produce suction artifacts for the endoscopist and promote reflux esophagitis.

C. **Endoscopy.** Esophagogastroduodenoscopy has become the primary method of examination of patients with upper GI hemorrhage because of its high diagnostic accuracy (85–95%) and low morbidity. Massive bleeding precludes adequate visualization, and thus the procedure should be performed when the lavage return becomes pinkish and clear. In patients in stable condition who have stopped bleeding, endoscopy can be done as an elective procedure within 24 hours. Early endoscopy has not been shown to change mortality in patients who have stopped bleeding (*N. Engl. J. Med.* 304:925, 1981), but this is not surprising, since endoscopy is mainly a diagnostic rather than a therapeutic modality. With the advent of therapeutic endoscopy (i.e., electrocautery) or more specific therapy, it is hoped that early diagnosis will improve survival. Upper endoscopy has a higher diagnostic accuracy when compared to the 22% localization with barium radiography as the initial diagnostic procedure (*Am. J. Dig. Dis.* 20:1103, 1975). Endoscopy may be most helpful in determining which of several potential lesions are actually bleeding and in predicting which patients may rebleed, as evidenced by a visible vessel in an ulcer crater. Diagnostic accuracy is highest if endoscopy is performed within the first 24 hours of bleeding and falls rapidly when performed after 48 hours. **Contraindications** include an uncooperative patient and life-threatening cardiac dysrhythmias.

D. **Arteriography.** When bleeding is so brisk that the stomach cannot be cleared adequately for complete examination by endoscopy, or when endoscopy is not diagnostic, selective abdominal angiography may localize the site of bleeding. Diagnostic success is likely only when the rate of bleeding is greater than 0.5–1.0 ml/minute at the time the procedure is performed. It is imperative that active assessment and treatment of blood loss continue uninterrupted during the procedure. Arteriography can follow endoscopy, but barium studies may prevent its performance for 24–48 hours. The procedure has the potential advantage of being both diagnostic and therapeutic, since, once a lesion is demonstrated, control of upper and lower GI bleeding may be achieved by selective arterial infusion of vasopressin. Although varices may be seen in the venous phase of arteriography, bleeding from varices is seldom documented by this method.

E. **Upper gastrointestinal barium radiography.** The discrepancy between radiographic and endoscopic findings in the early diagnosis of bleeding lesions is now well recognized, with endoscopy having a higher diagnostic yield. Superficial mucosal lesions, such as erosive gastritis and Mallory-Weiss tears, are rarely detected by single-contrast radiography. Furthermore, although a barium study may identify a lesion, it cannot confirm that the lesion is bleeding. Barium should not be given if early endoscopy or angiography is anticipated, since it will adhere to the mucosa for several hours and interfere with these examinations. In the evaluation of the nonbleeding patient in stable condition, when endoscopy is incomplete or prior to elective surgery, air-contrast barium x-ray studies can provide helpful information.

III. Therapy: upper gastrointestinal bleeding

A. **Peptic ulcer (duodenal, gastric, or anastomotic ulcer)**

1. **Medical therapy.** Cimetidine has not been shown to be of value in stopping ongoing bleeding, but once the active hemorrhage has ceased, cimetidine combined with hourly antacids may be beneficial in the prevention of rebleeding (*Gastroenterology* 80:1313, 1981). If rebleeding does not occur within 72 hours, the therapy may be switched to a standard regimen for the treatment of ulcer (see Chap. 14).

2. **Surgery** is generally considered the therapy of choice for continued bleeding or rebleeding from peptic ulcer disease. In the patient with exsanguinating hemorrhage, it may be necessary to proceed directly to the operating room without further diagnostic delay. Other considerations for surgery are:

a. Bleeding that requires 5 units or more of blood in 24 hours with continued circulatory instability. However, a set number of units should not be the only deciding factor for surgery; the overall assessment of the patient and the inability to maintain hemodynamic stability are also important.

b. Rebleeding from a gastric or duodenal ulcer that requires additional transfusion during the same hospitalization.

c. Difficulty in obtaining adequate amounts of compatible blood, a past history of GI bleeding, or evidence of a "visible vessel" in an ulcer crater (*N. Engl. J. Med.* 305:915, 1981) may influence the decision to perform early surgery.

3. Intraarterial vasopressin. Selective arterial infusion of vasopressin in the therapy of bleeding peptic ulcers has been generally ineffective, but it may be tried in the patient considered at high surgical risk (see sec. **B.2**).

4. Intravenous vasopressin. The **IV** route is **not** recommended in bleeding lesions other than esophageal varices, because vasopressin is ineffective in arterial bleeding and has no proved value in other bleeding lesions. Superior mesenteric artery pressure is not reduced as effectively as with intraarterial vasopressin (see sec. **B.1**).

B. Esophageal varices. When esophageal varices are the confirmed source of bleeding, ice-water lavage of the stomach may temporarily reduce bleeding. The suspicion that varices are present should not prevent passage of a nasogastric tube for the evaluation of GI bleeding.

1. Continuous peripheral IV infusion of low-dose vasopressin should be the initial therapeutic maneuver for bleeding varices. This appears to act by decreasing portal venous pressure. The formulation is 100 units of vasopressin in 250 ml of 5% D/W, resulting in 0.4 unit of vasopressin/ml. This can be delivered with a microdrip infusor via a peripheral vein on the following schedule: 0.3 unit/minute for 12 hours; 0.2 unit/minute for the next 24 hours; and finally, 0.1 unit/minute for an additional 24 hours. Control of bleeding varices by this method appears comparable to the arterial route (*Ann. Surg.* 186:369, 1977). An **alternative method** involving a short trial should quickly show whether or not vasopressin will be of any therapeutic efficacy (*Gastroenterology* 77:540, 1979). Begin at 0.3 unit/minute for at least 30 minutes, and, if this is ineffective, progressively increase the dose at 30- −60-minute intervals, up to 0.9 unit/minute, for a maximum 2- −4-hour trial period. These methods control bleeding from esophageal varices in 50% of patients. **Warning:** Since coronary artery vasoconstriction as well as decreased cardiac output can occur, this therapy should be used only with extreme caution in patients with vascular disease, especially coronary artery disease. Subcutaneous infiltration can cause ischemia and gangrene of the digits.

2. Intraarterial vasopressin. Intraarterial vasopressin, 0.1−0.4 unit/minute, through selective catheterization of the superior mesenteric artery, may be effective if continuous peripheral IV infusion of vasopressin has failed. The latter, however, should always be tried first.

3. Balloon tamponade of varices with the Sengstaken-Blakemore double-balloon tube or the **single intragastric Linton balloon tube** (Linton tube [Davol]) may be used when vasopressin is contraindicated or unsuccessful. The Sengstaken-Blakemore double-balloon tube has a gastric and an esophageal balloon, but morbidity and mortality secondary to pulmonary aspiration have attended its use; therefore, it should not be used unless modified by the addition of an accessory tube to permit continuous suction of fluid accumulating in the esophagus and pharynx. (For a complete discussion of the Sengstaken-Blakemore tube, see *Gastroenterology* 61:291, 1971.) The use of either tube should be undertaken only with the aid of personnel experienced in the use of such equipment. The procedure for use of the **Linton single intragastric balloon tube** is as follows:

a. A new tube should be used each time and checked for leaks by air inflation prior to use.

b. After the stomach has been thoroughly emptied of clots with a large-bore orogastric tube, the lubricated Linton tube is passed into the stomach, usually through the nose. After making certain it is in the stomach, by fluoroscopy if necessary, the only balloon (gastric balloon) is inflated with 700–800 ml of air. **Inflating the balloon in the esophagus can result in rupture.** A 1-kg weight is attached to the outside end of the tube to compress the balloon against the gastroesophageal junction.

c. The stomach is then lavaged with iced saline until clear, and the gastric tube is attached to suction. The esophageal lumen is also attached to intermittent suction; this connection should be taped to prevent inadvertent lavage of the esophagus.

d. The patient will require close physician and nursing supervision. As long as the required volume of air is in the gastric balloon, slippage up the esophagus would be unusual. If the balloon should become displaced into the pharynx, there is the danger of asphyxiation. Scissors should be kept at the bedside, so that the tube may be immediately transected and withdrawn.

e. Balloon tamponade should not be maintained for more than 48 hours, since it may result in necrosis of the gastroesophageal junction.

4. Endoscopic sclerosis of varices. After massive hemorrhage has been controlled by vasopressin or balloon tamponade, injection of a sclerosing agent into esophageal varices via an endoscope has been helpful. It has also been used to control active bleeding, but its safety and long-term usefulness need further evaluation. The incidence of recurrent bleeding is reduced, but no improvement occurs in overall survival (*Lancet* 2:552, 1980). Successful therapy requires repeated injection sclerotherapy to obliterate all varices. Complications include esophageal perforation, stricture, ulceration, and the possible formation of gastric varices.

5. Oral propranolol may be helpful in preventing recurrent GI bleeding in patients with cirrhosis and esophageal varices who are otherwise in good condition (*N. Engl. J. Med.* 305:1371, 1981). A dose necessary to reduce the heart rate by 25% is administered twice daily. Propranolol is not used for acute bleeding but to prevent rebleeding in a selected group of patients who have previously bled from varices.

6. Shunt therapy. Portacaval shunts are very effective in reducing portal pressure and preventing variceal hemorrhage. However, hepatic encephalopathy is a common complication of this form of shunt surgery and often replaces bleeding as the cause of death. Other surgical procedures, such as the distal splenorenal shunt, have been advocated to maintain hepatic circulation and decrease the incidence of encephalopathy following shunting.

a. Emergency portacaval shunt, when performed during active bleeding, carries a 25–50% mortality. Temporary control of bleeding by vasopressin infusion or esophageal tamponade prior to surgery may reduce this mortality.

b. Therapeutic portacaval shunts can be performed electively in patients who have a history of variceal bleeding. Worsening clinical status, including evidence of hepatic precoma, may be a contraindication to surgery. Patients with a serum albumin of less than 2 gm/dl, a bilirubin greater than 3 mg/dl, ascites, or a history of previous hepatic coma have approximately a 50% mortality. With minimal hepatic impairment the operative mortality is 10–15%. In patients with alcoholic liver disease the incidence of recurrent bleeding from varices is strikingly reduced following a therapeutic shunt, but the mortality from hepatic coma is increased proportionately. The results of controlled surgical trials suggest a slight decrease in overall mortality following a therapeutic shunt in such patients, but the decrease has not reached the level of statistical significance.

c. **Prophylactic portacaval shunt.** A prophylactic shunt should not be performed in a patient with varices that have not bled. Well-controlled trials in alcoholic cirrhosis have convincingly demonstrated that, although the incidence of hemorrhage is decreased, patients who undergo such a procedure have increased overall mortality, chiefly related to the occurrence of encephalopathy.

C. Hemorrhagic gastritis and stress ulcers

1. **Medical therapy.** Cimetidine has not proved to be of value during the active bleeding phase. Maintaining gastric pH at 7.0 with antacids has been reported, in uncontrolled studies, to stop bleeding from acute gastritis. Once bleeding has stopped, cimetidine plus hourly antacids may decrease the incidence of rebleeding during the 72-hour high-risk period.

2. **Prophylaxis for stress ulcer.** Antacids have been shown to be valuable in the prevention of bleeding from stress ulcers when given hourly to titrate the gastric pH above 3.5 (*N. Engl. J. Med.* 298:1041, 1978). Cimetidine has also been shown to be valuable in the prevention of stress ulcers when 300 mg q6h IV is used (*Lancet* 1:617, 1977). This dosage should be decreased to 300 mg q12h in patients with renal failure. These drugs will have their greatest prophylactic value in the seriously ill and in burn and trauma patients.

3. **Intraarterial vasopressin.** Selective arterial catheterization with vasopressin infusion is often effective in the control of GI bleeding. The left gastric artery is infused for most gastric mucosal lesions (e.g., erosive gastritis and stress ulcers). The vasopressin infusion begins at 0.2 unit/minute for 20 minutes, at which time the arteriogram should be repeated to confirm that there is no further extravasation. The infusion should be continued at this rate for 24 hours. Then, if the nasogastric aspirate is clear, vital signs are stable, and no further blood is required, the rate should be decreased to 0.1 unit/minute for another 12–16 hours. If the patient's condition remains stable, the vasopressin infusion can be stopped and the catheter kept patent with 5% D/W for an additional 8–12 hours. If bleeding does not recur, the catheter should be removed on the third day. Vasopressin infusion controls gastric mucosal hemorrhage in approximately 80% of the patients; recurrent bleeding occurs in 16%.

4. Surgery may be necessary in the management of bleeding stress ulcers unresponsive to arterial vasopressin, but the surgical mortality is very high.

D. Mallory-Weiss tear.
The great majority of patients with a tear at the esophagogastric junction will stop bleeding spontaneously and seldom rebleed. The nasogastric tube should not be left in place once the diagnosis has been made. Selective infusion of vasopressin into the left gastric artery has been successful for the patients that continue to bleed. Rarely, surgery to oversew the bleeding vessel may be necessary.

E. Aortoenteric fistula.
A fistula from an abdominal aneurysm or prosthetic aortic graft to the intestine can result in massive GI bleeding, but a smaller "herald bleed" can occur hours to weeks before the catastrophe. **Any patient with an abdominal aortic graft who presents with GI bleeding must be assumed to have a fistula until it is proved otherwise.** A normal arteriogram will not rule out aortoenteric fistula, while upper endoscopy can be helpful in eliminating

other diagnostic possibilities. Awareness of the diagnostic possibility and expedient surgical correction are necessary to prevent exsanguination.

IV. Diagnosis: lower gastrointestinal bleeding

A. Rectal examination, anoscopy, and/or sigmoidoscopy should be performed on all patients with lower GI bleeding. This is an obvious diagnostic approach that is often overlooked or "deferred."

B. Radioisotopic detection of GI bleeding with **technetium-99m sulfur colloid scintography** is a simple and practical screening test to evaluate patients with lower GI bleeding. Although this test can detect bleeding at rates as low as 0.05–0.1 ml/minute in animals, angiography detects bleeding in humans only if the rate exceeds 0.5 ml/minute. The sensitivity of sulfur colloid scintography may be greater than arteriography in detecting the site of lower bleeding (*AJR* 137:741, 1981). Visualization of the bleeding site is within the first 5 minutes after IV administration. Colonic bleeding may not be detected if it originates in a region superimposed on either the hepatic or splenic areas of uptake, which limits its usefulness in upper tract bleeding. This technique identifies the general anatomic location of bleeding, but more precise localization and determining the exact etiology will usually require further investigation such as arteriography or colonoscopy.

The **technetium-99m–labeled red blood cell scan** can localize bleeding that occurs intermittently or at very slow rates. It can detect as little as 5–70 ml of blood loss occurring within 24 hours after a single isotope injection (*Lancet* 2:852, 1977) and may be more sensitive than the sulfur colloid scan. In one study where both tests were performed, 40% of patients with a negative sulfur colloid scan had a positive-labeled red blood cell scan (*J.A.M.A.* 247:789, 1982).

C. Steps in diagnosis. The diagnostic plan in active lower GI bleeding, once the rectal examination has been performed, should be as follows:

1. A technetium-99m sulfur colloid scan will be the first diagnostic test in the majority of patients with active lower hemorrhage. The labeled red blood cell scan may be the initial test if bleeding is intermittent or slow.

2. If the sulfur colloid scan is negative and the bleeding has slowed, arteriography should be deferred. The scan can then be repeated when there is evidence of recurrent active blood loss, or one can obtain a labeled red blood cell scan.

3. A positive scan permits prompt arteriography (or colonoscopy if the bleeding has slowed) to define precisely the site of bleeding.

4. In patients with a negative scan but clinical evidence of continuing blood loss, an arteriogram should be performed, with special attention to the hepatic and splenic flexure areas.

D. Arteriography should be used in the diagnostic sequence described in **C**. As in upper bleeding, arteriography has the added advantage of permitting the infusion of arterial vasopressin to control bleeding as a primary therapy or in preparation for surgery. In recurrent acute bleeding that has ceased, angiography may still be helpful by demonstrating vascular anomalies or tumor vessels (*Surg. Clin. North Am.* 59:811, 1979).

E. Colonoscopy has met with only limited success in the evaluation of acute lower GI bleeding because of the inability to clear the colon of blood for adequate visualization. However, once the active phase of rectal bleeding has passed and if a barium enema is nondiagnostic, colonoscopy can have a significant diagnostic yield (*Ann. Intern. Med.* 89:907, 1978).

F. An air-contrast barium enema in lower GI bleeding can be performed with good colon preparation in the stable patient. Its use during acute lower GI bleeding will interfere with procedures that offer a higher diagnostic yield.

G. Lower and upper GI bleeding are sometimes difficult to differentiate, and, in such instances, nasogastric aspiration may be helpful. If there is any question as to the level of bleeding, upper endoscopy should be considered.

V. Specific lesions: lower gastrointestinal bleeding

A. Diverticulosis accounts for 70% of significant lower GI bleeding in which arteriography detects extravasation of contrast medium, yet bleeding occurs in only 3–5% of patients with diverticulosis. Bleeding will continue in 20% of patients, 20% will stop bleeding and then rebleed during the same hospitalization, and 60% will cease bleeding. For the group that continues to bleed, if arteriography locates the site, selective arterial vasopressin can stop the bleeding in 90%. Surgery may be necessary in patients with rebleeding during the same hospitalization, those that fail on vasopressin, or those with a proved history of a bleeding diverticulum.

B. Vascular abnormalities. Arteriovenous malformations (angiodysplasia) can cause both acute GI bleeding and self-limited, but chronic, recurrent GI bleeding. Arteriovenous malformations are usually found in the right colon, but lesions in the stomach and duodenum may occur. When the lesions are found to be actively bleeding by colonoscopy or arteriography, the therapeutic decisions are much more clear-cut than the more common occurrence of finding a lesion that is not bleeding at discovery. **Note:** Angiodysplasia of the colon is common in elderly patients even without GI bleeding (*Gastroenterology* 72:650, 1977). Prior to any surgical resection, other vascular dysplasias should be sought, since they are frequently multiple. Endoscopic electrocoagulation may be used on a smaller lesion if the suspicion is high that it represents the source of bleeding.

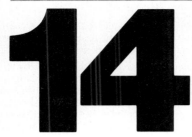 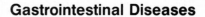

Gastrointestinal Diseases

Esophagitis

I. Reflux esophagitis

A. General considerations. Reflux of gastric contents through an incompetent lower esophageal sphincter can lead to esophageal inflammation and cause heartburn. In a small minority of patients this process results in bleeding or stricture formation. Hiatal hernias can often be seen on radiographs of patients with reflux esophagitis; however, the competency of the sphincter, not the presence of the hernia, determines whether acid will enter the esophagus. The medical therapy of patients with reflux is mainly aimed at reducing the quantity and acidity of the gastric contents available for reflux and, to a lesser extent, at pharmacologically elevating the **lower esophageal sphincter (LES) pressure.**

B. First-line therapy. The following regimen will achieve a reduction in symptoms for most patients (*Ann. Intern. Med.* 93:926, 1980):

   1. Bed blocks. During the daytime, gravity helps keep the stomach contents out of the esophagus. At night, the patient can receive some help from gravity by placing 4- –6-in. blocks under the head of the bed. Propping the patient's head up with pillows is ineffective and should not be substituted for bed blocks.

   2. Diet. Eating or drinking prior to retiring should be discouraged. Alcohol, chocolate, and coffee should be avoided, especially if the patient can correlate their use with increased symptoms. The obese patient may achieve a reduction in reflux symptoms by losing weight.

   3. Antacids. If the acid contents of the stomach can be neutralized, they will have a less damaging effect on the esophagus. The mainstay of reducing gastric acidity has been long-term antacid therapy. For patients whose symptoms are only mild and intermittent, 2 tblsp of liquid antacid at bedtime or with heartburn is sufficient. For patients with more severe reflux, antacids should be taken in the same dosages and on the same schedule as for peptic ulcer disease (see Peptic Ulcer Disease, sec. **I.A**).

   4. Smoking should be stopped.

   5. Anticholinergics decrease LES pressure and should not be used in patients with reflux.

C. Second-line therapy. For patients who have persistent symptoms on first-line therapy:

   1. Cimetidine. Gastric acid production can be reduced with cimetidine, 300 mg PO qid.

   2. Increased LES pressure. Either bethanecol or metoclopramide can be used to raise LES pressure. Bethanecol, 25 mg PO, is given 30 minutes before meals and at bedtime. This cholinergic agent should not be given to patients with asthma, bladder outlet obstruction, or ischemic heart disease. Metoclopramide, 10 mg PO, is given 30 minutes before meals and at bedtime.

D. Third-line therapy. Surgery is rarely indicated in reflux esophagitis, but it should be considered in patients with significant complications, including pulmonary aspiration, bleeding, and strictures not readily managed with bouginage. Intractability is another indication for surgery. However, the patient should have an adequate trial of aggressive medical therapy before surgery is recommended, and the existence of significant esophagitis should be documented by endoscopy and biopsy.

II. Candida esophagitis. **Candida** esophagitis is most common in patients with a malignancy, diabetes, or an impaired immune system. The usual presenting complaints are pain on swallowing and dysphagia. A barium swallow can frequently demonstrate findings suggestive of candidiasis. Endoscopy with biopsy is diagnostic. Treatment for mild disease is nystatin oral suspension, 250,000 units in water q2h.

Peptic Ulcer Disease

Estimates are that 5–10% of the general population will have a peptic ulcer during a lifetime. Peptic ulcer is a recurrent disease, and at least half of the patients will have a recurrence within 5 years. Duodenal ulcers are almost never malignant, but about 5% of gastric ulcers are cancerous. Endoscopic biopsy of all gastric ulcers is generally recommended to determine whether the ulcer is benign or malignant. The combination of an upper GI series plus endoscopy with biopsy and cytologic examination is more than 95% accurate in distinguishing benign from malignant ulcers. Patients with a gastric ulcer should have a follow-up GI series or endoscopy after 4 weeks of aggressive therapy. If the lesion is smaller but not fully healed, another GI series should be performed after an additional 4 weeks of therapy. If the ulcer is unchanged or larger at 4 weeks, or is not at least 90% healed at 8 weeks, malignancy should be suspected and surgery performed.

The goals of ulcer treatment include relief of pain, healing of the ulcer, and prevention of recurrence. Until recently, it was assumed that relief of pain correlated with ulcer healing. New studies have demonstrated that ulcer symptoms may resolve even though the ulcer is not healed.

I. Treatment

A. Antacids

1. **General comments.** Benign peptic ulcers, with rare exceptions, occur only if the stomach is capable of secreting HCl. The reduction of gastric acidity is the cornerstone of therapy in peptic ulcer disease. Gastric acidity can be effectively reduced with either antacids or cimetidine; there is no compelling reason to choose one over the other.

2. **Dosage and timing.** The proper timing of antacid administration is determined by the variations in gastric pH with time. The presence of food in the stomach causes an increase in gastric acid production, but food acts as a buffer. About 90 minutes after a meal, the food has emptied from the stomach, and the unbuffered gastric acid causes the ulcer patient to experience pain. If an antacid is taken 1 hour after eating, it will buffer the stomach acid for an additional 2 hours; but if it is taken in the fasting state, its buffering action is lost within 30 minutes. The proper dosage of antacid is that sufficient to buffer the stomach acid. Since it is impractical to monitor gastric pH constantly, one must estimate the proper dosage; 100 mEq of antacid 1 and 3 hours after eating and at bedtime should keep the gastric pH in an acceptable range (Table 14-1). Patients who cannot tolerate this antacid load should be given as much as can be tolerated.

Table 14-1. Antacid preparations

Antacid	Buffering capacity (mEq/15 ml)	Buffering capacity (ml/100 mEq)	Sodium content (mEq/15 ml)
$Al(OH)_3$			
Amphojel	20	75	0.9
$Al(OH)_3$ + $Mg(OH)_2$			
Maalox Therapeutic Concentrate	95	16	0.11
Maalox Plus[a]	40	37.5	0.18
Mylanta[a]	37.5	40	0.10
Mylanta-II[a]	75	20	0.15
Riopan	40	37.5	0.04
Gelusil[a]	34	44	0.10
Gelusil-II[a]	72	20	0.18
$CaCO_3$			
Tums tablet	19.5[b]		0.125[b]
$Al(OH)_3$ + $Mg(OH)_2$ + $CaCO_3$			
Camalox	54	26	0.33

[a]Contains simethicone.
[b]Per 2 tablets.

3. **The choice of antacid** is determined by buffering capacity, sodium content, and side effects. In general, liquid antacids are more effective than tablets. Magnesium hydroxide [$Mg(OH)_2$] is a potent antacid, but large, frequent doses can cause severe osmotic diarrhea. For this reason, magnesium hydroxide is combined with aluminum hydroxide [$Al(OH)_3$] in most popular preparations. For patients who have diarrhea while taking a magnesium hydroxide–aluminum hydroxide mixture, a constipating antacid, pure aluminum hydroxide, should be given with alternate doses. Magnesium-containing antacids are contraindicated in patients with severe renal disease. Aluminum hydroxide has only moderate buffering capacity and is mainly used to balance the laxative effects of the magnesium hydroxide. Aluminum hydroxide binds phosphate in the lumen and may cause hypophosphatemia. It also binds a number of drugs in the intestinal lumen, including tetracycline, thyroxine, and chlorpromazine, which may result in decreased absorption of these drugs. Calcium carbonate is an effective and well-tolerated antacid, but enough calcium may be absorbed in high doses to cause hypercalcemia and hypercalciuria; therefore, the dosage should not exceed 8 gm/day (16 tablets).

4. **Recommendations**

   a. **Acute therapy.** Patients with a new peptic ulcer should take 100 mEq of liquid antacid (see Table 14-1) 1 and 3 hours after meals and at bedtime. They should take another dose if awakened by pain at night. This regiment should continue for 4–6 weeks or longer if healing is not complete. Failure of therapy with antacids frequently is the result of inadequate dosage or improper timing.

   b. **Long-term therapy.** We do not recommend maintenance antacids after the initial course of therapy. Occasional episodes of pain can be treated with antacids as needed.

   c. **A recurrence** of significant ulcer symptoms should be treated as a new ulcer.

5. **Use as prophylaxis for GI bleeding.** Seriously ill patients, in intensive care units and elsewhere, are at high risk of the development of upper GI hemorrhage, most frequently from gastritis. Many of these patients have been treated prophylactically with either antacids or cimetidine to prevent hemorrhage. Two recent studies show that antacids are more effective than placebo or cimetidine for this purpose (*N. Engl. J. Med.* 302:426, 1980; *Surg. Gynecol. Obstet.* 153:214, 1981). Antacids are given by nasogastric tube in quantities sufficient to keep the gastric pH above 4.0. Maalox Therapeutic Concentration, 20 ml q2h, will keep the pH above 4.0 in the great majority of patients. Diarrhea is the only frequent side effect.

B. **Cimetidine**

1. **General comments.** Cimetidine blocks the H_2 histamine receptor. Its chief therapeutic effect in peptic ulcer disease is the inhibition of gastric acid synthesis. Cimetidine (300 mg) inhibits nocturnal acid secretion by 90–95% for 5–7 hours. It also effectively inhibits acid production in response to food, pentagastrin, and histamine. If 300 mg of cimetidine is given with a meal, it will inhibit gastric acid secretion in response to the meal by 70%.

2. **Use in duodenal ulcer disease.** Cimetidine is more effective than a placebo in promoting the healing and relieving the pain of a duodenal ulcer. A comparision of cimetidine and high-dose antacids has shown no difference in the rate of healing of duodenal ulcers (*Gastroenterology* 74:402, 1978). The use of full-dose antacids plus full-dose cimetidine is unnecessary, although cimetidine can be supplemented with antacids as needed for relief of pain.

3. **Use in benign gastric ulcer.** Most gastric ulcers heal without therapy. There is no evidence that cimetidine is better than antacids in treating gastric ulcer

(*Gastroenterology* 74:416, 1978). In fact, there is little evidence that either antacids or cimetidine is better than placebo.

4. **Use as prophylaxis for GI bleeding.** Cimetidine is now commonly used in an attempt to prevent upper GI bleeding in patients at high risk (patients with severe burns, on respirators, and following major surgery). Over the past few years, thousands of high-risk patients have been given cimetidine to prevent GI bleeding, and yet the evidence for its efficacy in this circumstance is meager. Recent studies suggest that antacids given in adequate dosage are superior to cimetidine in preventing bleeding (see **A.5**).

5. **Dosage.** The usual dosage of cimetidine is 300 mg PO qid (with meals and at bedtime); 300-mg ampules are available for IV use. The dosage should be reduced in renal failure to 300 mg bid.

6. The **toxicities** of short courses of cimetidine appear to be modest. Low incidences of agitation and confusion occur most commonly in older patients. There may be a small rise in creatinine that resolves when the drug is stopped. Chronic cimetidine administration has caused gynecomastia. The effects of long-term administration have not been fully evaluated. Cimetidine reduces hepatic blood flow and thus reduces the clearance of drugs whose metabolism and excretion are affected by liver blood flow (e.g., diazepam and propranolol). Potentiation of warfarin-type anticoagulants has been noted with concomitant cimetidine administration. Close monitoring of the prothrombin time is indicated when these drugs are given concurrently.

C. **Anticholinergics.** Anticholinergics are weak inhibitors of gastric acid secretion and no longer play a major role in the treatment of peptic ulcer disease.

D. **Diet.** There is no evidence that a bland diet improves symptoms or promotes ulcer healing. The patient should be instructed to avoid foods that cause epigastric discomfort. Late evening snacks should be avoided, since they stimulate gastric acid production at a time when the patient is asleep and unable to take antacids. Milk is a poor buffer, and its protein and calcium content promotes acid secretion.

E. **Hospitalization.** In refractory cases, short-term hospitalization may be necessary to institute optimal medical management or to remove the patient from a stressful home environment.

F. **Drugs, alcohol, and tobacco.** High-dose aspirin ingestion is associated with an increased incidence of gastritis and gastric ulcer and should be avoided in patients with an active or healed peptic ulcer. If aspirin must be given for therapeutic reasons (e.g., to patients with rheumatoid arthritis), it should be ingested in combination with an antacid. There is no convincing evidence that glucocorticoids cause ulcer disease, but their use should be limited, if possible, in patients with peptic ulcer disease. Other drugs, such as reserpine, indomethacin, or phenylbutazone, may cause epigastric distress, but there is no evidence that they cause peptic ulceration. Since alcohol in high concentrations damages the gastric mucosal barrier and can cause gastritis, it is contraindicated in patients with peptic ulcer disease. Cigarette smokers have a higher-than-expected incidence of peptic ulcer and delayed healing. Cigarette smoking should be avoided by patients with a history of peptic ulcer, especially by those with an active ulcer.

G. **Recurrence.** In most patients, peptic ulcers heal whether untreated or treated with cimetidine or antacids. However, in many patients, ulcer disease will eventually recur. The incidence of recurrence can be 50% or higher. No single satisfactory method is available for dealing with this problem. One reasonable approach to patients in whom ulcers recur only at long intervals and who present with the classic pain of peptic ulcer disease is to discontinue the antacids or cimetidine when the ulcer heals and restart therapy when symptoms recur. For the patient who has painless ulcers and in whom recurrent ulcers present with hemorrhage, it may be reasonable to continue cimetidine indefinitely or to consider surgery. Recurrent ulcers and the presence of other severe medical problems, which make the patient a poor surgical risk, may justify chronic maintenance cimetidine therapy. Cimetidine given in a dose of 400 mg at bedtime or 400 mg bid reduces the incidence of recurrence of duodenal ulcers (*Lancet* I:900, 1977; *Gut* 17:389, 1976). If cimetidine is discontinued after a long course of therapy, the rate of recurrence is high. The safety of long-term cimetidine usage has not been established.

II. Complications of peptic ulcer disease

A. Bleeding. See Chap. 13.

B. Gastric outlet obstruction occurs in about 5% of patients with peptic ulcer disease, particularly in those with duodenal ulcers situated close to the pyloric channel. Severe nausea and vomiting develop, which can lead to fluid deficits and metabolic alkalosis. A history of vomiting food that was ingested several hours previously is suggestive of outlet obstruction. The presence of a succussion splash 4 hours after eating is further evidence of pyloric obstruction. When this complication is suspected, a large nasogastric tube should be placed in the antrum of the stomach. If more than 400 ml is obtained from the tube within 30 minutes, the stomach is probably obstructed. If obstruction is present, nasogastric suction should be maintained for at least 72 hours to decompress the stomach. Dehydration, metabolic alkalosis, and hypokalemia can be corrected with saline and potassium supplementation. Only after this period should an upper GI series be performed. Although occasional patients respond to medical management alone, the problem tends to recur, and most patients will require surgery.

C. Perforation occurs in 5–10% of ulcer patients and necessitates emergency surgery. In a small percentage of patients, perforation occurs in the absence of previous symptoms of peptic ulcer. The site of perforation is usually along the anterior portion of the duodenal bulb. A plain upright film of the abdomen may aid diagnosis by showing the presence of free air under the diaphragm.

D. Penetration posteriorly into the pancreas is most common. The onset of penetration is often characterized by a change in symptoms (the pain becomes severe, continuous, and radiates to the back, and antacids no longer relieve it). These patients respond poorly to medical management, and most require an operation.

E. Intractability. Patients whose ulcers fail to heal and who still have symptoms after an intensive medical regimen (for 6 weeks) or who have frequent recurrences may be considered as candidates for gastric surgery. However, the physician should first be aware that significant problems can occur following gastric surgery (see sec. III) that may be as distressing to the patient as the original ulcer. An active ulcer must be documented radiologically or endoscopically before an operation is performed.

III. Morbidity following gastrectomy and vagotomy

A. Abdominal complaints. The most common complaint after gastric surgery is abdominal discomfort or vomiting after meals. Some of these patients may have surgically correctable problems, such as recurrent ulcer, obstructed afferent loop, or gastric outlet obstruction. The patient should be evaluated to see if these conditions exist. In most postgastrectomy patients with these complaints, however, no surgically correctable lesion exists. Their symptoms are due to rapid gastric emptying of a high osmotic load, resulting in distention of the jejunum and subsequent excessive secretion of water and electrolytes into the gut lumen and release of vasoactive substances (e.g., serotonin and bradykinin). The discomfort and vomiting may be accompanied by vasomotor symptoms (palpitations, sweating, dizziness). This symptom complex is call the **dumping syndrome.** An attempt should be made to treat the vomiting, pain, and vasomotor symptoms by altering the patient's diet. The patient is encouraged to eat six small meals a day that are relatively high in protein and low in available carbohydrate. Liquids with meals should be avoided. Anticholinergics may be useful in the relief of these complaints.

B. **Malabsorption.** Mild steatorrhea can occur after gastric surgery and is probably related to decreased transit time and inadequate mixing of food with bile and pancreatic secretions. Rarely, bacterial overgrowth secondary to afferent-loop stasis may lead to steatorrhea. Symptoms related to chronic malabsorption of calcium and vitamin D develop in a significant number of postgastrectomy patients. Over a period of years, metabolic bone disease, usually osteomalacia, will develop in at least 30% of patients with a Billroth II anastomosis. Calcium and vitamin D supplementation should be given (see Chap. 19).

C. **Anemia.** Postgastrectomy anemia typically develops slowly over a period of years and is secondary to deficiencies of folate, vitamin B_{12}, and especially iron. Iron-deficiency anemia is usually a result of dietary iron malabsorption, but blood loss from gastritis or marginal ulcer also contributes. Surgical reduction of gastric secretion of intrinsic factor rarely causes vitamin B_{12} malabsorption, since intrinsic factor normally is secreted in great excess, and, following surgery, enough usually remains for vitamin B_{12} absorption. When the cause of anemia is identified, appropriate iron, folate, or vitamin B_{12} replacement should be given.

D. **Diarrhea.** Mild diarrhea is a common problem following vagotomy. The patient should be evaluated for remediable conditions complicating postgastrectomy dysfunction (e.g., lactase deficiency or fat malabsorption); if none is found, a trial of symptomatic therapy with diphenoxylate, codeine, or tincture of opium is appropriate.

IV. **Zollinger-Ellison syndrome.** Zollinger-Ellison syndrome is caused by a gastrin-secreting non-β islet cell tumor of the pancreas or duodenum that results in marked gastric hypersecretion. Approximately two-thirds of Zollinger-Ellison tumors are malignant with respect to their biologic behavior or histologic appearance. Although this syndrome accounts for less than 1% of peptic ulcer disease, its consequences can be devastating if the diagnosis is not made. The most common presentation is a simple duodenal bulb ulcer, but large or multiple ulcers in the distal duodenum or jejunum, or recurrent ulceration after an adequate ulcer operation, should alert the physician to the possibility of this disease. Patients with Zollinger-Ellison syndrome almost always have the combination of gastric hypersecretion and a markedly elevated serum gastrin. The major morbidity and mortality of this syndrome do not come from the tumor itself but from the peptic ulcer disease caused by the hypergastrinemia.

Therapy is aimed at eliminating gastric acid secretion. Cimetidine can control the hypersecretory aspect of the syndrome (*Gastroenterology* 74:453, 1978) although total gastrectomy may be necessary. Unfortunately, neither gastrectomy nor cimetidine inhibits the growth of the underlying tumor, which is only rarely resectable.

Malabsorption

I. **Establishing the presence of malabsorption.** Malabsorption of nutrients (especially fat) can occur with any one of a variety of illnesses and should be considered in patients with unexplained weight loss, steatorrhea, or chemical abnormalities consistent with malabsorption. Once it is established that one nutrient is malabsorbed, studies should be done to determine whether other nutrients are also malabsorbed. **Fat malabsorption** is established with a 72-hour fecal-fat determination. On a diet of 100 gm/day of fat, the patient's stool should contain less than 6 gm/day of fat. The oral xylose absorption test (25 gm PO) is a good screening test for establishing the absorptive capacity of the intestine. Most diffuse diseases of the small bowel will result in abnormal xylose absorption. Serum calcium and magnesium levels should be monitored, since these minerals are also frequently malabsorbed in diffuse small-bowel disease. In diseases of the ileum, bile acids and vitamin B_{12} are not absorbed normally. Malabsorption of fat-soluble vitamins will lead to abnormally low serum carotene and prolonged prothrombin time (malabsorption of vitamin K).

II. **Specific diagnoses.** Once the diagnosis of malabsorption is established, the next step is to find the underlying cause. Barium radiographs of the small bowel may be abnormal in Crohn's disease, celiac sprue, blind loops, amyloidosis, and jejunal diverticula. Small-bowel biopsy by Crosby capsule is a valuable test in many kinds of diffuse small-intestine disease, including celiac sprue, giardiasis, Whipple's disease, and lymphangiectasia.

A. **Celiac sprue disease (gluten enteropathy).** Patients with celiac sprue disease are sensitive to gluten, a protein present in wheat, barley, rye, and possibly oats. The diagnosis is made by biopsy of the small intestine, which characteristically reveals complete absence of villi, and by the favorable clinical and histologic response to a gluten-free diet. However, since adherence to a gluten-free diet is difficult, the diagnosis should first be established by small-bowel biopsy. Careful dietary instruction is important, since gluten is present in many different types of food (e.g., ice cream, salad dressing, canned vegetables, instant coffee, mustard, beer, candy bars, hot dogs). In addition to dietary restriction, the patient may require iron, folate, calcium, and vitamin supplementation if these specific deficiencies are present (Table 14-2). Patients with sprue frequently have a secondary lactase deficiency and should be on a lactose-free diet until the small bowel recovers. (The following cookbook is available for the sprue patient: M. N. Wood, *Gourmet Food on a Wheat-Free Diet*. Springfield, Ill.: Thomas, 1972.)

B. **Lactase deficiency.** These patients have a selective deficiency of lactase, a brush-border enzyme that splits lactose into glucose and galactose. It is a common disorder and is present in 70–90% of adult blacks, Orientals, and American Indians, and in 10% of people of Western Europe ancestry. Temporary lactase deficiency may also occur as part of the clinical spectrum of other diseases of the small bowel, including viral and bacterial enteritis. Undigested lactose in the bowel lumen increases the osmolality of the intestinal contents and results in an osmotic diarrhea. This effect is further enhanced by the breakdown of lactose into organic acids by colonic bacteria. The symptoms of lactase deficiency (abdominal cramps, flatulence, and diarrhea) can be relieved by the elimination of dairy products from the diet. The diagnosis is usually confirmed by a **lactose tolerance test**: The patient ingests 50–100 gm of lactose, and blood glucose levels are obtained at 0, 15, 30, 60, and 120 minutes. A positive test is indicated by the onset of cramps and diarrhea and failure of the blood glucose to rise 20 mg/dl over the baseline.

Patients with lactase deficiency should be placed on a low-lactose diet and should avoid milk (including skim milk), butter, cream, ice cream, sour cream, yogurt, sherbert, cottage cheese, and cheese dips. Lactase deficiency is seldom absolute, and many of these patients retain enough lactase to tolerate small amounts of dietary lactose (e.g., as in highly processed cheese such as cheddar, Parmesan, and Roquefort).

C. **Bacterial overgrowth.** Any condition that causes intestinal stasis can result in bacterial overgrowth of the small intestine. Jejunal diverticula, scleroderma, afferent-loop obstruction of a Billroth II anastomosis, or partial small-bowel obstruction secondary to adhesions or Crohn's disease can all result in increased numbers of microorganisms in the small intestine. Deconjugation of bile salts by the excess bacteria causes fat malabsorption. The bacteria may also have a direct toxic effect on the mucosa itself. The organisms will compete for available vitamin B_{12} in the intestine, which can lead to megaloblastic anemia.

Table 14-2. Representative dosages for agents used in the management of patients with malabsorption syndrome

1. *Calcium:* Normal replacement is 1–2 gm/day. Calcium carbonate may be given as Titralac (400 mg calcium/5 ml) or OsCal (250 mg calcium/tablet).
2. *Magnesium:* Magnesium gluconate, 500 mg qid (each tablet contains 29 mg of magnesium).
3. *Iron:* Ferrous sulfate, one 320-mg tablet qid. Each tablet contains 64 mg of iron.
4. *Fat-soluble vitamins*
   Vitamin A: 25,000-unit tablets; for severe deficiency, 25,000–100,000 units/day; maintenance is 3000–5000 units/day.
   Vitamin D: Initial dose is 50,000 units 2–3 times per week. Dosage varies considerably, based on response as determined by serum and urinary calcium.
   Vitamin K: Vitamin K_1 (water miscible), 10 mg PO or IM qd, or vitamin K_3 (menadione), 10 mg PO qd.
5. *Folic acid:* 1–5 mg PO qd for 4–5 weeks is adequate to replenish stores and correct anemia; maintenance dose is 1 mg PO qd.
6. *Vitamin B_{12}:* 100–1000 μg/day IM for 2 weeks as a loading dose (if required). Maintenance dose is 100–1000 μg/month.
7. *Vitamin B complex:* Any multivitamin preparation that contains daily requirements (thiamine 1.6 mg, riboflavin, 1.8 mg, niacin 20 mg) should be administered bid.

1. The **diagnosis** is usually made by the history and can be confirmed by small-bowel intubation and anaerobic and aerobic culture of the aspirate. More than 10^7 microorganisms/ml usually indicates an overgrowth of bacteria.

2. **Treatment** consists of surgical correction of the intestinal abnormality, if possible, and administration of broad-spectrum antibiotics such as tetracycline, 250 mg PO qid. For long-term therapy it is usually advisable to give antibiotics intermittently (e.g., for 2 weeks out of the month).

D. **Ileal resection.** Bile salts and vitamin B_{12} are absorbed in the terminal ileum. Loss of more than 50 cm of this portion of intestine (as in Crohn's disease) will lead to malabsorption of bile salts; a somewhat greater loss is required for malabsorption of vitamin B_{12}. Unabsorbed bile salts pass into the colon, where they stimulate the secretion of water and electrolytes, resulting in diarrhea.

1. **Cholestyramine** (4 gm qid) will control diarrhea by binding bile salts in the intestinal lumen. However, patients who have had more than 100 cm of ileum resected will lose enough bile salts daily to result in fat malabsorption. The diarrhea in these patients may be caused by the irritant effect of hydroxy fatty acids on the colonic mucosa. Thus, these patients do not benefit from cholestyramine (it can aggravate steatorrhea by binding bile salts), but will have symptomatic improvement when put on a low-fat diet.

2. Most adults ingest 100–150 gm of fat daily, so that a 50% reduction (to 50–75 gm daily) will often reduce steatorrhea and provide a diet that patients with ileal resections of 100 cm or more can tolerate. Diets containing less than 40 gm/day of fat are unpalatable, and the patient will have difficulty in maintaining an adequate caloric intake. Medium-chain triglycerides (MCTs), which contain fatty acids 8–10 carbon atoms in length, can be used as an additional source of fat. Some of the MCT is absorbed intact and thus does not require pancreatic lipase. Although MCTs are relatively unpalatable, recipe books are available that include MCT oil among the ingredients in many different types of dishes. About 25–40 gm (2–3 tblsp) of fat can be ingested as MCT. Larger amounts of MCT will contribute to the diarrhea. These patients will require fat-soluble vitamins and calcium supplements in addition to parenteral vitamin B_{12} (see Table 14-2).

E. **Giardiasis.** The symptoms of *Giardia lamblia* infestation include explosive watery diarrhea, lower abdominal cramps, and occasionally fever, vomiting, and headaches. Although giardiasis rarely leads to malabsorption in immunocompetent persons, it is often present in the gut of hypogammaglobulinemic patients and is a cause of malabsorption in this group. The diagnosis can be made by identifying *G. lamblia* in the stool, from a duodenal aspirate, or on small-bowel biopsy. Quinacrine, 100 mg PO tid, or metronidazole, 250 mg PO tid, for 5 days is usually effective.

Inflammatory Bowel Disease

I. **Ulcerative colitis**

A. **General considerations.** Ulcerative colitis is a chronic disease of unknown cause characterized by remissions and exacerbations. Most patients can be treated medically as outpatients, but in a small proportion the disease runs a severe course and can be life-threatening. The predominant symptom of ulcerative colitis is bloody diarrhea. Proctoscopy is the most important examination for establishing the diagnosis and following the course of therapy. The mucosa of the rectum is edematous, hyperemic, and friable, with an exudate of mucus, pus, and blood. A barium enema is useful in determining the extent of involvement, but it can exacerbate the disease and should never be performed during an acute or relapsing phase of the illness. Patients can usually be followed medically for many years, but those with frequent relapses of fulminant disease will often come to surgery. Because the disease involves only the colon and rectum, total proctocolectomy is curative.

B. Sulfasalazine has two uses in the therapy of ulcerative colitis: as maintenance therapy to prolong the length of remission and, in combination with corticosteroids, to treat mild acute exacerbations of ulcerative colitis. Only a small percentage of the intact drug is absorbed by the small intestine, so that most of it reaches the colon, where it is metabolized by colonic bacteria to sulfapyridine and 5-aminosalicylate; sulfapyridine is absorbed and excreted in the urine, and 5-aminosalicylate is excreted in the feces. The mechanism by which sulfasalazine exerts its effect is unclear.

Side effects of the drug include nausea, vomiting, diarrhea, headache, fever, skin rash, hemolytic anemia, and, rarely, agranulocytosis. Skin rash is a hypersensitivity reaction and mandates discontinuance of the drug. Headache and nausea are toxic side effects and can usually be handled by reducing the dosage. Adverse reactions occur more commonly when 4 gm or more is administered daily, particularly in patients who are slow hepatic acetylators of the drug. For patients with active disease the recommended starting dosage is 1 gm/day, slowly increasing to 2–4 gm/day in 4 divided doses. Many patients will require maintenance therapy (2 gm/day) to prolong the length of remission.

C. Glucocorticoids are beneficial in obtaining remissions in patients with moderate or severe disease and may be given in conjunction with sulfasalazine. Oral prednisone, 40–60 mg/day, should be given for several weeks until the patient's symptoms improve and improvement is noted on proctoscopic examination. It can then be gradually tapered and discontinued over 2–3 months. There is no evidence that glucocorticoids are beneficial in maintaining remissions. When relapse occurs during sulfasalazine maintenance, glucocorticoids in full doses should again be employed and gradually tapered when remission is achieved. The activity of certain extracolonic manifestations, such as ocular lesions, skin disease, and arthritis, often parallels (although may precede or follow) the activity of the colonic disease and usually responds well to glucocorticoids. Patients who are refractory to outpatient management should be hospitalized and given hydrocortisone, 50–100 mg IV q6h. If the patient requires more than 15 mg of prednisone daily over a period of many months to keep the disease under control, a colectomy should be considered, since the morbidity of a colectomy may be less than that of prolonged high-dose glucocorticoids. Glucocorticoid enemas (50 mg hydrocortisone or 20 mg methylprednisolone qd) are particularly effective if the disease is limited to the rectum (ulcerative proctitis).

D. Azathioprine (up to 2 mg/kg/day PO) has a limited role in the management of ulcerative colitis and can be used in patients who are unresponsive to conventional medical management and are not surgical candidates. Azathioprine may also be used to reduce the maintenance dose of glucocorticoids in patients who are not surgical candidates.

E. Diet. Patients in remission have no specific dietary restrictions, but foods (such as milk products) recognized by the patient to cause abdominal cramping and flatulence should be excluded. A low-roughage diet decreases stool weight and often provides symptomatic improvement for patients in relapse. Elemental diets may also be useful during acute phases of the disease (see Chap. 11).

F. Anticholinergic and antidiarrheal drugs are often beneficial in decreasing abdominal pain and diarrhea. Such drugs include tincture of belladonna, tincture of opium, diphenoxylate, and codeine. They are contraindicated in severe cases.

G. Fulminant disease and toxic megacolon. An acute fulminant phase (either as a first attack or relapse) occurs in 5–10% of ulcerative colitis patients, with severe diarrhea, abdominal pain, hemorrhage, hypoalbuminemia, fever, sepsis, electrolyte disturbances, and dehydration. Toxic megacolon, in which the colon becomes atonic and dilates, develops in 1–2% of patients with ulcerative colitis. The **diagnosis** of toxic megacolon is made when the colon is dilated to a diameter of 6 cm or more (measured at the midtransverse colon), and systemic toxicity is present. **Treatment** includes the following:

1. Give nothing by mouth; start nasogastric suction to prevent further bowel distention.

2. Treat dehydration and electrolyte disturbances vigorously. Hypokalemia is frequent, and up to 200 mEq of K^+/day may be required. Blood transfusions should be given as needed. Total parenteral nutrition may be beneficial during this period (see Chap. 11).

3. **Broad-spectrum antibiotics** should be administered parenterally (e.g., cefoxitin, 2 gm IV q4h, and gentamicin, 1.7 mg/kg IV q8h).

4. Give **parenteral glucocorticoids** (100 mg hydrocortisone IV q6h).

5. **Do not use anticholinergic or narcotic drugs,** because they can precipitate or aggravate toxic megacolon.

6. Acutely ill patients not responding to intensive medical therapy within 48 hours must be considered for total colectomy. **Early surgical consultation** is the best procedure in severely ill patients.

H. **Cancer in ulcerative colitis.** Ulcerative colitis is associated with a tenfold greater incidence of adenocarcinoma of the colon than in the general population. The incidence of cancer is increased with the duration of disease (at 15 years the cumulative risk is 5–8%; at 25 years it is 25%). Carcinoma is more common in those with pancolitis and in those in whom ulcerative colitis develops in childhood. Regular proctoscopic and colonoscopic examinations with multiple biopsies are an important part of the management of patients with long-standing disease. Studies are now underway to identify the best methods of following ulcerative colitis patients for the development of cancer. At present, definitive recommendations for management cannot be made.

II. Crohn's disease

A. **General considerations.** Like ulcerative colitis, Crohn's disease is marked by periods of remission between exacerbations. The presentation, complications, and degrees of severity are varied and do not lend themselves to universal specific recommendations, only to general principles of management. Patients entering a period of active disease should be put on bed rest and their symptoms treated. In mild cases, diarrhea may be treated with tincture of opium or diphenoxylate. Intestinal obstruction requires decompression with a nasogastric tube (decompression, combined with fluid replacement, may allow intestinal edema and spasm to subside).

B. **Medical therapy**

1. Acute exacerbations can be treated with prednisone (40–60 mg PO qd). In more fulminant disease, glucocorticoids should be given parenterally (hydrocortisone, 50–100 mg IV q6h). Sulfasalazine (1 mg PO qd, slowly increasing to 2–3 gm/day in 4 divided doses) is effective in the treatment of acute exacerbations of colonic or ileocolic disease but not in the treatment of disease confined to the ileum. Sulfasalazine plus prednisone is no better than prednisone alone.

2. The role of azathioprine and its metabolite, 6-mercaptopurine, in the management of Crohn's disease is controversial. The evidence in support of a role for these drugs is slim, and they carry a significant morbidity, including an increased incidence of pancreatitis. Although these agents are not recommended as first-line drugs for the treatment of Crohn's disease, they may be

tried either when steroids have failed or in combination with steroids to allow a dosage reduction in steroids.

3. Preliminary studies indicate that **metronidazole** is useful in the treatment of perianal Crohn's disease. The oral dosage is 20 mg/kg/day (*Gastroenterology* 79:357, 1980). The safety of chronic metronidazole administration has not been established, and it is not approved by the FDA for this use.

4. Maintenance of **adequate nutrition** is a major part of therapy in Crohn's disease. Patients with ileitis frequently need parenteral vitamin B_{12} therapy. With specific oral replacement of calcium, magnesium, folate, iron, and other nutrients, absorption may be poor, and thus large doses of oral supplements may be needed. In patients with bile-salt deficiency due to ileal disease, substitution of MCTs for dietary fat will result in better absorption and diminished steatorrhea. In some cases a course of parenteral nutrition will be necessary to carry the patient through a severe phase of the illness (see Chap. 11).

C. **Surgery.** Most uncomplicated cases of Crohn's disease can be managed medically; surgery is generally reserved for the disease's complications: fistulas, obstruction, abscess, perforation, and bleeding. Surgery is required for the treatment of obstruction that does not respond to decompression and parenteral steroids.

Constipation

I. **General therapeutic considerations.** Factors predisposing to constipation must be recognized and treated. Many drugs induce constipation, including narcotics, aluminum hydroxide antacids, anticholinergics, iron supplements, and some antihypertensive agents. Conditions that cause pain on defecation (thrombosed external hemorrhoids, anal fissures, and anal strictures) predispose to constipation. A number of endocrine disorders, including diabetes, hypothyroidism, and hyperparathyroidism, may predispose to constipation. When constipation develops in a previously normal middle-aged or elderly person, colonic carcinoma must be excluded.

Constipation in hospitalized patients is a common problem, even for those whose bowel habits were normal at home. Prolonged immobilization, as in some orthopedic and neurologic patients, leads to constipation. Barium sulfate used in x-ray studies is constipating, as are many medications, especially analgesics. In addition, there are many hospital patients in whom straining at stool is especially undesirable (e.g., patients with myocardial infarction or recent abdominal surgery).

Patients who are **chronically constipated**, with no underlying illness, frequently benefit from an increase in the mass and moisture content of the stools. This can be achieved by increasing the fiber content of the diet or by giving bulk-forming agents. Dietary fiber can be increased with bran flakes or unprocessed bran, 2 tblsp/day, either spread on cereal or baked in bread and muffins. The most commonly used bulk-forming agent is psyllium (Metamucil), given PO as 1 tsp in water bid–tid.

II. **Laxative therapy**

A. **Contraindications** to laxatives include undiagnosed abdominal pain, intestinal obstruction, chronic constipation, and allergy. The incidence of allergy to phenolphthalein (Ex-Lax) in the general population may be 5–7%.

B. **Preparations of laxatives**

1. **Emollient laxatives.** Dioctyl sodium sulfosuccinate (Colace) and dioctyl calcium sulfosuccinate (Surfak) are surface-active wetting and dispersing

agents that soften the stool by allowing water and fat to penetrate the fecal mass. Since these agents promote the intestinal absorption of mineral oil, the two groups of agents should not be used concurrently. The **dosage** is 240 mg Surfak or 50–200 mg Colace daily.

2. Bulk-forming agents increase the moisture content and mass of the stool and thereby stimulate reflex peristalsis. Preparations include psyllium (Metamucil), 1–2 tsp in a glass of water bid, and methylcellulose, 1.0–1.5 gm bid–tid.

3. **Stimulant cathartics**

   a. **Castor oil** acts on the large intestine, producing prompt evacuation. Ordinarily, it is used only in bowel preparation for a special examination. The dose is 15–30 ml.

   b. **Bisacodyl (Dulcolax),** a structural analogue of phenolphthalein, stimulates peristalsis in the colon. It may be administered PO or as a suppository. The oral **dosage** is 2 or 3 5-mg tablets at bedtime; 10-mg rectal suppositories are available and act in 15–60 minutes.

   c. **Anthraquinone cathartics,** extract of cascara and extract of senna (Senokot), stimulate the colon and usually produce a single bowel evacuation 6–10 hours after administration. Senokot is useful in patients who take cathartics chronically. The **dosage** of cascara is 4–12 ml, generally given at bedtime; 1 tablet of extract of senna is given qd–bid.

4. **Saline cathartics** are relatively nonabsorbable salts that retain water in the lumen of the colon by osmotic forces:

   a. **Milk of magnesia.** Give 15–30 ml at bedtime.

   b. **Magnesium citrate solution.** Give 200 ml of a standard solution.

Diarrhea

The therapy of diarrhea consists in (1) correction of fluid and electrolyte disturbances (see Chap. 2), (2) treatment of the specific underlying disease, and (3) use of nonspecific antidiarrheal agents.

I. **Acute diarrhea.** Infectious agents (viral, bacterial, and parasitic), toxins, poisons, and drugs are the major causes of acute diarrhea.

A. **Drugs causing diarrhea include the following:**

   1. Laxatives. (Diarrhea caused by surreptitious phenolphthalein ingestion can be detected by adding base to the stool, which gives a red color.)

   2. Antacids containing magnesium hydroxide.

   3. Antibiotics that may cause diarrhea by inducing bacterial overgrowth or by causing pseudomembranous colitis.

   4. Digitalis, quinidine, and ganglionic blocking agents.

   5. Colchicine.

B. **Viral and bacterial infections.** The most common causes of diarrhea in this country are viral enteritis and infections with noninvasive bacteria, especially enterotoxigenic *Escherichia coli.* Infections with *Shigella, Salmonella, Campylobacter jejuni,* or *Yersinia* species are less common causes of diarrhea. **Most acute diarrheal episodes of viral or bacterial origin are self-limited and do not require specific therapy.** Patients should be on a clear liquid diet, and fluid status should be monitored carefully. If dehydration or electrolyte imbalance develops, parenteral fluids should be given. In *Shigella* and *Salmonella* gastroenteritis, diphenoxylate and other nonspecific antidiarrheal agents should not be used, since they may prolong the duration of the infection. For the role of antibiotics in the therapy of bacterial enteritides, see Chap. 10.

C. Parasites

1. **Amebiasis** is a frequent cause of acute or chronic diarrhea. The diagnosis may be made at sigmoidoscopy. Patients with rectal involvement will have discrete, shallow ulcers covered with exudate. Trophozoites may be seen on microscopic examination of scrapings from these ulcers. Treatment for asymptomatic intestinal infection is **diiodohydroxyquin** (650 mg PO tid for 20 days). Treatment for symptomatic disease is **metronidazole** (750 mg PO tid for 5–10 days) plus diiodohydroxyquin (650 mg PO tid for 20 days).

2. **Giardiasis** commonly presents as diarrhea, either acute or chronic (see Malabsorption, sec. **II.E**).

II. Chronic diarrhea.
Chronic diarrhea may be a sign of serious illness or a functional symptom. The proper approach depends on the clinical setting, and only general guidelines can be given.

A. Small stool versus large stool.
If the patient presents with a history of frequent small-volume stools associated with urgency and tenesmus, the site of the underlying disorder is most likely the distal colon. If the patient presents with a history of stools that are large in volume, the underlying disease **is usually in the small bowel** (especially if the stools are greasy or show other signs of malabsorption).

B. Classification of chronic diarrhea.
In many diarrheal illnesses there is both an osmotic and a secretory component to the diarrhea. Specific treatment for many of the diseases mentioned in **1–4** may be found in other sections of this chapter.

1. **Osmotic diarrhea** is caused by the accumulation of poorly absorbed solutes in the gut. These solutes may be drugs or ingested nutrients. The diarrhea usually stops with fasting. Typically, stool sodium and potassium do not account for all the stool osmolality. Causes of osmotic diarrhea include lactose (in lactase deficiency) and osmotic laxatives (e.g., milk of magnesia).

2. **Secretory diarrhea** is caused by an abnormal secretion of water and electrolytes into the intestinal lumen. In this condition, the effective osmotic pressure of the intestinal contents is the same as that of the plasma. Typically, the diarrhea persists despite fasting. There are numerous causes of secretory diarrhea, incuding bacterial enterotoxins, secretory hormones (e.g., vasoactive intestinal polypeptide), some laxatives, and dihydroxy bile acids (these occur with bile-acid malabsorption).

3. **Mucosal injury.** Many illnesses causing injury to the intestinal mucosa result in diarrhea, with both osmotic and secretory components. Diseases in which mucosal injury causes diarrhea include inflammatory bowel disease, celiac disease, lymphoma, and ischemic bowel disease.

4. **Deranged intestinal motility.** The most clearly defined example of deranged intestinal motility is irritable bowel syndrome.

III. Nonspecific antidiarrheal agents.
Nonspecific antidiarrheal agents are generally overused. **Their routine use in the treatment of all diarrheal states is not indicated.** In most acute diarrheas they are unnecessary. In chronic diarrhea they are not a substitute for treatment of the underlying illness. In *Salmonella* and *Shigella* infections, they may prolong the illness.

A. Bulk-forming agents.
See Constipation, sec. **II.B.2**.

B. Absorbents.
Kaopectate, 60–90 ml, is given qid.

C. Narcotic agents.
Realize the dangers and observe the necessary precautions if

used in patients with asthma, chronic lung disease, benign prostatic hypertrophy, or acute angle-closure glaucoma.

1. **Paregoric (camphorated tincture of opium).** The **dosage** is 4–8 ml after
   each liquid stool or qid.

2. **Deodorized tincture of opium.** The **dosage** is 0.5–1.5 ml tid or qid.

3. **Opium and belladonna.** The **dosage** is 30 mg of powdered opium and 15 mg
   of belladonna, 1 capsule tid or qid.

4. **Codeine.** The **dosage** is 16–64 mg bid–qid.

5. **Diphenoxylate hydrochloride (Lomotil)** is a meperidine congener. It effectively inhibits excessive GI motility. A 2.5-mg dose is approximately equivalent in antidiarrheal efficacy to 4 ml of paregoric. It has low analgesic activity and is free of parasympatholytic actions and addiction potential when
   used in the correct dosage range. Side effects are uncommon (nausea, dizziness, vomiting, and, rarely, pruritus and skin rashes). **It is contraindicated
   in patients with advanced liver disease.** Respiratory depression will occur
   with overdose and may be potentiated by phenothiazine derivatives, barbiturates, or imipramine-type antidepressants. Each diphenoxylate tablet or 5
   ml of the liquid contains 2.5 mg diphenoxylate hydrochloride and 0.025 mg
   atropine sulfate (a subtherapeutic amount added to discourage deliberate
   overdose). The **dosage** is 5 mg tid or qid until initial control of diarrhea is
   effected; then a maintenance dosage of 2.5 mg bid–tid is given.

Diverticular Disease

I. **Diverticulosis.** Diverticula are acquired herniations of colonic mucosa through the
muscular layers of the colonic wall, in close proximity to penetrating nutrient
arteries. Their occurrence increases markedly with age. Epidemiologic evidence
suggests that diverticulosis occurs more frequently in developed nations than in
third-world countries, since the populations in the former ingest a highly refined
diet that is low in dietary fiber. Most diverticula are asymptomatic and do not
require treatment. However, they can be the cause of profuse lower GI bleeding
that in most cases resolves spontaneously. Some of these patients may also suffer
from symptoms of irritable bowel syndrome and should be treated accordingly (see
Irritable Bowel Syndrome).

II. **Diverticulitis.** Diverticulitis is a complication of diverticular disease in which perforation of a diverticulum occurs. Left lower quadrant pain accompanied by fever
and chills, with laboratory evidence of inflammation, is the most common manifestation of acute diverticulitis. Occasionally, a left lower quadrant mass may be
present. Fistulas to the bladder, vagina, or skin may form from the diseased colon.
Patients should be given nothing by mouth; IV fluid replacement is necessary.
Nasogastric suction should be instituted if there are signs of bowel obstruction.
Ampicillin or tetracycline should be administered during the acute attack. Immediate surgical consultation is advisable, since operative intervention may be
required if complications arise. After the acute phase, a high-bulk diet should be
instituted to decrease colonic pressures, which theoretically will decrease recurrences. To expand stool volume, metamucil or bran is frequently used in addition to
a high-bulk diet.

Irritable Bowel Syndrome

Irritable bowel syndrome is the most common GI problem seen by physicians. It is a
diagnosis of exclusion. The patient complains of abdominal pain, which can be
steady or cramping, can involve any quadrant of the abdomen, and can radiate to

the back or chest. The pain will often be accompanied by constipation or diarrhea, or alternating constipation and diarrhea. A small group of patients will complain of diarrhea without abdominal pain. Lactase deficiency can present with a clinical picture resembling irritable bowel syndrome (diarrhea, cramps, flatulence, bloating). Patients with these complaints should have a lactose tolerance test. The symptoms of irritable bowel syndrome are probably related to increased colonic motor activity, but there is commonly an underlying psychiatric disorder, such as hysteria or depression. The altered bowel function should be **treated** with a diet high in bulk and consisting of fruits, vegetables, and wheat bran in the form of bran flakes or 2 tblsp unprocessed bran/day. Commercial bulk laxatives that contain psyllium (Effersyllium, Konsyl, Metamucil), 1–2 tsp PO bid, may be used instead of bran but are more expensive. The pain of irritable bowel syndrome is more difficult to treat. Anticholinergics, such as belladonna, 10–15 drops PO tid, or propantheline, 15–30 mg PO qid, may be tried. Often, combining an anticholinergic with a tranquilizer, such as diazepam, chlordiazepoxide, or with phenobarbital may be helpful. Psychiatric consultation or treatment with antidepressant medication may be appropriate in selected cases.

Pseudomembranous Colitis

Pseudomembranous colitis is now most commonly described as a sequela to antibiotic therapy, although it may be seen with severe underlying disease (e.g., ischemia) without antibiotics. Lincomycin, tetracycline, chloramphenicol, ampicillin, and particularly clindamycin have been associated with this disorder. Usually, 4–9 days after the start of antibiotics (although it may be longer), fever, cramps, and nonbloody diarrhea develop. Proctoscopic evaluation reveals characteristic yellow white, raised, plaquelike pseudomembranes. This syndrome is caused by an overgrowth of the colonic flora with toxin-producing *Clostridium difficile*. In patients with antibiotic-induced pseudomembranous colitis, this overgrowth should be treated by **discontinuing the offending antibiotic** and treating the patient with oral **vancomycin**. The recommended dosage for oral vancomycin is 125–500 mg PO qid, although most patients do well on 125–250 mg PO qid. Vancomycin is not well absorbed when given PO and is very effective in killing *C. difficile* in the colon (*Lancet* 2:226, 1978). Pseudomembranous colitis may recur when vancomycin is discontinued. This requires either another course of therapy with vancomycin or a trial on another agent. Some success has been reported with oral bacitracin, but its use is still investigational.

Pancreatitis

I. Acute pancreatitis

A. General considerations. Acute pancreatitis is generally associated with excessive alcohol consumption, gallstones, hyperparathyroidism, hyperlipoproteinemias types I, IV, and V, and with a number of drugs, including thiazides, oral contraceptives, isoniazid, furosemide, and azathioprine. The therapy of acute pancreatitis is largely empirical. Controlled studies of most aspects of the management of the disease are unavailable.

B. Pain relief. Meperidine (Demerol), 75–100 mg IM q4h, is probably the drug of choice. There are no data to show that narcotics exacerbate acute pancreatitis.

C. Diet. Patients with acute pancreatitis should be given nothing by mouth and should be placed on nasogastric suction. This should be continued until the patient is pain free and nausea and vomiting have resolved. After nasogastric suction has been stopped, the patient can be started on clear liquids and the diet slowly advanced.

D. Fluid managment. Maintenance of an adequate circulating blood volume is the most important aspect of the management of the patient with acute pancreatitis. Careful monitoring of input and output is critical. Fluid losses through vomiting, nasogastric suction, sweating, and pooling of fluid in the abdomen and retroperitoneum must be considered and treated. Hypocalcemia is a frequent finding and should be corrected with IV calcium gluconate. Hypomagnesemia may also occur in acute pancreatitis. Blood glucose levels should be monitored, since hyperglycemia has a tendency to develop in these patients. A few patients present with circulatory collapse; in these patients the maintenance of an adequate circulating blood volume is the greatest problem. Circulating volume may be increased by giving whole blood or plasma.

E. Antibiotics. There is no demonstrable benefit from the use of prophylactic antibiotics in acute pancreatitis. In febrile patients ($>2°C$ above normal), the likelihood of infection (pancreatic abscess, infected pseudocyst) is increased. Full culturing should be done in these patients, and a broad-spectrum antibiotic program should then be started (e.g., ampicillin, 1 gm q6h, and gentamicin, 1.7 mg/kg IV q8h).

F. Surgery. In a few patients with acute pancreatitis, surgery has a therapeutic role. Patients with cholangitis caused by an obstructed common bile duct need emergency surgery. Patients with pancreatic abscess or a life-threatening hemorrhagic pancreatitis may benefit from surgical drainage.

G. Anticholinergics. Although anticholinergics have long been used in the therapy of acute pancreatitis, no studies have clearly established their efficacy.

H. Underlying factors. Hyperparathyroidism, hyperlipoproteinemia, and other treatable causes of acute pancreatitis should be excluded.

II. **Chronic pancreatitis.** Chronic pancreatitis is usually associated with chronic alcoholism. As opposed to acute pancreatitis, chronic pancreatitis is not often associated with cholelithiasis. Abstinence from alcohol will frequently result in symptomatic improvement. Pain relief is a great problem in patients with chronic pancreatitis. They frequently require narcotics for pain relief, and addiction is common. The onset of severe malabsorption is marked by steatorrhea and weight loss. Malabsorption due to exocrine pancreatic insufficiency can be managed with oral enzyme supplements and a suitable diet (high in protein and carbohydrates and low in fat [50 gm/day]). Enzyme supplements in the form of Viokase (0.3-gm tablet) or Cotazym (0.3-gm tablet) may be given as 2–3 tablets taken at regular intervals 6–12 times a day. As steatorrhea diminishes with enzyme supplementation, the fat content of the diet may be increased. Since these enzymes are inactivated by gastric acid, they may be given in conjunction with a regimen of antacids or cimetidine if the clinical response to enzyme replacement is inadequate. Insulin-dependent diabetes frequently develops in these patients.

Common Anorectal Problems

I. **Hemorrhoids**

A. External thrombosed hemorrhoid presents with the sudden onset of a pain in the anus. On physical examination it appears as a tense, bluish lump covered with skin. If pain is severe, prompt relief can be obtained by excision of the thrombosed vein under local anesthesia. If pain is mild or has already started to resolve, the patient can be given oral analgesics, sitz baths, stool softeners, and topical emollients (see **B.1–3**).

B. Internal hemorrhoids commonly present with either bleeding or prolapsing mass that may or may not be reducible. Pain is usually not a prominent feature. Prolapsed internal hemorrhoids appear as masses separated by radial folds. The upper portions are covered with red mucosa. **Treatment** includes the following:

1. **Stool softeners** are useful to prevent straining at stool. Surfak, 240 mg/day, or Colace, 50–200 mg/day, are commonly used.

2. **Sitz baths** are useful for relief of inflammation and for hygiene. The patient sits in a tub of warm water for 15 minutes bid. Tucks pads (cotton soaked in witch hazel) also give some symptomatic relief.

3. **Ointments and suppositories** containing analgesics, emollients, and astringents are of only limited value.

4. **Surgery** is indicated if medical management fails.

II. **Anal fissure.** Anal fissure presents with the acute onset of anal pain during defecation. Physical examination reveals an elliptical tear in the skin of the anus, usually in the posterior midline. Anal fissures are commonly caused by the passage of a hard stool. Acute fissures usually heal in 2–3 weeks with stool softeners, analgesics, and sitz baths. Chronic fissures require surgical therapy.

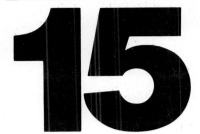

Anemia and Red Cell Transfusion

General Considerations

I. **Diagnostic approach.** Anemia may result from inadequate production of erythrocytes (due to deficiency states or primary bone marrow failure), excessive destruction of erythrocytes, loss of blood, or a combination of these factors. Precise diagnosis of the cause(s) of the anemia is the key to proper management. Apart from a thorough history and physical examination, the initial studies should be limited to the following:

A. **The hemoglobin and the hematocrit** provide an index to the severity of the anemia (except in acute blood loss). The hematocrit value reported by the Coulter counter is a calculated and corrected figure (RBC count × mean corpuscular volume [MCV], corrected for plasma trapping) and does not always correspond exactly to the classic spun hematocrit. The hemoglobin, on the other hand, is measured directly and hence is more reliable.

B. **The MCV,** which is determined directly by the Coulter counter, is routinely reported along with the blood count and should be used (together with the peripheral blood smear examination) to classify the anemia as microcytic, macrocytic, or normocytic. In some conditions (e.g., pernicious anemia) the abnormality in MCV will often precede the actual onset of the anemia by weeks or months. The other indices reported (mean corpuscular hemoglobin and mean corpuscular hemoglobin concentration) are calculated figures and are hence less reliable than the MCV.

C. **Inspection of the peripheral blood film** is the single most important diagnostic maneuver and should be done prior to the ordering of further laboratory studies. Evaluation of the size, shape, and color of the red cells, the presence of polychromatophilia (suggesting a high reticulocyte count), inspection of the white blood cells and platelets, and identification of any abnormal cells often will reduce the number of diagnostic possibilities.

D. **The reticulocyte count** provides a good indication of whether the anemia is due to diminished production or to excessive loss or destruction of red cells.

II. **Therapeutic approach.** Therapy should be specific. "Shotgun" therapy can obscure or delay an accurate diagnosis, preclude evaluation of the response to specific therapy, and sometimes harm the patient. Transfusion therapy should be used only when essential.

Inadequate Production of Blood

I. **Primary bone marrow failure (disordered proliferation or differentiation of stem cells).** Bone marrow failure results in inadequate delivery of erythrocytes, leukocytes, and platelets to the peripheral blood.

A. **Aplastic anemia** may be congenital (e.g., Fanconi's anemia) or acquired (associated with drugs, chemical agents, ionizing radiation, viral infection, immunologic abnormalities, or idiopathic). The anemia is generally normocytic, and the prognosis is determined largely by the severity of the associated leukopenia and thrombocytopenia. **Pure red cell aplasia** may be congenital (Blackfan-Diamond syndrome), idiopathic, or acquired. A thymona is associated with 30–50 percent of cases of the idiopathic variety. Marrow failure associated with other specific disease states is discussed in secs. **VI–VIII.**

B. **General principles of management**

1. **Recognition and removal of the cause** may lead to remission. A thorough history of exposure to drugs and chemicals should be obtained, keeping in mind that the offending agent may be in the patient's home or place of business. The patient must be instructed to avoid all potentially toxic chemicals and drugs.

2. **Transfusions** are usually not necessary unless the hemoglobin falls below 6–7 gm/dl. Chronic anemia is generally well tolerated. Some patients with angina or congestive heart failure (CHF) may require a higher hemoglobin concentration, but there is usually no significant benefit in raising the hemoglobin above 9–10 gm/dl. To minimize complications, transfusions should be given only when necessary. Sensitization to minor blood groups often occurs after repeated transfusions. If immune reactions to leukocyte, platelet, or serum protein antigens in the donor blood occur, buffy coat–poor, washed, or frozen washed, packed RBC transfusions may be of value (see Red Cell Transfusion, sec. **III.A**).

3. **Prevention of infection and bleeding** is important when there is significant leukopenia or thrombocytopenia. Toothbrushes should be soft and used gently. The stools should be kept soft. Electric razors are advisable. Scrupulous body hygiene may decrease the incidence of skin infections. Medications should be given orally whenever possible. Aspirin-containing analgesics can inhibit platelet function and should be avoided. Rectal manipulation (e.g., thermometers) should be avoided. Careful hand washing and the use of masks by personnel with upper respiratory infections constitute adequate reverse isolation procedures for hospitalized patients.

4. **Management of infection and hemorrhage.** Infections should be treated early and vigorously with antibiotics after appropriate cultures have been obtained. Rarely, hemorrhage due to thrombocytopenia may respond to low dosages of corticosteroids (e.g., prednisone, 10–20 mg/day) even though the platelet count does not improve. In the case of serious bleeding, hemostasis is usually achieved by transfusion of platelet concentrates.

C. **Specific treatment**

1. **Bone marrow transplantation.** The prognosis for patients with severe aplastic anemia (marked bone marrow hypoplasia, corrected reticulocyte count <1%, granulocytes <500/μl, platelet count <10,000/μl) is very poor. Recent results suggest that bone marrow transplantation may be the treatment of choice for younger patients with severe aplastic anemia. Tissue typing should be done **soon after diagnosis** in these patients and their family members, and those with HL-A–identical siblings should be referred to transplantation centers early in the course of the disease, preferably before any transfusions have been given (to avoid alloimmunization). In patients without a HL-A–identical sibling and in others with the less severe forms of hypoplastic anemia, the following conservative measures may be tried:

2. **Glucocorticoids** usually do not induce a remission in aplastic anemias. However, a reasonable trial of therapy (e.g., prednisone, 40–80 mg/PO/day for 4

weeks) is warranted. Following this, the dosage should be tapered to the lowest effective level or discontinued if no benefit is apparent.

3. **Androgens.** As many as 60% of children respond favorably to these drugs, but the results are less encouraging in adults. Nonetheless, an empirical trial of androgens usually is indicated, since the incidence of spontaneous remission is low, and the response to other modes of therapy, with the exception of bone marrow transplantation, has been disappointing. An adequate therapeutic trial should last 4–6 months. The dosage should be large (e.g., testosterone enanthate, 200–600 mg IM weekly; fluoxymesterone, 30–40 mg/day PO; oxymetholone, 2 mg/kg PO/day). In leukopenic or thrombocytopenic patients, IM injections should be avoided. Virilizing side effects are common and can be extremely distressing, especially in the young female patient. Rarely, cholestatic jaundice may occur. Combined treatment with androgens and glucocorticoids usually does not succeed when each agent alone has failed.

4. **Immunosuppressive drugs.** In pure red cell aplasia the use of cyclophosphamide, azathioprine, or 6-mercaptopurine may induce a remission. Thymectomy is advised if a thymoma is present. Occasional patients with idiopathic aplastic anemia may also respond to immunosuppressive agents. Glucocorticoid therapy can be beneficial in the Blackfan-Diamond syndrome.

II. **Megaloblastic anemias (disordered DNA synthesis).** Deficiencies of vitamin B_{12} and folate cause more than 95% of the megaloblastic anemias. Differentiation of pernicious anemia from other megaloblastic anemias is particularly important, because treatment of pernicious anemia must be continued for life, and because correction of the hematologic abnormalities of pernicious anemia may occur following large doses of folic acid, while neurologic damage progresses and may become irreversible. The most helpful diagnostic tests are serum vitamin B_{12} and folate levels and the Schilling urinary vitamin B_{12} excretion test.

A. **Treatment of vitamin B_{12} deficiency, including pernicious anemia**

1. **Transfusions** are seldom necessary, even when anemia is severe. They should be reserved for patients who cannot wait for the response to vitamin B_{12} therapy, e.g., patients with significant angina, CHF, postural hypotension, shock, or infection. Only packed RBCs should be used, and they must be given with caution. Partial exchange transfusions may avoid volume expansion; IV diuretics may be required as well.

2. **Vitamin B_{12}.** The minimum daily vitamin B_{12} requirement is 2.5–5.0 µg. Initial therapy consists of 100–1000 µg IM daily for 2 weeks to replenish body stores. Then 100–1000 µg IM is administered once monthly for the patient's lifetime. Oral vitamin B_{12}–intrinsic factor preparations and liver extracts are not recommended for the treatment of pernicious anemia unless the patient is sensitive to the parenteral form. (As part of the Schilling test, a "flushing" dose of 1 mg of B_{12} is routinely given; thus, a therapeutic test is simultaneously begun.)

3. **Response to therapy.** Within 8 hours after specific treatment is started, the bone marrow begins a transformation to normoblastic morphology, which may be complete within 48 hours. Serum bilirubin and lactic dehydrogenase concentrations fall rapidly. Serum iron may fall to subnormal levels (to diagnose concomitant iron deficiency, one must demonstrate persistent low serum iron or diminished marrow iron stores after several weeks of therapy). Rarely, hypokalemia develops soon after B_{12} therapy is begun, and fatal dysrhythmias can result. Reticulocytosis begins on the second or third day and is maximal on the fourth to twelfth day. Symptomatic improvement may occur within 1–3 days. Significant expansion of the plasma volume, as well as an increase in the red cell mass, may occur during the period of reticulocy-

tosis, resulting in hypervolemia that may precipitate CHF. The response to vitamin B_{12} may be attenuated by active infection, renal disease, tumor, ingestion of alcohol, or iron deficiency.

B. Treatment of folic acid deficiency. Folic (pteroylglutamic) acid deficiency may be due to dietary inadequacy, malabsorption (sprue, regional enteritis), inhibition of absorption (phenytoin, birth control pills), increased requirements (chronic hemolysis, pregnancy, hyperthyroidism, chronic exfoliative dermatitis), or interference with utilization (antimetabolites, triamterene, alcohol). The minimum daily requirement of folate is 50–100 μg; pregnant women require 300–400 μg/day. Folic acid is available in a 1-mg tablet and in an injectable form containing 5 mg/ml; folic acid is also present in many multivitamin preparations in amounts ranging from 0.1–1.0 mg. A dosage of 1–5 mg of folate/day PO for 4–5 weeks is usually adequate to replenish body stores and correct the anemia; even patients with malabsorption may absorb enough of this oral dosage to respond appropriately. Therapy should be continued until the underlying cause of the deficiency is removed or corrected (e.g., correction of diet, termination of pregnancy, end of lactation, cessation of antagonistic drugs, control of hemolysis). Therapy may be required indefinitely for patients with malabsorption, continuing dietary inadequacy, or chronic hemolysis. Proper dietary instructions should be given.

III. Iron-deficiency anemia (disturbance of heme synthesis)

A. Iron requirements. The normal adult human body contains 2–6 gm of iron. Adult men and postmenopausal women normally lose about 1 mg of iron daily in sweat, urine, desquamated skin, and stools. Iron assimilation normally balances iron loss. The average diet in the United States contains an estimated 6 mg of iron/1000 cal, only 5–10% of which is absorbed. Thus, the normal diet provides only basal iron requirements. Absorption, however, may increase to 20% or more during iron deficiency. Menstruating women may lose an average of 30 mg of iron per menstrual period; pregnant women lose an estimated 700 mg of iron in each full-term pregnancy, and lactating women lose about 0.5 mg/day in milk. Blood donation is sometimes overlooked as a source of iron deficiency (each unit of blood contains about 250 mg of iron).

B. Diagnosis of iron deficiency. As iron deficiency develops, iron stores decrease, as reflected by diminished, then absent, stainable marrow hemosiderin. The serum iron concentration then falls, transferrin levels increase (transferrin saturation falls to 15% or lower), sideroblasts disappear from the marrow, and a mild normocytic normochromic anemia develops. Only after this sequence do the classic features of the hypochromic microcytic anemia of severe iron deficiency develop, with the MCV less than 80 μ^3, serum iron less than 40 μg/dl, total iron-binding capacity greater than 400 μg/dl, saturation of transferrin less than 10%, and depletion of tissue levels. Thus, the **most sensitive diagnostic studies** for detection of early or mild iron deficiency are (1) determination of the percentage saturation of transferrin, and (2) iron stains of the bone marrow aspirate (not of the biopsy specimen). **Serum ferritin levels** usually reflect marrow iron stores but are useful only if they are low (<10 ng/ml). Falsely elevated values (in the presence of iron deficiency) can be seen in inflammatory conditions. The most common cause of iron deficiency is excessive blood loss due to heavy menstrual bleeding, multiple pregnancies, or GI bleeding. If the cause is not obvious, a careful search must be made for the source of blood loss, and other causes must be considered, such as dietary inadequacy, malabsorption, frequent blood donation, recurrent hemoptysis, or urinary loss of iron in prosthetic heart valve hemolysis or paroxysmal nocturnal hemoglobinuria.

C. Treatment. The goals of treatment include the correction of the anemia and the replenishment of iron stores. The optimal supplemental dosage of iron should provide enough iron to support a maximal hemoglobin increase (50 mg of ferrous iron/day). Oral therapy is preferred.

1. **Oral administration. Since only ferrous iron is efficiently absorbed, ferrous salts should be used**; ferric salts (in many liquid preparations) are expensive and not recommended. Iron is primarily absorbed in the duodenum; sustained-release and enteric-coated preparations are generally poorly dissolved in gastric and duodenal secretions and may be largely lost in the stool. Inexpensive and efficacious iron preparations, such as ferrous sulfate (0.32-gm tablet qid) and ferrous gluconate (0.32-gm tablet 6 times/day), supply the 50 mg of ferrous iron needed for optimal marrow response, assuming 20% absorption. Nausea and diarrhea may occur in 20–25% of patients treated with optimal doses of iron. Dose-related GI side effects may be minimized by using suboptimal therapy or by increasing the daily dose of iron gradually (1 tablet the first day, 2 the second day, etc.). Food (especially eggs and cereals) and antacids reduce GI side effects but also interfere with the absorption of iron. To replenish depleted body iron stores, administration of iron should continue for 4–6 months after hemoglobin has returned to normal. Patients should be told that the stools will become black. The guaiac test is not affected, but orthotoluidine may give a false-positive reaction. **Remember:** The major reason that iron-deficient patients fail to respond to oral therapy is failure to take the iron.

2. **Parenteral administration** of iron should be reserved for those unable to tolerate or absorb adequate amounts of oral iron: e.g., patients with malabsorption syndromes; some patients who have ulcerative colitis, regional enteritis, or intestinal shunts; and occasionally the grossly unreliable patient. Extensive chronic blood loss may also necessitate parenteral therapy if oral replacement cannot keep up with the losses. The total amount of iron required, including replenishment of marrow stores, may be calculated as follows:

   Gm iron required = (normal Hgb − patient's Hgb) × 0.255

   Iron dextran (Imferon) is a stable complex of ferric hydroxide and low-molecular-weight dextran (5000–10,000) supplied as a dark brown solution containing 50 mg iron/ml. The dosing schedule is controversial and the package insert should be read carefully. IV administration is less painful than IM injection.

   Complications of parenteral administration are infrequent but potentially serious. **Anaphylaxis,** which is not dose-related, usually occurs immediately, although it has occurred several hours after administration. Appropriate treatment of anaphylaxis should be instituted at the first evidence of such a reaction. **Delayed reactions** characterized by lymphadenopathy, fever, myalgias, arthralgias, and malaise may be dose-related. These reactions usually occur 12–48 hours after administration and they may persist for several days. Mild analgesics will relieve most symptoms.

D. **Response** to therapy, manifested by a maximal increase in reticulocyte count, occurs in 7–12 days. An increase in hemoglobin should be noted by 2 weeks; by 2 months the level should be normal. There is little difference in the time course of the response to oral and parenteral iron administration unless malabsorption is present.

IV. **Thalassemia (disturbances of globin synthesis).** The thalassemias are characterized by genetically determined underproduction of at least one of the normal globin peptide chains (most commonly the beta chain). **β-Thalassemia trait** produces mild to moderate hypochromic microcytic anemia that may be confused with iron deficiency anemia. Generally, no treatment is required, although such patie have increased folic acid requirements and may need supplementation. As a co quence of intensive transfusion programs, **homozygous thalassemia (th semia major)** patients are now surviving into adulthood. Multiple transfu result in iron overload, which ultimately leads to CHF, dysrhythmias, and h failure. The use of prolonged SQ infusions of iron-chelating agents to preve overload is under investigation. Although the technique can increase iro tion and result in negative iron balance, its efficacy in preventing or r organ dysfunction due to excessive iron deposition is unclear. The use of (young red blood cells) to increase the survival of transfused blood (and thereby decrease the frequency of transfusion) is also under investigation. Splenectomy is useful when the spleen is so large that it causes mechanical pressure symptoms or when hypersplenism is documented, but it can predispose to fulminant pneumococcoal sepsis, especially in young patients. Immunization with polyvalent pneumococcal vaccine (Pneumovax) several weeks prior to splenectomy is recommended.

V. Sideroblastic anemia. Sideroblastic anemia is characterized by normal or increased transferrin saturation, hypochromic microcytic RBCs, and increased marrow iron, with a defect in iron utilization (at the level of heme biosynthesis) manifested by ringed sideroblasts. It may be hereditary, idiopathic, drug induced (isoniazid, cycloserine), or associated with collagen vascular disease, carcinoma, malabsorption, or chronic alcoholism; it can precede myeloproliferative disorders such as acute leukemia. The drug-induced forms may respond to drug withdrawal. Some patients may respond to large doses of pyridoxine (50–200 mg PO qd), or folic acid (5 mg PO qd), or both. Refractory cases should be managed with a trial of androgens (see sec. **I.C.3**) and the judicious use of transfusions. Iron overload can be a significant problem in some cases. Corticosteroids and splenectomy are not indicated.

VI. Anemia of chronic disease. The anemia of chronic disease is characterized by hemoglobin levels of 7–10 gm/dl, decreased serum iron **and** iron-binding capacity (i.e., a normal or increased transferrin saturation), and increased marrow iron stores. The underlying mechanisms include diminished reutilization of iron from hemoglobin catabolism, impaired RBC production, and decreased RBC survival. This type of anemia is associated with chronic infections, collagen vascular diseases, inflammatory bowel disease, lymphomas, and metastatic malignancies. It does not respond to the administration of iron or other hematinic agents, although a transient increase in hemoglobin production may occasionally be seen after iron therapy. Hemoglobin values usually return to normal if successful treatment of the underlying disease is possible.

VII. Anemia of renal disease. Both decreased RBC survival and marrow failure can occur in the anemia of renal disease. Red blood cell survival (inversely proportional to BUN levels) improves with dialysis. Marrow failure may respond to androgen therapy, and a trial with these agents is warranted if there is a significant transfusion requirement. Other frequent contributing factors include bleeding (with resultant iron deficiency), and folate deficiency secondary to hemodialysis or poor nutrition.

VIII. Myelofibrosis, myeloproliferative disorders, and other myelophthisic anemias. Anemia can result from infiltration of the bone marrow by metastatic carcinoma, lymphoreticular malignancies, granulomatous disorders, primary hematologic malignancies, or idiopathic myelofibrosis. A leukoerythroblastic peripheral blood picture is characteristically seen. The primary aim of therapy is to improve the underlying disease. No specific treatment is available for idiopathic myelofibrosis. In general, treatment is supportive, with the judicious use of blood transfusions. Androgens, though of transient benefit in some patients, can cause cholestatic jaundice, hyperuricemia, or fluid retention. Corticosteroids may be valuable when hemolysis contributes to the anemia or when thrombocytopenia is severe. Occasional responses to high doses of pyridoxine have been reported. When massive splenomegaly, severe anemia, and obvious marrow failure are present, it is often difficult, even with measurement of ^{51}Cr–tagged RBC survival, to determine the degree of contribution of the hypersplenism to the anemia.

Some patients improve significantly (reduction in spleen size, decreased hypermetabolic symptoms and transfusion requirements) following a course of therapy with busulfan (2–4 mg PO qd as a starting dosage). This dosage is lower than that administered in chronic myelocytic leukemia, because leukopenia is more easily produced in myelofibrosis. An occasional patient who is a poor operative risk may benefit transiently from irradiation of the spleen; radiation must be administered cautiously in small doses to minimize the risk of persistent, refractory pancytopenia.

Splenectomy may be considered in patients who have significant hemolysis, mechanical pressure, severe thrombocytopenia felt to be due to splenic sequestration, or recurrent, painful infarctions. After splenectomy, the liver may enlarge gradually and can become enormous. Thrombocytosis of significant degree (>1 million/μl), seen early in the course of myelofibrosis or as a "rebound phenomenon" after splenectomy, may be reduced by myelosuppressive drugs such as busulfan.

IX. Anemia of pregnancy. The hemoglobin concentration begins to decrease after the eighth week of gestation and becomes stationary between the sixteenth and twenty-second weeks; this physiologic "anemia" occurs because plasma volume increases to a greater degree than does the total RBC volume. More severe anemia (hemoglobin <10 gm/dl) usually reflects iron deficiency. The prophylactic administration of iron (ferrous sulfate, 320 mg PO qd) during pregnancy is recommended. Megaloblastic anemia of pregnancy is less common in this country than is iron-deficiency anemia. Nonetheless, it should be prevented by routine prophylaxis with folate (1 mg PO qd) during pregnancy.

Abnormal Red Blood Cell Destruction: Hemolytic Anemias

Increased rates of RBC destruction may be due to **intracorpuscular** defects of the red cell (often hereditary), to a variety of **extracorpuscular** influences (e.g., drugs, antibodies, hypersplenism), or to a combination of the two types of abnormalities. If RBC destruction is not severe and the bone marrow can compensate, red cell counts can remain normal, and an elevated reticulocyte count may be the only clue to the ongoing hemolysis. Anemia results when the hemolytic process is severe or the bone marrow production of RBCs is not compensatory. Identification of the type of hemolytic anemia is essential for effective management.

I. Hereditary spherocytosis (abnormal shape, normal hemoglobin). Hereditary spherocytosis is characterized by spherocytic erythrocytes, increased osmotic fragility, autohemolysis, and excessive destruction of erythrocytes in the spleen. The anemia can be cured permanently by **splenectomy**, although the RBC defect persists. Splenectomy should be deferred past early childhood because of the increased susceptibility of children to severe bacterial infection after this operation. However, even if the anemia is only mild, splenectomy should be performed later in almost all affected children and young adults because of the frequent complications of gallstones and of aplastic or hemolytic crises. At surgery, accessory spleens should be carefully sought and removed; cholecystectomy may be performed at the time of splenectomy if indicated. Aplastic crises may occur prior to splenectomy, but usually no therapy other than blood transfusion is required; recovery occurs in about 10 days. Similar problems can be seen in other less common hereditary RBC abnormalities, such as elliptocytosis and pyropoikilocytosis. Management is similar to that in hereditary spherocytosis but must be individualized, since the severity of hemolysis can be variable.

II. Hereditary enzyme deficiencies resulting in increased red blood cell destruction. These anemias are caused by a variety of specific, genetically determined biochemical defects of red cells. Splenectomy is valueless in this group of disorders (except for amelioration of the anemia of pyruvate kinase deficiency), as are corticosteroids. The most common disease in this group is glucose 6-phosphate dehydrogenase (G-6-PD) deficiency. Over 150 G-6-PD isoenzyme variants have been described that have varying clinical significance. In the usual variety (A-), an X-linked recessive trait in 10–13% of American blacks, G-6-PD activity is normal in reticulocytes but diminishes progressively in aging cells. The older cells, with the least G-6-PD activity, are more subject to hemolysis under oxidant stress and are selectively destroyed. The hemolytic reaction ceases when only young cells (normal G-6-PD) remain. Therefore, soon after an episode of hemolysis, assays of G-6-PD activity may show normal findings, and the diagnosis may be missed. In a less common variety, usually seen in whites, G-6-PD activity in all cells is extremely low. Hemolytic episodes under oxidant stress are severe, not self-limited, and are occasionally fatal; even heterozygous females may be clinically affected.

An increasing number of drugs and chemicals have been reported to precipitate hemolysis in these patients. A few commonly used drugs that cause hemolytic episodes include antimalarials, chloramphenicol, nitrofurans, para-aminosalicylic acid, sulfonamides, sulfones, and water-soluble vitamin K analogues. These must be avoided in susceptible patients. In addition, fava beans, febrile disease states, diabetic ketoacidosis, hepatitis, and other acute or chronic illnesses have been associated with hemolysis. Chronic hemolysis may also occur in the absence of any apparent stress.

III. Sickle cell anemia (anemias due to abnormal globin). Generally, patients heterozygous for hemoglobins A and S (sickle trait) with less than 50% hemoglobin S have no symptoms. However, such patients may have sickle crises if exposed to low oxygen concentrations, e.g., severe pneumonia or flying in unpressurized aircraft. There is no specific therapy for homozygous sickle cell anemia; complications of the disease must be treated as they arise. Maintenance of adequate hemoglobin levels and tissue oxygenation, however, may reduce the incidence of certain complications.

A. Painful crises. The frequency of painful crises may be reduced in some patients by prophylactic partial exchange transfusions given at about 6-week intervals to maintain the population of normal RBCs at 15–40%. Such a prophylactic program should be attempted only in (1) the few sickle cell patients who are having frequent crises and frequent hospitalizations and (2) pregnant patients, especially in hemoglobin S-C disease, in which transfusions may substantially reduce the high maternal and fetal mortality and morbidity. Otherwise, prolonged prophylactic transfusion programs are seldom practical and carry the risk of isoimmunization, hepatitis, and iron overload. There is conflicting evidence as to whether partial-exchange transfusions shorten the duration of painful crises; certainly, 1- or 2-unit exchanges are not worthwhile.

1. During painful crises the following measures are essential:

   a. Analgesics should be given as required.

   b. Nasal oxygen should be administered.

   c. Acidosis should be corrected.

   d. Fluid balance should be maintained by vigorous oral or IV fluid replacement.

2. Many different agents have been tried over the years for the management or prevention of sickling crises. Although several such agents are effective in vitro, none has as yet achieved practical usefulness because of excessive toxicity or lack of significant benefit in vivo.

B. Aplastic crises are less common than painful crises; they usually occur in children and may be fatal if not recognized and treated with transfusion. Marrow function usually returns within several days, but aplasia may persist as long as 2–3 weeks. **Folic acid,** 1 mg PO qd, is useful, particularly in periods of stress (e.g., infections).

C. Complications. Certain **infections,** particularly pneumococcal disease and *Salmonella* osteomyelitis or septicemia, occur with increased frequency in patients with sickle cell disease. The use of a polyvalent vaccine has been shown to decrease the incidence of pneumococcal infections. **Chronic leg ulceration** usually requires bed rest, careful local care, and occasionally antibiotics. **Hematuria** can occur, sometimes even in the heterozygous individual. Surgical procedures can be associated with an increased morbidity and mortality; the importance of carefully administered **anesthesia** and maintenance of oxygenation cannot be overemphasized. If the risk of hypoxia is high, preoperative exchange transfusions should be considered. **Radiographic studies** that involve the injection of hypertonic contrast material should be avoided if at all possible.

IV. **Paroxysmal nocturnal hemoglobinuria.** Paroxysmal nocturnal hemoglobinuria is a rare acquired disease in which the red cells are abnormally sensitive to lysis by complement. It is frequently seen in association with myeloproliferative disorders or aplastic anemia. The diagnosis is made by positive sucrose hemolysis and acid hemolysis (Ham test).

Therapy is directed at prevention and management of the **three major complications:** aplastic or hemolytic crises, thrombosis, and infection. Intravenous infusion of 1000 ml of 6% low-molecular-weight dextran may help to control hemolysis as a temporary measure during crises, but hemorrhagic manifestations and allergic reactions may occur after repeated infusions. When transfusions are required, packed RBCs should be used, because infusion of plasma has been associated with massive hemolysis. In some patients, washed or frozen red cells may be required. Splenectomy is seldom useful unless massive splenomegaly and hypersplenism are present; postsplenectomy thrombocytosis may increase the tendency to thrombosis. Oral administration of **androgens** (e.g., fluoxymesterone, 20–30 mg/day, or oxymetholone, 2 mg/kg/day) may stimulate erythropoiesis and reduce hemolysis. **Corticosteroids** are not of proved benefit, but may be tried in difficult cases. **Folic acid,** 1 mg qd, should be given PO when there is evidence of ongoing hemolysis. **Oral anticoagulants** may decrease the incidence of thrombotic complications; however, heparin has been reported to increase hemolysis and should be avoided. Because of the loss of hemoglobin and hemosiderin in the urine, patients may become iron deficient. Iron should then be given, although such therapy may transiently increase hemolysis.

V. **Mechanical damage.** Intravascular hemolysis often occurs in patients with **prosthetic heart valves,** particularly aortic valve prostheses. Although most cases of severe anemia are associated with regurgitation from a defective valve and may be improved by repair or replacement, in some cases there is no demonstrable malfunction. Through loss of hemosiderin in the urine, all patients with significant anemia become iron deficient and require iron-replacement therapy, occasionally in massive IV doses. Severely ill patients with significant anemia may benefit from tranfusion to restore normal hematocrit values to reduce the heart rate and decrease shearing forces. Because of increased red cell production and turnover, the folate requirement is usually increased, and folate therapy is warranted.

VI. **Microangiopathic hemolytic anemia.** Microangiopathic hemolytic anemia occurs in the disseminated intravascular coagulation syndrome, thrombotic thrombocytopenic purpura, widespread neoplasms, vasculitis, sepsis, preeclampsia or toxemia of pregnancy, and certain snakebites. Treatment is directed to the underlying disorder.

VII. **Autoimmune hemolytic anemia (red blood cell destruction mediated by antibodies).** Included in the category of autoimmune hemolytic anemia (AHA) is a heterogeneous group of disorders characterized by the presence on the surface of the patient's red cells (and sometimes in the plasma) of one or more immunoglobulins that are detectable by a positive reaction with antihuman globulin (Coombs') serum. The anemia may be subdivided into secondary AHA and idiopathic AHA. **Secondary AHA** is related to an identifiable underlying disease or drug (neoplastic hematopoietic diseases such as chronic lymphocytic leukemia; collagen vascular disease; drugs, such as penicillin, quinine, and methyldopa; and other conditions, such as carcinoma, sarcoidosis, primary atypical pneumonia, infectious mononucleosis, and ovarian teratoma). **Idiopathic AHA** comprises the 20–40% of cases in which no underlying disease or associated disorder can be demonstrated. The coating immunoglobulins most commonly consist of IgG reacting with red cells at body temperature (warm antibodies) or, less frequently, IgM optimally reacting at 4–10°C (cold antibodies that usually bind complement). The latter may occur as idiopathic chronic cold agglutinin disease or in association with infections, such as primary atypical pneumonias or infectious mononucleosis. Paroxysmal cold hemoglobinuria is a rare syndrome caused by an IgG cold hemolysin. It may be idiopathic, or it may occur in association with a variety of viral infections or latent syphilis.

A. **Therapy in idiopathic AHA** should be specifically directed at decreasing the rate of RBC destruction. Very rarely, patients will recover spontaneously.

1. **Glucocorticoids** are the drugs of choice. The initial dosage is usually 60–100 mg of prednisone PO qd, and the trial should be continued for 1–3 weeks. If improvement occurs, the corticosteroid dosage should be reduced slowly over a 6- –8-week period, then discontinued or kept at the minimal dosage necessary to maintain remission. On occasion, small doses of corticosteroids must be administered indefinitely. About 15% of patients given corticosteroids in adequate dosage will have a permanent remission; 70% will have partial or complete remission, with relapses when corticosteroids are reduced or discontinued; and 15% will have no benefit. The use of ACTH confers no advantage over corticosteroids.

2. **Splenectomy** is considered for patients who do not respond to corticosteroids or who require high-dose corticosteroids (>10–20 mg prednisone/day) for 6 months or longer. Although ^{51}Cr-labeled RBC survival studies may be useful in demonstrating decreased RBC survival, the lack of increased sequestration over the spleen does not necessarily imply that splenectomy will fail. About 50% of patients have a complete permanent remission after splenectomy; in 20%, remission is followed by relapse, and 30% do not respond favorably, although resumption of corticosteroid therapy may be of value.

3. **Immunosuppressive drugs.** Patients who fail to respond to corticosteroids and splenectomy may benefit from agents that suppress antibody formation (e.g., azathioprine, cyclophosphamide).

4. **Blood transfusion** should be avoided if possible, since the benefit from transfusion is transient because of rapid destruction of transfused cells. Typing and cross matching may become extremely difficult; minor blood group sensitization is not uncommon and may aggravate the hemolytic process; and finally, tissue iron overload may occur with repeated transfusions. However, blood transfusion must be administered as a lifesaving measure in acute situations in which severe anemic hypoxia or circulatory failure is imminent.

   The major problems result from the masking of significant alloantibodies in the patient's serum. Therefore, compatibility tests are carried out on a large number of donor units to select those that give the weakest reactions in vitro. In cases in which no compatible in vitro cross match can be obtained, "in vivo cross match techniques" may be performed. This is done by labeling a small aliquot of the least incompatible unit with 10–15 μCi of ^{51}Cr and determining the survival of the transfused cells in the patient over a period of time. Alternatively, a sample of blood is drawn 30 minutes after injection of 15–20 ml of the most compatible unit and the plasma inspected for evidence of visible hemolysis. These procedures should be carried out in close consultation with the blood bank personnel.

5. **Plasmapheresis** has been tried, with promising but variable success in decreasing the antibody titer in AHA. However, this expensive and time-consuming measure should be used only in selective circumstances.

6. Patients with AHA should receive **folic acid** (1 mg/day) routinely.

B. Therapy in symptomatic AHA should be directed at control of the underlying process, although more specific measures, as described in **A**, may become necessary (see p. 278).

C. Patients with idiopathic cold agglutinin disease tend to respond poorly to corticosteroids or splenectomy, but chlorambucil may be useful. Such patients should avoid exposure to low temperatures.

VIII. Hypersplenism. Hypersplenism may be primary or secondary and frequently results in a decrease of all the formed elements of the blood. Secondary causes of hypersplenism include all causes of massive splenomegaly, e.g., infections and portal hypertension. In most cases the definite diagnosis can be made only in retrospect, when removal of the spleen results in improvement of the anemia or pancytopenia.

Anemia Due to Blood Loss

Acute blood loss can result in anemia, and the cause is usually obvious. However, it should be kept in mind that the site of the bleeding can be occult, e.g., ruptured ectopic pregnancy, and that the hemoglobin and hematocrit may not accurately reflect the severity of the blood loss until fluid shifts have occurred (2–12 hours). **Chronic blood loss** usually results in iron-deficiency anemia (see Inadequate Production of Blood, sec. **III**, p. 272).

Nosocomial anemia is a surprisingly frequent complication of prolonged hospitalization, especially in intensive care units. Anemia results because of the frequent bloodletting for numerous investigations. Furthermore, since the patient is often suffering from some underlying serious ailment, an appropriate reticulocytosis may not occur. Awareness of this problem is the key to both its prevention and to the avoidance of unnecessary investigation when it does occur.

Red Cell Transfusion

The following section deals with the uses, dangers, and complications of red cell transfusions. The use of other blood components, such as plasma, granulocytes, and platelets, is discussed in Chaps. 16 and 17.

I. Indications. Acute blood loss sufficient to produce significant hypovolemia is the **only** indication for the use of fresh **whole blood** in adults. In all other instances, specific blood component therapy is recommended. When transfusion is necessary in the treatment of **chronic anemia,** packed RBCs should be used. In certain situations (see sec. **II**), washed or frozen RBCs may be preferable.

II. General approach to transfusion reactions. In all instances of suspected reactions to blood transfusions, the following steps should be taken immediately: **Stop the transfusion and keep the IV line open.** Check to make absolutely sure that the blood the patient received was indeed the blood intended for that patient. Make an evaluation of the type of reaction that is occurring (see sec. **III**), and proceed with the appropriate diagnostic and therapeutic maneuvers.

III. Complications and dangers of blood transfusions

A. Fever without hemolysis is probably the most common transfusion reaction. Febrile reactions may be produced by a sensitivity reaction to donor white cells (less often to platelets or plasma proteins) in patients who have received multiple transfusions. When such a reaction occurs, the transfusion should be stopped and antipyretics administered. If the reaction does not subside promptly, or if other symptoms supervene, a more serious reaction, such as one of those outlined in **B** and **C,** should be considered and investigated. In such an instance, it is unwise to continue transfusing the same unit. Rarely, febrile reactions may result from contamination of transfusion equipment with pyrogenic material.

In patients who **frequently** have febrile reactions, buffy coat–poor or washed, packed RBCs (which are relatively poor in white cells and platelets) can be used. Washed frozen RBCs can also be used but are more expensive.

B. Allergic reactions manifested by urticaria, itching, or wheezing are relatively common. Anaphylactic reactions, with laryngeal edema or vascular collapse, are rare. When an allergic reaction is detected, the transfusion should be stopped and an antihistamine (diphenhydramine maleate, 50 mg) given IV. For the more severe reactions, epinephrine and steroids may be required. Severe anaphylactic reactions may occur in patients who are **IgA deficient** (about 0.1% of the general population).

C. Acute hemolytic reactions due to RBC incompatibility are serious; diagnosis and therapy must be prompt.

    1. Clinical manifestations of hemolysis include the following: **Phase I (immediate) symptoms,** which may begin after 50 ml or less of blood have been given, include a throbbing headache, severe lumbar pain (almost pathognomonic), precordial pain, dyspnea, anxiety, and restlessness. Physical signs include flushed face, then cyanosis; distended neck veins; initial slowing of the pulse, followed by a rapid, thready beat; diaphoresis and cold, clammy skin; and then profound shock, usually within an hour. Consumption coagulopathy (disseminated intravascular coagulation) can cause bleeding. Hemolytic reactions may occur with few or no symptoms in obtunded or anesthetized patients. A slight, diffuse oozing of blood at the operative site sometimes may be the only clue. **Phase II (interval)** lasts for several hours to days, during which the patient appears symptomatically improved. Objectively, however, there is hemoglobinemia, hemoglobinuria, and occasionally jaundice. Oliguria and anuria may supervene. **Phase III (acute renal failure)** is not an invariable concomitant of intravascular hemolysis and hemoglobinuria and may as well reflect prior renal disease or a period of hypotension or acidosis. With proper management, many patients survive acute renal failure.

    2. Investigative procedures. As soon as a hemolytic transfusion reaction is suspected, the following investigative and therapeutic procedures should be carried out:

        a. Stop the transfusion and save the remaining donor blood for further testing.

        b. Carefully, to avoid hemolysis, draw a sample of venous blood from the arm opposite the site of the transfusion, and collect one clotted and two anticoagulated (citrated) tubes. The clotted sample, one anticoagulated sample, and the donor blood are returned to the blood bank to be typed and cross-matched again. A hemolytic antibody is sought by direct and indirect Coombs' tests.

        c. The presence of free hemoglobin in the recipient's plasma is sought by examining the supernatant of a citrated sample after gentle centrifugation, by either simple inspection or quantitative methods. Pink plasma indicates at least 20 mg of free hemoglobin/dl. If more than 6 hours have elapsed before the sample is drawn, increased bilirubin and methemalbumin and decreased or absent haptoglobin levels may be measured.

        d. A sample of urine is inspected for free hemoglobin.

    3. Treatment should begin immediately. If a hemolytic transfusion reaction is even remotely suspected, **stop the blood transfusion at once** without awaiting further symptoms. Keep the IV line open.

a. **Phase I.** Mannitol (25 gm) is infused IV over a 5-minute period as soon as the reaction occurs or is suspected; urine flow should be maintained over 100 ml/hour. The initial dose of mannitol may be repeated, but no more than 100 gm should be given in any 24-hour period. If hypotension develops, hypovolemia must be corrected; normal saline or plasma expanders, such as human plasma protein fraction, are suitable for this purpose. If necessary, compatible fresh whole blood may be given. **Caution:** The same error(s) that led to the transfusion reaction in the first place may be duplicated in the preparation of blood for emergency transfusion. Therefore, further attempts at blood transfusion should be deferred until compatibility can be assured. Vasopressor drugs may be necessary, but they may be ineffective or even harmful (diminished renal blood flow) in the presence of hypovolemia. If there is no response to mannitol, the fluid regimen must be modified. If bleeding complicates a hemolytic transfusion reaction, disseminated intravascular coagulation should be suspected and documented by appropriate laboratory determinations (see Chap. 16).

b. **Phase II.** In the presence of oliguria, limit fluid intake to insensible losses plus other fluid output. Maintain adequate nutrition and electrolyte balance. Fluids that contain potassium should not be administered orally or parenterally.

c. **Phase III.** The management of acute renal failure is discussed in Chap. 3.

4. **Delayed transfusion reactions** are mild hemolytic reactions that are noticed 7–21 days after a transfusion, usually because of a drop in the hematocrit. A serologically detectable incompatibility usually is not found on reexamination of the original pre-cross-match serum, but the offending antibody frequently can be identified in the patient's serum at the time of or within 10 days following the reaction. Many of these antibodies belong to the Rh and Kidd systems and seem to represent anamnestic responses. Occasionally, frank hemoglobinemia and hemoglobinuria occur, rarely with reversible renal shutdown. Delayed transfusion reactions may sometimes be confused with the onset of autoimmune hemolytic anemia.

D. **Cardiac failure.** Patients with borderline cardiac compensation should be given packed RBCs cautiously while the central venous pressure is monitored. It may be advisable to administer digoxin to such patients before transfusion or to administer concurrently an IV diuretic, e.g., furosemide, 40 mg.

E. **Potassium intoxication.** When whole blood is stored, potassium leaks from the red cells. At 10 days the plasma K^+ concentration reaches 15 mEq/liter; after 21 days it is about 21 mEq/liter. The K^+ concentration is highest in the plasma immediately around the sedimented RBCs; thus, resuspension and recentrifugation of old blood and use of the packed cells may reduce the risk of hyperkalemia. When transfusions must be given to patients with hyperkalemia or renal insufficiency, fresh RBCs or RBCs stored less than 5 days should be used.

F. **Bacterial contamination** of blood, although extremely rare with modern blood collection and storage techniques, produces severe reactions (characterized by chills, high fever, vomiting, bloody diarrhea, delirium, and marked hypotension) that are often fatal. If such a reaction is suspected, the transfusion should be stopped immediately; the remaining donor blood should be sent for culturing. A small sample of lightly centrifuged donor plasma should be gram-stained for immediate microscopic examination, which is frequently positive. Appropriate antibiotics and supportive care should be given.

G. **Complications of massive transfusion**

1. **Excessive bleeding** following massive transfusion, exchange transfusion, or extracorporeal circulation is related to the decrease in the number of compe-

tent circulating platelets (due to poor platelet viability in stored blood) and dilution of coagulation factors (V and VIII, which are in low concentrations in stored blood). To avoid this complication, every fourth or fifth unit administered within a 12- –18-hour period should be freshly obtained. Alternatively, 1 unit of fresh-frozen plasma should be given with every 5 units of packed RBCs. Platelet transfusions may also be required.

2. **Acidosis and hyperkalemia** may be prevented by the administration of 1 ampule of sodium bicarbonate (44.6 mEq) for each 5 units of stored blood.

3. **Hypothermia** can result from rapid transfusions of large volumes of blood at 4°C and can precipitate dangerous ventricular tachyarrythmias. This can be prevented by the use of an approved blood-warming device.

4. **Complications resulting from microaggregates** of platelets, leukocytes, and fibrinogen may be significant. Therefore, a 20- –40-μ blood filter is usually recommended when massive transfusions are given.

5. **Citrate intoxication** is extremely rare. It may occur in infants receiving exchange transfusion with citrated whole blood and in normal adults given more than 2000 ml of citrated blood or plasma in 30 minutes or less. In adults with severe liver disease, citrate intoxication may develop with smaller amounts of blood. The clinical manifestations usually are secondary to hypocalcemia and may present as hypotension, decreased cardiac output, or tetany (positive Chvostek's and Trousseau's signs). The ECG may demonstrate a prolonged Q–Tc interval. If more than 2000 ml of blood must be given rapidly, the administration of calcium gluconate, 10 ml of a 10% solution given slowly IV, should be considered.

H. **Transmission of hepatitis.** Prospective studies indicate that clinical or serologic evidence of hepatitis will develop in 5–10% of recipients after transfusion. The use of paid commercial donors, multiple transfusions, and pooled plasma fractions all increase the risk of hepatitis infection. Mandatory screening of donors with sensitive serologic tests for HBsAg has successfully decreased the incidence of hepatitis B but has been accompanied by the recognition that non-A, non-B hepatitis now accounts for 85–90% of posttransfusion hepatitis.

I. **Other infectious agents** may occasionally be transmitted by blood transfusion. Cytomegalovirus or Epstein-Barr virus infections may simulate typical serum hepatitis or produce other syndromes. Malaria, microfilarial diseases, trypanosomiasis, and spirochetal infections are problems in areas of the world where these diseases are endemic.

J. **Transfusion hemosiderosis.** A large number of transfusions given over a long period to a patient who is not bleeding will lead to accumulation of large stores of iron, since each 500 ml of blood contains 200–250 mg of iron.

K. **Air embolism** is very rare with the widespread use of plastic blood-donor bags. When air embolism occurs, the administration tubing should be clamped and the patient turned on the left side with head down and lower extremities elevated. It has been stated that normal adults can tolerate as much as 200 ml of air IV, but as little as 10 ml may be fatal in seriously ill patients.

L. **Noncardiac pulmonary edema** appears to be a hypersensitivity response and may be associated with the presence of leukoagglutinins in donor (common) or recipient (rare) plasma. This reaction is characterized by the abrupt development of numerous pulmonary infiltrates, fever, chills, dyspnea, and a nonproductive cough. Symptoms usually clear within 48 hours; however, severe reactions may require supportive measures, including oxygen, vasopressors, antihistamines, and high doses of corticosteroids. This reaction should be differentiated from similar symptoms caused by circulatory overload. The donor involved should be advised against further blood donation.

M. Other rare complications of blood transfusion include **graft-versus-host disease** (in immunosuppressed patients) and posttransfusion purpura.

IV. Emergency transfusions. There is seldom enough delay in typing and cross matching to warrant the administration of blood that is not crossed-matched. The administration of saline or plasma expanders while blood is being prepared is less dangerous than the administration of unselected type O Rh-negative (universal donor) blood. In rare situations, as in acute blood loss with severe shock, it may be necessary to transfuse the blood before proper cross matching can be done. Determination of group and type can be performed in about 5 minutes; for emergency transfusions, group-specific and type-specific blood that is not cross-matched is preferred over universal donor blood that is not cross-matched. If one cannot wait for group-specific and type-specific blood, O Rh-negative packed RBCs of measured low titers of anti-A and anti-B can be used. After a patient has been given many units of O Rh-negative blood, it may be preferable to continue the transfusions during that episode with O Rh-negative blood; switching to A blood if the recipient is found to be type A, for example, may result in hemolysis of the A blood by the accumulation of anti-A antibodies added during the O Rh-negative blood transfusions. In a serious emergency, if the recipient is a man or a nulliparous woman who has not received blood transfusions in the past, it is possible to use O Rh-positive blood in the manner just described if universal donor blood is not available. Although hemolysis may occur after a few days (if the recipient should be Rh-negative) because of production of anti-Rh antibody, such hemolysis is relatively gradual and not life-threatening.

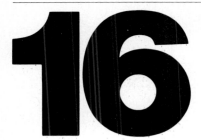

Bleeding Disorders

I. General considerations. Most episodes of abnormal bleeding are diagnosed from a careful history and physical examination. Hemorrhage may be due to a discrete vascular lesion or to a disorder of the hemostatic system. When a discrete vascular lesion (e.g., a wound), is not obvious, hemostatic screening tests are performed, routinely comprising the prothrombin time (PT), the partial thromboplastin time (PTT), and the platelet count. These tests, coupled with the history and physical examination, either help in the diagnosis of the disorder or direct further studies.

A. History and physical examination. Special emphasis should be placed on the following historical details: the amount, course, and previous history of bleeding; the ingestion of aspirin, over-the-counter medications, alcohol, or oral anticoagulants; transfusion history; family history of bleeding disorders; and response to hemostatic stress (e.g., dental extraction and surgery). The appearance of bleeding or hematomas hours after injury suggests a coagulation factor deficiency. Histories of isolated instances of easy bruising are common and should be pursued only if other features suggestive of a bleeding disorder are present.

Physical examination aids in quantitation of bleeding, because orthostatic changes in pulse and blood pressure indicate an acute blood loss of at least 10% of blood volume. Petechiae suggest a platelet or vascular abnormality. Palpable purpura most often arises in leukocytoclastic vasculitis. Deep hematomas or hemarthroses imply a coagulation factor defect.

B. Laboratory studies confirm the clinical diagnosis. Studies of major clinical import are outlined in **1–3**.

1. Peripheral smear. Each cell line should be examined sequentially for morphologic or numerical change. The presence of fragmented RBCs and schistocytes suggests disseminated intravascular coagulation (DIC), although these are seen in a minority of cases. Normally, at least 10 platelets/oil-immersion field are seen. Blood smears prepared from finger sticks may exhibit inhomogeneous platelet distribution; therefore, a number of fields should be examined before concluding that thrombocytopenia or thrombocytosis is present. The WBC morphology may suggest leukemia as an underlying cause of bleeding.

2. Platelet studies. The template bleeding time is an in vivo test of platelet function; normal values are 3–8 minutes. The template bleeding time is prolonged in thrombocytopenia ($<100,000/\mu l$), vascular disorders, and platelet functional defects. The finding of a prolonged bleeding time combined with a normal platelet count should prompt an additional search for a history of ingestion of aspirin-containing compounds or nonsteroidal anti-inflammatory agents. Because bleeding times in thrombocytosis may not correlate with bleeding diathesis (see sec. **II.B**), the test is less useful when evaluating thrombocytosis.

3. Coagulation tests must be interpreted in the setting of each institution's capabilities. Reagents and techniques vary, as do corresponding normal

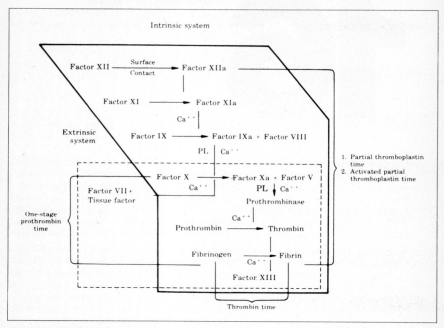

Fig. 16-1. A modified coagulation scheme. The solid frame encompasses the intrinsic system; the broken frame, the extrinsic system. Brackets indicate the sequence of reactions estimated by the indicated coagulation test. PL = phospholipid; a = activated.

values and the sensitivity of assays. A clean venipuncture with blood drawn directly into the anticoagulant and prompt processing are essential. If the hematocrit is abnormally elevated, relative amounts of blood and anticoagulant may require adjustment for meaningful results; consult the laboratory personnel prior to obtaining samples to avoid error. A simplified clotting scheme is presented in Fig. 16-1. The major coagulation tests are as follows:

a. **Prothrombin time** measures the "extrinsic system" (Fig. 16-1). Reported values must be related to a control and are often expressed as a percentage by comparison with dilutions of normal plasma; i.e., a PT of 20% is equivalent to that of a 1 : 5 dilution of normal plasma. Because of the asymptotic nature of the standard curve, large variations in a prolonged PT may result in small percentage changes; therefore, one must evaluate the actual PT (in seconds) as well as its percentage equivalent. A prolonged PT indicates a deficiency in one or more of the extrinsic system factors or implies the presence of an inhibitor.

b. **Partial thromboplastin time and activated partial thromboplastin time (PTT and aPTT)** measure the "intrinsic system." The PTT depends on glass activation of factor XII, whereas in the activated PTT, kaolin or Celite is employed for this purpose. All coagulation factors except platelet factor 3, factor XIII, and factor VII are measured by this test.

The test is also sensitive to the presence of heparin and circulating anticoagulants. **The performance of a PTT on a 50 : 50% mix of normal plasma and the patient's plasma may differentiate a factor deficiency from the presence of a circulating anticoagulant (inhibitor).** If the PTT remains long or is not completely corrected, an inhibitor is present. Correction to normal usually implies factor deficiency, but the presence of a mild (low-titer) inhibitor is not excluded. A similar maneuver can be done with the PT.

c. **Thrombin time (TT)** measures the time required for a standard thrombin solution to clot plasma. It is prolonged by hypofibrinogenemia (<90 mg/dl), by the presence of circulating anticoagulants (primarily, fibrin degradation products and heparin), and by dysfibrinogenemias (e.g., liver diseases, hereditary disorders). Performance of a TT in the presence of a certain concentration of protamine sulfate (a "corrected TT") can differentiate the presence of heparin from that of other circulating anticoagulants, the latter most often being fibrin degradation products. "Correction" of the TT with a 50 : 50% mix of normal plasma and the patient's plasma in most cases can distinguish dysfibrinogenemias and hypofibrinogenemias from the presence of circulating anticoagulants.

d. **Fibrinogen** may be assayed as the highest dilution of plasma in which a clot is seen after addition of thrombin (normal is 1 : 64 or higher), or it may be quantitated by a number of methods. In general, a clinically significant hypofibrinogenemia implies a level of less than 100 mg/dl. The blood of patients with hereditary dysfibrinogenemia characteristically shows marked differences in fibrogen levels when assayed simultaneously by immunologic and functional methods.

e. **Fibrin degradation products** circulate in abnormal amounts in the plasma of patients with DIC and primary fibrinolytic states and can be quantitated in a number of ways, all time-consuming. The test is useful in diagnosing and following patients with these disorders. A "corrected TT" or a TT performed on a 50 : 50% mix of normal plasma and the patient's plasma may provide rapid but less definitive evidence of the presence of fibrin degradation products (see **c**).

f. **Individual factor assays** may be performed as required. If a coagulation factor deficiency is causing hemorrhage, the PT, or PTT, or both will be prolonged, except in the case of a factor XIII deficiency, which requires a specific fibrin-stabilizing factor assay. **The normal range for clotting factor activity is 50–150% of normal.**

4. **Basic approach to coagulation tests.** The history and physical examination usually disclose a reason for prolongation of PT or PTT, or both. The most frequently observed abnormality usually is an unexplained isolated prolongation of PTT. After the PTT is measured again to exclude technical problems, a 50 : 50% mix with normal plasma is performed to help differentiate inhibitors (circulating anticoagulants) from factor deficiency. If the PTT is corrected, deficiency of factor VIII, IX, XI, or XII is present (see Fig. 16-1). Similarly, an isolated prolonged PT that is corrected by a 50 : 50% mix indicates factor VII deficiency. This follows, since deficiency of any additional or other factors would prolong the PTT as well.

II. Quantitative platelet disorders

A. **Thrombocytopenia** is the most common cause of abnormal bleeding.

1. **Classification.** Thrombocytopenia results from either decreased platelet production or increased peripheral utilization (destruction or sequestration). A bone marrow examination is the necessary first step in a logical approach to the differential diagnosis. It should be performed virtually in all instances with the exceptions of known chronic idiopathic thrombocytopenic purpura (ITP) or recently administered myelosuppressive chemotherapy. Normally, approximately eight megakaryocytes are found per bone spicule. Decreased numbers suggest decreased platelet production; normal or increased numbers imply increased platelet consumption. Further etiologic distinctions are derived from the history, physical findings, therapeutic trial, or by exclusion.

2. **General therapeutic considerations.** In general, platelet counts in excess of 50,000/μl are not associated with significant bleeding problems, and severe spontaneous bleeding is rare in patients with platelet counts higher than 20,000/μl in the absence of coagulation factor abnormalities. All patients with thrombocytopenia should be instructed to avoid trauma and to seek early treatment when such trauma occurs. Intramuscular injections and rectal thermometers should be avoided, as should drugs known to inhibit platelet function (e.g., salicylates). In severe cases, toothbrushes, abrasive food, enemas, and constricting garments should be avoided. However, patients vary in their ability to tolerate thrombocytopenia, and such restrictions may be individualized.

3. **Platelet transfusions** should be reserved for patients experiencing serious hemorrhage related to thrombocytopenia or should be used as an adjunct to major surgery to prevent serious postoperative bleeding. Platelet transfusions also may be used as prophylactic therapy in certain chronic thrombocytopenic states (e.g., aplastic anemia). Prophylactic platelet transfusions are employed during induction and consolidation therapy of acute leukemia. Platelet counts should be maintained above 20,000/μl at all times during chemotherapy-induced thrombocytopenia. Whenever possible, profoundly immunocompromised patients should receive **irradiated blood products** to prevent inadvertent lymphoid engrafting with subsequent graft-versus-host disease.

   a. If long-term platelet support is anticipated, the patient and all full-blooded siblings should undergo **HL-A typing,** although this may not be technically possible in leukemic patients with high numbers of circulating blasts.

   b. Donor platelet survival will depend on such factors as the age of the transfused platelets, the underlying conditions present in the recipient (e.g., fever, infection, hepatosplenomegaly), and, if the patient has been previously transfused, the degree of alloimmunization. The normal half-life of infused platelets should be about 4 days.

   c. Platelet transfusion is initiated with 6–10 units of leukocyte-reduced random donor platelets. An average unit contains about 10^{11} platelets.

   d. A **platelet count** should be obtained 1 hour after infusion to measure the increment achieved by transfusion. An initial transfusion into a nonimmunized recipient should raise the platelet count by about $10,000/\mu l/M^2/10^{11}$ platelets transfused. We consider a poor increment to be a 1-hour increase of less than $5000/\mu l/M^2/10^{11}$ transfused platelets.

   e. Single-donor **HL-A-matched platelets** should be employed if poor increments are noted after three consecutive transfusions with random donor products.

   f. **Complications** of platelet transfusion include fevers, chills, and transmission of hepatitis. Fever is usually due to leukoagglutinin reactions, but bacterial contamination also should be considered.

4. **Specific therapeutic situations**

   a. The diagnosis of **idiopathic (autoimmune) thrombocytopenic purpura** should be made only after exclusion of all other causes of thrombocytopenia. It exists in two forms: (1) an acute self-limited form, often seen in children following viral infections and occasionally seen in adults as well and (2) a chronic recurrent disorder not necessarily associated with an obvious initiating event.

      (1) The acute form is probably not benefited by any therapy. The chronic form should be initially treated with prednisone (1.5 mg/kg/day),

which is continued until the platelet count is above 100,000/μl and then is slowly tapered.

(2) Rapid recurrence, lack of response to corticosteroid therapy (approximately 1 week of treatment), inability to withdraw corticosteroids, or late relapse should lead the physician to consider splenectomy. Life-threatening hemorrhage at presentation precludes a corticosteroid trial and mandates emergency splenectomy. A careful search for accessory spleens should be made at the time of operation.

(3) Persistence of disease following splenectomy may be expected in up to 20% of patients. These patients should be treated with prednisone, 1.5 mg/kg/day, with or without immunosuppressive agents (e.g., azathioprine, 200 mg/day). Dosages of both drugs should be slowly tapered to the minimum necessary to prevent undue risk of hemorrhage. Alternatively, weekly IV vinca alkaloids have been employed.

(4) Patients with chronic ITP frequently do not have significant hemorrhage despite profound thrombocytopenia. Treatment of the patient refractory to most of the measures outlined should be initiated for increasing hemorrhagic manifestations and **not** for worsening thrombocytopenia per se.

b. Immune thrombocytopenias and hypersplenism. In general, immune thrombocytopenia associated with such diseases as systemic lupus erythematosus (SLE), chronic lymphocytic leukemia, and lymphoma respond to the treatment program outlined for ITP. Therapy also must be directed at the underlying disease. In cases of presumed splenic platelet sequestration, the approach to splenectomy must be tempered by the fact that operative morbidity and mortality are increased in these patients. Splenectomy should be reserved for patients with unmanageable bleeding from thrombocytopenia. When the decision is difficult, a markedly shortened platelet survival and evidence of selective splenic sequestration of injected ^{51}Cr-labeled platelets increase the likelihood that splenectomy may benefit the patient, although a failure to find sequestration does not exclude such a benefit.

c. Transfusion-associated purpuras. An abrupt thrombocytopenia may follow massive transfusion or extracorporeal circulation and is due to dilution or mechanical removal of platelets. It lasts 3–5 days and may be treated with platelet transfusion. Posttransfusion purpura is a rare condition, occurring primarily though not exclusively in multiparous P1^{A1}-negative women approximately 7 days after a blood transfusion. The problem is largely self-limited, but if therapy becomes necessary, cautious partial-exchange transfusion with whole blood or plasmapheresis is the treatment of choice. Platelet transfusions and corticosteroids are not beneficial.

d. Drug-induced thrombocytopenias are secondary to decreased platelet production (from thiazide diuretics, ethanol, estrogens) or increased platelet destruction, primarily on an immunologic basis. Although a wide variety of drugs has been implicated as causing thrombocytopenia, only a few (e.g., quinine, quinidine, digitoxin, thiazides, ethanol, estrogens, heparin) have been shown to have more than a very rare association with thrombocytopenia.

Drug-induced thrombocytopenia is diagnosed by noting temporal relationships between the onset of drug administration and the onset of thrombocytopenia and between the cessation of drug administration and recovery from thrombocytopenia (occasionally requiring weeks). **All drugs should be discontinued in patients with thrombocytopenia** unless the thrombocytopenia is known not to be drug related, or the drug is essential to the patient's welfare. Once the thrombocytopenia has resolved, necessary drugs may be readministered cautiously, one at a time.

   e. **Thrombotic thrombocytopenic purpura** is a rare syndrome characterized by the presence of a microangiopathic hemolytic anemia, thrombocytopenia, fever, renal abnormalities (usually mild), and protean neurologic findings. Its prognosis has improved over the past 5 years coincident with the addition of plasmapheresis, plasma infusion, and whole blood exchange transfusion to other therapies. Attempts to organize multicenter randomized studies aimed at factoring out ineffective but traditional treatments have failed. We currently recommend a combination of plasmapheresis and antiplatelet agents as initial therapy; the former has been tested at multiple centers and is free of volume overload problems, whereas the latter is relatively innocuous and probably effective. Because of case reports of platelet transfusions preceding sudden neurologic deteriorations, these are best avoided.

B. Thrombocytosis can be associated with platelet dysfunction and bleeding or predispose to thrombosis. An arbitrary clinical "danger level" of greater than 1 million/μl has been cited, although bleeding times may be prolonged or normal in this setting. Approximately one-third of patients with thrombocytosis in general medical centers will be found to have a malignancy. Other associated conditions are much less common; for instance, only 5% of patients with thrombocytosis will be found to have an underlying myeloproliferative disorder. Bleeding with thrombocytosis should prompt a search for a localized lesion before thrombocytosis is presumed to be causal.

A patient with diffuse hemorrhage, thrombocytosis, and no other underlying coagulation abnormality should undergo plateletpheresis while a search for the cause of the thrombocytosis and long-term therapy are instituted. Similarly, patients with active GI hemorrhage, thrombocytosis, prolonged bleeding time, and no clear-cut localized lesions should be considered for plateletpheresis. For long-term control, reduction of the megakaryocytic mass by intermittent courses of alkylating agents is recommended.

III. Qualitative platelet disorders. A number of congenital and acquired defects in platelet function have been described. Their clinical presentations vary, and their therapy is not well established. Therapy of the acquired defects should be directed at the underlying disorder. Platelet transfusions should be utilized in such situations as preparation for emergency surgery.

IV. Coagulation factor disorders

A. Inherited disorders

   1. **Hemophilia.** Congenital deficiencies of factor VIII or IX (hemophilia A and B respectively) are X-linked recessive disorders. Hemophilia A is about 5 times more frequent than B. The clinical presentations of the defects are similar and vary in proportion to the degree of factor deficiency as determined by in vitro clotting assays. Patients with mild to moderate factor deficiencies may not have their first serious bleeding episode until adult life.

      a. The **treatment** of factor VIII deficiency (hemophilia A) is usually accomplished by infusion of one of a variety of factor VIII concentrates. The amount infused varies according to the severity and location of the hemorrhage and must be tailored to the individual patient. Minor cuts, scratches, and superficial ecchymoses usually require no therapy. Uncomplicated hemarthroses or symptomatic hematomas in noncritical areas can be treated initially by achieving a factor VIII level of approximately 50% of normal, then repeating this dose q12h for 2–4 days. Life-threatening hemorrhage, hematomas in critical areas (e.g., the neck), and major surgery require initial achievement of a factor VIII level of approximately 100%, followed by administration of about one-half the initial dose q8h for 1–2 days and q12h thereafter for 3–5 days following cessation of bleeding.

One unit of factor VIII activity is equal to the activity present in 1 ml of normal human plasma; therefore, 1 unit/ml of factor VIII activity will correspond to 100% activity as measured by in vitro assays. One may estimate a patient's plasma volume at 41 ml/kg of body weight and thereafter calculate the amount of factor VIII necessary by applying the following equation (assume the initial VIII concentration is 0.0%):

Units factor VIII required = (desired factor VIII concentration − initial factor VIII concentration) × plasma volume

Prior to factor VIII infusion, patients should be premedicated with diphenhydramine HCL, 50 mg IV, to avert urticarial reactions. Following the initial therapy, factor VIII levels should be monitored daily and therapy adjusted to attain a factor VIII concentration of about 50% immediately after infusion for minor bleeding episodes and about 80% for major bleeding episodes.

Administration of **cryoprecipitate,** 10–15 bags initially (1 bag of cryoprecipitate usually contains 100–150 units of factor VIII), for hemarthrosis is an acceptable alternative to factor VIII concentrates. It is less expensive and carries a relatively low risk of hepatitis transmission, but amounts of factor VIII vary per bag, so that the response is less predictable. **Under no circumstances should aspirin be given to patients with coagulation factor deficiency. This error is most often made in the prescription of aspirin-containing analgesic combinations.**

Hemarthrosis is the most frequently encountered problem in the adult patient with hemophilia. The duration of the episode and the extent of hemorrhage and subsequent joint deformity may be minimized if replacement therapy is initiated as soon as possible. The clear advantage of home treatment programs is related to these facts. Joint immobilization by an Ace bandage or "soft" casting is mandatory. Arthrocentesis should be considered only if severe pain and swelling are present, a postinfusion factor VIII level is therapeutic, and the affected joint affords easy access. Factor VIII dosages are calculated by using the equation previously given.

b. **Inhibitors** to factor VIII are present in 10–20% of hemophiliac patients. Under no circumstances should a patient with a factor VIII inhibitor undergo arthrocentesis; all such patients should be hospitalized for therapy. Successful treatment of patients with inhibitors has been reported with the following modalities: (1) massive intermittent doses or continuous infusion of factor VIII, (2) prothrombin complex concentrates, and (3) immunosuppressive therapy. Immunosuppressive therapy is generally felt to be most effective in nonhemophiliac inhibitor management.

c. **Factor IX deficiency** is treated using guidelines similar to those given for hemophilia A, with the exception that transfused factor IX has a considerably longer half-life (18–30 hours for factor IX versus 12 hours for factor VIII) and therefore need not be given as often. Minor hemorrhage usually is controlled with plasma (15–20 ml/kg body weight). **Prothrombin complex concentrates** containing factor IX are available for the treatment of more severe hemorrhage.

2. **von Willebrand's disease** is an autosomal dominant hereditary disorder characterized by a variable decrease in factor VIII activity, a prolonged bleeding time, and abnormal ristocetin platelet aggregation. In contrast to patients with hemophilia A, patients with von Willebrand's disease may show a prolonged progressive rise in factor VIII activity following transfusion of

plasma, cryoprecipitate, or other factor VIII concentrates. In general, bleeding episodes in patients with von Willebrand's disease are more easily controlled than bleeding episodes in patients with hemophilia A. Furthermore, major events such as surgery do not present so severe a risk to patients with von Willebrand's disease as they do to hemophiliac patients. Treatment of hemorrhage may be initiated with 10–15 ml/kg/day of plasma or its equivalent. Platelet transfusion should be given for brisk bleeding as well. Bleeding time and factor VIII activity must be monitored. Further therapeutic guidelines are not well established, but drugs that interfere with platelet function should be avoided.

3. **Other inherited defects.** Patients with hemophilia A, hemophilia B, and von Willebrand's disease constitute more than 90% of all patients with severe hereditary bleeding defects. The remaining factor deficiencies are treated with infusions of plasma fractions rich in the specific component desired.

B. **Acquired disorders**

1. **Vitamin K deficiency.** Vitamin K is a cofactor for the gamma glutamyl carboxylation of factors II, VII, IX, and X. Noncarboxylated factors exhibit markedly decreased enzymatic activity in vitro. Therefore, in vitamin K deficiency, fibrin generation is impaired, and a hemorrhagic diathesis results. Conditions associated with vitamin K deficiency include obstructive liver disease, malabsorption syndromes, conditions that alter a patient's normal intestinal flora, and nutritional deficiencies. The PT usually is an adequate measure of the activity of the vitamin K–dependent factors in these circumstances. Therapy depends on the severity of the hemostatic defect. Serious hemorrhage requires treatment with plasma transfusion (15–20 ml/kg, then 5–8 ml/kg q8–12h); mild defects can be corrected with parenteral vitamin K_1 (see Use of Anticoagulants, sec. **III.D**). Vitamin K will not correct these hemostatic defects in the presence of severe hepatocellular disease.

2. **Coagulopathies associated with liver disease.** Severe liver disease causes deficiencies in a number of coagulation factors (I, II, V, VII, and IX–XI). Severe bleeding in a patient with liver disease presents a very difficult therapeutic problem. Replacement therapy with fresh-frozen plasma is recommended. All such patients should receive parenteral vitamin K_1 (10 mg SQ qd for 3 days), although the majority will not respond.

This situation may also be complicated by the concomitant presence of DIC (see **3**). The diagnosis of DIC in a patient with liver disease can be extremely difficult. It may be aided by the presence of a microangiopathic blood smear and decreased levels of factor VIII, both usually normal in liver disease uncomplicated by DIC.

3. **Disseminated intravascular coagulation** is the consequence of intravascular activation of the coagulation system, with resultant consumption of coagulation factors and platelets. It can be acute or chronic and may vary greatly in clinical severity. Laboratory findings in DIC usually include thrombocytopenia, a microangiopathic blood smear, hypofibrinogenemia, an elevation in fibrin degradation products, a prolonged TT, and decreased levels of factors V and VIII. The following conditions account for most of the cases: **infections** (e.g., gram-negative sepsis, meningococcemia, Rocky Mountain spotted fever); **shock**; obstetric complications; **malignant diseases** (e.g., carcinoma of the prostate, lung, and other organs, acute leukemia, and especially promyelocytic leukemia); complications of surgery (e.g., extracorporeal circulation, prostate surgery); transfusion reactions; anaphylaxis; SLE; extensive tissue damage; giant hemangiomas; and snakebite.

Treatment of the underlying condition is the major therapeutic approach to DIC. Heparin should **not** be used in this syndrome unless the bleeding is unmanageable by replacement with fresh-frozen plasma, platelets, or other hemostatic factors (*Blood* 60:284, 1982).

4. **Circulating anticoagulants** present in patients with hemophilia A have been discussed in **A.1**. The spontaneous generation of anti–factor VIII antibodies in nonhemophiliac patients also has been reported. Other forms of circulating anticoagulants have been demonstrated in SLE and in the dysproteinemic states, but they are usually not associated with clinically severe bleeding, and therapy may be directed at the underlying condition. Rarely, a severe bleeding episode will necessitate measures similar to those employed in hemophiliac patients with anti–factor VIII antibodies.

V. **Vascular purpura or "easy bruising."** Vascular purpura or easy bruising seen in the presence of a normal platelet count and normal coagulation studies should suggest the presence of one of the following: (1) senile purpura; (2) purpura simplex; (3) infectious purpura (e.g., meningococcemia, Waterhouse-Friderichsen syndrome, certain viral infections); (4) fat embolism; (5) cryoglobulinemia or macroglobulinemia; (6) amyloidosis; (7) allergic purpura (e.g., Henoch-Schönlein purpura, certain drugs); (8) scurvy; (9) Cushing's syndrome; (10) hereditary hemorrhagic telangiectasia; (11) autoerythrocyte sensitivity; and (12) factitious purpura. Therapy is directed toward the underlying condition.

Thrombosis

I. **Arterial occlusion.** The early recognition and institution of treatment of arterial occlusion is essential. In general, most peripheral occlusions require surgical intervention (e.g., embolectomy, resection). If embolectomy yields evidence of "red" thrombus formation only (i.e, no atheroembolic nidus is present), an origin in the left atrium or paradoxical embolization is suggested. Long-term anticoagulation with warfarin drugs is indicated in such patients (see Use of Anticoagulants, sec. **III**). In addition, patients at increased risk of arterial embolization related to mitral valve disease with left atrial enlargement or prosthetic heart valves are candidates for long-term anticoagulant prophylaxis with warfarin drugs. Indications for acute anticoagulation for emboli in the cerebral circulation are presented in Chap. 22.

II. **Venous thrombosis.** Superficial venous thromboses generally are controlled by local therapy consisting of heat, elevation, and rest. Deep venous thromboses (DVT) present more difficult diagnostic and therapeutic problems and pose a significant danger to the afflicted patient. Physical signs are notoriously unreliable in DVT; venography should be employed to confirm the diagnosis before patients are committed to long-term anticoagulation. Initial therapy for deep venous thrombosis should include the local measures mentioned, plus anticoagulation with heparin (see below). The patient who shows evidence of stable or resolving disease may be switched to warfarin therapy gradually (over about 6 days). Warfarin is continued for an additional 2–6 months, depending on the relative risks of embolism and hemorrhage in each individual patient. A recurrence of venous thrombosis while the patient is receiving adequate warfarin therapy necessitates heparin therapy for about 14 days, followed again by a warfarin drug. The use of custom-made elastic stockings and the avoidance of activities or postures that promote venous stasis may reduce recurrences.

Low-dose heparin therapy may be of use in preventing DVT in certain high-risk patients. These would include obese patients undergoing major abdominal surgery, patients in congestive heart failure, and, in general, clinical situations requiring 5 days or more of strict bed rest. Relative contraindications to heparin therapy (Table 16-1) must always be kept in mind.

Current regimens for low-dose heparin include 5000 units injected SQ q8–12h. A highly concentrated heparin (about 20,000 units/ml) should be used and should be injected rapidly SQ through a 25-gauge needle, followed by pressure over the injection site to minimize hemorrhage. Laboratory monitoring is not necessary. Therapy should be continued while the patient remains bedfast. If thrombosis occurs, a low-dose heparin regimen is **not** effective in preventing propagation of the fibrin clot, and a standard anticoagulation regimen must be utilized.

Table 16-1. Relative contraindications to anticoagulation

Active bleeding or bleeding tendencies (e.g., active peptic ulcer, hemophilia)
Severe hypertension
Cerebrovascular hemorrhage
Central nervous system or ophthalmic surgery
Pericarditis, vasculitis, bacterial endocarditis
Pregnancy (contraindications primarily relate to warfarin drugs)
Inadequate laboratory facilities
Unsatisfactory patient cooperation

Use of Anticoagulants

I. **General considerations.** A decision to employ anticoagulants always involves weighing the risk of potential hemorrhage secondary to the anticoagulants and the risk of thrombosis or embolism in the absence of anticoagulants. Prior to the initiation of anticoagulant therapy, patients must be carefully screened for the presence of relative contraindications to therapy (see Table 16-1), because the failure to detect such contraindications could prove fatal. Their stringency varies, and in the final analysis a decision to employ anticoagulant therapy must always be individualized.

II. **Heparin.** Heparin is the drug of choice for acute anticoagulation. It is a naturally occurring sulfated mucopolysaccharide that acts by markedly potentiating the action of a plasma alpha-2 globulin, antithrombin III (heparin cofactor). Because antithrombin III has activity against thrombin, Xa, IXa, and XIa, heparin administration will result in the prolongation of the PT, PTT, and TT. Heparin is metabolized in the liver and excreted in the urine; patients with hepatic or renal disease may be unduly sensitive to the drug.

    A. **Preparations.** Heparin sodium injection USP is available in solutions containing 1000, 5000, 10,000, 20,000, or 40,000 USP units/ml. The dosage is prescribed in units rather than in milliliters.

    B. **Administration.** The major complication of heparin therapy is bleeding. **Continuous IV infusion** is the administrative method of choice because of the reduced incidence of bleeding complications when compared to intermittent administration. Heparin therapy should be initiated by a bolus injection of 5000 units as a loading dose, followed by 1000–2000 units/hour by mechanical infusion pump. Except when fluid restriction is absolutely required, **the concentration of infused heparin should not exceed 20,000 units/liter of IV fluid;** mechanical pump failure during infusion of a more concentrated solution can lead to massive overdosage. Heparin therapy should be monitored by the PTT. Specific therapeutic values should be established for each laboratory; usually, these range between 1½–2½ times the control. Initially, the PTT should be measured q4h and the infusion rate adjusted accordingly. Once a steady dosage schedule is established, once-daily monitoring is sufficient.

    C. **Precautions.** Patients receiving heparin should avoid trauma and report promptly any episode of bleeding or melena. Anatomic areas at risk should be examined regularly (e.g., the CNS, optic fundi, surgical wounds). It is advisable to determine the hematocrit periodically and to examine the stool for occult blood. Symptoms suggesting hemorrhage (e.g., sudden onset of flank or back pain) should prompt immediate determination of the PTT and hematocrit, and the heparin infusion should be discontinued until the possibility of hemorrhage is eliminated. Documented bleeding should be ascribed to drug toxicity, and heparin should be stopped, although the possibility that a localized lesion is responsible for bleeding should also be entertained. Severe hemorrhage may be counteracted by protamine sulfate administration (see **E**).

D. Toxicity. Hemorrhage constitutes the primary toxicity of heparin. Other side effects are relatively uncommon. Acute, reversible thrombocytopenia has been reported following administration of heparin. Hypersensitivity or anaphylactic reactions are extremely rare.

E. Antidote. Heparin is not detectable in a normal patient's plasma 4 hours after cessation of therapy. If anticoagulation must be reversed more rapidly (a rare occurrence), **protamine sulfate** will effectively neutralize heparin. It is administered in a dilute solution of 2 mg/ml made by diluting 5 ml of a 1% solution (50 mg) with 20 ml of saline. Protamine sulfate must be given very slowly, i.e., no more than 50 mg over a 10-minute period and no more than 200 mg within 2 hours.

The dosage varies with the amount of heparin presumed circulating at the time of protamine sulfate administration. Immediately following an injection of heparin, 1.0–1.5 mg of protamine sulfate will be needed to antagonize 100 units of heparin; 30 minutes following heparin injection, only 0.5 mg protamine/100 units of heparin will be needed. In the continuous infusion setting, assume that half the preceding hourly dose must be neutralized. Quantities greater than 100 mg should be used only in very extreme circumstances. Protamine itself has anticoagulant properties; therefore, conservative estimates of the amount of protamine needed must be used. The exact neutralizing dose can be best judged by a protamine titration test if facilities are available. Otherwise, neutralizing effect should be monitored with a PTT immediately after drug administration.

III. Warfarin drugs. Warfarin drugs act in the liver, interfering with the vitamin K–dependent gamma glutamyl carboxylation of factors II, VII, IX, and X. These agents provide a less rapid anticoagulation than that achieved with heparin, but they are much more convenient for long-term outpatient use. Following initiation of therapy, vitamin K–dependent clotting factor activities will decline at varying rates, factor VII having the shortest half-life. The PT will become prolonged at about 48 hours, but a week may pass before all the vitamin K–dependent factors are at therapeutically beneficial levels.

A. Preparation and administration. Sodium warfarin can be given orally or parenterally. Therapy generally is initiated with a warfarin dosage of 10–15 mg/day for 3–5 days, followed by a maintenance dosage of 2–15 mg/day. The maintenance dosage is determined by following the patient's PT (usual therapeutic range, about 20% or 1½–2½ times the control). Once a steady state has been reached, it is necessary to check the PT only about every 2 weeks during prolonged therapy (see **C**).

B. Precautions. The precautions noted for heparin (see sec. **II.C**) apply equally to the warfarin drugs.

C. Drug interactions and toxicity. A steady state of anticoagulation with warfarin drugs is highly dependent on liver function and vitamin K intake and absorption. Anything that will affect the former (e.g., hepatitis) or the latter (e.g., alterations in normal bowel flora, decreased food intake) will alter the patient's coagulation status. Such alterations, if not recognized and corrected, may lead to fatal hemorrhagic or thrombotic episodes. A large variety of drugs also interact with the warfarins in vivo to modify their effects (Table 16-2).

Outside of hemorrhage, toxic effects are rare. Occasional anorexia, nausea, vomiting, diarrhea, urticaria, purpura, or alopecia may occur. A hemorrhagic vasculitis (resulting in skin necrosis, especially over the breast) has also been observed and may be fatal; immediate cessation of the drug is indicated.

Table 16-2. Some agents that interact in vivo with warfarin drugs

Increase prothrombin time	Decrease prothrombin time
Antibiotics	Barbiturates
Quinine, quinidine	Glutethimide
Chloral hydrate	Griseofulvin
Clofibrate	Rifampin
Phenylbutazone	Ethchlorvynol
Propylthiouracil	Estrogens (?)
D-Thyroxine	
Mefenamic acid	
Salicylates (large doses)	
Anabolic steroids	
Glucagon	
Nortriptyline	
Disulfiram	
Sulfinpyrazone (?)	

   D. Antidote. Following cessation of warfarin therapy, the PT gradually will return to normal. This may be hastened by the parenteral administration of vitamin K. **Phytonadione** (vitamin K_1) is the drug of choice. Intravenous administration of 20 mg will return the PT to normal within 6–12 hours, independent of the amount of warfarin ingested. When given IV, vitamin K_1 must be given very slowly (not more than 1 mg/minute) to avoid precipitating a hypotensive episode. Smaller amounts are often useful in controlling minor hemorrhagic episodes. A "rebound" hypercoagulable state following abrupt discontinuance of warfarin or after vitamin K therapy probably does not occur, but vitamin K therapy may make renewed oral anticoagulation very difficult for a number of days after it is given. For this reason, patients with prosthetic heart valves requiring obligate anticoagulation who are overanticoagulated and bleeding are more easily treated by infusion of 1–2 units of fresh-frozen plasma (FFP).

IV. Fibrinolytic enzyme therapy. Fibrinolytic enzyme therapy (streptokinase and urokinase) has been released for treatment of "massive" pulmonary embolism and DVT. To date, no change in immediate mortality has been seen, although accelerated resolution of emboli and lowering of pulmonary capillary blood volumes and diffusing capacities suggested greater resolution of emboli with thrombolytics than with heparin. However, one finds it difficult to ascribe **clinical** significance to these findings, given the extremely low incidence of cor pulmonale as a sequela of pulmonary embolism (*N. Engl. J. Med.* 289:56, 1973). Bleeding complications are more frequent, more severe, and more difficult to reverse than with heparin therapy. Therefore, at this time, it appears prudent to restrict fibrinolytic enzyme therapy to patients who meet the following criteria: (1) well-documented pulmonary embolism (unequivocal V/Q scan or pulmonary arteriogram) and (2) demonstration of cardiovascular or respiratory compromise, either hypotension with signs of pulmonary hypertension or marked $(A-a)O_2$ gradient with an inability to oxygenate.

Fibrinolytic treatment of patients with DVT has not decreased the incidence of pulmonary embolism, although a preliminary report suggests that postphlebitic complications may be fewer (*Br. J. Surg.* 66:838, 1979). We cannot recommend fibrinolytic therapy for DVT other than in the setting of a clinical study.

Contraindications to fibrinolytic therapy include surgery, parturition, liver or kidney biopsy, or a diagnostic procedure involving arterial puncture in the preceding 10 days (other contraindications are detailed in Table 16-1).

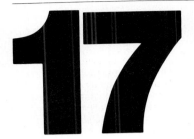

Chemotherapy in Malignant Disease

Effective treatment of malignancy requires accurate diagnosis and staging, appropriate therapy, intensive supportive care, and proper management of complications. The following sections discuss chemotherapeutic drugs, complications of drug administration, the supportive care of the patient, and common or emergent problems in medical oncology. Methods of diagnosis and indications for the use of specific therapies are beyond the scope of this chapter.

Chemotherapeutic Drugs

Chemotherapeutic drugs are employed for the palliation, induction of remission, or cure of malignant disorders. They also are used in adjuvant settings to decrease the risk of subsequent metastases in patients who have undergone "curative" surgery, presumably by eliminating occult micrometastases. In addition, chemotherapeutic drugs are used for the treatment of autoimmune disorders and for the treatment of organ rejection in transplantation. A clearly defined **goal of therapy** should be outlined before any chemotherapeutic drug is used.

The following section provides a brief description of the drugs available for use in cancer therapy. (For additional details the reader is referred to R. T. Dorr and W. L. Fritz, *Cancer Chemotherapy Handbook*. New York: Elsevier, 1980.) Because the toxicities of drug combinations are not necessarily predicted by the toxicities of the individual agents, original reports should be reviewed prior to administration. The recommended dosage schedule should be followed precisely because the efficacy and toxicities of drug combinations may be schedule dependent. Dosage reduction tables should be employed for patients with myelosuppression or altered metabolic and excretory pathways. Chemotherapeutic drugs have a low therapeutic ratio and are potentially lethal; a complete blood count should be obtained on the day of treatment and periodically following therapy.

I. **Alkylating agents.** Alkylating agents form covalent bonds with guanine residues, resulting in abnormal nucleotide pairing and cross linking of DNA strands. Most alkylators kill both resting and dividing cells.

A. **Mechlorethamine (nitrogen mustard)** most often is used in combination with other drugs for the treatment of Hodgkin's disease. It is available in 10-mg vials and is reconstituted with sterile water. Mechlorethamine is a powerful vesicant; protective gloves and eyeglasses should be used during preparation, and skin exposure should be treated immediately with copious quantities of water or 2% sodium thiosulfate solution. Mechlorethamine should be administered IV immediately after reconstitution through the side port of a freely running infusion of 5% D/W. Hydrocortisone sodium succinate, 100 mg, may be added to the 5% D/W infusion to ameliorate the chemical thrombophlebitis associated with mechlorethamine administration.

Dose-limiting granulocytopenia and thrombocytopenia are maximal 2–3 weeks after administration, and marrow recovery usually is complete in 4–6 weeks. Other toxicities include anorexia, nausea, vomiting, alopecia, amenorrhea, impaired spermatogenesis, fever, headache, diarrhea, weakness, dermatitis, mucosal ulceration, and bone marrow suppression.

B. Chlorambucil (Leukeran) usually is used for the treatment of chronic lymphocytic leukemia. Chlorambucil is available as a 2-mg tablet; the usual initial dosage is 6–14 mg PO daily for 3–6 weeks. Toxicity may be enhanced in patients receiving barbiturates. Dose-limiting neutropenia and thrombocytopenia usually are rapidly reversible, but irreversible marrow toxicity may occur. Blood counts should be followed weekly, and the dosage should be reduced as the peripheral leukocyte and platelet counts fall. Mild nausea and impaired spermatogenesis can occur. Hepatotoxicity, exfoliative dermatitis, pulmonary fibrosis, and allergic febrile reactions have been reported. Prolonged treatment with chlorambucil increases the risk of acute nonlymphocytic leukemia.

C. Busulfan (Myleran) is an alkylating agent used for the treatment of symptomatic chronic myeloid leukemia. Busulfan is available as a 2-mg tablet; the usual dosage is 4–8 mg PO daily until the white count falls to approximately 20,000/μl.

The incidence of nausea and vomiting is low. Delayed and prolonged marrow suppression usually is dose related, although some patients will experience pancytopenia after even small doses. Frequent blood counts minimize the risk of potentially fatal marrow aplasia. Other toxicities include alopecia, glossitis, sterility, impotence, amenorrhea, gynecomastia, and skin hyperpigmentation. Long-term therapy has been associated with irreversible pulmonary fibrosis and a wasting syndrome characterized by anorexia, weight loss, and hypotension.

D. Melphalan (Alkeran) has a spectrum of activity similar to that of nitrogen mustard and is used for the treatment of multiple myeloma and ovarian cancer. Melphalan is available as a 2-mg tablet; the usual dosage is 0.25 mg/kg PO daily for 4 days, repeated at intervals of 4–6 weeks. The incidence of nausea, vomiting, and alopecia is very low. Hematologic toxicity is frequent, with thrombocytopenia being more common than leukopenia. Prolonged treatment with melphalan increases the risk of acute nonlymphocytic leukemia.

E. Cyclophosphamide (Cytoxan) is an immunosuppressant and antineoplastic drug. It is available as a 50-mg tablet and in vials containing 100, 200, and 500 mg of drug. The drug may be reconstituted for IV administration with normal saline, 5% D/W, or sterile water for injection (SWI).

When administered PO, the drug should be taken early in the day and the patient instructed to maintain a large fluid intake. High-dose therapy requires IV hydration at a rate of 150–250 ml/hour and monitoring of fluid balance. Water intoxication secondary to an antidiuretic hormone–like effect of cyclophosphamide metabolites may develop; the peak of this effect occurs 6–8 hours after a large IV dose. Furosemide administration may be necessary to maintain urine output when this effect occurs.

Leukopenia is the usual dose-limiting toxicity of cyclophosphamide. Other toxicities include nausea, vomiting, thrombocytopenia, and hemorrhagic cystitis. Many patients experience reversible alopecia.

II. Antimetabolites. Antimetabolites interfere with the synthesis of essential cell components by competing with natural enzyme substrates or by contributing to the synthesis of abnormal cell constituents. They exert their major activity during the S phase (DNA synthesis) of the cell cycle, and, in general, their greatest toxicity occurs in tissues that have a high growth fraction, e.g., gastrointestinal mucosa.

A. Methotrexate interferes with DNA synthesis through the inhibition of dihydrofolate reductase. This inhibition can be bypassed by the administration of folinic acid (calcium leucovorin). Methotrexate is absorbed orally and is bound to albumin; its displacement by sulfonamides, tetracycline, phenytoin, or salicylates may enhance toxicity. Its distribution into an effusion with later reentry into the circulation may produce serious toxicity. Most of the drug is eliminated by the kidneys, and dosage should be reduced in the presence of renal insufficiency. Salicylates and probenicid may inhibit renal tubular secretion of methotrexate and prolong its serum half-life. Patients receiving methotrexate should not take other drugs without consulting their physician.

1. The drug is supplied in tablet, liquid, and powder form.

    a. Preservative-protected liquid: 5 mg and 50 mg

    b. Preservative-free powder: 20 mg, 50 mg, 100 mg, and 250 mg

    c. Preservative-free liquid: 50 mg, 100 mg, and 200 mg

    d. Tablets: 2.5 mg

    The powder and liquid may be reconstituted with normal saline or SWI.

2. Methotrexate is used in the treatment of many malignant and benign disorders, including acute lymphocytic leukemia, breast cancer, choriocarcinoma, and psoriasis. A variety of dosage schedules have been employed, ranging from daily low-dose oral therapy to intermittent high-dose IV therapy with leucovorin "rescue." The latter is investigational and potentially dangerous and should be employed only by physicians familiar with this method.

3. **Toxicities** include leukopenia, thrombocytopenia, diarrhea, and ulcerative stomatitis. Therapy should be withheld until these toxicities abate. Alopecia, anemia, hepatotoxicity, dermatitis, pneumonitis, nausea, and vomiting can occur. High-dose therapy can cause nephrotoxicity.

4. **Folinic acid (calcium leucovorin)** may be used to treat overdosage or minimize toxicity. The usual dosage is 3–6 mg IV q6h for 3 days. If possible, a safe serum methotrexate level (i.e., $<5 \times 10^{-8}$ M) should be documented before discontinuing folinic acid. Folinic acid is absorbed from the GI tract, although oral administration is not at present approved by the FDA.

5. **Intrathecal methotrexate** is used for treatment of malignant meningitis. Either the 20-mg vial of preservative-free powder or the 50-mg vial of preservative-free liquid may be used. A dose of 12 mg/M^2 (not to exceed 15 mg) is drawn into a sterile syringe and diluted with preservative-free saline to a volume of 5 ml. A lumbar puncture is performed, and 5–10 ml of cerebrospinal fluid (CSF) is removed for appropriate laboratory studies. The syringe containing the methotrexate is attached to the lumbar puncture needle, and an additional 5 ml of CSF is withdrawn. Then, the mixture of methotrexate solution and CSF is slowly injected into the spinal canal.

    Side effects of intrathecal methotrexate include fever, nausea, vomiting, mild stomatitis, and headache. Intrathecal methotrexate may potentiate the myelosuppression induced by concurrent systemic chemotherapy; this may be minimized by the administration of folinic acid (calcium leucovorin), 6 mg IV q6h for 8 doses beginning 12 hours after intrathecal therapy.

B. **6-Mercaptopurine** is a purine antagonist used in the treatment of acute leukemia. It is available as a 50-mg tablet. The usual dosage is 75–100 mg/M^2 PO qd; both hepatic and renal impairment necessitate dosage reductions. Because 6-mercaptopurine is degraded by xanthine oxidase, **only 25% of the standard dosage should be administered to patients receiving allopurinol.**

    The most common **toxicities** are leukopenia and thrombocytopenia. Anorexia, nausea, vomiting, stomatitis, and diarrhea occur in some patients. Cholestatic jaundice, hepatic necrosis, dermatitis, and drug fever have been reported.

C. **Azathioprine (Imuran)** is an imidazolyl derivative of 6-mercaptopurine with a similar mechanism of action. Azathioprine is not used in the conventional treatment of any neoplasm but is used widely as an immunosuppressant in the treatment of chronic active hepatitis, inflammatory bowel disease, allograft rejection, and collagen vascular disorders. Azathioprine is available as a 50-mg tablet and in a 20-ml vial containing 100 mg of injectable sodium salt. Both hepatic and renal impairment require dosage reductions. Azathioprine is degraded by xanthine oxidase; **only 25% of the standard dosage should be administered to patients receiving allopurinol.**

Toxicities of azathioprine include delayed bone marrow suppression, fever, oral ulcerations, alopecia, pancreatitis, and cholestatic jaundice. Prolonged administration of azathioprine may increase the risk of lymphoma and acute nonlymphocytic leukemia.

D. 6-Thioguanine has a spectrum of activity similar to that of 6-mercaptopurine. It is not metabolized by xanthine oxidase, however, and allopurinol administration does not affect its activity. 6-Thioguanine is available as a 40-mg tablet and should be administered between meals. Toxicities resemble those of 6-mercaptopurine.

E. 5-Fluorouracil undergoes enzymatic conversion to an active pyrimidine metabolite that inhibits thymidylate synthetase. It is used in the treatment of carcinoma of the GI tract, bladder, and breast. 5-Fluorouracil is available in 10-ml ampules containing 500 mg of the drug in aqueous solution. It may be administered by IV push or diluted with 5% D/W or normal saline and administered by IV infusion. A wide variety of dosage schedules have been employed.

Toxicities of 5-fluorouracil include anorexia, nausea, stomatitis, diarrhea, and myelosuppression. Cerebellar dysfunction, alopecia, dermatitis, tearing, and increased skin pigmentation have been reported.

F. Cytosine arabinoside is a pyrimidine antagonist used in the treatment of acute leukemia. Vials containing 100 or 500 mg of drug may be reconstituted with 5% D/W or normal saline. The usual daily dosage is $100-200$ mg/M^2 SQ or IV q12h or by continuous IV infusion. Patients with liver dysfunction should receive lower dosages.

Severe myelosuppression usually occurs $12-14$ days after initiation of treatment and may persist for several weeks. Other toxicities include nausea, vomiting, diarrhea, and abdominal pain. An influenzalike syndrome of fever, rash, and arthralgias has been reported.

III. Vinca alkaloids. Vinca alkaloids bind to microtubular proteins and arrest cell division in metaphase, although their exact mechanism of antineoplastic activity is not known. Vinca alkaloids are excreted by the biliary system; patients with hepatobiliary disease require dosage reduction.

A. Vincristine is used for the treatment of leukemia, lymphoma, and solid tumors. It is available in vials containing 1 or 5 mg of powder. Each vial is supplied with an ampule of saline diluent. The dosage is $1-2$ mg/week IV. **Extravasation** causes severe local tissue necrosis.

Vincristine can cause severe, irreversible **neurologic toxicity.** Maximal neurologic dysfunction can occur as late as 4 weeks after a single injection. Neurologic dysfunction may be minimized by reducing dosage at the earliest sign of weakness or severe paresthesias. Mild paresthesias, loss of deep tendon reflexes, and neuritic pain are common and are **not** indications for discontinuing the drug. Muscle weakness, hoarseness, ptosis, diplopia, constipation, abdominal pain, ileus, urinary retention, myalgias, and jaw pain have been reported. Alopecia may occur in some patients but often is reversible even with continuance of the drug. Marrow toxicity usually is minimal.

B. Vinblastine has a mechanism of action and mode of excretion similar to that of vincristine, but the two drugs are not cross-resistant. Vinblastine is used in the treatment of lymphoma, breast cancer, and testicular cancer. Vinblastine is available in vials containing 10 mg of drug. The vials are reconstituted with 10 ml of normal saline. The usual dosage is 3–5 mg/M² IV at intervals greater than 1 week. **Extravasation** causes severe local tissue necrosis. Hepatobiliary disease may require dosage reduction. Marrow toxicity is more prominent than with vincristine and occurs 5–10 days after therapy. Neurologic toxicity is less common than with vincristine.

IV. **Antitumor antibiotics.** Antitumor antibiotics are products of microbial fermentation. No generalizations can be made concerning their mechanisms of action or pharmacokinetics.

A. **Doxorubicin (Adriamycin)** inhibits both DNA replication and RNA synthesis. It is available in vials containing 10 mg or 50 mg of drug. It is reconstituted with SWI and administered IV. **Extravasation** causes tissue necrosis. The usual dosage is 50–70 mg/M² IV every 3 weeks, but many other schedules are utilized. Doxorubicin undergoes hepatic transformation; 50% of the usual dose should be administered if the serum bilirubin is greater than 1.5 mg/dl, and 25% of the usual dose is administered if the serum bilirubin is greater than 3.0 mg/dl. The urine may turn a red color as a result of renal excretion of doxorubicin metabolites.

Toxicities include severe myelosuppression, alopecia, cardiac toxicity, stomatitis, anorexia, and diarrhea. Hypersensitivity reactions and hyperpigmentation are infrequent complications. Radiation toxicity may be potentiated in patients concurrently receiving doxorubicin, and a "recall" phenomenon may be seen when doxorubicin is administered after radiation therapy.

Cardiac toxicity can limit the total doxorubicin dosage. Dysrhythmias may be observed shortly after doxorubicin administration, and lethal congestive heart failure has been observed in patients receiving prolonged therapy. The latter seldom occurs with a total dosage of less than 550 mg/M² unless cyclophosphamide or mediastinal radiotherapy has been administered; in these circumstances, the maximum cumulative dosage should not exceed 450 mg/M².

Most noninvasive attempts to identify patients at high risk of cardiomyopathy during doxorubicin therapy are unsuccessful; the ECG, systolic time intervals, and echocardiogram are not sensitive in predicting tolerance to additional doxorubicin. Preclinical toxicity is detected more reliably by transvenous endomyocardial biopsy and perhaps by exercise radionuclide ventriculography (*Cancer* 46:1109, 1980).

B. **Daunorubicin** shares many properties with doxorubicin, including DNA intercalation, hepatic transformation, and production of cardiac toxicity. Daunorubicin is often used in combination with cytosine arabinoside for the treatment of acute nonlymphocytic leukemia. The usual dosage is 45 mg/M² IV daily for 3 days. **Extravasation** causes tissue necrosis. Toxicities are similar to those of doxorubicin.

C. **Bleomycin** is a mixture of glycopeptides used in the treatment of lymphoma, testicular carcinoma, and some epidermoid tumors. Bleomycin is available in vials containing 15 mg (15 units) and is reconstituted with SWI, normal saline, or 5% D/W. The usual dosage is 10–20 units/M² IV, IM, or SQ weekly or twice weekly. Renal impairment requires dosage reduction.

Anaphylactoid reactions have been observed, especially in patients with lymphoma. These usually occur within 6–15 hours after initial infusion and consist of hypotension, mental confusion, fever, chills, and wheezing. Treatment is symptomatic and includes the use of antihistamines, corticosteroids, and pressor agents. The manufacturer recommends that a test dose of 2 units or less be administered for the first 2 doses. If no acute reaction occurs, the regular dosage schedule may be followed.

The chronic use of bleomycin has been associated with a progressive, potentially fatal form of pulmonary fibrosis. Symptomatic dyspnea and inspiratory rales usually precede radiographic changes. No specific treatment is recommended other than discontinuance of the drug. The risk of pulmonary fibrosis can be minimized by careful clinical observation and limitation of total dosage to 400 units. Severe skin reactions, mucositis, alopecia, nausea, and fever may occur.

D. Mitomycin C selectively inhibits DNA synthesis and its mechanism of action may be similar to that of the alkylating agents. Mitomycin C is used for the treatment of malignancies of the breast and GI tract. It is supplied in 5-mg and 20-mg vials and may be reconstituted with SWI, 5% D/W, or normal saline. Delayed myelosuppression limits IV administration to 6–8-week intervals. **Extravasation** causes tissue necrosis. Renal toxicity has been reported, and extreme caution should be excercised when administering the drug to patients with renal impairment. Gastrointestinal disturbances and alopecia are common. Lethargy, weakness, and confusion also have been observed.

E. Actinomycin D is used in the treatment of testicular carcinoma, sarcoma, and melanoma. The drug is given IV by a variety of dosage schedules. **Extravasation** causes severe tissue necrosis. Other toxicities include radiation "recall," myelosuppression, nausea, vomiting, alopecia, stomatitis, diarrhea, and skin rashes.

F. Mithramycin is used infrequently as a chemotherapeutic agent because of its unpredictable and potentially life-threatening toxicities. These include a severe hemorrhagic diathesis, hepatic dysfunction, hypocalcemia, neurologic reactions, and fever. At lower dosages, mithramycin is used for the treatment of hypercalcemia, but it should be administered only by those experienced in its use. The usual dosage is 15–25 µg/kg IV every 3–7 days. Mithramycin should be administered by IV infusion over 4–6 hours. **Extravasation** causes tissue necrosis.

V. Miscellaneous agents

A. Procarbazine inhibits DNA, RNA, and protein synthesis. The most commonly used regimen employing procarbazine is MOPP therapy for Hodgkin's disease. In this regimen, the 50-mg capsules are administered PO in monthly cycles at a dosage of 100 mg/M^2 daily for 2 weeks. To minimize side effects the daily dose may be escalated by increments of 50 mg until the recommended daily dose is achieved. Renal or hepatic impairment may require dosage reduction.

Procarbazine is a monoamine oxidase inhibitor; caution should be exercised when the drug is administered concurrently with barbiturates, narcotics, decongestants, phenothiazines, antihypertensives, tricyclic antidepressants, or foods with high tyramine content. Concurrent alcohol ingestion can cause a disulfiramlike effect. Other toxicities include myelosuppression, peripheral neuropathy, somnolence, agitation, and psychoses. A transient influenzalike syndrome has been observed but generally is limited to the first course of therapy.

B. Nitrosoureas (BCNU and CCNU) alkylate DNA and interfere with other enzymatic processes. Their high lipid solubility allows for passage across the blood-brain barrier. Nitrosoureas are used in the treatment of GI malignancy, myeloma, and lymphoma. BCNU is dissolved in ethanol, mixed with saline, and administered IV. It may cause giddiness, flushing, confusion, and phlebitis. Local irritation is minimized if the infusion rate and ethanol concentration are reduced. CCNU is administered PO. Myelosuppression occurs 3–4 weeks after nitrosourea administration. Nausea, vomiting, hepatic dysfunction, renal failure, and cumulative dose-related pulmonary toxicity have been observed.

C. Hydroxyurea is used acutely for the rapid reduction of high peripheral blast counts in acute leukemia (see Common or Emergent Clinical Problems, sec. I) or intermittently for the treatment of chronic myeloid leukemia. Hydroxyurea is supplied as a 500-mg capsule. Caution should be exercised when administering the drug to patients with hepatic or renal dysfunction. Toxicities include myelosuppression, nausea, vomiting, stomatitis, skin rash, alopecia, and drowsiness.

D. **Dacarbazine (DTIC)** is a purine analogue with alkylating properties. It is used in the treatment of melanoma, sarcoma, and Hodgkin's disease. Dacarbazine is available in 100- and 200-mg vials and is reconstituted with SWI, 5% D/W, or normal saline. The drug is incompatible in solution with hydrocortisone. Dacarbazine is administered by IV push or by slow IV infusion. **Extravasation** causes tissue necrosis.

Myelosuppression is the most serious toxic effect. Virtually all patients experience anorexia, nausea, and vomiting. Fever, myalgias, malaise, alopecia, facial flushing, and facial paresthesias have been observed.

E. **Cis-diamminedichloroplatinum(II) (DDP)** inhibits DNA, RNA, and protein synthesis and may act as an alkylating agent. It is used in the treatment of carcinoma of the testes, head and neck, bladder, and ovary. The drug is supplied in 10- and 50-mg vials and reconstituted with SWI. The usual dosage is 20 mg/M^2 IV daily for 5 days or 50–100 mg/M^2 IV once monthly.

Regardless of dosage schedule, it is imperative to ensure adequate renal function prior to therapy and to establish a brisk diuresis by means of IV hydration. Some physicians use parenteral furosemide or mannitol to enhance urine flow. In-hospital protocols usually employ prolonged hydration and slow infusion of DDP. For example, IV hydration can be initiated on the night prior to therapy, and furosemide, 40 mg IV, can be administered immediately prior to initiation of chemotherapy. The reconstituted DDP solution is added to 2 liters of 5% dextrose in ½ normal saline with mannitol (25 gm/liter) and administered over 6–8 hours. Outpatient protocols employ brief and intense hydration, aggressive use of diuretics, and more rapid administration of DDP. The infusion rate of DDP should never exceed 1 mg/minute.

Toxicities of DDP include severe nausea, vomiting, renal dysfunction, tinnitus, high-frequency hearing loss, and marrow suppression. Anaphylaxis is a rare complication. Nephrotoxicity generally limits therapy.

F. L-**Asparaginase** administration rapidly depletes blood asparagine levels and inhibits protein synthesis. The drug is used for the treatment of acute lymphocytic leukemia. Patients who experience anaphylaxis or other allergic reactions to the standard preparation obtained from *Eschereschia coli* may be treated with enzymes from *Erwinia carotovora*. Other toxicities include clotting abnormalities, liver dysfunction, CNS depression, and hyperglycemia. Fatal hemorrhagic pancreatitis can occur.

G. **Tamoxifen** is an estrogen antagonist used in the treatment of breast carcinoma. The recommended dosage is 10–20 mg PO bid. Nausea, vomiting, hot flashes, visual blurring, and thrombocytopenia have been reported with this drug. A transient flare of bone pain and hypercalcemia may be observed after initiation of the drug and may be associated with an antitumor response.

Administration of Chemotherapeutic Drugs

I. **General considerations.** All drugs should be stored, diluted, and administered in accordance with information provided in the package insert. Chemotherapeutic drugs should be carefully prepared and administered only by qualified personnel. When possible, veins in the antecubital fossa, wrist, dorsum of the hand, and arm ipsilateral to a mastectomy site should be avoided.

II. **Extravasation of drugs.** Extravasation of drugs may result in severe local tissue necrosis (Table 17-1). The risk of drug extravasation is minimized by proper admin-

Table 17-1. Drugs commonly associated with severe local tissue necrosis

Actinomycin-D	Mithramycin
Dacarbazine	Mitomycin C
Daunomycin	Streptozocin
Doxorubicin	Vinblastine
Mechlorethamine	Vincristine

istration through a freshly started, patent IV line. Early treatment of extravasation may lessen tissue damage (*Cancer Treat. Rev.* 7:17, 1980).

When extravasation occurs, the following procedures should be followed:

A. Stop the injection immediately, and withdraw 5 ml of blood through the IV needle to remove some of the offending drug; then remove the IV needle.

B. Attempt to withdraw additional drug by SQ aspiration using a 27-gauge needle.

C. Read the package insert, and institute appropriate recommendations.

D. Infuse 100 mg of hydrocortisone SQ.

E. Apply warm compresses for at least 1 hour.

F. Apply 1% hydrocortisone cream to the area, and cover with a sterile dressing.

Supportive Care

The administration of large dosages of drugs with low therapeutic ratios places the already ill patient at risk of serious complications secondary to drug therapy. Intensive, wide-ranging support is necessary to minimize these complications and to increase the probability of a successful outcome. Detailed discussions regarding the psychologic, economic, and medical aspects of patient support are available in textbooks of oncology. An approach to several common medical complications of malignancy or chemotherapy will be discussed in secs. I–VI.

I. **Emesis.** Emesis is often the most disabling side effect of chemotherapy but may be ameliorated through the proper use of antiemetic drugs (*Ann. Intern. Med.* 95:352, 1981). **Antiemetic drugs should be administered prior to chemotherapy and on a regular basis rather than prn.**

Phenothiazines frequently are efficacious but may be inadequate against strongly emetic agents, such as DDP, doxorubicin, and dacarbazine. Concurrently administered antihistamines or benzodiazapenes sometimes may be valuable through their sedative effects. Metoclopramide may be effective in the prevention or relief of nausea and vomiting in some patients refractory to phenothiazines. Corticosteroids, haloperidol, tetrahydrocannabinol, droperidol, and domperidone have been used on an investigational basis in patients refractory to phenothiazines.

II. **Analgesics.** Analgesics should be administered to the cancer patient in severe pain without undue concern over addiction. Oral drugs should be used whenever possible. Although "Brompton's cocktail" has been used widely, **morphine sulfate elixer** (10 mg/5 ml) may provide equal analgesia with fewer side effects and less cost. The initial dosage is 10 mg PO q6h and should be escalated until the desired level of analgesia is achieved. Stool softeners may be necessary to minimize the constipating side effects of morphine. A more extensive list of analgesics is provided in Chap. 1.

III. **Infections.** Infections are a major cause of morbidity and mortality in patients treated with intensive myelosuppressive chemotherapy. Bacterial infections are most common, but infections due to fungi, pneumocystis, and viruses also occur frequently. Complications due to infection may be minimized by their prevention, rapid identification, and early treatment.

A. Patients should be **isolated** from known sources of infection, and everyone in contact with the patient should adhere to a vigorous hand-washing protocol. Routine mask and gown isolation is of limited value. Strict aseptic techniques should be employed when performing invasive procedures. Intravenous catheters should be changed regularly and at the first sign of inflammation.

B. **Patient hygiene** should be carefully maintained, with special attention directed toward cutaneous, oral, and rectal areas. Electric razors are advisable. Toothbrushes should be soft and used gently. Elective dental extraction should be considered prior to chemotherapy in patients with severe caries or periodontal disease. Stools should be kept soft. Rectal irritation and subsequent rectal abscess formation can be minimized by avoiding rectal temperature taking, suppositories, enemas, and unnecessary digital examinations.

C. The use of **prophylactic antimicrobials** in the neutropenic patient is controversial. Trimethoprim-sulfamethoxazole may reduce the incidence of acquired infections in patients with severe granulocytopenia; however, when infections subsequently arise, they generally are caused by organisms resistant to this antimicrobial combination (*Ann. Intern. Med.* 95:555, 1981). **Nystatin** oral suspension (10 ml "swish and swallow" qid) should be administered to minimize fungal colonization of the GI tract.

D. **Rapid identification of infection** can minimize morbidity. **Fever** in the neutropenic host should be assumed to be due to infection until proved otherwise. Appropriate cultures should be obtained immediately and more aggressive diagnostic procedures instituted when necessary.

E. **Empirical antimicrobial therapy** should be instituted when infection is suspected:

1. Use of an aminoglycoside and a semisynthetic penicillin active against *Pseudomonas* is recommended because of the high incidence of gram-negative bacillary infections in neutropenic patients.

2. Culture results, clinical setting, and local susceptibility patterns may suggest the addition of an antistaphylococcal antimicrobial.

3. **Fungal infections** occur frequently in neutropenic patients receiving broad-spectrum antibiotics. The morbidity of these infections and the difficulty encountered in their diagnosis argue for the early addition of empirical antifungal therapy. We recommend the institution of amphotericin B in the following clinical settings:

   a. Fever without a documented source that persists for more than 72 hours after the institution of appropriate antibiotics

   b. A new fever of unknown source that occurs during treatment with broad-spectrum antibiotics

   c. Documentation or a strong suspicion of fungal infection

F. **Specific antimicrobial therapy** is indicated when a documented source of infection is identified. Guidelines concerning the use of antimicrobials may be found in Chap. 10.

G. Monitoring of **serum antimicrobial levels** is necessary to document the adequacy of therapy.

IV. **Transfusion therapy.** Transfusion is often necessary during periods of prolonged marrow suppression. Whenever possible, profoundly immunocompromised patients should receive **irradiated blood products** to prevent inadvertent lymphoid engrafting and subsequent graft-versus-host reactions.

A. The gradual onset of **anemia** commonly is due either to marrow suppression from chemotherapy or marrow replacement by neoplastic cells. A precipitous decline in the hemoglobin concentration suggests hemorrhage or hemolysis and warrants immediate attention. Transfusion is required when symptoms occur or when the hemoglobin concentration falls below 8 gm/dl. Specific guidelines for red cell transfusion may be found in Chap. 15.

B. **Thrombocytopenia** may be due to inadequate production of platelets, increased consumption of platelets (e.g., disseminated intravascular coagulation), or sequestration (e.g., hypersplenism). Intramuscular injections and drugs that impair platelet function should be avoided. We favor elective transfusion to maintain a platelet count above $20,000/\mu l$ when thrombocytopenia is due to inadequate platelet production. When prolonged thrombocytopenia is anticipated, patients should undergo **histocompatibility typing** prior to treatment, so that matched products can be provided if allosensitization to random donor platelets occurs. An additional discussion of platelet transfusion can be found in Chap. 16 (see p. 288).

C. **Granulocyte transfusions** improve survival of patients with prolonged, severe granulocytopenia (i.e., <500 granulocytes/μl) and gram-negative septicemia (*N. Engl. J. Med.* 296:701, 1977). In this setting, granulocyte transfusions should be instituted as soon as septicemia is documented and continued daily until granulocyte recovery occurs. The routine use of granulocyte transfusions for the treatment of septicemia due to gram-positive organisms or fungi remains investigational. The prophylactic use of granulocyte transfusions is discouraged.

Complications of granulocyte transfusion include leukoagglutinin reactions with manifestations ranging from fever and rigors to a fulminant respiratory distress syndrome. The administration of amphotericin B in patients receiving granulocyte transfusions may be associated with an increased incidence of respiratory distress (*N. Engl. J. Med.* 304:1185, 1981).

V. **Metabolic disturbances.** Metabolic disturbances may be present prior to treatment or may occur during therapy. The rapid proliferation or destruction of neoplastic cells may lead to rapid changes in the concentration of metabolic products. Anticipation and identification of these changes are desirable because the gradual correction of minor metabolic abnormalities is less hazardous than the acute intervention often necessary with more severe disturbances.

A. **Hyperuricemia** is common in patients with leukemia or lymphoma and may be exacerbated by chemotherapy-induced tumor lysis. Uncorrected hyperuricemia can cause uric acid nephropathy and renal failure. Patients with malignancies characterized by chemotherapy responsiveness, large tumor mass, and high cell turnover should receive **allopurinol** as early as possible prior to the initiation of chemotherapy. The usual dosage is 600 mg PO initially, followed by 300 mg PO daily. Renal impairment may require a lower dosage. Vigorous hydration (e.g., 3 liters/M^2/24 hours in patients with normal cardiac and renal function) is employed to establish and maintain a brisk diuresis.

B. **Hyperphosphatemia** may occur as part of a tumor lysis syndrome (*Medicine* [Baltimore] 60:218, 1981). Reciprocal depression of serum calcium may lead to neuromuscular irritability and tetany. Because of the tendency toward renal tubular calcium phosphate precipitation in the presence of alkaline urine, bicarbonate and acetazolamide therapy should not be employed routinely unless chemotherapy must be instituted prior to normalization of the serum uric acid level with allopurinol.

C. **Hyperkalemia** can result from tumor lysis but must be distinguished from the pseudohyperkalemia found in patients with extreme leukocytosis. The latter phenomenon results from leukocyte lysis in the sample tube.

D. Hypercalcemia may be due to the presence of extensive bony metastases or to the production of humoral factors. Long-term control of hypercalcemia usually requires successful therapy of the underlying neoplasm. Treatment of acute hypercalcemia is discussed in Chap. 19.

VI. Disseminated intravascular coagulation. Disseminated intravascular coagulation (DIC) is frequently observed in patients with acute promyelocytic leukemia and its microgranular variant. Measurements of coagulation should be done prior to chemotherapy in all patients with acute leukemia, because intensive blood component support and heparin therapy may be necessary if DIC is present. Measures of coagulation should include the prothrombin time (PT), activated partial thromboplastin time (aPTT), fibrinogen level, fibrin degradation products (FDP), platelet count, and thrombin time. Treatment of DIC with heparin rarely is indicated in malignancies other than acute promyelocytic leukemia.

Common or Emergent Clinical Problems

I. Leukostasis. Leukostasis may be observed in patients with acute leukemia or in the blast crisis of chronic myeloid leukemia and requires urgent treatment (*Blood* 60:279, 1982). Peripheral blood blast counts greater than 50,000/μl are associated with a high incidence of leukostasis and intracerebral hemorrhage. Similar extreme elevations of the more mature cells seen in chronic lymphocytic leukemia or chronic myelogenous leukemia usually do not cause leukostasis.

While awaiting a response to definitive antileukemic chemotherapy, rapid lowering of the blast counts can be achieved with **oral hydroxyurea** (see Chemotherapeutic Drugs, sec. **V.C**). The initial dose is 3 gm PO, followed by 1 gm PO every hour until the blast count has been reduced to less than 50,000/μl. Alternatively, 10 gm PO may be administered initially and the same dose repeated in 24 hours if the blast count remains elevated. **Leukapheresis** provides a more rapid method of blast reduction and is recommended when the facilities are available.

II. Malignant meningitis. Malignant meningitis is a complication of many neoplastic diseases, including leukemia, lymphoma, and solid tumors. When examination of the CSF demonstrates malignant cells, intrathecal methotrexate generally is the preferred treatment (see Chemotherapeutic Drugs, sec. **II.A.5**). Cytosine arabinoside and thiotepa also have been employed in the treatment of patients who have not responded to intrathecal methotrexate therapy. Cranial irradiation is indicated in most settings. Placement of an Ommaya reservoir should be considered if prolonged intrathecal therapy is anticipated.

III. Intracranial tumors. Intracranial tumors may respond poorly to systemic chemotherapy because standard doses of most drugs (except procarbazine, nitrosoureas, and corticosteroids) do not cross the blood-brain barrier. Radiation therapy is the treatment of choice. Dexamethasone, 6–10 mg PO q6h, should be administered to reduce cerebral edema. Dexamethasone should be continued as long as cerebral edema persists.

IV. Spinal cord compression. Spinal cord compression is a medical emergency and requires immediate neurosurgical consultation. **Back pain** is frequently the earliest sign of cord compression and requires careful evaluation. The probability of a successful outcome is increased if treatment is instituted prior to the onset of more extensive neurologic deficits. Although treatment must be individualized, high-dose corticosteroids and radiation therapy may be as effective as laminectomy (*Ann. Neurol.* 3:40, 1978).

V. Malignant pleural effusions. Malignant pleural effusions due to lymphoma, breast cancer, or ovarian cancer may respond to systemic chemotherapy. Refractory effusions usually require closed-tube thoracostomy. Instillation of nitrogen mustard, tetracycline, bleomycin, or other sclerosing agents should be considered only after complete drainage is accomplished. Additional details are provided in Chap. 9.

VI. Superior vena cava obstruction. Superior vena cava obstruction can be due to a variety of malignant and nonmalignant disorders and may develop rapidly or insidiously. Histologic identification of the cause is essential, particularly if a malignancy is suspected. In emergent situations caused by malignancy, radiation therapy usually is required. Treatment with nitrogen mustard or other drugs may be a reasonable alternative for rapidly responsive tumors (e.g., small-cell carcinoma of the lung and malignant lymphoma).

VII. Neoplastic cardiac tamponade. Neoplastic cardiac tamponade must be distinguished from pericarditis due to mediastinal radiation therapy or infection. Treatment usually consists of drainage plus pericardotomy or irradiation. Elective pericardiocentesis should be performed only by experienced physicians who possess the skills necessary to manage its potentially fatal complications.

Thyroid Disease

Evaluation of Thyroid Function

When the history and physical examination provide an incentive for laboratory evaluation of thyroid function, the clinician must choose from a wide variety of tests. Knowledge of the mechanisms of thyroid hormone production, distribution, and metabolism is essential for a proper choice of tests and a correct interpretation of the results.

Hypothalamic thyrotropin-releasing hormone (TRH) stimulates the synthesis and release of pituitary thyroid-stimulating hormone (TSH), which activates thyroidal iodine uptake, synthesis, and release of thyroxine (T_4) and triiodothyronine (T_3). Circulating thyroid hormones exert negative feedback effects at the level of the pituitary, to decrease TSH secretion. They may also have effects on the hypothalamus.

T_4 is produced exclusively in the thyroid gland. However, 80% of T_3 production is through 5'-monodeiodination of T_4 in peripheral tissues; only 20% results from thyroid secretion. In hyperthyroidism there is usually increased thyroid production of both T_4 and T_3. In hyperthyroid patients, the proportion of total T_3 production derived from thyroid secretion is greater than normal, and their peripheral T_3 concentrations are usually more abnormally raised than their T_4 concentrations. Occasionally, hyperthyroid patients will have abnormalities only in peripheral T_3 concentrations (**T_3 toxicosis**).

T_4 is also 5'-deiodinated peripherally to 3,3',5'-triiodothyronine (reverse T_3, rT_3), which is biologically inactive and not measured in T_3 assays. Over 95% of rT_3 is produced peripherally. Of T_4 peripherally deiodinated in the normal adult, approximately 40% is converted to T_3 and 60% to rT_3. During acute or chronic illness, or fasting, the activity of 5'-deiodinase may decrease, resulting in decreased production of T_3 and decreased 5'-deiodination of rT_3. This is reflected in decreased peripheral T_3 concentrations and increased peripheral rT_3 concentrations. Propylthiouracil (PTU) inhibits extrathyroidal conversion of T_4 to T_3 and increases rT_3 concentrations. Glucocorticoid administration may also decrease serum T_4 concentrations and increase rT_3 concentrations. A "**high T_4 syndrome**" has been reported to occur in thyrotoxic persons with a coincident nonthyroidal illness and in nonthyrotoxic hospitalized psychiatric patients, acutely ill patients, and elderly patients. Such patients have elevated levels of circulating T_4 and normal or decreased levels of T_3.

All forms of thyroid hormone are present in plasma as free molecules, but 99.98% of T_4, 99.8% of T_3, and 99.5% of rT_3 circulate bound to the proteins thyroxine-binding globulin (TBG), thyroxine-binding prealbumin (TBPA), and albumin. Thyroxine normally leaves the blood with a half-life of 6–7 days; T_3, with a half-life of 1–2 days.

The **serum T_4 concentration** measured by competitive protein-binding assay or by radioimmunoassay is the most useful and widely available test of thyroid function.

The total T_4 concentration is, as one would expect, greatly influenced by the quantity of binding protein present in plasma; **free T_4** provides a more accurate assessment of thyroid function, especially when alterations in binding are suspected. **Thyroxine-binding globulin and thyroid hormone binding** are increased in pregnancy, with estrogen therapy, in acute hepatic disease, with chronic narcotic use, in acute intermittent porphyria, and on a genetic basis. They are decreased by androgens, nephrotic syndrome, hypoproteinemia, chronic hepatic disease, or on a genetic basis. Neither inorganic iodide nor iodine-containing radiographic contrast materials are measured in T_4 or free T_4 determinations. Heparin has been shown to increase free T_4 temporarily (*J. Clin. Endocrinol. Metab.* 32:633, 1971). **Total T_3** is measured by radioimmunoassay, and **free T_3** can be measured by equilibrium dialysis techniques, although facilities for its measurement are not widely available.

Free T_4 concentrations can be estimated indirectly by measuring and correcting for alterations in plasma T_4 and T_3 binding capacity. This is done by measuring the competition between T_4 and T_3 binding components in plasma and a binding resin for radiolabeled T_3. A high **T_3 resin uptake (RT$_3$U)** reflects low plasma binding capacity for T_4 and T_3, and a low uptake reflects the opposite. In hyperthyroid states, binding sites are more saturated than normal, and the RT$_3$U is high. TBG is increased in hypothyroidism, providing an increased binding capacity for T_3 and T_4, and the RT$_3$U is low. It is possible to consider the T_4 determination and the RT$_3$U together, and, in doing so, estimate the concentration of free thyroid hormone (Free T_4 Index).

In severe prolonged illness, the level of circulating T_4 may fall to subnormal levels despite clinical euthyroidism. This **euthyroid "sick" state** (*Ann. Intern. Med.* 90:905, 1979) apparently results from decreased thyroid hormone binding to plasma proteins. In such patients, the Free T_4 Index is usually low, RT$_3$U high, free T_4 and TSH normal.

Plasma TSH is measurable by radioimmunoassay. An elevated TSH is usually indicative of primary hypothyroidism. Undetectable TSH levels may be found in normal or hyperthyroid subjects. Although extremely rare, TSH-secreting pituitary tumors may result in elevated TSH with hyperthyroidism; TSH may be measured before and at defined intervals after thyrotropin-releasing hormone (TRH) administration **(TRH test)**. The responses of TSH to TRH are blunted in hyperthyroidism. Most patients with primary hypothyroidism will have a quantitatively increased TSH response to TRH administration, while those with secondary hypothyroidism will have a response that is characteristic of euthyroid patients or quantitatively decreased from normal. Patients with tertiary or hypothalamic hypothyroidism respond normally or supranormally to TRH. Euthyroid men over 40 may exhibit a blunted response, as may patients taking aspirin.

The **in vivo uptake of radioiodine (RAIU),** usually measured 24 hours after radioiodine administration, is often elevated in hyperthyroid states. It is subject to variation as a result of alterations in iodine intake. As well as being ingested in food, iodine may be ingested in various drugs, especially cough and cold remedies, or it may be absorbed through the skin from topical preparations. Organic iodine-containing compounds, such as radiographic dyes, bind to serum proteins and slowly release iodine over a prolonged period of time. Low RAIU values occur in patients with acute thyroiditis or as a result of exogenous thyroid hormone or iodide administration.

Many thyroid function tests may be altered by **phenytoin (Dilantin).** Euthyroid patients receiving phenytoin may have decreased T_4, T_3, and free T_4 values, and the RT$_3$U may be normal or increased. The TSH levels are usually normal, as are the TRH test findings. These patients are probably euthyroid and should be treated as such unless they are obviously clinically hypothyroid, have an elevated TSH, or have an increased TSH response to TRH.

Hypothyroidism

Hypothyroidism may be due to ablation (surgical or medical) or inflammation of the thyroid gland (primary hypothyroidism), a failure of the pituitary to secrete an adequate amount of TSH as a result of intrinsic pituitary disease (secondary hypothyroidism), or insufficient hypothalamic stimulation (tertiary hypothyroidism). Hypothyroidism may also result from therapeutic neck irradiation (e.g., mantle irradiation for Hodgkin's disease). The presence of a goiter in the hypothyroid patient suggests chronic thyroiditis in adult patients or defects in thyroid hormone synthesis in children. Patients who are hypothyroid due to destruction of thyroid tissue may not have a goiter. Plasma TSH will distinguish primary from secondary or tertiary disease. If TSH is low, TRH stimulation should be done to distinguish secondary from tertiary hypothyroidism. With evidence of secondary or tertiary hypothyroidism, a formal visual field evaluation should be done and radiographic studies of the sella turcica obtained to search for a pituitary or hypothalamic tumor. It should be recalled that considerable pituitary enlargement may occur in some patients with long-standing hypothyroidism, and that this does not necessarily represent a pathologic pituitary tumor. Primary hypothyroidism may be associated with immunologic adrenocortical destruction (Schmidt's syndrome), and secondary hypothyroidism is frequently associated with decreased adrenal function that may be clinically inapparent. **Treatment of the hypothyroidism without adrenal replacement therapy in such circumstances may precipitate adrenal crisis.**

I. **Preparations of thyroid hormones.** Table 18-1 lists commonly used preparations.

   A. **Natural preparations**

   1. **Thyroid USP (desiccated thyroid, thyroid extract)** is a dried, defatted powder of animal thyroid glands standardized according to iodine content. Since some manufacturers do not standardize their tablets according to bioassay, biologic activity per grain may vary considerably. For this reason, synthetic preparations may be more predictable than natural preparations. The use of desiccated thyroid has been reported to result in elevated T_3 levels accompanied by thyrotoxic symptoms and normal or low T_4 levels, which may mislead the clinician (*Am. J. Med.* 64:284, 1978).

   2. **Thyroglobulin (Proloid)** is a purified animal thyroid extract that conforms to the USP standards for iodine content and is subjected to bioassay.

   B. **Synthetic preparations**

   1. **Sodium levothyroxine (thyroxine, T_4) (L-thyroxine) (Synthroid)** is the sodium salt of the natural isomer of T_4. The potency is dependable. Since

Table 18-1. Preparations of thyroid hormones

Preparation	Tablet sizes	Usual adult daily replacement dose
Thyroid USP (desiccated thyroid)	16, 32, 65, 100, 130, 200, 260, and 325 mg	100–300 mg
Thyroglobulin (Proloid)	16, 32, 65, 100, 130, 200, and 325 mg	100–300 mg
Sodium levothyroxine (T_4) (Synthroid)	25, 50, 100, 200, 300, and 500 μg	100–200 μg
Sodium liothyronine (T_3) (Cytomel)	5, 25, and 50 μg	50–100 μg

most T_3 is produced peripherally, thyroid replacement with T_4 alone is adequate therapy. **Levothyroxine is the preferred drug for thyroid replacement therapy under most circumstances.**

2. **Sodium liothyronine (triiodothyronine, T_3) (Cytomel)** is not bound to plasma proteins as avidly as is T_4, and its circulating half-life is shorter. For this reason it is generally given in divided doses. Because of decreased protein binding and the increased potency of T_3 in suppressing TSH secretion, measurements of circulating T_4 are low in patients taking T_3, and hypothyroidism is best excluded by the finding of a normal or low TSH. T_3 may be useful in hypothyroidism when urgent treatment is required.

3. **Combinations of T_4 and T_3** offer no advantage over preparations of T_4 alone and are more expensive.

II. **Treatment of hypothyroidism.** The objective of treatment is the restoration of the normal metabolic state. Preparations of T_4 are usually given once a day. Among the earliest objective effects of treatment are diuresis and decreased puffiness, followed later by cardiotonic effects, increased appetite, and decreased constipation. Measurement of plasma T_4 and TSH may be used to monitor therapy. A full replacement dose (but not excessive) of thyroid hormone should ultimately be given if well tolerated. This is usually accomplished by 100–200 µg/day of L-thyroxine.

A. **Hypothyroidism in the medically stable patient.** There is no need to restore normal metabolism rapidly in a patient who has probably been hypothyroid for a long time. Precipitation of angina or cardiac dysrhythmias are potential serious complications of treatment, especially in elderly patients or those with underlying heart disease. In such patients, gradual replacement of thyroid hormone should be **initiated with 25–50 µg of L-thyroxine/day or its equivalent;** the dose is increased by 25–50 µg at intervals of 2–3 weeks until full replacement dosage is achieved (100–200 µg/day).

Because its half-life is shorter than that of T_4, T_3 has been used initially to treat hypothyroidism when underlying heart disease is suspected. It is reasoned that undesired side effects will disappear more rapidly than those of T_4 after the drug is stopped. It must be remembered, however, that the onset of the effect of T_3 is more abrupt than that of T_4, and for this reason it may be more likely to precipitate angina.

B. **Situations requiring rapid treatment of hypothyroidism.** Trauma, surgery, and infection are poorly tolerated by the hypothyroid patient and may lead to myxedema coma. When trauma or infections occur, or when nonelective surgery is necessary, hypothyroidism should be corrected as rapidly as is compatible with a reasonable risk. Treatment with liothyronine, 50–100 µg/day in divided doses, should begin immediately. If the oral route is undependable, 100–200 µg/day of levothyroxine can be given IV. Obviously, slower thyroid replacement is preferable in less serious states or with surgery that can be safely delayed. If rapid thyroid replacement is poorly tolerated, the risks of further thyroid therapy must be balanced against the risks of hypothyroidism.

C. **Myxedema coma** is the most severe complication of hypothyroidism. It is usually characterized by signs of myxedema, unresponsiveness, hypotension, bradycardia, hypoventilation, hyponatremia, and occasionally seizures. Hypothermia, which may be unrecognized because the thermometer is not shaken down sufficiently, is usually present. Treatment should be initiated as soon as the clinical diagnosis is made and appropriate blood samples for thyroid hormone measurement have been obtained. Mortality may approach 50%. **Intravenous therapy should be used,** since GI absorption of drugs or absorption from IM sites may be undependable. **Therapy** may be regarded as consisting of three aspects:

1. **Maintenance of vital functions**

   a. **Hypoventilation** may lead to carbon dioxide retention, which contributes to narcosis. Arterial blood gases should be measured and aggressive pulmonary toilet and assisted ventilation implemented if required.

   b. **Hypotension** may respond poorly to pressor agents until thyroid hormone has been replaced. Volume repletion with isotonic fluids should be carried out.

   c. **Hypothermia** should not be treated with external heat, since this may exacerbate circulatory failure by increasing oxygen requirements and decreasing peripheral vascular tone.

   d. **Hyponatremia,** due to impaired free water clearance, will usually be corrected with improvement of the patient's metabolic status. Administration of hypotonic fluids should be avoided.

   e. **Hypoglycemia** may require IV glucose for correction.

   f. **Symptoms of hypoadrenocorticism** may be precipitated by the rapid administration of thyroid hormone, and they can be prevented by the IV administration of 300–400 mg of hydrocortisone sodium succinate over 24 hours, followed by rapid tapering as the patient's condition improves.

   g. **All CNS depressants** should be avoided.

2. **Replacement of thyroid hormone.** A single dose of 200–500 μg (0.2–0.5 mg) of sodium levothyroxine given IV will usually restore the peripheral pool of thyroxine to normal and make thyroxine available for metabolic use. This may be followed by 50–200 μg/day IV until oral preparations can be tolerated. Alternatively, liothyronine, 50–100 μg initially, followed by 50 μg/day or 25 μg BID, may be given by nasogastric tube. The dosage may be modified in patients who are unusually large or small and should definitely be decreased in elderly patients or in those who may have coronary artery disease. Such patients should receive no more than 100 μg of levothyroxine/day.

3. **Treatment of precipitating factors.** Underlying infection should be looked for and treated if present. **Patients who are euthyroid "sick" must be carefully distinguished from patients with myxedema coma, since the former should not receive thyroid replacement therapy.**

Hyperthyroidism

Hyperthyroidism is most commonly due to **Graves' disease** (diffuse toxic goiter). Less common causes include nodular toxic goiters (single or multiple adenomas), acute thyroiditis, or the ingestion of excess thyroid hormone. Far less common causes include iodine-induced thyrotoxicosis (jodbasedow), thyroid carcinoma, TSH-secreting pituitary adenomas, hydatid mole or choriocarcinoma, and ovarian teratomas containing thyroid tissue (**struma ovarii**). The presence of ophthalmopathy or pretibial myxedema is restricted to patients with Graves' disease.

The treatment of hyperthyroidism will depend, at least in part, on the cause, which must be determined in each case. The following discussion will generally be directed toward the hyperthyroidism of Graves' disease; exceptions for the other causes of hyperthyroidism will be noted.

I. **General therapeutic considerations.** Specific therapy is influenced by the cause and severity of the hyperthyroidism, the age of the patient, the presence of complicating features, and the preferences of patient and physician.

A. Cause of the hyperthyroid state

1. **Graves' disease** is characterized by spontaneous remissions and exacerbations. There is no evidence that any form of therapy hastens the appearance of remission or alters the natural course of the disease. Drug therapy is designed to control the secretion of thyroid hormone or to counteract its peripheral effects until remission occurs spontaneously. Radioiodine and surgery, by destruction or excision of thyroid tissue, reduce the capacity of the thyroid gland to secrete hormone. Graves' disease may be managed by any of the three modalities.

2. **Single and multiple toxic adenomas** produce hyperthyroidism that is usually not characterized by remissions. Therefore, surgery or radioiodine is the preferred treatment.

3. A functioning **thyroid carcinoma** should be removed surgically. If this is not possible, radioiodine therapy is recommended.

4. **Iodine-induced thyrotoxicosis** may occur after administration of potassium iodide (SSKI) or organic iodides (e.g., intravenous pyelogram dye) to patients with multinodular goiter, quiescent Graves' disease, or toxic adenoma. Iodine-induced thyrotoxicosis is usually mild and remits spontaneously, requiring only symptomatic treatment; however, severe thyrotoxicosis requiring antithyroid drug therapy has been reported.

5. Hyperthyroidism in **choriocarcinoma** or **hydatid mole** is due to secretion of thyrotropic materials by the tumor or mole. The resulting thyrotoxicosis is usually mild and can be controlled prior to surgery by antithyroid drugs or propranolol.

B. Age of patient.
After two decades of follow-up, radioiodine therapy for thyrotoxicosis has not been shown to be associated with an increased incidence of leukemia or thyroid cancer. Radioiodine should probably not be used, however, in women of childbearing age, unless medical or social reasons require its use, because of the potential for genetic abnormalities in their offspring. Radioiodine is the preferred therapy in older patients, especially in those who are poor surgical risks.

C. Severity of the hyperthyroidism.
Mild hyperthyroidism may be treated with radioiodine without any adjunctive therapy. More severe hyperthyroidism should be brought under control with drugs before treatment with radioiodine or surgery, if either is planned.

D. Complicating features

1. **Pregnancy.** Untreated thyrotoxicosis in pregnancy is associated with an increased incidence of prematurity. The use of radioiodine is contraindicated in pregnancy; therefore, surgery or antithyroid drug treatment should be used. Surgery may be done during the second trimester, but should be avoided during the first or third trimester because of the risk of inducing abortion or premature labor. Since the antithyroid drugs propylthiouracil (PTU) and methimazole (Tapazole) readily cross the placenta, the aim of therapy with these drugs during pregnancy should be to administer the smallest dose compatible with the near-normal metabolic state. This will place the fetus at minimal risk from both maternal hyperthyroidism and antithyroid drug–induced goiter or cretinism. The maternal T_4 should be maintained in the slightly supranormal range; and, since measurement of total T_4 during pregnancy may be complicated by increases in maternal thyroid hormone–binding capacity, the **free T_4** measurement is probably the most satisfactory laboratory index to follow. Control of therapy is complicated, since hyperthyroidism tends to become less severe in late pregnancy. Since thyroid hormones cross the placenta poorly, the use of antithy-

roid drugs combined with thyroid hormone to prevent fetal hypothyroidism is not warranted.

Pregnant hyperthyroid women can be treated with PTU without interfering with subsequent development in their offspring. Propranolol (Inderal) and iodides should not be used for long-term treatment of hyperthyroidism during pregnancy, but they may be used on a short-term basis (1–7 days) if rapid control of hyperthyroidism is necessary.

    2. Compression symptoms or **disfigurement** from a large goiter are indications for **surgery.**

  E. Personality and preference of the patient. Patients who cannot be relied on to take medication regularly may be treated with radioiodine or surgery, but the substantial incidence of hypothyroidism following these forms of therapy and the possible future need for thyroid hormone replacement should be considered.

II. General therapeutic measures

  A. Hospitalization is necessary only in severe cases such as impending thyroid storm or when hyperthyroidism is complicated by congestive heart failure, thyrotoxic periodic paralysis, or other threatening conditions.

  B. Sedation. Nervousness, hyperactivity, and irritability may be controlled by tranquilizers such as phenobarbital (30–60 mg tid–qid), chlordiazepoxide 10–20 mg qid), or diazepam (5 mg qid). These symptoms also respond well to propranolol, 10–40 mg qid.

  C. Nutrition. Vitamin supplements are desirable because of increased requirements. Weight gain may result from continued high caloric intake after the hyperthyroidism is brought under control; this should be avoided.

  D. Dysrhythmias and congestive heart failure. Hyperthyroidism may cause atrial fibrillation, sinus tachycardia, or congestive heart failure (CHF). Standard digitalis or diuretic therapy for CHF or dysrhythmias is usually adequate, but an expected response may not be obtained until the hyperthyroidism is corrected. Sinus tachycardia and other supraventricular dysrhythmias generally respond to propranolol.

III. Specific therapeutic measures. As noted, three types of therapy are used to treat hyperthyroidism: antithyroid drugs, radioiodine, and surgery.

  A. Drug therapy

    1. Drugs that inhibit hormone formation or release

      a. Thiourea derivatives act by interfering with the organification of iodide to form iodotyrosines and with the coupling of iodotyrosines to form T_4 and T_3. Propylthiouracil also potently inhibits peripheral deiodination of T_4 to T_3 and thus may be of clinical benefit more quickly than methimazole. Thioureas are well absorbed and, because they are secreted in milk, should not be given to nursing mothers.

        (1) Preparations and dosage. Either one of the thiourea derivatives may be used to treat hyperthyroidism. The usual starting dose for **PTU,** which is available only in 50-mg tablets, is 150 mg q6–8h. **Methimazole** is available in 5- and 10-mg tablets and, because of its longer half-life, can be given bid–tid. The usual starting dose is 30–60 mg/day. The dosages of both thioureas should be adjusted according to the severity of the disease, the urgency of control, and the responsiveness of the patient. Because these drugs act by preventing the formation of thyroid hormone, no effect will be observed until the gland becomes depleted of stored hormone, which may take 2–3 weeks. A normal metabolic state can usually be achieved by 6 weeks, at which time it may be possible to decrease the dose by about one-third. Daily doses of PTU up to 1500 mg or 150 mg of methimazole may be required.

(2) Assessment and duration of treatment. The clinical course and the serum T_4 are the best guides to the adequacy of therapy. The thyroid gland often becomes smaller if remission of the underlying disease occurs. Enlargement may be due to intensification of the hyperthyroidism (low TSH) or to iatrogenic hypothyroidism (high TSH). It is important to distinguish between the two.

A major difficulty in the drug management of Graves' disease is determining the appropriate time to withdraw drug therapy. The practice at our institution has been to continue treatment for 1–2 years or until euthyroidism can be maintained in the absence of therapy. It has been suggested that antithyroid drugs be discontinued 3–6 months after euthyroidism has been achieved, or that they be discontinued as soon as euthyroidism has resulted (*N. Engl. J. Med.* 297:173, 1977). It must be remembered that premature withdrawal of the drug may be followed by an exacerbation of the hyperthyroidism that is difficult to control. Gradual drug withdrawal over several weeks or more has been suggested as a solution for this potential problem.

(3) Toxicity is approximately equal with PTU and methimazole. Toxic reactions may be dose related. Reactions such as skin rashes, fever, arthralgias, diarrhea, hepatitis, and salivary gland enlargement occur in 3–5% of patients. **Agranulocytosis,** the most severe complication of thiourea therapy, which is seen in 0.2–0.5% of patients, can occur at any time but is usually reversible. If not detected early, it can lead to lethal infection. Its onset is usually sudden, so that periodic WBC counts are of little value in guarding against it. Granulocytopenia, which may be seen in hyperthyroidism or during drug treatment, should not be confused with agranulocytosis. The patient should be advised to report evidence of infection (e.g., fever, sore throat, furunculosis), and the drug should be discontinued until the WBC count has been obtained.

Mild skin rashes generally respond to antihistamines without discontinuation of the drug, or to changing from one thiourea to the other. All structurally related drugs should be avoided, however, in patients who have experienced a major toxic reaction to one of the thioureas.

b. Iodide inhibits thyroid hormone synthesis (Wolff-Chaikoff effect) when its intrathyroidal concentration increases, but the hyperfunctioning thyroid may escape from this effect after 3 or more weeks. The major therapeutic effect of iodide is its prompt inhibition of thyroid hormone release from the hyperfunctioning gland. Iodide alone does not adequately control hyperthyroidism for long periods, and its use should be **confined to the treatment of thyroid storm** or to the preparation of the thyroid gland for surgery. Given tid, 1–2 drops of SSKI provide more than enough iodide; higher doses may increase the potential for toxic side effects (acneform rash, salivary gland swelling, gynecomastia).

c. Lithium blocks the release of hormone from the thyroid gland and can be used to treat hyperthyroidism; however, the incidence of toxic side effects, such as tremor, nausea, hyponatremia, and dysrhythmias, makes it less desirable than the thioureas for this purpose. Euthyroid patients receiving lithium for mania may exhibit normal or decreased T_4, and many will have an increased TSH response to TRH. If such patients are chemically hypothyroid, they should receive thyroid replacement as their clinical state warrants.

2. **Drugs that control the peripheral manifestations of hyperthyroidism.** **Propranolol** is a beta-adrenergic blocking agent that improves or abolishes tachycardia, tremor, nervousness, and excess sweating in hyperthyroid patients. It does not influence thyroid hormone secretion but does decrease the peripheral conversion of T_4 to T_3. Propranolol can be used to control the symptoms of hyperthyroidism until a thiourea or radioiodine can take effect. In addition, it has been used to prepare patients for surgery (*N. Engl. J. Med.* 298:643, 1978). Although propranolol is usually contraindicated in low output CHF, its use may result in improvement of the high output CHF and tachycardia of thyrotoxicosis. Treatment is begun with 10 mg qid, and the dosage is increased until control of symptoms is achieved (usually 40–60 mg qid; however, doses of up to 120 mg qid have been used).

B. **Radioactive iodine**

1. **Dosage.** Radioiodine (^{131}I) limits secretion of thyroid hormone by destroying thyroid tissue. The major long-term side effect of radioiodine therapy is hypothyroidism, which occurs in 5–25% of patients within the first year and in approximately 3% each year thereafter. Dosages of radioiodine for the treatment of Graves' disease vary from 40–200 μCi/gm of estimated thyroid weight. Many centers currently use a dose of 80–160 μCi/gm. Higher doses of radioiodine result in a greater likelihood of cure but earlier and more frequent onset of hypothyroidism. Lower doses result in less hypothyroidism but a greater incidence of treatment failure that necessitates re-treatment with radioiodine or drug therapy, or both. The incidence of hypothyroidism occurring 2 years or more after radioiodine treatment may not be dose dependent.

   Multinodular toxic goiters and toxic nodules usually require larger total doses of radioiodine, often as much as 20–50 mCi.

2. **Considerations in the use of radioiodine**

   a. **Radiation thyroiditis.** Transient exacerbation of hyperthyroidism occurs 1–2 weeks after administration of radioiodine due to leakage of thyroid hormone into the circulation from damaged follicles. This is rarely a significant clinical problem but may present a danger to patients with cardiac or other serious medical disease. The larger the mass of hyperfunctioning tissue, the larger the amount of stored hormone that can potentially be released. To **prevent** hyperthyroidism from radiation thyroiditis, hormone stores can be depleted prior to radioiodine therapy by pretreatment with PTU or methimazole until euthyroidism is achieved. The antithyroid drugs are then withdrawn 3 days prior to ^{131}I therapy and may be reinstituted 2–3 days following therapy. Once radiation thyroiditis has occurred, antithyroid drugs are of no benefit, and propranolol should be given to counteract the peripheral manifestations of thyroid hormone excess.

   b. **Latency of response.** Because the effects of radioiodine are slow to appear, frequently requiring 2–3 months and occasionally as long as 6 months to become maximal, severe hyperthyroidism and CHF should be treated with thioureas and propranolol until a euthyroid state is achieved. If no response is seen after 6 months, the patient should be reevaluated and the radioiodine treatment repeated.

   c. **Iodide administration** prior to radioiodine should **not** be used, since it will raise the plasma inorganic iodide concentration and thus lower the fraction of the dose of ^{131}I taken up by the thyroid.

   d. **Intrathyroidal hemorrhage** has been reported to occur in patients taking anticoagulants. The prothrombin level should therefore be greater than 20% before treatment.

e. To avoid ^{131}I administration during **pregnancy,** some have recommended that the drug be administered to women only during the menses.

3. Complications of therapy. Lifelong follow-up evaluation of patients treated with ^{131}I is important. **Hypothyroidism** must be recognized and treated. Visits should be frequent during the first year following treatment.

After radioiodine therapy, clinically euthyroid patients may demonstrate elevated TSH values with normal or slightly low T_4 values. It is not clear whether or not these patients require thyroid supplementation. Prophylactic administration of thyroid hormone following either radioiodine or surgical therapy for thyrotoxicosis is not advisable, since it may cause morbidity by its additive effects in the event of persistent or recurrent hyperthyroidism. Rarely, hypoparathyroidism has been reported after the administration of large doses of radioiodine.

C. Surgical treatment. Subtotal thyroidectomy is an effective means of treating hyperthyroidism; the incidence of relapse is generally less than 10%. If the hyperthyroidism recurs, another method of treatment is used, because further surgery is technically difficult and is associated with an increased incidence of complications.

1. Preparation for surgery. Most surgeons prefer to operate on euthyroid patients. A **thiourea** drug should be administered in the usual dosage to control the hyperthyroidism and continued until the time of surgery. **Iodide** (SSKI, 1–2 drops tid) can be given concurrently for 1–2 weeks prior to surgery to increase the firmness of the thyroid gland and decrease its vascularity.

2. Complications of thyroidectomy include the risks of anesthesia as well as hemorrhage into the operative site, with tracheal obstruction and postoperative thyroid storm, which is very rare with proper preoperative preparation of the patient. Damage to the recurrent laryngeal nerve occurs in 1–4% of patients. This is usually unilateral and results in only minimal voice changes; but, if it is bilateral, airway obstruction may develop postoperatively. The incidence of **hypothyroidism** is 10–30% in the first year postoperatively and an additional 1–2%/year thereafter; therefore, careful lifetime follow-up is essential. The temporary occurrence of postoperative hypothyroidism is common for the first few months, and therapy should be withheld if possible for the first 6 months. **Hypoparathyroidism** occurs in up to 4% of patients. Although usually transient and mild, it may be permanent. Tetany may occur in the first postoperative week. The serum calcium should be rechecked in all patients 3–6 months after surgery.

IV. Management of thyroid storm

A. General comments. Thyroid storm is a medical emergency in which organ system decompensation occurs due to a severely hyperthyroid state. It may develop spontaneously, but more often it is precipitated by infection or other stress (e.g., surgery after inadequate preparation of the patient for the operative procedure). Hyperpyrexia, diarrhea, dehydration, tachycardia and dysrhythmias, and CNS abnormalities are usually present. The syndrome may progress rapidly to coma, shock, and death. Prompt treatment is essential and cannot be delayed for laboratory confirmation of hyperthyroidism.

B. Treatment is directed toward four objectives.

1. Control of the synthesis and release of thyroid hormone

a. Sodium iodide inhibits hormone release and should be given by slow IV infusion (1–2 gm/24 hours), starting 1–3 hours **after** thiourea administration. When the patient can take fluids by mouth, SSKI, 5–10 drops q8h, may be substituted. Following recovery from thyroid storm, iodide should be discontinued over a period of 2–3 weeks.

    b. Methimazole, 30–40 mg, or **PTU,** 300–400 mg, should be given PO or by nasogastric tube to prevent synthesis and accumulation of hormone stores. Because of its peripheral effect on decreasing T_4 conversion to T_3, **PTU** is the drug of choice. The initial dose of thiourea should be repeated q8h and decreased as necessary following recovery.

  2. Reversal of peripheral effects of hyperthyroidism. Propranolol should be given IV (1 mg/minute, with careful monitoring of the patient's ECG and vital signs, up to 10 mg), or PO, or by nasogastric tube (40–80 mg q6h).

  3. Restoration and maintenance of vital functions

    a. Hydrocortisone sodium succinate (100 mg IV q6h) or its equivalent is used to treat the relative adrenal insufficiency that may occur in severe thyrotoxicosis. It may also act by decreasing peripheral conversion of T_4 to T_3. Corticosteroid therapy should be tapered as the hyperthyroidism is controlled.

    b. Fluids, electrolytes, and vasopressor agents should be used as necessary to treat dehydration, electrolyte imbalance, and hypotension.

    c. Acetaminophen and a cooling blanket may be used to lower the temperature, which may exceed 42°C (105°F).

    d. Nutritional requirements should be met with IV glucose if necessary. Vitamins should be given.

    e. Oxygen therapy may be required.

    f. Congestive heart failure should be treated with digitalis and diuretics as needed.

  4. Precipitating factors, such as infections, should be identified and treated.

Ophthalmopathy of Graves' Disease

The ophthalmopathy of Graves' disease may precede, accompany, or follow hyperthyroidism or may be seen in the absence of recognizable thyroid disease. Ophthalmopathy (true exophthalmos) must be distinguished from the stare and lid retraction that accompany hyperthyroidism. In ophthalmic Graves' disease, there is an increase in retrobulbar tissue within the orbit and infiltration of extraocular muscles. Involvement may be primarily unilateral. Patients may present with pain, lacrimation, photophobia, blurring of vision, or diplopia. As the amount of retrobulbar tissue increases, the globe is pushed forward. The tissue may compress the optic nerve and vascular supply of the retina, with resultant loss of vision. Global adhesions or shortening of the inferior rectus muscle, which is the first eye muscle to be affected, initially leads to loss of superior temporal gaze. Eventually, upward and lateral gaze are impaired, but downward eye movement is usually preserved. Chemosis and periorbital edema may result from obstruction of the drainage from the orbit. Formal measurement of visual fields and evaluation of extraocular muscle function should be included in the evaluation of exophthalmos. The extent of the proptosis can be measured by an exophthalmometer; the distance from the lateral orbital rim to the anterior corneal surface is measured. Normal measurements rarely exceed 20 mm, and the difference between the two eyes is normally not greater than 1 mm.

I. Course. Graves' ophthalmopathy usually progresses from mild or moderate proptosis to stabilization, with subsequent slow regression. Only a few patients with ophthalmopathy progress to the point where vision is threatened. A **classification** of the eye changes in Graves' disease proposed by The American Thyroid Association includes the following six categories: (1) mild proptosis without other changes;

(2) early involvement of soft tissue; (3) proptosis; (4) extraocular muscle involvement; (5) corneal involvement; (6) optic nerve involvement.

II. Treatment. The treatment of Graves' ophthalmopathy must be flexible. **One must correct hyperthyroidism to control noninfiltrative ophthalmopathy optimally.** The progression of the eye disease should determine whether vigorous therapy is needed immediately or can be withheld while awaiting spontaneous improvement.

A. Mild exophthalmos. The eyes should be protected from irritation; sunglasses and 0.5–1.0% methyl cellulose eyedrops may be helpful. Elevation of the head of the bed while the patient sleeps at night may improve drainage of fluid from the orbit. Diuretics are sometimes beneficial. Guanethidine eyedrops in a 5% solution (1 gt qid) may be useful for relieving symptoms secondary to lid retraction and exposure.

B. Rapidly progressive or severe exophthalmos associated with the appearance of chemosis, conjunctivitis, or visual impairment is a poor prognostic sign and requires more vigorous therapy.

1. Tarsorrhaphy may be used to extend the lid when proptosis is so marked that the eye remains exposed during sleep.

2. Corticosteroids in high doses (120–200 mg prednisone/day) are occasionally of benefit in patients with rapidly progressive disease. If improvement occurs, the dose should be reduced gradually to the lowest effective maintenance level. If no improvement occurs within 4 weeks, corticosteroids should be withdrawn.

3. Orbital decompression is the most reliable method of relieving severe exophthalmos. **Indications** for decompression include corneal exposure and ulceration, progressive loss of visual acuity or visual fields, severe chemosis or orbital edema, and cosmetic restoration of stabile exophthalmos.

4. Muscle surgery to correct imbalances of extraocular muscles and to lyse adhesions should be performed after the exophthalmos has stabilized. **As is the case with all of the surgical procedures just described, this operation should be performed by experienced specialists.**

Thyroiditis

I. Acute Thyroiditis. Acute thyroiditis is a self-limited inflammation of the thyroid gland of unknown etiology. There may be pain (occasionally referred to the ear), swelling, and tenderness in the thyroid, accompanied by fever and malaise. In mild cases there may be no overt signs of inflammation. The disease often follows a typical sequence, consisting of an initial period of hypermetabolism associated with decreased RAIU, elevated T_4, suppressed TSH, and diminished TSH response to TRH. The erythrocyte sedimentation rate (ESR) is usually increased. Elevations of thyroglobulin reflect the disruption of thyroid follicles, and T_4 elevations result from leakage of stored hormone. A period of euthyroidism follows, which may in turn be followed by a period of transient chemical or clinical hypothyroidism. A return to a state of normal thyroid function is usually observed from 1–2 weeks to several months following the initial presentation. Most cases of acute thyroiditis can be managed with propranolol for symptoms of hypermetabolism and aspirin for pain; corticosteroids (40 mg prednisone daily) are required when the illness is severe. They should be gradually withdrawn over a period of 6–8 weeks but not before the RAIU has returned to normal, so as to prevent relapse.

Painless thyroiditis should be considered when a nontender goiter or normal-sized thyroid gland is associated with thyrotoxicosis, low RAIU, normal or slightly elevated ESR, absent or low antithyroid antibodies, and recovery within weeks. Propranolol is the only treatment required.

II. **Hashimoto's thyroiditis.** Hashimoto's thyroiditis is a common thyroid disorder characterized by a painless goiter that frequently progresses to hypothyroidism. Histopathologically, there is a combination of diffuse lymphocytic infiltration, obliteration of thyroid follicles, and fibrosis. Hashimoto's thyroiditis may coexist with pernicious anemia or other diseases with a presumed autoimmune basis. The disease presents with hyperthyroidism in a small percentage of cases and may be treated with any of the modalities used to treat Graves' disease. It is most common in women in the middle decades of life. Antibodies directed against various thyroid antigens are characteristically present in very high titer; TSH is often elevated, and full replacement doses of thyroid hormone are used to suppress goiter formation. Patients with Hashimoto's thyroiditis may become myxedematous if given iodides or lithium.

III. **Suppurative thyroiditis.** Suppurative thyroiditis is an uncommon disorder and is due to infection of the thyroid gland with pyogenic organisms. *Staphylococcus aureus, Streptococcus hemolyticus,* and pneumococci are the most common infecting organisms, but precise identification of the pathogen (needle aspiration) is necessary for optimal antibiotic treatment. The disease is characterized by severe pain, tenderness, and thyroid swelling. Dysphagia, fever, and malaise are often present. The disease may respond to antibiotic administration alone, but surgical excision of an abscess or surgical drainage is often required for definitive treatment. Thyroid function is usually normal.

Thyroid Nodules

I. **General principles.** Enlargement of the thyroid gland in euthyroid patients should suggest the possibility of cancer. Few goiters, however, harbor cancer, and few patients with thyroid cancer die as a result of the disease. It is possible to integrate observations from a wide variety of sources and list a set of general principles regarding thyroid nodules and cancer.

A. The incidence of cancer is higher in solitary nodules than in multinodular goiters.

B. A solitary nodule that is "cold" on scan is more likely to harbor a cancer than one that takes up radioiodine ("hot"). Since a nodule that accumulates isotope during a sodium pertechnetate scan may present as a cold nodule during iodine scan (*J.A.M.A.* 228:866, 1974), the latter is preferred for cancer screening if facilities are available. The incidence of malignancy in cold nodules is 10–25%.

C. A nodule in a younger patient is more likely to contain cancer than one in an older patient.

D. A nodule is more likely to be malignant in males than in females.

E. A history of irradiation of the neck, face, or mediastinum during childhood markedly increases the risk of malignancy in a nodule.

F. Malignant nodules are likely to be firm or hard. A thyroid nodule firmly fixed to the trachea or surrounding tissues is highly suggestive of cancer. Regional cervical lymphadenopathy may be the result of metastases from a thyroid cancer.

II. **Evaluation of the nodule.** In addition to the considerations listed in sec. I, a sonogram may help differentiate cystic from solid masses. Cystic nodules, however, may harbor cancer. Needle biopsy of the thyroid may be performed, but this technique is subject to sampling error and requires specialized expertise in surgery and pathology for proper performance and interpretation. **Surgical excision** is therefore both a diagnostic and therapeutic modality, and the decision to operate is usually based on clinical judgment and experience.

III. Management. In the absence of obvious signs of malignancy (unusual hardness, rapid growth, lymph node involvement, or metastases), the following can be used as a guide to therapy:

A. Multinodular goiter should be treated with suppressive doses of T_4 (200 µg/day) or T_3 (75–100 µg/day) for as long as they are well tolerated by the patient. Progression of a goiter after 3–6 months of therapy is an indication for surgery.

B. Solitary nodule. A judgment must be made based on the considerations that have been presented, the ability of the patient to withstand surgery, and the wishes of the informed patient. Most physicians would agree, however, that surgical excision should be performed on all single cold nodules in men under 60 and women under 40 years of age.

IV. Surgery. Surgery should consist of excisional biopsy and, if cancer is present on the frozen section, total or near-total thyroidectomy, along with excision of adjacent lymph nodes. A radical neck dissection is not usually necessary. Postoperative treatment with suppressive doses of T_4 and T_3 and/or ablative doses of radioiodine may be indicated, depending on the operative findings and characteristics of the cancer.

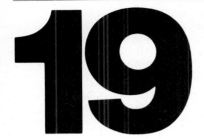

Mineral, Parathyroid, and Metabolic Bone Disorders

Serum Mineral Disorders

I. Calcium. The serum calcium concentration is maintained primarily by the combined actions of parathyroid hormone (PTH) and vitamin D. **Parathyroid hormone** is released in response to a decrease in serum ionized calcium and elevates the serum calcium concentration by increasing net bone resorption, promoting renal tubular calcium reabsorption, and stimulating intestinal calcium absorption largely through regulation of vitamin D metabolism. In addition, PTH decreases serum phosphate by reducing renal tubular resorption of phosphate (TRP). Thus, in states of PTH excess, the percentage of TRP* will be inappropriately low (<80%) for the level of serum phosphate. At normal serum phosphate levels (3.5–5.0 mg/dl), the TRP on a fasting urine sample normally ranges between 80–90%. However, when the serum phosphate is 2.5 mg/dl or less, the TRP should be over 90%.

Vitamin D stores are derived from ingestion of vitamin D_2 and D_3 and from cutaneous production of vitamin D_3, a process that is stimulated by solar ultraviolet irradiation. Vitamins D_2 and D_3 are equipotent in humans. Since vitamin D is fat soluble, normal intestinal absorption of vitamin D depends on normal fat absorption. Vitamin D is initially converted in the liver to 25-hydroxycholecalciferol (25-OHD), which is then converted to 1α, 25-dihydrocholecalciferol (1,25 [OH]$_2$D) in the kidney. Renal conversion to 1,25(OH)$_2$D is stimulated by PTH and by reduced PO_4 levels. Vitamin D metabolite deficiency can be the result of inadequate intake and decreased production, reduced intestinal absorption, decreased hepatic or renal functional mass with reduced conversion of vitamin D to its active metabolites, or increased rates of hepatic catabolism and excretion. In vitamin D–deficiency states, intestinal calcium absorption is decreased, leading to reduced serum calcium levels and secondary hyperparathyroidism.

Approximately 45% of serum calcium is bound to protein, primarily albumin, and is in equilibrium with the ultrafilterable calcium that constitutes the remaining 55% (5% complexed and 50% ionized). Decreases in serum protein concentrations cause proportional changes in the total serum calcium—approximately 0.8 mg calcium/dl for each decrease of 1 gm/dl in serum albumin. Acidosis increases the ionized fraction of calcium, while alkalosis decreases it. Thus, in severe alkalosis, signs of tetany may be present (e.g., hyperventilation syndrome), since the ionized fraction of calcium primarily determines its membrane effects. **Remember:** Hyperkalemia and hypomagnesemia potentiate the cardiac and neuromuscular irritability produced by hypocalcemia, and vice versa.

A. Hypocalcemia. The most common cause of reduced **total** serum calcium concentration is hypoalbuminemia. However, the ionized calcium is normal in this condition, and no treatment is indicated. Common causes of **true** hypocalcemia (reduced total and ionized calcium) include vitamin D deficiency, acute pancreatitis, magnesium deficiency, hyperphosphatemia, hypoparathyroidism,

---

*TRP = 1 − (U/P phosphorus/U/P creatinine) × 100, where U/P = urine-to-plasma ratio.

pseudohypoparathyroidism, and renal tubular acidosis. The fasting plasma phosphate is normal or low in most cases of vitamin D deficiency and calcium malabsorption and is increased in most hypocalcemic patients with hypoparathyroidism or renal insufficiency who have adequate phosphate intake. The common **early symptoms** of hypocalcemia are circumoral paresthesias and tetany, the latter manifested by carpopedal spasm and positive Chvostek's and Trousseau's signs. The patient may also manifest mental instability, confusion, and seizures. The ECG may demonstrate a prolonged Q–T interval.

1. **Acute management.** Acute symptomatic hypocalcemia is a medical emergency requiring the prompt administration of 10–20 ml 10% calcium gluconate (100–200 mg calcium) IV over 10–15 minutes. Subsequent calcium needs may be titrated with an IV drip of calcium gluconate (600–800 mg calcium/1000 ml 5% D/W) until these requirements can be met with oral calcium supplements. Serum magnesium levels should be checked, especially in patients with chronic alcoholism or malabsorption. If severe hypomagnesemia is present (serum magnesium concentration 0.8 mEq/liter or less), magnesium replacement may rapidly restore serum calcium levels (see sec. **III.A**).

   Postoperative hypoparathyroidism may develop after surgery on the parathyroid glands or surrounding area; often, it is transient and mild. Symptomatic hypocalcemia generally appears 24–48 hours after surgery. If the patient has tetanic symptoms or if the serum calcium is below 7.0 mg/dl, a calcium gluconate infusion should be used to maintain serum calcium in the range of 8.0–8.5 mg/dl during the immediate postoperative period. The adequacy of therapy can be estimated at the bedside by monitoring Chvostek's or Trousseau's sign (carpal spasms occur after occlusion of the arterial pulse for up to 5 minutes with a blood pressure cuff). However, frequent monitoring of serum calcium levels is essential for optimal management.

   When regular oral intake is started, the patient should be maintained on a low-phosphorus diet (reduced milk product and meat intake) and the serum calcium maintained with calcium supplementation. Generally, 1.5–3.0 gm of elemental calcium will be required. A suitable, convenient preparation of oral calcium is **calcium carbonate** (e.g., Titralac, 400 mg Ca^{2+}/5 ml or 170 mg Ca^{2+}/tablet; Dicarbosil, 500 mg Ca^{2+}/tablet, and Os-Cal, 250 and 500 mg Ca^{2+}/tablet). If hypocalcemia and hyperphosphatemia persist 10–14 days after parathyroid surgery, the addition of a vitamin D preparation may be necessary (see **2**).

2. **Chronic hypocalcemia.** Effective management requires proper diagnosis of the underlying disorder. Treatment is directed toward increasing intestinal absorption; this can be achieved to some extent by increasing calcium intake.

   a. **Calcium** supplementation is necessary to achieve a total daily calcium intake of 1500–3000 mg (see **1**).

   b. **Vitamin D** must be used in chronic hypocalcemia to enhance intestinal calcium absorption when calcium supplementation alone is inadequate. The serum calcium and 24-hour urinary calcium excretion should be monitored at frequent intervals. The **therapeutic goal** is to restore serum calcium to near-normal levels (>8.0 mg/dl) while minimizing hypercalciuria (<4 mg/kg/day). In patients with hypocalcemia secondary to hypoparathyroidism severe hypercalciuria often develops with attempts to normalize serum calcium. In this situation, the degree of hypercalciuria may limit the level of serum calcium that is acceptable. No vitamin D preparation should be given unless serum phosphate levels have been restored to normal by dietary phosphorus restriction and the use of phosphate-binding antacids (e.g., Basaljel, Amphojel, Dialume). Vitamin D requirements are variable and depend on the age of the patient, the severity of the disease, and the calcium intake. The usual starting dosage in patients with hypoparathyroidism is 50,000 units/day of vitamin D_2 or D_3, which may be gradually increased to 200,000 units or more in resistant patients.

Patients with hypoparathyroidism are occasionally resistant to vitamin D_3 therapy. They may, however, respond to more potent analogues of vitamin D (e.g., **dihydrotachysterol; 1α, 25-dihydroxycholecalciferol [calcitriol]**; or **25-hydroxycholecalciferol [calcifediol]**). Compared with vitamin D_3 therapy, these analogues (1) are more potent, (2) have quicker onset of action, and (3) have a greater tendency to induce hypercalciuria but a shorter duration of toxicity (should it occur). **Caution:** Since these agents are extremely potent (especially 1α, 25-dihydroxycholecalciferol), therapy should be initiated with low doses (0.2–0.4 mg/day of dihydrotachysterol, 0.25 μg/day of 1α, 25-dihydroxycholecalciferol, or 50 μg/day of 25-hydroxycholecalciferol), and subsequent dosage increments should be given at intervals of 2–3 weeks, depending on laboratory findings. Some patients with hypoparathyroidism may require 1α, 25-dihydroxycholecalciferol doses in excess of 1–2 μg/day. The dosage of the vitamin D preparations and oral calcium supplements should be reduced as the desired level of serum calcium is approached and should be discontinued (at least temporarily) if toxicity develops.

B. **Hypercalcemia** is caused by hyperparathyroidism, neoplastic disorders, thiazide diuretics, acute immobilization, vitamin D intoxication, sarcoidosis and other pulmonary granulomatous diseases, the milk-alkali syndrome, hyperthyroidism, and acute adrenal insufficiency. Symptoms of hypercalcemia include anorexia, nausea, vomiting, abdominal pain, constipation, polyuria, dehydration, psychosis, obtundation, and finally coma. The most important therapeutic measure is the promotion of renal calcium excretion. Restriction of calcium intake should be instituted simultaneously.

1. **Saline.** Adequate hydration is critical. Urinary calcium excretion is enhanced by saline infusion, since sodium competitively inhibits tubular resorption of calcium. Assuming that cardiac function is normal, alternating normal and half-normal saline should be rapidly infused (250–500 ml/hour) until the central venous pressure is 10 cm H_2O; this results in a calcium diuresis and reduction in serum calcium in virtually all patients. Furosemide should be given IV in frequent small doses (20–40 mg q2h) to prevent volume overloading and increase calcium excretion. Urinary sodium, potassium, and water losses must be replaced to allow for continued calciuria and natriuresis. Overzealous use of furosemide without adequate water and electrolyte replacement will lead to volume depletion, and the serum calcium will invariably rise.

2. **Glucocorticoids** may be useful adjunctive therapy for hypercalcemia associated with lymphomas, multiple myeloma, non-PTH-secreting tumors metastatic to bone, and vitamin D intoxication. Large initial dosages of hydrocortisone (250–500 mg q8h) are followed by long-term maintenance prednisone (10–30 mg/day). The onset of action is slow (several days). The mechanism of action involves a combination of decreased intestinal calcium absorption, decreased bone turnover, and decreased renal tubular resorption.

3. **Calcitonin** will temporarily lower the serum calcium levels by 1–3 mg/dl and may be particularly effective in cases of severe hypercalcemia due to excessive PTH production. Skin testing with 1 MRC unit (0.10 ml of a 1:10 dilution of calcitonin SQ) should always precede administration. The usual dosage is 4 units/kg of body weight SQ or IM q12–24h. Calcitonin should be used only if rehydration and salt loading have proved ineffective. It is not suited for long-term therapy for hypercalcemia, but its hypocalcemic effects may be prolonged when combined with glucocorticoids or mithramycin.

4. **Mithramycin** is a cytotoxic antibiotic used for the treatment of embryonal tumors of the testis. A predictable side effect has been hypocalcemia produced by inhibition of bone resorption. Other side effects, including thrombocytopenia and renal and hepatic damage, have limited its use. It has been most commonly used in refractory hypercalcemia secondary to malignancy. The effective dose is 15–25 μg/kg given by slow IV infusion over 4–6 hours. A fall in serum calcium is seen within 12 hours, and the effect lasts for 3–7 days. Repeat doses are given at intervals of 3 or more days as required to maintain serum calcium below 12 mg/dl. Although toxicity is rarely seen at this dosage, mithramycin should not be used routinely in the treatment of most hypercalcemic patients.

5. **Phosphate supplementation** may be useful in certain circumstances after volume loading has achieved its maximal effect. The major mode of action is alteration of calcium-phosphate equilibrium toward deposition in the bone and soft tissues and reduction of intestinal calcium absorption. Due to the risk of severe metastatic calcification, phosphate therapy should be limited primarily to patients with **reduced** serum phosphate levels (e.g., primary hyperparathyroidism) and should **never** be used in patients with preexisting hyperphosphatemia (e.g., vitamin D toxicity). Either **Phospho-Soda** (600 mg phosphorus/5 ml), 1 tsp PO tid–qid, or **Neutra-Phos** (250 mg phosphorus/capsule), 2–3 capsules PO tid–qid as tolerated, may be used. Neutra-Phos is somewhat less likely than Phospho-Soda to cause severe diarrhea. If the patient is unable to take oral medications, phosphate may be given as a 100-ml retention Fleet enema bid. Intravenous phosphate administration, however, should be used with **extreme caution** in the treatment of hypercalcemia, since its use has been associated with severe soft tissue calcification, renal cortical necrosis, and fatal shock.

6. **Long-term management of hypercalcemia** includes treatment of the underlying disease as well as direct measures to control serum calcium levels. General measures include a low-calcium (400-mg) diet, maintenance of hydration and mobilization, and, when feasible, a salt intake of 8–10 gm/day. Phosphate supplementation may be of benefit.

   Chronic management of hypercalcemia in malignancy poses a special problem. Two forms of hypercalcemia associated with cancer have been recognized: One form is associated with neoplastic invasion of bone, and the other is associated with tumor-produced PTH-like and non-PTH-like stimulants of osteolysis. The former process is associated with normal or elevated TRP and serum PO_4 and with undetectable PTH levels. Prednisone, 10–30 mg/day, may suppress the production of osteolytic factors sometimes associated with these tumors (especially in myeloma) and thereby help control serum calcium. Patients with tumors secreting PTH present with hypophosphatemia and a low TRP (below 80%); PTH levels may or may not be elevated, depending on the particular radioimmunoassay. Tumor irradiation or chemotherapy usually results in a prompt reduction in serum calcium levels. When hypercalcemia persists, phosphate supplementation with Neutra-Phos, 2 capsules PO tid–qid, or Phospho-Soda, 5 ml PO tid–qid, may be useful. Prostaglandin-mediated hypercalcemia has been implicated in some solid tumors. A trial of prostaglandin inhibitors for 3 days is occasionally successful (e.g., **aspirin**, 600–1200 mg PO tid, or **indomethacin**, 50 mg PO tid. Dichloromethylene diphosphonate, at present investigational, is also beneficial in the hypercalcemia of malignant disease. **Mithramycin** may also be given (see **4**).

II. **Phosphorus.** Phosphorus is the most abundant intracellular anion, with about 80% of the total body phosphorus located in bone. Serum phosphorus levels (normal range for adults is 2.8–4.5 mg/dl) may not reflect total body stores, and rapid shifts of phosphorus between body compartments can occur. Therefore, the best guide to the treatment of phosphorus disorders is frequent monitoring during treatment.

Phosphate ion concentrations should be expressed in millimoles/liter; elemental phosphorus, in milligrams/dl (1 mmol of phosphate contains 31 mg of phosphorus, and 1 mmol of phosphate/liter equals 3.1 mg phosphorus/dl).

A. Hypophosphatemia can result from hyperalimentation, nutritional recovery after starvation, treatment of diabetic ketoacidosis, malabsorption, overuse of phosphate-binding antacids, alcohol withdrawal, diuretic phase of acute tubular necrosis, and prolonged respiratory alkalosis.

   1. Complications of severe hypophosphatemia (<1 mg/dl) include muscular weakness, rhabdomyolysis, neurologic abnormalities (e.g., paresthesias), hemolysis, platelet dysfunction, and cardiac failure (*Arch. Intern. Med.* 137:203, 1977).

   2. Treatment of hypophosphatemia depends on its degree of severity and associated symptoms.

   a. For mild to moderate hypophosphatemia (1.0–2.5 mg/dl), oral phosphate supplementation is usually adequate. This can be accomplished with **Neutra-Phos** (mixture of sodium and potassium phosphate, containing 250 mg phosphorus and 7 mEq each of sodium and potassium per capsule) or **Phospho-Soda** (each milliliter contains 129 mg phosphorus and 4.8 mEq sodium with no potassium). The usual dosage is 2 capsules of Neutra-Phos or 5 ml of Phospho-Soda bid–tid. The amount of oral phosphate that can be given is often limited by the development of diarrhea.

   b. For patients with mild to moderate hypophosphatemia who cannot tolerate oral intake, or for patients with severe hypophosphatemia (<1.0 mg/dl), IV phosphorus repletion is required. Only general guidelines can be given regarding the initial doses of IV phosphorus replacement (*Ann. Intern. Med.* 89:941, 1978): For severe hypophosphatemia, an initial phosphorus dose of 2.5–5.0 mg/kg of body weight given IV over 6–8 hours is appropriate; mild to moderate hypophosphatemia will require less. Additional dosages will be dependent on the new serum phosphorus level and the patient's clinical status. To minimize risks, the maximum IV dose of phosphorus should not exceed 7.5 mg/kg of body weight/6–8 hours.

   c. Convenient parenteral preparations of phosphorus include **Na phosphate** (each milliliter contains 93 mg phosphorus and 4 mEq sodium) and **K phosphate** (each milliliter contains 93 mg phosphorus and 4 mEq potassium).

   d. Hypophosphatemia is a frequent complication of diabetic ketoacidosis, and replacement should begin with the initiation of therapy. Potassium and phosphate replacement can be combined by the addition of 5 ml of potassium phosphate to 1 liter of IV fluid, providing approximately 22 mEq of potassium and 15 mmol (466 mg) of phosphorus/liter.

   These recommendations are only for the treatment of hypophosphatemia in patients with **normal renal function,** and caution is needed in repleting phosphorus in patients with renal insufficiency. Recommendations for phosphorus therapy during hyperalimentation are given in Chap. 11.

   3. The **hazards** of parenteral phosphorus administration include hypocalcemia, metastatic calcification should hyperphosphatemia develop, hypotension, and the potential for electrolyte or fluid abnormalities from the accompanying cations (Na^+ and K^+). **Calcium and phosphorus preparations cannot be given together in the same IV infusion.**

B. Hyperphosphatemia generally results from renal insufficiency (the main cause), hypoparathyroidism, increased catabolism, certain neoplastic diseases (leukemia, lymphoma), and administration of vitamin D metabolites. The main complication of hyperphosphatemia is metastatic calcification (*Clin. Nephrol.*

7:138, 1977). **Treatment** includes dietary phosphorus restriction and the use of phosphate-binding antacids (see Chap. 3, sec. **V.H**).

III. Magnesium. The serum magnesium level is normally 1.4–2.2 mEq/liter. Although control of magnesium metabolism is not well understood, many of the factors that regulate calcium homeostasis influence magnesium as well. However, body stores of magnesium are considerably less than the calcium stores, and the level of serum magnesium is less tightly controlled. Therefore, a prolonged deficiency in magnesium absorption or an increased magnesium intake in the face of decreased renal excretion can lead to significant alterations in serum magnesium levels. Disorders in serum magnesium concentration produce symptoms both by direct membrane effects and indirectly through alterations in calcium metabolism.

A. Hypomagnesemia occurs commonly in malabsorption syndromes (especially after small-bowel intestinal bypass surgery), in chronic alcoholism, severe diarrhea, and following prolonged parenteral feeding or nasogastric suction. It has also been observed following parathyroid surgery in patients with chronic hyperparathyroidism and in primary hyperaldosteronism, diabetic keto-acidosis, hyperthyroidism, chronic mercurial diuretic therapy, during and after aminoglycoside and cis-diamminedichloroplatinum therapy, and in states of diuresis (following acute tubular necrosis or obstruction, hyperosmolar states, or saline administration).

1. The **major signs and symptoms** include weakness, muscle fasciculations, tremors, personality changes, vertigo, and convulsions. Convulsions constitute a severe complication and are frequently associated with a fatal outcome. Hypocalcemia, due to cation shifts and an inappropriately low PTH response, occurs frequently in severe magnesium depletion. Many of the presenting signs and symptoms in such patients are due to the hypocalcemia per se. Magnesium administration will rapidly reverse the symptom complex caused by hypocalcemia, as well as the symptoms associated with hypomagnesemia.

2. Magnesium replacement may be accomplished by the IV, IM, or oral routes; the IV route should be reserved for patients requiring immediate control of seizures or tetanic contractures. In such cases, 1–2 gm of magnesium sulfate (8–16 mEq Mg^{2+}) as a 10% solution may be given IV over 15 minutes. If a favorable clinical response occurs, further parenteral therapy should be given IM in dosages of 1 gm q4–6h, depending on the serum magnesium level and clinical status of the patient. When repeated doses are to be given parenterally, the patellar reflexes should be tested before each dose; if they are absent, no more magnesium is to be given. Oral magnesium therapy to prevent depletion when excessive losses are continuous may be given as **magnesium oxide,** supplied in 10-grain tablets that provide 35 mEq of magnesium; 1–2 tablets/day should be adequate for most patients.

B. Hypermagnesemia is almost exclusively seen in patients with severe renal failure who have been treated with a magnesium-containing antacid (e.g., Mylanta, Maalox) or a laxative (e.g., milk of magnesia). Mild degrees of hypermagnesemia are seen with far-advanced renal disease but are usually asymptomatic. With elevation of the serum magnesium level to 3–5 mEq/liter, hypotension, nausea, and vomiting usually occur. With further elevation to 7 mEq/liter, drowsiness, hyporeflexia, and muscular weakness are noted. When the level reaches 12–15 mEq/liter, coma supervenes, and respiratory depression is frequent. Cardiac abnormalities are also noted with extreme elevations of serum magnesium and include prolongation of the Q–Tc interval, atrioventricular block, and cardiac arrest.

Treatment, other than removing the source of excess magnesium, is usually not necessary for mild elevations. Administration of calcium gluconate IV will temporarily reverse the symptoms resulting from severe hypermagnesemia. Definitive therapy may occasionally require peritoneal dialysis or hemodialysis.

Parathyroid Disease

I. **Primary hyperparathyroidism.** Primary hyperparathyroidism has a broad clinical spectrum, ranging from biochemical abnormalities in an asymptomatic patient to the more classic presentations of hypercalcemic symptoms, kidney stones, and bone disease.

A. **Characteristic findings** include persistent hypercalcemia, hypophosphatemia, a reduced TRP, and a tendency toward hyperchloremic acidosis. Alkaline phosphatase is elevated in perhaps 75% of patients. The 24-hour urine calcium excretion may be low, normal, or elevated, depending on the balance between the filtered calcium load and tubular calcium resorption. Subperiosteal resorption (most easily seen in the phalanges) may be demonstrable radiographically. The diagnosis is confirmed by radioimmunoassay for PTH. Assays with specificity for the carboxy-terminal region of the PTH molecule provide the best separation between the normal and the hyperparathyroid state.

It is important to differentiate between primary hyperparathyroidism and ectopic tumor production of PTH. Such tumors account for 2–5% of all cases of hyperparathyroidism; approximately one-third are lung (squamous cell) carcinomas, one-third, renal cell carcinomas, and one-fourth, urogenital carcinomas. Therefore, normal findings on a chest radiograph, abdominal plain film, intravenous pyelogram, urinalysis, and pelvic examination exclude more than 90% of such tumors and constitute an adequate evaluation for ectopic PTH production unless definite localizing signs of malignancy are present.

B. **Surgical treatment.** The criteria we use for parathyroid exploration in patients with presumed primary hyperparathyroidism include the following: (1) a serum calcium averaging more than 1.0 mg/dl above the upper limits of normal; (2) kidney stone formation; (3) deteriorating renal function; (4) hypercalciuria; (5) radiologically evident bone disease; or (6) symptoms of hypercalcemia. Following parathyroid surgery the serum calcium should be checked q8h for several days and then daily for 3–4 days to detect significant hypocalcemia.

C. **Medical treatment.** Only patients who do not meet operative criteria or who are poor operative risks should be managed conservatively on a regimen that includes a low-calcium diet, hydration with 3–4 liters of fluid/day, and a high salt intake (8–10 mg/day) as tolerated. Thiazide diuretics should be avoided, since they will further elevate serum calcium by reducing urinary calcium excretion. Phosphate supplementation with Phospho-Soda, 5 ml tid–qid, or Neutra-Phos, 2 capsules tid–qid, may reduce serum and urine calcium. However, phosphate should not be used in patients with persistent urinary tract infections and an alkaline urine because of the increased risk of calcium-phosphate stone formation.

II. **Hypoparathyroidism.** Hypoparathyroidism results from either decreased PTH secretion (surgical removal, idiopathic hypoparathyroidism) or decreased end-organ responsiveness to PTH (pseudohypoparathyroidism). Lenticular cataracts, basal ganglia calcifications, epidermal lesions, and cutaneous candidiasis are often seen in long-standing hypoparathyroidism. Typical somatic features (round face, short stature, shortened metacarpals) are commonly seen in patients with pseudohypoparathyroidism. Biochemical findings are identical in both forms of hypoparathyroidism: hypocalcemia, hyperphosphatemia, and a TRP approaching 100%. Pseudohypoparathyroidism can be distinguished from hypoparathyroidism by the lack of a phosphaturic response to PTH and elevated serum PTH levels. However, the management of both forms is similar. **Treatment** of hypoparathyroidism is that of the associated hypocalcemia as previously outlined (see Serum Mineral Disorders, sec. **I.A.2**).

Serum magnesium should be checked and supplemental magnesium administered if indicated. Occasionally, the use of thiazide diuretics (hydrochlorothiazide, 50 mg bid) may reduce the hypercalciuria associated with vitamin D and calcium therapy and promote the elevation of serum calcium.

Metabolic Bone Disease

I. **Osteopenia.** Bone is in a constant dynamic state of turnover and maintenance of normal bone metabolism requires (1) adequate mineral intake, absorption, and retention; (2) normal levels of biologically active vitamin D metabolites; and (3) normal parathyroid function. Since bone is by far the largest body reservoir of mineral and buffering capacity, maintenance of normal extracellular fluid (ECF) ionized calcium and pH levels not infrequently occurs at the expense of bone mineral content. Mineral and bone homeostasis can be disrupted by (1) decreased vitamin D intake, absorption, or activation; (2) decreased mineral absorption or retention; (3) disorders of PTH production or response; (4) administration of drugs or hormones that disrupt normal regulatory systems; and (5) disorders of endogenous hormone production.

Osteopenia (decreased bone mass as detected radiographically, by bone densitometry or by bone biopsy) results when the rate of bone resorption exceeds formation. Normal bone formation requires adequate protein availability for matrix synthesis and adequate supplies of calcium and phosphorus to mineralize the matrix. Insufficient mineral availability, due to vitamin D deficiency or renal tubular phosphate resorption defects, leads to a deficiency of mineralized matrix known as **osteomalacia.** A parallel loss of bone mineral and bone protein matrix (due to aging, immobilization, premature menopause, or hormonal or genetic factors) results in **osteoporosis.** A chronic increased PTH effect on bone produces **osteitis fibrosa.** Often, several varieties of histologic change are seen in a given patient with osteopenia.

Osteopenia is a clinical-radiologic diagnosis; once it is diagnosed, a thorough evaluation is indicated to determine the cause. A careful history, which may reveal such conditions as premature menopause, anticonvulsant drug or corticosteroid therapy, malabsorptive symptoms, or a myopathy that suggests hypophosphatemia, often provides critical clues as to the proper diagnostic approaches. In the absence of specific clues the **diagnostic procedures** that follow are useful.

A. **General evaluation**

1. Generalized malignancy (e.g., myeloma) as a cause of osteopenia should be reasonably excluded. A bone scan may be helpful here.

2. Selected bone radiographs, in addition to suggesting the decreased bone density of osteopenia, may provide useful diagnostic findings: rachitic epiphyseal changes (in children); pseudofractures, especially in the proximal long bones or pelvis (osteomalacia in adults); or subperiosteal resorption, especially in hand radiographs (hyperparathyroidism).

3. Serum T_4, A.M. and P.M. plasma cortisols, and 24-hour urinary free cortisol excretion are useful in excluding osteopenia-producing endocrinopathies.

4. Fasting morning serum calcium (total and ionized), phosphorus, and alkaline phosphatase with fractionation should be determined at least 3 times; 24-hour urinary calcium excretion and TRP should be determined twice. (**Note:** Thiazide therapy reduces urine calcium excretion to one-half to two-thirds of original levels.)

5. Measurements of serum PTH (preferably with carboxy-terminal specific radioimmunoassays) and of 25-hydroxycholecalciferol (25-OHD) should be obtained if possible.

6. Measurement of serum electrolytes and demonstration of adequate urine acidification (pH <5.4 in the morning urine or after a NH_4Cl load) test for distal renal tubular acidosis.

7. Histologic analysis of undecalcified sections of bone (bone biopsy) is diagnostic of the **type** of osteopenia in most instances.

B. Types of osteopenia

  1. Osteomalacia (decreased mineralized matrix) is generally due to vitamin D deficiency, renal phosphate leak, malabsorption, or anticonvulsant therapy (e.g., phenytoin, phenobarbital).

    a. Diagnosis. Vitamin D deficiency is suggested by hypocalcemia, hypophosphatemia, an elevated alkaline phosphatase, a reduced TRP (<80%), and reduced 24-hour urine calcium excretion (<80 mg). A careful dietary and drug therapy history should be obtained. The diagnosis is confirmed by demonstrating a reduced serum 25-OHD level. Serum PTH levels may be mildly elevated. Iliac crest **bone biopsy** with tetracycline labeling is often useful. Gastrointestinal function studies (D-xylose excretion, 72-hour stool fat, and small-bowel mucosal biopsy when necessary) should be done when **malabsorption** is suspected (see Chap. 14, Malabsorption).

    Osteomalacia secondary to **renal phosphate leak** is suggested by persistent hypophosphatemia in the presence of a normal serum and 24-hour urine calcium and normal serum 25-OHD levels; % TRP is markedly reduced, and serum PTH is normal (as opposed to the definite PTH elevations seen in hyperparathyroidism). This syndrome may occur as an isolated lesion or in combination with renal glucose, uric acid, and amino acid leaks or the full Fanconi syndrome. Vitamin D–resistant rickets is a renal phosphate leak existing from birth, resulting in rickets, osteomalacia, long-bone deformity, and stunted growth. Physical and x-ray findings are characteristic.

    b. Treatment. The aim of treatment of vitamin D deficiency is to restore serum calcium levels to normal, thereby ensuring that mineral availability has been normalized. In the rare case of **dietary deficiency,** vitamin D, 50,000 units/day for 1–2 months, followed by a normal diet (400 units vitamin D and 800 mg calcium per day), is adequate. In **fat malabsorption syndromes,** treatment of the primary disorder is combined with calcium supplementation (1600–2400 mg/day) plus vitamin D, 50,000 units 3–7 times weekly, or more as required. Careful monitoring of serum and urine calcium is important, since improved absorption following treatment of the primary disease can easily lead to vitamin D intoxication. The osteomalacia in patients with increased hepatic vitamin D catabolism due to **anticonvulsant drug therapy** is treated with vitamin D, 50,000 units/day, with calcium supplementation for 3–6 months until serum mineral and 25-OHD levels are normal. At that point, prophylactic therapy with vitamin D, 800–2000 units/day (2 standard multivitamin tablets) plus adequate calcium intake is instituted.

    Isolated renal phosphate leaks, whether congenital or acquired, are treated with phosphate, 1800–2400 mg/day in divided doses (Phospho-Soda, 1 tsp qid, or Neutra-Phos, 2–3 tablets qid), plus vitamin D, 50,000 units/M^2/day. Treatment must continue for life. In the case of **renal tubular acidosis,** akalinization plus calcium, 1000–1500 mg/day, plus vitamin D, 50,000–100,000 units/week, is instituted. Once bone mass has been restored, vitamin D can usually be discontinued while alkalinization is maintained.

  2. Osteoporosis

    a. Diagnosis. Osteoporosis is essentially a clinical diagnosis of exclusion, with all mineral levels being normal. It is suggested by a family history of easy fractures, a previous history of prolonged or total immobilization, or premature menopause. Osteoporosis is most common in postmenopausal white women. In this population, careful evaluation to exclude other causes must be undertaken (see **A**). The diagnosis is confirmed by bone biopsy.

  b. Treatment of osteoporosis remains unsatisfactory. The mainstay of treatment is dietary calcium supplementation (1–2 gm calcium/day) and adequate mobilization. Regular exercise may prevent osteoporosis or slow its progression. It is reasonable to add vitamin D_2 or D_3 (50,000 units, 1–2 times/week for 2–4 months). Although sodium fluoride has been advocated, its general use cannot be recommended at this time. Estrogen therapy, if initiated within 1–2 years after menopause, may be effective in preventing progressive bone loss. There is a risk of uterine cancer with the use of exogenous estrogens, and this therapy should be reserved for selected patients. If estrogen therapy is used, it should be combined with the progestin in a cyclic fashion (e.g., **conjugated estrogen**, 0.625 mg/day, first to twenty-first day of each month, with the addition of **medroxy-progesterone**, 10 mg/day on the sixteenth to the twenty-first day of each month). Gynecologic examinations should be performed at least yearly as long as this form of therapy is continued.

3. Osteitis fibrosa

  a. Diagnosis. Osteitis fibrosa is the result of increased PTH activity (primary or secondary hyperparathyroidism). The diagnosis of hyperparathyroidism is discussed under Parathyroid Disease, sec. **I.A.**

  b. Therapy. The osteopenia of primary hyperparathyroidism can be treated only by surgical removal of the abnormal parathyroid tissue. Following normalization of PTH levels, a significant improvement in bone mass occurs over 12–18 months. Medical management alone (low-calcium diet, hydration, phosphate supplements) improves the biochemical findings, but does not appear to increase bone mass. In isolated calcium malabsorption in older persons (24-hour urine calcium <50 mg, normal fat absorption, normal serum 25-OHD levels), vitamin D, 50,000 units 1–3 times/week, plus calcium, 750–1000 mg/day, should be given. A satisfactory response is indicated by maintenance of 24-hour urine calcium in the range of 120–200 mg.

4. Glucocorticoid-induced osteopenia

  a. General considerations and diagnosis. Glucocorticoid-induced osteopenia is a mixture of osteoporosis that is due to direct inhibition of bone formation and osteitis that is due to decreased calcium absorption with secondary hyperparathyroidism. It can occur in anyone chronically receiving the equivalent of 7.5 mg/day or more of prednisone. Typical x-ray findings include diffuse osteopenia, vertebral compression fractures, and aseptic necrosis of the femoral or humoral heads. Serum and urine chemistries and 25-OHD levels are usually normal. The serum PTH may be mildly elevated. Bone biopsy is confirmatory.

  b. Treatment. General measures include maintenance of the highest possible level of physical activity in order to stimulate bone formation; a reduction of the glucocorticoid dosage to the lowest possible levels (often by adding nonsteroid anti-inflammatory drugs); and maintenance of a diet adequate in protein, vitamin D, and calcium. Recent evidence suggests that suppression of the secondary hyperparathyroidism that results from glucocorticoid-induced calcium malabsorption can reduce the loss of bone mass. An appropriate regimen is calcium, 750–1000 mg/day, plus vitamin D, 50,000 units 2–3 times/week or 25-hydroxy vitamin D. Urine calcium should be monitored periodically to avoid hypercalciuria (>4 mg/kg/day).

II. Paget's disease. Paget's disease is a disorder of bone remodeling marked by extremely high bone turnover rates and a tendency to bone overgrowth, leading to progressive bone deformity and nerve-compression symptoms. The process may involve only one bone or may be widespread, involving virtually the entire skeleton. The diagnosis is made by the characteristic radiographic appearance of the bone lesions. Bone biopsy is indicated only in the rare patient in whom the radiographic findings raise the possibility of malignancy.

A. Symptoms are produced by the following: (1) muscular strain resulting from the postural changes produced by severe bowing of the femur and tibia; (2) bone periosteal stretching produced by exuberant bone overgrowth; (3) joint deformity resulting from involvement of periarticular bone, especially in the hip; (4) nerve-root compression from vertebral overgrowth; and (5) narrowing of cranial ostia, with compression of cranial nerves, especially the second and eighth cranial nerves. Additionally, high output cardiac failure resulting from increased blood flow to bone is occasionally seen in older patients with widespread disease. The bone alkaline phosphatase is often extremely high, closely paralleling the disease activity and extent of involvement. Serum and urine calcium levels are generally normal but can become significantly elevated when a patient with widespread involvement is put on bed rest. Such patients should be mobilized as much as possible and maintained on enforced hydration and a high-salt diet as tolerated. The use of thiazide diuretics should be avoided.

B. Treatment is indicated only in patients with bone pain, hypercalcemia, hypercalciuria with recurrent renal calculi, and high output cardiac failure.

  1. The vast majority of patients with active disease can receive adequate symptomatic relief from mild analgesic therapy, e.g., aspirin (650 mg 3–5 times/day), indomethacin (25 mg tid–qid), or ibuprofen (1600–2400 mg/day).

  2. In the patient in whom further therapy is indicated despite adequate mobilization, diphosphonates, calcitonin, or mithramycin may be tried.

   a. Diphosphonates are stable analogues of pyrophosphate that inhibit the growth and dissolution of hydroxyapatite crystals and directly impair osteoclast function. Etidronate disodium diphosphonate (EHDP) is the disodium salt of diphosphonic acid. A dosage of 5 mg/kg of body weight/day for 6 months is beneficial for the relief of pain, suppression of serum alkaline phosphatase, and improvement of bone histology. Higher dosages lead to osteomalacia. The EHDP is stopped at 6 months, followed occasionally by prolonged remissions off the medication. If relapses occur, EHDP may be reinitiated. Diarrhea is occasionally reported but is generally mild.

   b. Calcitonin appears to reduce bone resorption, with secondary diminution in the osteoclastic activity (*Ann. Intern. Med.* 95:192, 1981). A skin test of 1 MRC unit SQ prior to administration of a full dose of calcitonin is important. The usual starting dosage for adults is 100 MRC units/day SQ. A response is indicated by a reduction in serum bone alkaline phosphatase and 24-hour urinary hydroxyproline excretion over several months. Bone pain should decrease over this interval. If an adequate response is achieved, the dosage may be lowered to 50 MRC units/day or less and given in combination with analgesic therapy. When marked symptomatic relief occurs, calcitonin often can be discontinued for periods of months, during which the patient remains relatively asymptomatic. With the recurrence of severe pain, calcitonin can be reinstituted, and a relatively rapid response ensues. Resistance to calcitonin may occur and is not overcome by increasing the dosage above 100 MRC units/day.

   Common **side effects** of calcitonin include nausea, anorexia, vomiting, flushing of the face for 1–2 hours after injection, and skin rashes. However, side effects usually are not severe and do not require cessation of the drug.

c. **Mithramycin,** 15–25 μg/kg of body weight, administered 1–2 times/week by slow IV infusion over 4–6 hours, has been reported to produce rapid symtomatic relief, improvement in biochemical variables, and a reduction in the high output cardiac state. Because of significant potential toxicity associated with mithramycin, it should be reserved for selected patients unresponsive to other forms of therapy.

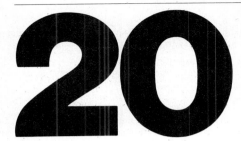

Diabetes Mellitus and Hyperlipidemia

Diabetes Mellitus

I. Diagnosis and classification

A. Diagnostic criteria. Current diagnostic criteria for diabetes mellitus (DM) are more stringent than in the past (*Diabetes* 28:1039, 1979). Criteria for gestational DM are given in sec. **X**. The diagnosis of DM should be made only if one of the following conditions is met:

1. Polyuria, polydipsia, and weight loss are present along with unequivocal elevation of plasma glucose (PG).

2. The fasting PG is ≥140 mg/dl on more than one occasion.

3. An oral glucose tolerance test is diagnostic on more than one occasion. Normal values are a fasting PG <115 mg/dl and a 2-hour PG <140 mg/dl, with all earlier PGs <200 mg/dl. The diagnosis of DM requires that the PG be > 200 mg/dl in both the 2-hour sample and at least one earlier sample. The test is performed in the morning after an overnight fast and should be preceded by unrestricted physical activity and a daily carbohydrate intake of at least 150 gm; 75 gm of glucose is given, and the PG is measured at half-hour intervals for 2 hours.

   An oral glucose tolerance test should not be performed if the fasting PG is diagnostic or if factors that impair glucose tolerance are present. These factors include the stress of illness, trauma, or surgery; certain drugs, such as thiazides, oral contraceptives, and glucocorticoids; physical inactivity; and carbohydrate restriction. (At least one of these factors is present in almost all hospitalized patients.) Since the benefit of establishing the diagnosis of asymptomatic DM is not clear, we do not perform an oral glucose tolerance test as a routine procedure.

B. Impaired glucose tolerance. This category comprises patients whose glucose tolerance lies between normal values and those diagnostic of DM. In this group the incidence of chronic complications of DM is low, and overt DM develops at an annual rate of only 1–5%. A substantial number have normal glucose tolerance with repeated testing. Older terms for impaired glucose tolerance, such as latent and chemical DM, should be abandoned.

C. Classification. Three major categories are recognized.

1. **Insulin-dependent, or type I, DM** (IDDM) comprises the majority of cases in children and young adults, although it can develop at any age. These patients require injected insulin to prevent ketoacidosis and sustain life.

2. **Non-insulin-dependent, or type II, DM** (NIDDM) usually occurs after age 40, although some young people also have this form. Ketoacidosis does not develop in these patients (except rarely, under severe stress of illness), but

they may need insulin to control symptomatic hyperglycemia. The majority are obese, and hyperglycemia usually improves with weight loss.

3. **Diabetes associated with other conditions,** including drugs, pancreatic disease, Cushing's syndrome, acromegaly, insulin-receptor abnormalities, and a variety of genetic syndromes.

II. Approach to therapy

A. **Education.** The first step in therapy is education, since successful treatment of DM depends on the informed patient, able to make day-to-day therapeutic decisions with a physician's advice. Individual instruction by the physician, diabetes nurse specialist, and dietician is most important. The diabetes education programs operated by many hospitals may be helpful. A number of useful publications are available, including *Diabetes Forecast,* a lay journal published by the American Diabetes Association.

Early education should emphasize practical daily management, including dietary recommendations, techniques of monitoring control, and what to do in case of illness. If insulin is used, the patient must know how to measure and inject it and how to recognize, prevent, and treat hypoglycemia. Later, most patients can learn more about the nature, treatment, and complications of diabetes. Foot care and the effects of exercise are particularly important. Education of family members should include the signs and treatment of hypoglycemia.

B. **Goals of therapy.** There are two distinct goals in the treatment of DM.

1. Prevention of the symptoms of hyperglycemia and glycosuria. This can be achieved with conventional techniques in almost all patients.

2. Maintenance of near-normal PG throughout the day (i.e., tight control) is now feasible in many patients with the use of multiple insulin injections and blood glucose (BG) monitoring. There is substantial, but not conclusive, evidence that late complications are due to the metabolic abnormalities of DM and that tight control will reduce their incidence (*Diabetes Care* 2:499, 1979). We believe that for each patient the physician should attempt to maintain the strictest control of PG possible without severe or frequent episodes of hypoglycemia.

C. **Choice of therapy.** The following are general guidelines for selecting among the three major therapeutic methods, i.e., diet, insulin, and oral hypoglycemic agents:

1. **IDDM.** By definition, this group requires treatment with insulin. Careful attention to diet is also necessary.

2. **Obese NIDDM.** Restriction of caloric intake is of prime importance. Often, glucose intolerance improves before substantial weight loss occurs. If symptoms persist after an adequate trial of caloric restriction (at least several weeks), therapy with insulin or oral hypoglycemic agents is necessary. Oral agents have been used widely in this group of patients. Although the report of the University Group Diabetes Program (UGDP) that treatment with tolbutamide is associated with increased risk of cardiovascular death has been disputed for over a decade, and an unequivocal resolution of the controversy is not in sight, this UGDB finding has not been refuted. Furthermore, though oral agents initially reduce hyperglycemia in most patients with NIDDM, after 5 years of follow-up in the UGDP study, average PG levels were the same in patients treated with tolbutamide and those treated with diet alone. Thus, there is little evidence of long-term benefit and some reason to suspect increased risk with the use of these drugs. While a dogmatic recommendation is not warranted, it is our practice to use **insulin** to treat patients with symptomatic NIDDM that cannot be controlled with diet alone.

3. **Nonobese NIDDM.** In this group, diet alone will not achieve satisfactory control, and additional therapy is required. The considerations in the choice between insulin and oral hypoglycemic agents discussed in **2** apply to this group as well.

D. **General care**

1. **Identification.** An identification tag or bracelet with medical information (e.g., Medic Alert) is essential, especially for patients treated with insulin or sulfonylureas.

2. **Atherosclerosis.** Diabetes mellitus is an important risk factor for atherosclerotic disease, and every effort should be made to reduce other risk factors, particularly smoking, hypertension, and hyperlipidemia.

3. **Exercise** may enhance physical and psychologic well-being, and favorably affect plasma lipoprotein levels. In patients with well-controlled DM, exercise lowers PG by enhancing glucose uptake into muscle and by accelerating absorption of injected insulin from an exercised extremity. Patients should take extra carbohydrate prior to exercise and inject insulin in the abdomen on days when exercise is planned. Since exercise exacerbates hyperglycemia and ketosis in poorly regulated DM, it should be recommended only after adequate control of DM. The possibility of underlying cardiovascular disease should be evaluated before a program of vigorous exercise is initiated.

4. Vaccination against influenza and pneumococcal infection is recommended.

III. **Monitoring diabetic control**

A. **General principles**

1. **Choice of technique.** The therapy of DM requires assessment of the degree of control of PG. A variety of methods is available, and the choice depends on the type of DM, the therapy used, the stability of control, and the desired degree of control.

   Insulin-treated patients require the most frequent and accurate monitoring, usually with several tests each day. In this group, the use of home BG monitoring is increasing and is essential if tight control is sought. In patients treated with diet or oral hypoglycemic agents, the aim of monitoring is to detect a major deterioration in control, and testing the urine for glucose once daily is usually adequate.

2. **Frequency of testing** should be determined by the probability of rapid, major changes in control. The frequency should be greatest after changes in therapy and in periods of stress or illness. In the latter setting, tests for urine ketones should also be performed.

3. **Education.** The patient must be taught the purpose and technique of monitoring and how to record results. Convenient books (e.g., *Clinilog*) simplify recording test results and insulin doses. Unless correct techniques are used and results accurately recorded, monitoring is worthless.

B. **Urine glucose tests**

1. **Products**

   a. **Clinitest** (tablets that use a copper reduction reaction) is the most accurate method, especially with high urine glucose concentrations, and has been considered the method of choice for IDDM. However, there is little value in accurately quantifying poor control, and for many of these patients, home BG monitoring is preferable. Clinitest is the most cumbersome and expensive urine glucose test; the tablets are very toxic if swallowed, and a variety of drugs (including penicillins, cephalosporins, isoniazid [INH], barbiturates, levodopa, salicylates, and probenecid) can produce false-positive results.

  b. Glucose oxidase strips (Diastix, Tes-Tape) offer the advantage of convenience and are the preferred method in patients with **NIDDM.** They tend to underestimate high glucose concentrations and are inhibited by ketones, levodopa, and high doses of salicylates or vitamin C. Accurate timing is required to obtain valid results. Diastix are somewhat easier to read, although Tes-Tape is slightly cheaper.

 2. Technique. Tests should be performed before meals and at bedtime. Double-voided specimens (obtained by voiding 30 minutes earlier and testing the second voided specimen) best reflect the concomitant BG. Results should be recorded as percentage values (i.e., gm/dl). "Plus" values should be abandoned because they are ambiguous (they correspond to different glucose concentrations with each product).

 3. The disadvantages of urine glucose tests are: (1) They are inconvenient, especially if the double-voiding technique is used; (2) they correlate poorly with the concomitant PG even when properly performed; (3) they are virtually useless in conditions with marked alteration of renal glucose threshold (renal failure, pregnancy) or impaired bladder emptying; and (4) they do not distinguish between normal PG levels and hypoglycemia.

C. Urine ketone tests. All diabetic patients should test for ketonuria in periods of stress or illness, since its presence indicates the need for close attention by the physician.

 Ketones can be measured by **Acetest** tablets or **Ketostix** (both use the nitroprusside reaction, which detects only acetoacetate and acetone). Ketostix are subject to deterioration with exposure to air, while Acetest tablets are stable. Use of the combined strip, **Keto-Diastix** (which costs twice as much as Diastix) for routine testing is unnecessary and wasteful.

D. The **plasma glucose** (PG) concentration is 15% greater than that of whole blood. Measurements of PG are primarily used to manage hospitalized patients during acute illness. Intermittent-fasting PG measurements provide some indication of control in patients with NIDDM, but in IDDM the fasting PG indicates little about glucose levels during the remainder of the day.

E. Home blood glucose monitoring

 1. Products. Two basic methods are available.

  a. Glucose oxidase reagent strips (Chemstrip bG and others) can be read by visual comparison with a standard color chart. This is the most convenient and least expensive home BG monitoring method.

  b. Reflectance meters (Glucometer, Stat Tek, and others) can be used to measure the color change on a reagent strip with somewhat greater accuracy than by visual comparison with standards. The meters are expensive and require periodic calibration. Portable, battery-powered instruments are now available.

 2. Technique. With both methods, a drop of capillary blood is placed on the reagent area of the strip, left for exactly 60 seconds, and then removed. The color change indicates the BG level.

 3. Advantages. Home BG monitoring is preferable to urine glucose testing in (1) pregnancy, (2) patients with unstable or "brittle" diabetes, (3) patients in whom urine tests are completely unreliable (e.g., with renal failure or neurogenic bladder), and (4) patients in whom tight control is attempted.

F. Glycosylated hemoglobin (Hb). Hemoglobin A_1c is the most abundant glycosylated Hb, constituting about 4% of Hb in normal persons. Hemoglobin A_1 comprises HbA_1c along with several other minor Hb components. Since the rate of glycosylation is proportional to the prevailing glucose concentration, the level of HbA_1 or HbA_1c is an index of the average PG during the preceding several weeks. Periodic determinations indicate the overall adequacy of the therapeutic regimen.

Chromatography is most widely used to measure HbA_1. Falsely elevated values are seen in uremia and in the presence of HbF; falsely low values are seen with HbS, HbC, and certain other variants. Glycosylated Hb levels are reduced in hemolytic anemias. Recent poor control may increase the apparent level in some assays.

IV. Diet. The objectives of dietary treatment differ with the type of diabetes, the presence of obesity, and the use of other forms of treatment. Hence, there is no single "diabetic diet." Special "diabetic" or "dietetic" foods (with the exception of artificially sweetened soft drinks) are expensive and unnecessary (*Annu. Rev. Med.* 30:155, 1979).

A. General considerations

   1. The physician must choose the appropriate dietary objectives and communicate them to the patient and dietitian.

   2. To achieve compliance, the patient must understand the purpose of the diet. A dietitian should be consulted to help design a diet that takes into account the patient's social and economic circumstances, food preferences, and eating habits and requested to instruct the patient and family members in its use. Sample menus and pamphlets alone will not work.

   3. The diet should be the simplest plan that will achieve the objectives for that patient. Many patients with NIDDM require only caloric restriction, and more complex requirements only jeopardize compliance.

   4. The appropriate caloric intake should be determined as outlined in Chap. 11. Meals usually each contain 20–40% of calories and snacks 10%.

   5. The nutrient composition of the diet should be specified.

      a. Carbohydrate (CHO) (4 kcal/gm). The former practice of restricting CHO does not contribute to control of PG. Carbohydrate should constitute 45–60% of calories, mainly as starch, while glucose and sucrose are restricted.

      b. Protein (4 kcal/gm) should make up 12–20% of calories in adults, with a minimum intake of 0.5 gm/lb of desirable body weight. In children and pregnant women, protein should constitute 20% of calories.

      c. Fat (9 kcal/gm) constitutes the remainder of the calories. While it has not been proved that a diet designed to lower plasma **cholesterol** will delay progression of atherosclerosis, we advocate that all patients follow a prudent diet consisting of (1) reduction of total fat intake to 30–35% of caloric intake; (2) reduction of saturated (animal) fat to less than 10% of calories; (3) provision of 10% of calories as polyunsaturated (vegetable) fat; and (4) reduction of cholesterol to 300 mg/day or less.

   6. **Alcohol** may be used in moderation but must be recognized as a source of calories (7 kcal/gm). It impairs hepatic gluconeogenesis and can lead to hypoglycemia in the fasting person. Alcohol can also augment the hypoglycemic effect of insulin and sulfonylureas and thus should always be taken with food. Diabetic patients with neuropathy or hypertriglyceridemia should avoid its use altogether. Some patients treated with sulfonylureas experience disulfiram (Antabuse)-like reactions.

   7. **Saccharin** remains the standard artificial sweetener, despite animal studies that suggest carcinogenicity. The position of the American Diabetes Association is that saccharin's benefit to diabetic patients as an aid in restriction of calories and sugar outweighs its potential risks.

8. Fiber. An increase in dietary fiber has been reported to lower postprandial glucose levels in diabetic patients, but its place in the treatment of DM is not yet established.

B. Diet in IDDM

1. Consistency. Insulin-treated diabetic patients have a fixed pattern of plasma insulin levels to which food intake must correspond to prevent hypoglycemia. Accordingly, consistency from day to day is the most important aspect of diet including (1) timing of meals, (2) distribution of caloric content between meals, (3) distribution of nutrients in each meal, and (4) amount and timing of exercise.

Exchange lists allow flexibility in the choice of food while maintaining the amount of calories and nutrients constant. Each meal contains a specific number and type of exchanges. The use of exchanges is described in *A Guide for Professionals: The Effective Application of Exchange Lists for Meal Planning,* which can be obtained from the American Diabetes Association, 2 Park Ave., New York, N.Y. 10016.

2. Caloric intake should aim at achieving and maintaining desirable body weight. Since these patients are not often obese, caloric restriction is seldom appropriate.

3. A bedtime snack should be eaten to prevent nocturnal hypoglycemia. Some patients require midmorning and midafternoon snacks.

4. If an acute illness diminishes appetite, the patient should try to maintain fluid and caloric intake with regular (not diet) soft drinks, soups, and juices. Insulin must be continued. If vomiting prevents intake or if ketonuria develops, IV fluids will be required.

C. Diet in NIDDM

1. In the obese person, caloric restriction will reduce, and in some cases eliminate, hyperglycemia. Supplemental vitamins are given if the daily intake is less than 1200 kcal.

2. If the patient is not obese and the diet is nutritionally adequate, limitation of cholesterol and saturated fat intake is the only dietary modification indicated.

3. If insulin is used to control hyperglycemia, the dietary principles appropriate for IDDM must be applied.

V. Insulin

A. Insulin preparations are listed in Table 20-1. The major characteristics of an insulin product are species source, concentration, degree of purity, and time course of action.

1. Species source. Most commercial insulin is a mixture of beef and pork insulin. Porcine insulin is closer in structure to human insulin than is bovine and is less antigenic in most patients. Preparations made from a single species are available and used in patients with allergy or immunologic resistance to insulin (see **3.b**). Biosynthetic human insulin produced with recombinant DNA techniques is currently undergoing clinical trials to determine its role in therapy.

2. Concentration. U-100 (100 units/ml) should be prescribed for all patients except those with very large insulin requirements, for whom U-500 insulin is available.

3. Purity

a. Single-peak insulin. Formerly, USP insulin contained substantial impurities. Proinsulin content (an index of insulin purity) was greater than

Table 20-1. Insulin preparations

Classification	Preparation[a]	Action after subcutaneous injection (hr)[b]		
		Onset	Peak effect	Duration
Rapid-acting	Regular	$\frac{1}{2}$–1	3–6	6–10
	Semilente	$\frac{1}{2}$–1	4–6	12–16
Intermediate-acting	NPH	$1\frac{1}{2}$–3	6–12	18–24
	Lente	1–3	6–12	24–28
Long-acting	PZI	4–6	14–24	36+
	Ultralente	4–6	18–24	36+

[a]New single component (purified) insulin products have a variety of trade names but fall into one of these categories.
[b]The times given are approximations and in some patients may be substantially prolonged.

10,000 parts per million (ppm). Gel filtration removes high-molecular-weight impurities, resulting in single-peak insulin, with less than 3000 ppm of proinsulin. Improved single-peak insulin with less than 50 ppm of proinsulin now constitutes almost all insulin sold in the United States.

   b. **Single-component (purified) insulin.** Further purification by ion exchange chromatography yields single-component insulin, which contains less than 10 ppm of proinsulin. Although purified pork insulin is the least antigenic insulin preparation, there are no data at present to justify treating the majority of patients with this costly product. Current **indications for purified pork insulin are:** (1) persistent insulin allergy, (2) immunologic insulin resistance, (3) insulin lipodystrophy, and (4) situations in which the need for insulin is likely to be temporary (e.g., during surgery or pregnancy), since intermittent therapy predisposes to allergy and resistance. Because the insulin requirement may fall when switching from single-peak to single-component insulin, it is prudent to reduce the dosage 10–20% to minimize the risk of hypoglycemia.

4. **Time course**
   a. **Rapid-acting insulins.** Regular insulin can be mixed with either NPH or Lente in any proportion. In some patients, antibody binding prolongs the effect of regular insulin, producing a peak effect at 4–8 hours and a duration of up to 24 hours. Only rapid-acting insulin can be given IV.

   b. **Intermediate-acting insulins.** The separate effect of regular insulin is somewhat better preserved when it is combined with NPH than with Lente. Lente is preferred in the occasional patient allergic to protamine.

   c. **Long-acting preparations** are seldom prescribed because of their propensity to produce nocturnal hypoglycemia. They may be useful in providing basal insulin requirements in patients treated with multiple injections of regular insulin. Protamine zinc and regular insulin cannot be mixed in the same syringe.

B. **Insulin regimens.** One of several basic patterns of insulin administration will succeed in the great majority of patients. The initial choice of regimen depends on the type of diabetes and the degree of control sought. The PG response is monitored and treatment adjusted accordingly. (In this and the following sections, NPH refers to intermediate-acting insulin.)

   1. Patients with NIDDM treated with insulin to control symptomatic hyperglycemia usually respond well to a single injection of NPH insulin before breakfast.

2. Patients with IDDM in whom the goal is prevention of symptoms can occasionally be treated with a single morning injection of NPH. Most patients, however, require a split-dose regimen with two injections of NPH, with or without regular insulin. When appropriately adjusted, such regimens usually provide two-thirds of the total NPH dose in the morning.

3. If tight control of PG is sought, a split-dose regimen with combined injections of NPH and regular insulin is essential, and control must be monitored with home BG monitoring. Nocturnal hypoglycemia often requires that the second injection of NPH be moved from before dinner to late in the evening. An alternative regimen consists of a daily injection of long-acting insulin to provide basal requirements, with regular insulin injected before each meal. This regimen has the advantage that the time of meals may be varied.

4. Portable insulin infusion pumps are being tested to determine their role in achieving tight diabetic control. Although commercially available, the indications for these devices have not been determined, and their use is considered investigational.

C. **Initiation of insulin treatment**

1. **Education.** The patient must be taught to measure and inject insulin properly. Monitoring technique and diet should be reviewed and day-to-day consistency in insulin, diet, and exercise emphasized.

2. **Hospitalization** is indicated for patients who are severely hyperglycemic, ketoacidotic, or otherwise seriously ill; it is also advisable in pregnant patients. Other patients may be hospitalized to facilitate teaching. Fine regulation of control, however, must be accomplished on an outpatient basis during usual daily activity.

D. **Adjustment of insulin dosage**

1. **Rate of adjustment.** The interval between dosage changes should be at least 2–3 days, since the full effect of an increase in dosage takes this long to appear, and more rapid changes may lead to hypoglycemia. Because there is variability in the day-to-day PG response to a given dose of insulin, adjustment should be made on the basis of patterns of urine or blood glucose that persist over several days rather than on the results of a single day. Changes should be made in only one dose of insulin at a time.

   Early in therapy, dosage increments should be 5–10 units. As satisfactory control is approached, increments should be reduced to 2–5 units.

2. **Initial adjustments.** In most patients, therapy is begun with a morning injection of 10–20 units of NPH, and the urine or blood glucose is measured before meals and at bedtime. The time of maximal fall in glucose (glucose nadir) is noted; this is usually in the late afternoon but occasionally is delayed until the evening. The dose of NPH is gradually increased until the glucose nadir is in a satisfactory range.

3. **Further adjustments.** Once the glucose nadir is in a satisfactory range, further adjustments are based on the diurnal pattern of blood or urine glucose levels. Only one adjustment should be made at a time, as outlined in **a–d**.

   a. If **fasting hyperglycemia** is present, a second injection of insulin is necessary. NPH, 5–10 units, is given before dinner, and the morning dose of NPH is reduced by a similar amount. The evening dose is gradually increased until the fasting urine or blood glucose is under control. If nocturnal hypoglycemia develops before the fasting glucose level is satisfactory, it can usually be avoided by giving the second dose of NPH at bedtime rather than before supper.

   b. If **late morning hyperglycemia** is present, regular insulin (about 5 units) is added to the morning NPH and adjusted until glucose levels before lunch are satisfactory. Usually, the dose of NPH must be adjusted downward to avoid afternoon hypoglycemia.

c. If there is **late evening hyperglycemia,** regular insulin (about 5 units) should be given before supper and adjusted until glucose levels before bedtime are controlled. A bedtime snack is essential to prevent nocturnal hypoglycemia.

d. A **hypoglycemic episode** is usually due to delay or omission of a meal or an unusual amount of exercise. If unexplained hypoglycemia is severely symptomatic or occurs consistently, the insulin dose with maximal effect at the time of hypoglycemia (see Table 20-1) should be reduced by 2- −5-unit decrements until hypoglycemia no longer occurs.

E. Problems with control

1. **Evaluation.** There are a number of causes of poor control, with frequent episodes of hypoglycemia, hyperglycemia, or both (sometimes termed "brittle" diabetes). Management of such patients requires careful attention to the details of insulin administration, the consistency of meals and exercise, the symptoms of hypoglycemia, the factors that affect sensitivity to insulin, and emotional problems. Home BG monitoring may be useful.

2. **Causes**

a. **Errors in management** include incorrect techniques of measuring or injecting insulin, inconsistency in eating and exercise habits, inaccurate performance of monitoring tests, failure to recognize an abnormal renal threshold for glucose, and omission of insulin when intercurrent illness is present.

b. Factors that affect **insulin absorption** include the site of injection (absorption is fastest from the abdomen, less rapid from the deltoid area, and slowest from the anterior thigh); exercise of the injected limb (which accelerates absorption); and injection of fibrotic areas from which absorption may be poor.

c. Factors that **increase insulin requirements** include weight gain, infection, the pubertal growth spurt, pregnancy, inactivity, Cushing's syndrome, acromegaly, hyperthyroidism, and high levels of insulin-binding antibodies (see **F.3**).

d. Factors that **reduce insulin requirements** include weight loss, increased exercise, renal failure, adrenal insufficiency, hypopituitarism, and malabsorption.

e. **Excessive insulin dosage (Somogyi effect).** Hypoglycemic episodes can lead to rebound hyperglycemia. If the hypoglycemia is asymptomatic, this sequence may lead to an increase in insulin dosage and exacerbation of the problem. This syndrome should be suspected when (1) urine tests negative for glucose are followed within a few hours by marked glycosuria or ketonuria; (2) there are wide fluctuations of PG over a few hours, unrelated to meals; and (3) symptoms of nocturnal hypoglycemia (e.g., sweating, morning headaches) are present.

Confirmation of this syndrome requires frequent PG measurements. Patients may be hospitalized for hourly samples over a 24-hour period, but if the patient is trained in home BG monitoring, frequent blood glucose measurements at home are preferable. A measurement at 3 A.M. will reveal most instances of nocturnal hypoglycemia. If hypoglycemia is found, the insulin dose should be reduced gradually.

f. **Emotional factors.** The contribution of psychologic and environmental disturbances to instability of control is difficult to assess. Resolution of stressful situations may improve control, but management of emotional problems may require psychiatric consultation.

F. Side effects

1. **Hypoglycemia** may result from excess insulin, omission or delay of meals, or exercise.

   a. **Manifestations** include tremor, diaphoresis, tachycardia, and hypothermia. Neurologic findings include confusion, abnormal behavior, seizures, and coma. Nocturnal hypoglycemia is often asymptomatic but may cause night sweats, difficulty awakening, morning headache, and nightmares. Propranolol should be used with caution, because it impairs recognition of and recovery from hypoglycemia.

   b. **Prevention** includes consistency in time and content of meals, avoidance of large changes in insulin dose, and ingestion of additional carbohydrate before exercise. Patients should learn to recognize early symptoms and always have concentrated carbohydrate available. Every insulin-treated patient should wear a Medic Alert Tag.

   c. **Treatment** is administration of carbohydrate by mouth; 10–20 gm (e.g., 1–2 cups of milk) is usually adequate, and larger amounts may lead to hyperglycemia. In a patient too obtunded to swallow safely, nothing should be given by mouth. If the patient is in a medical facility, 50 ml of 50% dextrose should be given IV. If IV dextrose cannot be given immediately, 1 mg of glucagon should be given SQ or IM. All patients should have glucagon, and a family member should know how to inject it.

2. **Allergy**

   a. **Local reactions** commonly occur soon after initiation of therapy and consist of pruritus, pain, or induration at the injection site. They usually subside spontaneously, but if they persist, therapy should be changed. Since some patients are allergic to protamine, NPH should be switched to Lente. If this does not succeed, purified pork insulin should be tried. Rarely, desensitization is required.

   b. **Systemic reactions,** such as urticaria, angioedema, and anaphylaxis, are rare and usually occur in patients with a history of interrupted insulin use. Treatment is desensitization with purified pork insulin (*Med. Clin. North Am.* 62:663, 1978).

3. **Insulin resistance** is usually defined as a requirement for more than 200 units/day for more than 2 days in the absence of ketoacidosis (*Diabetes Care* 2:283, 1979).

   a. Causes include obesity, infection, and glucocorticoid or growth hormone excess, but the most common cause of insulin resistance, as previously defined, is a high concentration of insulin-binding antibodies. Such antibodies develop in almost all patients treated with insulin, but in immunologic insulin resistance, the serum insulin-binding capacity is usually greater than 30 units/liter.

   b. Therapeutic approaches to immunologic resistance include: (1) changing to purified pork insulin; (2) use of multiple injections of regular insulin rather than intermediate-acting preparations (U-500 insulin may be especially useful); (3) glucocorticoid therapy (prednisone, 60 mg PO qd, with tapering as insulin requirements decrease); and (4) use of sulfated insulin, a chemically modified and less antigenic preparation (*Diabetes* 27:307, 1978).

4. **Lipodystrophy**

   a. **Lipoatrophy** (loss of subcutaneous fat at the site of insulin injection) is seen less commonly with present single-peak insulins. It responds to daily injection of purified pork insulin into the affected areas.

Table 20-2. Sulfonylureas

Generic and brand name	Daily dosage range (mg)	Duration of action (hr)	Dose frequency	Route of elimination
Tolbutamide (Orinase)	500–2000	6–12	bid–tid	Hepatic
Tolazamide (Tolinase)	100–750	12–24	qd–bid	Hepatic and renal
Acetohexamide (Dymelor)	250–1500	12–24	qd–bid	Hepatic and renal
Chlorpropamide (Diabinese)	100–500	up to 60	qd	Hepatic and renal

    b. Insulin hypertrophy consists of masses of adipose tissue that develop at injection sites, usually in patients who do not rotate sites. The masses gradually disappear if injection in these sites is avoided.

VI. Sulfonylureas. Sulfonylureas are now the only oral hypoglycemic agents available (Table 20-2).

    A. Indications. Sulfonylureas should be used only in symptomatic patients with NIDDM in whom diet has failed to control hyperglycemia. Efforts at weight loss in the obese must continue. Sulfonylureas are started at low dosages and gradually increased until symptoms are controlled and the fasting PG is 110 mg/dl or less.

    B. Response to therapy. Only 60–75% of appropriately selected patients respond adequately. Failure to control hyperglycemia after 4 weeks of therapy is termed *primary failure;* these patients require insulin to control symptoms. Of patients who respond initially, 5–30% will subsequently cease to respond and require insulin. This is termed *secondary failure,* and its incidence appears to increase with duration of therapy.

    C. Contraindications. Sulfonylureas should not be used in (1) IDDM, (2) hepatic or renal dysfunction, (3) pregnancy and lactation, and (4) children. Sulfonylureas may not control diabetes during severe stress, such as major surgery or infection. There is no evidence of benefit in asymptomatic patients.

    D. Side effects

        1. Hypoglycemia is most common with chlorpropamide and may be severe and prolonged even with the short-acting agents. Predisposing factors include age over 50 years, hepatic or renal disease, alcohol use, and fasting. A variety of drugs potentiate the hypoglycemic effects of the sulfonylureas, including salicylates, sulfonamides, phenylbutazone, methyldopa, clofibrate, chloramphenicol, bishydroxycoumarin, and monoamine oxidase inhibitors. Patients with sulfonylurea-induced hypoglycemia should be admitted to the hospital, since treatment may require infusion of large amounts of dextrose for several days.

        2. Hyponatremia may occur in patients taking chlorpropamide. Other sulfonylureas do not have this effect.

        3. A disulfiram (Antabuse)-like reaction, with flushing, headache, nausea, and tachycardia, occurs in some patients after ingestion of alcohol.

        4. Other toxic reactions include rashes, GI symptoms, blood dyscrasias, and cholestatic jaundice.

VII. Diabetic ketoacidosis

    A. Prevention. During an acute illness, patients must (1) test their urine for ketones; (2) continue insulin even if anorexia and nausea lead to diminished eating; (3) take fluids containing sugar and salt; and (4) contact their physician promptly if vomiting or ketonuria develops. These measures will prevent most episodes of diabetes ketoacidosis (DKA) or ensure their early treatment.

B. General management. Treatment requires (1) replacement of fluid and electrolyte deficits, (2) sufficient insulin to reverse the metabolic abnormalities, and (3) prompt recognition and management of precipitating illnesses and complications. The key to successful therapy is frequent and careful observation of the patient's clinical and biochemical status, with modification of therapy when appropriate.

1. Diagnostic studies

   a. Serial measurements. To assess the response to treatment, a flow sheet of clinical findings and biochemical values must be kept. Initially, vital signs, mental status, fluid intake, and urine output should be recorded at half-hour intervals. Plasma glucose, sodium, potassium, bicarbonate, and the anion gap should be measured hourly. Rapid determination of blood glucose with Dextrostix and a reflectance meter facilitates management. As the patient's condition approaches normal, the interval between observations is gradually increased.

   b. Serum ketones should be estimated by the nitroprusside reaction (Acetest tablets). Serum is diluted 1 : 1 with water and applied to a crushed tablet. This test detects acetoacetate but not the predominant ketoacid, beta-hydroxybutyrate, and the result is thus only qualitative. Rarely, a false-negative test may occur in states of low cellular redox potential (e.g., hypoxia, lactic acidosis), in which all ketoacid is in the form of beta-hydroxybutyrate. Repeated determinations of serum ketones are useless; the anion gap provides the best estimate of ketoacid concentration.

   c. Other studies should be done initially but repeated only if circumstances indicate. These include plasma creatinine, blood urea nitrogen, calcium, phosphorus, osmolality, and arterial blood pH, PO_2, and PCO_2. (Serum creatinine measured by automated methods may be spuriously elevated.) An ECG, chest x ray, urinalysis and urine culture, and, in most cases, blood cultures should be obtained.

2. Precipitating factors. The following precipitating factors must be sought:

   a. Infection is most common, and cultures should be obtained from any site suggested by the history or examination. Infected patients with DKA often have no fever, and leukocytosis is common in the absence of infection. Thus, a high index of suspicion is necessary, and, if there is clinical evidence of infection, antibiotics should be given while culture results are awaited.

   b. Other common **precipitating factors** include omission of insulin, myocardial infarction, pancreatitis, stroke, trauma, and surgery.

3. Aspiration of gastric contents is a threat in the comatose patient. Endotracheal intubation for protection of the airway, followed by nasogastric suction, is indicated in this situation.

4. Bladder catheterization should be avoided if possible but is indicated if the urine output cannot be determined otherwise.

5. Abdominal pain is common in young patients with DKA. Its cause is unknown, but it usually subsides within 6–8 hours after therapy is begun. If the patient is older than 40 years, if acidosis is not severe, or if pain persists, a primary abdominal disorder should be suspected. Hyperamylasemia is very common in DKA and does not correlate with abdominal pain.

6. Oral intake should be resumed as soon as the patient is fully conscious and able to tolerate a liquid diet. Much of the electrolyte deficit can be replaced by the oral route more safely than by the IV route.

C. Fluid and electrolytes. Patients with DKA are severely depleted of water and electrolytes.

1. Volume

   a. The first priority of treatment is rapid restoration of intravascular volume. One liter of 0.9% NaCl is given in the first half-hour, and further therapy is determined by the patient's response. Generally, 0.9% NaCl is continued at approximately 1 liter/hour until heart rate, blood pressure, and urine output indicate that severe depletion of intravascular volume has been alleviated. This usually requires no more than 2–3 liters.

   b. Further therapy consists of the administration of hypotonic solutions, since osmotic diuresis produces loss of water in excess of electrolytes. A 0.45% NaCl solution is given with the aim of replacing the fluid deficit within 12–24 hours. In practice, this is usually accomplished by giving 1 liter of 0.45% NaCl q2–4h. When the PG is 300 mg/dl or less, all IV fluids should contain 5% dextrose, to prevent hypoglycemia. Intravenous fluids should be continued until oral intake is well established.

   c. The adequacy of fluid replacement must be judged by frequent clinical assessment. In patients at increased risk of congestive heart failure, clinical criteria may not be sufficiently sensitive, and direct monitoring of central venous or pulmonary artery pressures is indicated.

   d. The use of 0.9% NaCl may lead to mild hypernatremia and hyperchloremia during the course of therapy, but this is seldom of clinical consequence. If plasma sodium exceeds 155 mEq/liter, 0.45% NaCl or 5% dextrose should be substituted.

2. Potassium. The initial plasma potassium concentration is usually normal or elevated but invariably falls with therapy, sometimes to levels that produce lethal dysrhythmias or paralysis. Most of the potassium should be administered as the chloride salt, although part may be given as the phosphate (see **4**). Plasma potassium must be monitored frequently and the rate of administration adjusted accordingly. Monitoring of the ECG for evidence of hypo- or hyperkalemia is valuable in guiding replacement; it is essential if (1) severe hypo- or hyperkalemia is present, (2) renal failure is present, or (3) plasma potassium measurements cannot be readily made. Once oral intake is established, the remaining potassium deficit should be replaced by this route.

   a. If the initial potassium level is normal or high and the patient is not uremic, potassium replacement is begun with 20–40 mEq KCl/liter after adequate urine output is established. Generally, this should begin with the second liter of IV fluid.

   b. Initial hypokalemia indicates unusually severe depletion; replacement must begin immediately, with 40 mEq KCl in the first liter of IV fluid. If oliguria is present, the amount should be reduced, since 20–50% of administered potassium is normally excreted in the urine.

3. Bicarbonate is required only in patients with (1) an arterial pH less than 7.1 or (2) an arterial pH less than 7.2 associated with hypotension or shock. Sodium bicarbonate, 2 ampules (88 mEq), is diluted in 1 liter of 0.45% NaCl and given over 1 hour. This is repeated until the pH is greater than 7.2 and the patient is no longer in shock.

4. Phosphate. Plasma phosphate is usually normal or elevated initially and falls during treatment. Some investigators advocate IV phosphate administration in the therapy of DKA. The practical benefit of such therapy has not been shown, and its use in DKA can produce hypocalcemia (with tetany), hypomagnesemia, and metastatic calcification. In most patients, oral phosphate replacement is adequate. If IV phosphate is used, the infusion rate should not exceed 16 mmol (equal to about 24 mEq of the usual potassium phosphate preparation) over 6 hours, and plasma calcium and phosphate levels should be monitored frequently. (Obviously, potassium phosphate alone cannot be used to replace potassium deficits.) **Contraindications** to IV phosphate include: (1) hypercalcemia, (2) hyperphosphatemia, and (3) renal failure.

D. Insulin. Vigorous debate over insulin regimens for DKA has served to emphasize that careful monitoring of the patient's clinical and biochemical status is more important than the choice of initial insulin regimen.

1. The goal of insulin treatment of DKA is correction of acidosis, and it should be continued until the anion gap is normal. Since this takes longer than correction of hyperglycemia, 5% dextrose should be added to IV fluids when the PG reaches 300 mg/dl, to prevent hypoglycemia. Some patients with DKA present with a PG less than 300 mg/dl, in which case IV dextrose must be given from the outset.

2. **Method.** In the treatment of DKA, IV infusion or IM injection of insulin is preferred. If the patient is hypotensive, the IV route should be used. Subcutaneous insulin should not be used because of unpredictable absorption.

   a. **Continuous IV infusion.** An initial IV loading dose of 20 units of regular insulin is given, followed by 10–15 units/hour. Regular insulin, 100 units, is diluted in 500 ml of 0.45% NaCl (20 units/dl), and 100 ml of the solution is allowed to run through the tubing prior to connecting it to the patient. This eliminates the need to add albumin to prevent insulin binding to the IV apparatus. The infusion is begun at 50–75 ml/hour, regulated by an infusion pump. If the response is inadequate, the dosage should be increased as outlined in **3,** after excluding mechanical problems with the infusion apparatus.

   b. **Intramuscular insulin.** An initial IV loading dose of 20 units of regular insulin is given along with 10–15 units IM; 5–10 units is then given IM hourly. If the response is inadequate, the dosage should be increased as outlined in **3.**

3. **Insulin resistance.** Regardless of regimen, some patients will prove to be resistant to the initial insulin dosage. This will quickly become apparent if the patient is monitored frequently. If the PG concentration does not fall by 75–100 mg/dl in the first 2 hours, or if it does not steadily decline thereafter, the insulin dosage should be doubled; if necessary, the dosage is increased further until a response is seen. In rare patients, hyperglycemia but not ketoacidosis has responded, emphasizing the need to monitor plasma bicarbonate and the anion gap. Failure of hyperglycemia to respond implies inadequate fluid replacement as well.

4. Complications of insulin therapy include hypoglycemia and hypokalemia. Frequent monitoring of PG and potassium is necessary for their prevention.

5. After correction of DKA, SQ insulin must be given to control hyperglycemia and prevent recurrent ketosis. A simple method is to give one-half to two-thirds of the patient's usual dosage of intermediate-acting insulin SQ (10–20 units in patients with newly diagnosed diabetes), beginning the first morning after admission, even if DKA has not completely resolved. Electrolytes and PG are measured at 4- –6-hour intervals, and additional regular insulin is given as needed. A regular diet is begun as soon as tolerated, and the dosage of insulin is adjusted as described in sec. **V.D.**

E. Complications of DKA

1. **Shock** is usually the result of severe volume depletion and should be treated by vigorous fluid replacement with 0.9% NaCl; monitoring of central venous or pulmonary artery pressure is indicated. Acidosis should be treated with bicarbonate (see **C.3**) if arterial pH is <7.2. If shock is refractory to volume replacement, other causes should be suspected, including myocardial infarc-

tion, sepsis, hemorrhagic pancreatitis, GI hemorrhage, or mesenteric infarction.

2. **Lactic acidosis.** Mild increases in plasma lactate are common and resolve with fluid replacement. Severe lactic acidosis is usually associated with shock and requires vigorous administration of fluids and bicarbonate.

3. **Cerebral edema** is a rare complication of DKA, most often seen in children and adolescents. Usually occurring within 4–16 hours of initiation of therapy, it is marked by the development of headache, obtundation, and papilledema. Therapy with mannitol and glucocorticoids is recommended.

VIII. Hyperosmolar nonketotic coma

A. **Clinical findings.** Typical patients with hyperosmolar nonketotic coma are elderly, with NIDDM (often undiagnosed), and present with obtundation, severe dehydration, and shallow respirations without the odor of acetone. Seizures and focal neurologic abnormalities are common. These patients usually have underlying disease, most often renal failure. Precipitating factors include those listed in sec. **VII.B.2**, as well as a variety of drugs, including diuretics, glucocorticoids, and phenytoin. Marked hyperglycemia, hyperosmolarity, and azotemia are present, but the serum nitroprusside reaction is at most weakly positive.

B. **Therapy.** Treatment of hyperosmolar nonketotic coma is identical to that of DKA. Average fluid and electrolyte deficits are greater in the former (the mean volume deficit is about 9 liters), and their correction is the first priority of therapy. Since patients are usually elderly and often have renal failure, monitoring of central venous or pulmonary artery pressures is frequently indicated. Precipitating conditions, underlying disease, and complications must be carefully sought.

IX. Management of diabetes in the surgical patient

A. **General principles.** The stress of surgery exacerbates the metabolic abnormalities of DM, and careful attention to PG control is necessary. Elective procedures should be postponed until satisfactory control is achieved, and operations should be scheduled for early morning.

The goals of treatment are (1) prevention of hypoglycemia and ketoacidosis by maintaining the PG between 150 and 250 mg/dl and (2) maintenance of fluid and electrolyte balance. The key to achievement of these goals is frequent assessment of PG and plasma electrolytes. Additional regular insulin is given if PG exceeds 300 mg/dl, and the rate of glucose infusion is increased if PG is less than 150 mg/dl.

B. The choice of therapy is guided by the patient's usual treatment and the extent of surgery, but all regimens require frequent PG measurements and appropriate modification of therapy. Rapid bedside methods of BG determination facilitate management. **Sliding-scale methods of insulin administration based on urine tests should be abandoned.**

1. Patients treated with diet alone may not require specific therapy, but small doses of regular insulin should be given if the BG exceeds 300 mg/dl. If temporary insulin therapy is needed, purified pork insulin should be used to minimize the future risk of insulin allergy or resistance (see sec. **V.A.3.b**).

2. In patients treated with sulfonylureas, the drug should be omitted on the day of surgery. For minor operations, insulin need be given only if the PG exceeds 300 mg/dl. For major operations, 15–20 units of NPH insulin should be given on the morning of surgery and 5% dextrose infused at approximately 125 ml/hour. Additional regular insulin should be given as necessary.

3. In insulin-treated patients undergoing minor procedures, the administration of the morning insulin may be delayed until the procedure is completed and the patient is fed, with reduction of the dose by about one-third. For major

surgery, a 5% dextrose infusion should be instituted prior to surgery, and one-half the usual daily insulin dosage should be given as NPH insulin SQ. Additional regular insulin is given as indicated by frequent PG measurements, and 150–200 gm/day of dextrose should be administered IV. As long as the patient is unable to eat, NPH insulin in the preceding dosage may be given daily and supplemented with regular insulin if the PG exceeds 300 mg/dl.

   4. Emergency surgery in a patient with ketoacidosis should be delayed for several hours if possible, until volume depletion and acidosis can be corrected. If delay is impossible, therapy should be pursued vigorously during and after surgery.

X. Diabetes and pregnancy

A. Diagnosis. Diabetes in pregnancy is divided into gestational DM, in which the onset occurs during pregnancy, and pregestational DM, in which the onset antedates conception (see *Diabetes Care* 1:49, 1978). During pregnancy, fasting PG ranges from 60–80 mg/dl, but the PG response to oral carbohydrate is greater than in the nonpregnant state. Accordingly, diagnostic criteria for gestational DM differ from those for nonpregnant patients. If two or more of the following PG values (mg/dl) are exceeded on an oral glucose tolerance test, the diagnosis of gestational DM is made: fasting PG, 150; 1 hour, 190; 2 hours, 165; 3 hours, 145. If risk factors for gestational DM are present (e.g., family history of DM, history of stillbirth or high-birth-weight baby, obesity), an oral glucose tolerance test should be performed in the first trimester and, if normal, repeated in the second trimester.

B. Therapy

   1. Diet must provide adequate calories to meet the nutritional needs of pregnancy, generally about 300 kcal more than the calculated requirement. Since ketosis is clearly detrimental to the fetus, caloric restriction is not appropriate.

   2. Insulin. Strict control of PG reduces the incidence of fetal complications. The precise fasting PG at which insulin therapy is indicated is controversial, but lies between 105–115 mg/dl. Most patients with gestational DM can be well controlled with one or two injections of NPH per day, but patients with pregestational DM almost always require two injections of both regular and NPH insulin. Insulin requirements often decrease in the first trimester, increase after the twenty-fourth week, and fall suddenly postpartum.

   3. Monitoring. Urine tests are often misleading, since the lowered renal glucose threshold may result in glycosuria even with a normal PG. Therefore, home BG monitoring is particularly useful in pregnancy. The goal of therapy is a BG at or below 100 mg/dl throughout the day, except for brief periods after meals.

XI. Chronic complications

A. Retinopathy is divided into two forms: (1) background (microaneurysms, intraretinal hemorrhages and exudates) and (2) proliferative (abnormal new vessels anterior to the retina). The major threat to vision is neovascularization, with preretinal and vitreous hemorrhage or retinal detachment.

   1. Prevention. Hypertension is associated with an increased incidence of retinopathy and must be vigorously treated. There is evidence indicating that tight diabetic control may reduce the incidence of retinopathy.

   2. Treatment. Photocoagulation reduces the rate of visual loss due to proliferative retinopathy but must be performed before irreversible damage occurs. Hence, all diabetic patients should be examined by an ophthalmologist annually, those with proliferative changes more often. Vitrectomy may restore vision in some patients with blindness due to vitreous opacification.

B. Nephropathy is characterized by proteinuria followed by progressive renal failure and hypertension; in some patients the nephrotic syndrome develops. Treatment of hypertension slows the decline in glomerular filtration rate.

   1. Treatment of renal failure. Conservative therapy includes (1) a diet restricted in protein, sodium, and potassium; (2) control of hypertension; (3) treatment of fluid overload with diuretics; (4) correction of contributing factors, such as urinary infection and obstruction due to bladder dysfunction; and (5) adjustment in insulin dosage, since requirements often decrease when uremia develops.

   Hemodialysis in DM has been associated with a high morbidity and mortality. Transplantation is the preferred therapy for end-stage renal failure.

   2. Hyperkalemia out of proportion to the degree of renal dysfunction may occur. Defects in renin, aldosterone, and insulin secretion have been implicated. If hyperkalemia is severe (e.g., plasma potassium >6.0 mEq/liter), it can be reduced with fludrocortisone, 0.05–0.1 mg PO qd.

   3. Diabetic patients, especially those with azotemia, are prone to the development of **radiographic contrast–induced acute renal failure.** Alternative diagnostic procedures should be used when possible. If contrast administration is necessary, patients should be well hydrated, and serum creatinine and urine output should be monitored for several days afterward.

C. Neuropathy

   1. Peripheral neuropathy affects sensory function more often than motor function. Common manifestations are symmetric paresthesias, hypesthesia, pain, and loss of tendon reflexes. Care must be taken to prevent injury to hypesthetic areas, especially the feet.

   Treatment of neuropathic pain is often unsatisfactory. Improved control of PG sometimes helps. Phenytoin, 100 mg tid, may be tried; any response will be apparent within 1 week. Analgesics, including narcotics, may be required.

   2. Autonomic neuropathy

      a. Orthostatic hypotension is usually worst in the morning, and hence patients should arise from bed carefully. Symptoms may respond to fludrocortisone, 0.1–0.3 mg PO qd, along with a liberal salt intake, but this therapy may precipitate congestive heart failure.

      b. Impotence is common in diabetic men. Coincidental psychologic, pharmacologic, and endocrine causes should be considered, since there is no specific treatment for neurogenic impotence. However, satisfactory results have been obtained with penile prostheses in some patients.

      c. Neurogenic bladder due to impaired bladder sensation and loss of the detrusor reflex leads to urinary retention, often complicated by infection. Treatment includes voiding q3–4h during the day, with manual pressure if needed, cholinergic agents such as bethanechol 10–20 mg PO qid, and antibiotics if infection is present. More severe cases may require intermittent catheterization or surgery on the bladder neck.

      d. Gastrointestinal manifestations. Although the pathogenesis of diabetic **diarrhea** is unknown, bacterial overgrowth of the small intestine has been implicated in some cases, and a trial of tetracycline, 250 mg PO qid, is indicated. Most patients will require symptomatic therapy with opiates. Other causes of diarrhea, including celiac disease, should be sought. Impaired gastric emptying may produce recurrent vomiting. In a few cases, this has responded to metoclopramide, 10 mg PO before meals.

D. The diabetic foot. Neuropathy, vascular insufficiency, and infection all contribute to foot problems. Prevention is crucial, with careful foot cleaning and nail care, well-fitting shoes, daily inspection for injury, and prompt medical atten-

Table 20-3. Plasma lipids: 95th percentile values (mg/dl)

Age (yr)	Men Cholesterol	Men LDL Cholesterol	Women Cholesterol	Women LDL Cholesterol
15–19	197	130	203	137
20–24	218	147	228	159
25–29	244	165	229	164
30–34	254	185	238	156
35–44	269	187	249	173
45–54	277	200	277	193
55–64	276	207	295	217
>65	275	198	293	214

tion to any problems. Patients should never attempt to remove calluses or ingrown toenails themselves. Ulcers may respond to bed rest, debridement, and antibiotics; podiatric appliances to relieve local pressure may be useful.

Hyperlipidemia

The plasma cholesterol (C) concentration, particularly the low density lipoprotein cholesterol (LDL-C) is directly correlated with the risk of atherosclerotic cardiovascular disease. High density lipoprotein cholesterol (HDL-C), on the other hand, is inversely correlated with the risk of atherosclerotic cardiovascular disease. Plasma triglycerides (TG) also correlate with arteriosclerotic cardiovascular disease risk, and in some patients, such as those with diabetes, renal failure, or familial hypertriglyceridemia, TG may be an independent risk factor.

I. Diagnosis and classification

A. Definition. A practical definition of hyperlipidemia is a LDL–C level greater than the 95th percentile for age and sex (Table 20-3) or a TG level greater than 200 mg/dl.

Although C values tend to remain constant, TG levels fluctuate considerably and should be measured only after a 12- –14-hour fast, by which time chylomicrons have been cleared in normal persons. Lipids should be measured while the patients are on their usual diet and taking no medications that might influence plasma lipid levels. Sampling should not be performed within 6 weeks of a major illness (e.g., myocardial infarction), since plasma TG may be elevated and plasma C depressed for a time afterward. Because plasma lipid levels may fluctuate and because the diagnosis of hyperlipidemia may lead to lifelong treatment, elevated levels should be amply documented by at least three measurements at intervals of several weeks.

B. Characterization of hyperlipidemia as elevation of chylomicrons, very low density lipoproteins (VLDL) or LDL can be done using measurements of total plasma C and TG, HDL-C, and observation of a fasting plasma sample refrigerated overnight. Lipoprotein electrophoresis is not necessary.

1. **Chylomicrons** are detected as a cream layer on top of the refrigerated plasma.

2. **VLDL.** Elevated VLDL levels are indicated by elevated plasma TG (if chylomicrons are absent) or turbidity of the refrigerated plasma.

3. **LDL.** Since LDL contains most of plasma C, isolated C elevation usually indicates LDL excess. If TG levels are elevated but less than 400 mg/dl, the LDL-C level can be estimated:

LDL-C = total C − (TG/5 + HDL-C)

where TG/5 represents the C contained in VLDL.

4. The major disorder not detected by this method is familial dysbetalipoproteinemia (type III hyperlipoproteinemia), in which remnant particles accumulate in plasma. Both TG and C are usually elevated, and isoelectric focusing of VLDL is required for diagnosis.

C. **Classification.** Hyperlipidemias may be divided into primary disorders (which may be familial or sporadic) and secondary disorders (Table 20-4). Recognition of the latter is important, since treatment of the underlying disease usually corrects the hyperlipidemia.

Another common classification divides hyperlipidemia into six phenotypes based on the pattern of lipoprotein elevation. However, classification according to this scheme is not necessary for selection of therapy.

II. Drugs used to treat hyperlipidemia

A. **Bile acid sequestrants** (cholestyramine and colestipol) are anion-exchange resins that bind bile acids within the intestine and lower LDL: they may produce a rise in VLDL.

1. **Dosage.** The initial dosage of cholestyramine is 4 gm (1 packet) PO bid with meals, gradually increasing to 8–16 gm PO bid. The powder can be mixed with a variety of liquids to enhance its palatability. Colestipol is given in a similar fashion; the dosage is 15–30 gm PO daily in 2 doses.

2. **Side effects** include constipation, nausea, and abdominal cramps. The resins interfere with absorption of digoxin, thyroxine, warfarin, phenylbutazone, and chlorothiazide.

B. **Clofibrate** lowers VLDL levels. LDL levels usually fall but they may rise in some patients. The World Health Organization trial has raised serious doubts about the use of clofibrate (*Br. Heart J.* 40:1069, 1978). The clofibrate-treated group had an incidence of cardiovascular death similar to that of the controls and a significantly increased incidence of death from noncardiovascular causes. The drug is contraindicated in the presence of impaired renal or hepatic function.

1. The **dosage** is 1 gm PO bid.

2. **Side effects.** LDL-C may rise, in which case the drug should be stopped. The incidence of symptomatic gallstones is increased. Dysrhythmias, nausea, diarrhea, leukopenia, alopecia, impotence, and abnormalities in liver function tests may be observed. A myopathic syndrome is sometimes seen, most often in patients with renal failure. Clofibrate potentiates the effects of warfarin, phenytoin, and tolbutamide.

C. **Nicotinic acid** lowers both LDL and VLDL. It is most often used as a secondary drug in patients with LDL excess.

1. **Dosage.** The initial dosage is 100 mg PO tid with meals, gradually increasing to 1–3 gm tid.

2. **Side effects.** Flushing and pruritus are prominent. These effects usually abate over several weeks and can be minimized by gradually increasing the dosage. Nausea and diarrhea are reduced by taking the drug with meals. Other side effects include hepatotoxicity, dysrhythmias, hyperglycemia, hyperuricemia, activation of peptic ulcer, acanthosis nigricans, and hyperpigmentation.

Table 20-4. NIH classification of hyperlipoproteinemia

Phenotype	Lipoproteins elevated	Clinical consequences	Major secondary causes
I	Chylomicrons	Pancreatitis, eruptive xanthomas, lipemia retinalis	Poorly controlled diabetes, dysglobulinemias
IIA	LDL	Premature CAD, tendon xanthomas	Hypothyroidism, nephrotic syndrome, biliary obstruction, dysglobulinemias
IIB	LDL + VLDL	Premature CAD	Same as IIA
III	Remnants (chylomicron and VLDL degradation products)	Premature CAD and PVD, palmar and tuberous xanthomas	Hypothyroidism, alcoholism, dysglobulinemias, poorly controlled diabetes
IV	VLDL	Premature CAD	Diabetes, alcoholism, glucocorticoids, estrogens, renal failure
V	Chylomicrons + VLDL	Pancreatitis, eruptive xanothomas, lipemia retinalis	Alcoholism, poorly controlled diabetes, dysglobulinemias

CAD = coronary artery disease; PVD = peripheral vascular disease.

D. Neomycin lowers LDL levels when given PO. Although it is poorly absorbed, toxic blood levels may occur in patients with impaired renal or hepatic function or with inflammatory bowel disease. Its use is contraindicated in these conditions.

1. The **dosage** is 0.5–2.0 gm PO daily in divided doses.

2. **Side effects.** Deafness and renal failure may occur if blood levels are too high. Diarrhea, abdominal cramps, antibiotic-associated enterocolitis, and candidiasis may occur. Digoxin absorption is impaired.

E. Probucol is a recently introduced drug that lowers LDL and HDL. Little is known about its long-term effects.

1. **The recommended dosage** is 500 mg PO bid.

2. **Side effects.** Diarrhea, flatulence, nausea, and abdominal pain may occur.

F. D-Thyroxine lowers LDL. It shares the metabolic effects of the L-isomer to some extent. It is contraindicated in the elderly and in those with known heart disease. D-Thyroxine should be used only in younger patients with LDL excess in whom a bile acid sequestrant alone is inadequate.

1. **Dosage.** The initial dosage is 1 mg PO qd and is increased by increments of 1 mg/day at monthly intervals to a maximum of 4–8 mg qd.

2. **Side effects** include angina and myocardial infarction in patients with coronary disease, the effects of thyroid hormone excess, glucose intolerance, and hepatotoxicity. The effect of warfarin is potentiated.

III. Therapy

A. Rationale. Treatment of chylomicron excess can eliminate eruptive xanthomas and prevent pancreatitis. In most other forms of hyperlipidemia, the aim of therapy is to reduce the risk of atherosclerotic cardiovascular disease, based on the hypothesis that reduction of elevated lipid levels will lower this risk. Although there is evidence to support this hypothesis, it is still unproved, and thus the treatment of hyperlipidemia in asymptomatic patients should be undertaken only after careful consideration. In those at high risk of coronary artery disease (because of family history, diabetes, hypertension, or smoking) and with definite elevation of plasma LDL–C or TG, we feel that therapy aimed at reducing lipid levels is indicated.

B. Diet should always be the initial treatment and should be given an adequate trial (at least several months) before the addition of drug therapy.

1. **Most hyperlipidemias can be treated with a single basic diet** that includes (1) caloric restriction in the obese; (2) restriction of fat intake to 30–35% of calories; (3) restriction of saturated fat to 10% of calories; (4) restriction of C from the average United States intake of 500–750 mg/day to 300 mg or less; and (5) provision of up to 10% of calories as polyunsaturated fat. Patients with elevated VLDL should avoid alcohol.

2. **Isolated chylomicron excess** is treated by restriction of dietary fat to less than 30 gm/day. Medium-chain TGs may be substituted. The aim of therapy in this condition is prevention of abdominal pain and pancreatitis by maintaining plasma TG below 1000 mg/dl.

C. Drug therapy should be initiated only if lipid levels remain clearly elevated after an adequate trial of diet. Drugs should be continued only if they produce a substantial effect on lipid levels (e.g., a further reduction of 15%) without major side effects.

1. **VLDL excess.** The role of drug therapy is in doubt at present, since the evidence that VLDL is an independent risk factor for atherosclerotic cardiovascular disease is debated. Clofibrate has been widely used. Nicotinic acid will also reduce VLDL levels. These patients should avoid estrogens.

2. **LDL excess.** Cholestyramine or colestipol are the drugs of choice. If they do not adequately lower the plasma C, nicotinic acid may be added. Other secondary drugs are neomycin, probucol, clofibrate, and D-thyroxine. Drug therapy is often required in familial hypercholesterolemia.

3. **Familial dysbetalipoproteinemia** (type III hyperlipoproteinemia). If hyperlipidemia persists despite diet, clofibrate or nicotinic acid usually produces a good response.

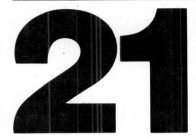

Arthritis and Related Disorders

Rheumatoid Arthritis

Rheumatoid arthritis (RA) is a systemic disease of unknown etiology with symmetric inflammation of synovial tissues as the dominant clinical manifestation. The course is variable but tends to be chronic and progressive. No curative therapy is available, but most patients can benefit from a combined program of medical, surgical, and rehabilitative services. Management has three goals: (1) suppression of inflammation in the joints and other tissues; (2) maintenance of joint function and prevention of deformities; and (3) repair of joint damage when such repair will relieve pain or improve function.

I. **Medical management**

A. **Salicylates,** of which **acetylsalicylate (aspirin)** is the prototype, are inhibitors of prostaglandin synthesis. They are anti-inflammatory as well as antipyretic and analgesic and sometimes are the only drugs required in patients with RA. Serum salicylate levels should be monitored; therapeutic serum levels are 15–25 mg/dl. Gastric irritation may be minimized by taking tablets after food or with antacids. Buffered preparations offer little advantage. **Enteric-coated tablets** cause less GI bleeding, but their absorption is variable, necessitating careful monitoring of serum levels during long-term administration. Combinations of aspirin with other drugs (phenacetin, antihistamines, acetaminophen, caffeine) have not been shown to be more effective than aspirin alone.

Magnesium salicylate, choline salicylate, choline magnesium trisalicylate, and **salsalate** are nonaspirin salicylate derivatives that may cause less GI distress than aspirin. In addition, choline magnesium trisalicylate and salsalate have long serum half-lives, permitting less frequent administration. They are more expensive than aspirin and may not be as effective.

1. **Indications** for salicylates are most conditions in which analgesic, antipyretic, or anti-inflammatory effects are desirable: osteoarthritis, traumatic arthritis, bursitis, ankylosing spondylitis, Reiter's syndrome, and psoriatic arthritis. They are often the first drugs chosen to treat RA.

2. **Metabolism.** Salicylates are metabolized by the liver and excreted by the kidneys. Alkalinization of the urine, as can occur with antacid or chronic buffered aspirin use, can significantly increase the rate of excretion.

3. **Administration.** Oral preparations and adult dosages of both aspirin and nonaspirin salicylates are listed in Table 21-1. For children with juvenile rheumatoid arthritis (JRA) weighing 25 kg or less, dosages of 90–130 mg/kg/day in 4–6 divided doses will achieve salicylate levels of 20–30 mg/dl; for children weighing more than 25 kg, a total daily dosage of 2400–3600 mg in divided doses is generally sufficient. Aspirin is also available as **rectal suppositories** for selected patients, but rectal absorption is erratic, and repeated use can cause rectal irritation. Serum salicylate levels should be drawn early (day 3 or 4) in the course of high-dose salicylate therapy (2–3 hours after the

Table 21-1. Nonsteroidal anti-inflammatory agents

Generic name	Trade name	Tablet size (mg)	Starting dose	Maximum daily dosage
Acetylsalicylate[a]	Aspirin	325	650–1300 q4–6h	[b]
Magnesium salicylate	Mobidin	600	600–1200 tid–qid	[b]
Choline salicylate	Arthropan liquid	1 tsp = 650	650 q4–6h	[b]
Choline magnesium trisalicylate	Trilisate	500, 750; 1 tsp = 500	1000–1250 bid; 2000–2500 qd	[b]
Salsalate	Disalcid	500	1000 tid or 1500 bid	[b]
Fenoprofen calcium	Nalfon	200, 300, 600	300–600 qid	3200
Ibuprofen	Motrin	300, 400, 600	400 qid	2400
Naproxen[a]	Naprosyn	250, 375, 500	250–375 bid	1000
Indomethacin	Indocin	25, 50, 75	25 tid; 75 qd	200
Tolmetin sodium[a]	Tolectin	200, 400	400 tid	2000
Sulindac	Clinoril	150, 200	150 bid	400
Meclofenamate sodium	Meclomen	50, 100	50 tid–qid	400
Phenylbutazone	Butazolidin	100	100 tid	600[c]
Oxyphenbutazone	Tandearil	100	100 tid	600[c]
Zomepirac sodium	Zomax	100	100 q6–8h	600
Naproxen sodium	Anaprox	275	275 q6–8h	1375
Piroxicam	Feldene	10, 20	20 qd	20

[a]See Rheumatoid Arthritis, secs. **I.A.3** and **I.B.1,3** for pediatric doses.
[b]Determined by measurement of serum salicylate level.
[c]See Rheumatoid Arthritis, sec. **I.B.6**.

last dose) to determine the achievement of a steady state. Thereafter, levels may be used periodically to determine patient compliance, to adjust the salicylate dose to a new steady state, or to confirm suspected toxicity.

4. **Contraindications.** Idiosyncratic reactions to salicylates occur, especially in patients with a history of asthma and nasal polyps. Salicylates must be avoided or given cautiously to such patients. Salicylates should be used carefully in patients with hyperuricemia; low dosages of aspirin (1.0–2.5 gm/day) are uricoretentive; high dosages (3–5 gm/day) are uricosuric. Salicylates can nullify the effect of probenecid and sulfinpyrazone and should not be given with these drugs. When salicylates are given with nonsteroidal anti-inflammatory drugs, the serum levels of these agents may be reduced; thus, combined use is not recommended. Because salicylates may reduce vitamin K–dependent clotting factors and thus potentiate warfarin, their use is contraindicated in patients taking anticoagulants.

5. **Side effects.** Gastrointestinal dysfunction (dyspepsia, nausea, vomiting, minimal GI blood loss) is the most common side effect. Massive bleeding and peptic ulceration are uncommon. Central nervous system toxicity (tinnitus, deafness, vertigo, irritability, incoherent speech, anorexia, diplopia, hallucinations, stupor, convulsions, coma, psychosis) tends to occur with high serum levels, particularly in the elderly. Reversible elevations of serum transaminases and alkaline phosphatase are occasionally seen with salicylate levels in the therapeutic range, especially in JRA and systemic lupus erythematosus (SLE). A reversible aspirin-induced depression of renal function (creatinine elevation of up to 1 mg/dl) has been seen in patients with SLE and RA, as well as in some normal persons. Uncommonly, even small amounts of aspirin can cause hypersensitivity reactions, including rhinitis, urticaria, angioedema, bronchial asthma, and vasomotor collapse. Caution must be used in patients with bleeding tendencies or coagulation defects, since platelet aggregation is irreversibly decreased by aspirin. Serum levels of 40–90 mg/dl are toxic and lead to salicylism with hyperventilation, respiratory alkalosis, metabolic acidosis, fever, coma, and ultimately dehydration, renal failure, and cardiovascular collapse (see Chap. 23).

B. **Other nonsteroidal anti-inflammatory drugs** (NSAIDs). These reversible prostaglandin synthesis inhibitors, discussed in **1–7**, are as effective as salicylates in treating various rheumatic diseases and can also be used to treat acute crystal-induced arthritis. These drugs, like salicylates, are antipyretic, analgesic, and anti-inflammatory, but they generally have fewer GI side effects and less ototoxicity than aspirin and are administered less frequently. All except fenoprofen, whose absorption is decreased when combined with food, should be administered PO with or after food to minimize GI irritation. Clinical experience suggests that patient response to an individual NSAID may be variable and at times unpredictable. Thus, if one drug is not effective during a 2- –3-week clinical trial, another should be tried. These drugs are considerably more expensive than aspirin.

The chief **side effects** of these agents are mild dyspepsia, nausea, and occasional headaches. Generally, patients sensitive to aspirin are also sensitive to these drugs. Reversible elevations of serum transaminases and inhibition of platelet aggregation can occur. Rarely, nephrotic syndrome and reversible renal failure, as well as cases of Stevens-Johnson syndrome, hemolytic anemia, aplastic anemia, vasculitis, and aseptic meningitis, have been reported in patients taking NSAIDs. These agents can cause salt retention, leading to edema or worsening of congestive heart failure. The NSAIDs should not be used in combinations with each other or with aspirin. Preparations and adult dosages are given in Table 21-1.

1. **Fenoprofen, ibuprofen,** and **naproxen** are propionic acid derivatives that are highly bound to plasma proteins. They can displace and increase the

toxicity of such drugs as the hydantoins, sulfonamides, and sulfonylureas. Propionic acid derivatives can be used with oral anticoagulants of the warfarin type, but careful monitoring of the prothrombin time is necessary whenever one of these drugs is started or stopped. Ibuprofen and tolmetin (see **3**) may be less likely to interact with anticoagulants. Naproxen may be used in children at a recommended dosage of 10 mg/kg/day in 2 divided doses.

2. **Indomethacin** is an indolacetic acid derivative. One-third to one-half of patients taking indomethacin experience untoward symptoms, and about 20% must discontinue its use. Gastrointestinal toxicity, including peptic ulceration and hemorrhage, can be more severe than with most other NSAIDs; thus, the drug should be avoided in patients with a prior history of ulcer disease. Central nervous system effects occur more commonly in the elderly and may include severe headache, dizziness, depression, hallucinations, and even seizures. Rarely, aplastic anemia, hemolytic anemia, leukopenia, and thrombocytopenia have been reported. The drug is contraindicated in pregnant and nursing women and in children under 14 years of age. Warfarin may be used without a dosage change, although prothrombin times should be checked periodically. A large bedtime dose (50–100 mg) may be effective in decreasing morning stiffness in RA patients. A sustained-release capsule is available for daily, single-dose therapy.

3. **Tolmetin** is a pyrrole chemically similar to indomethacin but with fewer GI and CNS side effects. It is approved for use in children (2 years and older). For children, the recommended starting dosage is 20 mg/kg/day in 3–4 divided doses; maintenance dosages range from 15–30 mg/kg/day. Dosages of warfarin anticoagulants are generally not altered by the use of tolmetin.

4. **Sulindac,** an indene acetic acid derivative, is structurally related to indomethacin but has less severe and less common adverse effects. Rash, pruritus, stomatitis, and hypersensitivity reactions have been reported. In most studies, no interaction with warfarin anticoagulants or oral hypoglycemic agents has been found. The drug is not recommended for use during pregnancy or lactation or for use in children.

5. **Meclofenamate sodium** is an anthranilic acid salt. Adverse GI effects, including a high incidence of severe diarrhea, and blood dyscrasias have been reported; thus, it is not a first-line choice among the NSAIDs. It is not recommended during pregnancy.

6. **Phenylbutazone** and **oxyphenbutazone** are more effective in the treatment of ankylosing spondylitis, traumatic tenosynovitis, bursitis, and acute gout than in the treatment of RA. However, their toxicity in comparison with other NSAIDs usually precludes their long-term use, because these drugs can cause severe bone marrow suppression (leukopenia, agranulocytosis, thrombocytopenia, aplastic anemia). **Physicians are obligated to obtain complete blood counts and platelet counts during a course of therapy,** although these determinations cannot always predict the development of blood dyscrasias.

   Severe GI side effects, including peptic ulceration, have also been associated with the use of these drugs. Both drugs prolong the prothrombin time in patients on warfarin anticoagulants and may potentiate the hypoglycemic effects of insulin and oral hypoglycemic agents.

   Initial recommended dosages vary with the severity of the inflammation. The total daily dosage should not exceed 600 mg, except for acute gout, for which 800 mg may be used during the first 24 hours only, followed by rapid tapering. Both drugs should be discontinued within 7–14 days.

7. Other NSAIDs include **naproxen sodium, zomepirac sodium,** and **mefenamic acid,** all of which have been marketed as having greater analgesic than anti-inflammatory effects. As a result, these agents and the prop-

ionic acid derivatives have been used for dysmenorrhea. **Naproxen sodium** is similar to naproxen and shares its toxicities. **Zomepirac sodium** is chemically related to tolmetin and has been approved for the relief of mild to moderately severe pain. Some studies have equated its analgesic effects to PO narcotics. Newer NSAIDs (e.g., **piroxicam**, an oxicam derivative) are available for daily, single-dose therapy. **Piroxicam** has toxicities similar to the other NSAIDs; it is not recommended for use in pregnant or nursing women.

C. Gold salts

1. **Indications.** Gold salts should be considered in patients with active synovitis who do not respond to conservative management, including salicylates or other NSAIDs. Patients who present with rapidly progressive, erosive arthritis are also candidates for immediate gold therapy. Gold is generally more effective than NSAIDs and may alter the natural history of RA by retarding the progression of bony erosions and joint-space narrowing. Thus, gold is considered a remitting agent, as opposed to the NSAIDs, which only relieve symptoms. About two-thirds of patients with RA who receive therapeutic amounts of gold show significant improvement. However, the drug is difficult to use because it requires frequent injections and close clinical and laboratory observation to monitor potentially serious toxicity. It has also been used successfully in JRA and psoriatic arthritis.

2. **Metabolism.** Water-soluble gold salts are absorbed rapidly from IM sites and reach maximal plasma concentrations in a few hours. The salts are deposited throughout the body, primarily in the reticuloendothelial system (liver and spleen), the renal tubules, and sites of inflammation such as the synovia. Excretion is primarily renal and is very slow; 85% of each dose is retained for at least 1 week. Measuring serum levels has not proved useful in predicting benefit or toxicity.

3. **Administration.** Gold salts are given by deep IM injection. **Gold sodium thiomalate (Myochrysine)** is an aqueous solution of the drug; **gold thioglucose (Solganal)** is a suspension in oil that slows absorption. The initial adult dose should be 50 mg. If this is tolerated without adverse effects, 50 mg should be given weekly thereafter. In children with JRA, the starting dose is 0.8–1.0 mg/kg (up to 50 kg). Improvement is gradual and continuous but is not seen until the cumulative dose has reached 400–800 mg. A NSAID should be continued for the symptomatic treatment of the arthritis while gold is introduced, and withdrawn slowly only after the gold has produced improvement. If no improvement occurs after a cumulative dose of 1000 mg, the drug should be discontinued.

In improved patients, the frequency of 50-mg injections can be reduced to every 2 weeks after 800–1000 mg of gold has been given. If this is well tolerated and improvement is maintained after 4 more doses, reduction to 50 mg every 3 weeks for 4 doses and ultimately to 50 mg/month can usually be accomplished. The dose of gold can often be reduced to 25 mg every 4 weeks in good responders who stay on the drug for long periods. If a relapse occurs as dosage intervals are increased, the preceding shorter dosage interval should be reinstituted until the relapse remits. If gold is discontinued, the disease usually flares within a few months and is often refractory to reinitiation of the drug. Therefore, good responders who do not have adverse effects are maintained indefinitely on monthly gold injections. Nevertheless, synovitis refractory to gold administration occurs in many patients after a few years of good response, and a major change in drug therapy is then required.

An oral gold preparation **(Auranofin)** is now available. In single or 2 divided doses of 2–9 mg/day, oral gold appears as effective as injectable gold in the treatment of RA and may cause less serious renal and hematologic toxicity; however, GI toxicity, including abdominal pain and diarrhea, is more common than with injectable gold.

4. Contraindications and side effects

a. Gold is contraindicated in patients with known gold allergies or in those who have had a severe toxic reaction. Although some toxicity is seen in over 50% of patients, it necessitates discontinuing the drug in less than 15%. Undesirable reactions can occur at any time during therapy, but toxicity usually does not appear until after 300–500 mg of gold salts have been administered. The most common manifestation of gold toxicity is **dermatitis,** often heralded by pruritus or eosinophilia. **Stomatitis** can accompany the rash or can occur alone. The injections should be stopped until the skin and mucous membrane lesions improve. A small test dose can then be given, and, if this is tolerated, therapy can be continued as previously outlined.

b. Gold **nephropathy,** probably occurring by an immune mechanism, is usually first manifested by proteinuria or microscopic hematuria. A urinalysis should be performed before each gold injection. If urinary abnormalities appear, therapy should be interrupted until the urine is normal and then reinstituted at small doses. If the abnormalities recur, gold must be stopped. Nephrotic syndrome is a severe reaction necessitating permanent discontinuance of therapy. It is usually reversible, and advancement to renal failure is rare.

c. The most serious side effects of gold are **hematologic:** thrombocytopenia, leukopenia, agranulocytosis, and aplastic anemia. The physician must obtain complete blood and platelet counts frequently, even though such testing will not detect all patients in whom a major hematologic complication will develop. For the first few months of therapy, hemograms should be done before each gold injection. If no changes occur after 3–4 months, the tests can be done at 2- –4-week intervals and ultimately at 6- –8-week intervals. **Management** of severe gold toxicity has included the administration of glucocorticoids, chelating agents (e.g., dimercaprol [BAL]), or both, but there is little evidence that either of these therapies has influenced the outcome of this life-threatening problem.

d. "**Nitritoid reactions,**" consisting of flushing, sweating, dizziness, and syncope, can occur soon after an injection but are rare and usually can be avoided by using oil-based gold thioglucose. Transient increased stiffness, arthralgias, and myalgias occasionally seen after gold injections can also be ameliorated by use of the thioglucose preparation. Rarely, reversible cholestatic jaundice and syndromes of reversible diffuse pulmonary injury and ulcerative intestinal disease have been reported with gold therapy.

D. D-Penicillamine (Cuprimine, Depen) is the D-isomer of 3-mercaptovaline.

1. Indications. Penicillamine is an effective remitting agent in the treatment of RA. However, because of potentially severe adverse effects, its use is restricted to patients who do not benefit from more conservative management, who have rapidly progressive, erosive synovitis, or who cannot take gold therapy for logistic reasons or toxic reactions. Penicillamine therapy requires careful monitoring of multiple clinical and laboratory parameters, as well as a reliable patient who will report for frequent follow-up visits.

2. Metabolism. Penicillamine is rapidly absorbed from the GI tract and excreted in the urine.

3. Administration. Penicillamine, available in 125- and 250-mg capsules (Cuprimine) and in a scored 250-mg tablet (Depen), is given PO once daily between meals to avoid chelation with dietary metals. Significant toxicities in early reports of penicillamine use have been reduced with a "go low, go slow" dosage schedule: 250 mg is given qd for 4–8 weeks, followed by a 125- –250-mg increase in daily dose every 4–8 weeks until clinical improvement occurs or until a daily dose of 750 mg is reached. Improvement is usually not seen before 3–6 months of treatment. If no response is seen at a daily dosage of 750 mg for 2–3 months, an increase to 1000 mg/day can be tried, although the incidence of adverse reactions greatly increases at this dosage.

Patients who manifest improvement without toxicity are maintained on penicillamine indefinitely. If the patient's condition is stable, the daily dose may be reduced by 125 mg every 3–6 months to attain the lowest dosage that will maintain a good response. Concomitant NSAID therapy should be continued and only tapered when penicillamine produces a good response. **Gold and penicillamine should not be used together.**

4. **Contraindications and side effects.** Some patients with a previous history of penicillin allergy, especially anaphylaxis, may also be sensitive to penicillamine. They should have a skin test prior to the initiation of penicillamine therapy to determine their current allergic status. Densensitization may be required.

   a. **Rash** is the most common side effect of treatment. A generalized eruption occurring in the first weeks of therapy will usually disappear when the drug is withdrawn and often does not recur when the drug is reintroduced at lower doses. Rashes seen after months of therapy are often pruritic, may resemble pemphigus, and require discontinuance of the drug. Restarting penicillamine after this reaction is dangerous. When a rash occurs with fever, rechallenge should be avoided.

   b. Alterations of taste **(hypogeusia)** are common in the first months of therapy but will usually abate even if therapy is continued. Treatment of this symptom with zinc is not effective and may interfere with the penicillamine therapy. **Stomatitis,** sometimes severe, can occur. It often resolves when the drug is discontinued and may not recur when the drug is reinstituted at a low dose. Cholestatic jaundice, dyspepsia, nausea, vomiting, skin changes (wrinkling, yellowing, blistering with scarring), and impairment in wound healing have been rarely reported.

   c. Life-threatening **hematologic complications** include leukopenia, agranulocytosis, aplastic anemia, and, most commonly, thrombocytopenia. Such reactions are usually reversible if the drug is discontinued immediately. Hemograms and platelet counts should be obtained weekly for 1–2 months, biweekly for 3–4 months, and at least monthly thereafter. Because counts can drop precipitously despite close monitoring, patients should be alerted to the signs of potential complications.

   d. **Proteinuria** can occur in up to 15% of patients on penicillamine therapy. It usually begins after 6–12 months of treatment and may require up to 2 years to resolve if it is necessary to stop therapy. If proteinuria exceeds 2 gm/day, or if hematuria develops and persists for a few weeks, the drug should be discontinued. The dose of penicillamine should never be increased in the presence of proteinuria, and some authors advocate a decrease of at least 125 mg/day in dosage when any degree of proteinuria develops.

   e. Penicillamine is teratogenic and should not be used during pregnancy.

   f. Rarely, several **autoimmune syndromes,** including myasthenia gravis, Goodpasture's syndrome, polymyositis, SLE, and fibrosing alveolitis, have been reported in association with penicillamine therapy.

E. **Hydroxychloroquine (Plaquenil)** is an antimalarial agent with moderate antiinflammatory effects that is useful in the treatment of RA as well as discoid and systemic lupus erythematosus.

   1. **Indications.** Hydroxychloroquine is used in patients with RA who fail to respond to more conservative NSAIDs, in some patients with moderate dis-

ease before gold or penicillamine are tried, or in patients who are unable to take gold or penicillamine (also see Systemic Lupus Erythematosus, sec. **I.C**).

2. **Metabolism.** Hydroxychloroquine is well absorbed from the GI tract and deposited in many tissues. The drug and its metabolites undergo slow renal excretion.

3. **Administration.** Therapy is usually initiated with one 200-mg tablet daily, although higher dosages (400–600 mg daily) can be used for 2–3 weeks in patients with very active arthritis. The response to this drug is slow, requiring 6 weeks to 6 months for beneficial effects. Long-term administration of more than 400 mg/day should be avoided because of eye toxicity (see **4**).

4. **Contraindications and side effects.** Hydroxychloroquine should not be used in patients with porphyria, glucose 6-phosphate dehydrogenase (G-6-PD) deficiency, or significant hepatic or renal impairment. It is also contraindicated in children and pregnant women. The most common **side effects** are allergic skin eruptions and GI disturbances. Serious **ocular effects** were often reported when higher dosages of the drug were used but are rare with current dosage recommendations. Hydroxychloroquine can be deposited in the cornea, leading to blurred vision or the appearance of halos around lights, a complication that is reversible if the drug is stopped promptly. More important, retinal deposition can lead to irreversible damage, although blindness is rare. Because subjective evaluations of visual changes will not detect early retinal lesions, every patient taking the drug must be seen by an ophthalmologist at 6-month intervals for a complete examination, including color vision testing and static visual fields. At the first sign of any visual impairment, especially reduced sensitivity to red light, the drug should be stopped. Rare complications of therapy include myopathy, neuropathy, ototoxicity, bone marrow suppression, emotional changes, and bleaching of the hair.

F. **Glucocorticoids.** Although glucocorticoids are not curative and probably do not alter the natural history of RA, they are the most potent anti-inflammatory drugs available.

1. **Indications.** Patients with RA who continue to have active synovitis in many joints despite a sufficient trial of NSAIDs, gold, penicillamine, or hydroxychloroquine are candidates for systemic glucocorticoid therapy. In addition, patients who have severe constitutional symptoms, such as fever, weight loss, anemia, vasculitis, and neuropathy, should also receive glucocorticoids. An occasional patient, incapacitated by arthritis and at risk of complications from immobility, can also be treated in an attempt to control the disease while waiting for slower-acting remitting agents to take effect. Once an arthritis patient is treated with glucocorticoids, it is often difficult to discontinue them entirely. Therefore, the smallest effective dosage should be used.

2. **Metabolism.** See Systemic Lupus Erythematosus, sec. **II.B.**

3. **Systemic administration.** The various glucocorticoid preparations are discussed under Systemic Lupus Erythematosus, sec. **II.** When used in non-life-threatening situations, an attempt should be made to start the patient on **alternate-day therapy** (a cumulative 2-day dose given q48h in the morning). This regimen lowers the incidence of some undesirable side effects—with the exception of cataract development and osteopenia—from that seen with equivalent dosages of daily steroids. Patients may not tolerate the flare of disease likely to occur on the "off" day, but the advantage in safety is considerable if such a regimen will suffice. Glucocorticoid preparations used in alternate-day therapy must be short acting to obtain these beneficial effects (see Table 21-2).

"Pulse-dose" glucocorticoid therapy (1 gm methylprednisolone given IV over 30–40 minutes each day for 1–3 days) may control a flare in patients

Table 21-2. Glucocorticoid preparations

Generic name	Trade name	Tablet size (mg)	Relative anti-inflammatory potency	Relative mineralo-corticoid potency	Approximate equivalent dose (mg)	Usual starting dose (mg/day) Moderate illness	Severe illness
Short-acting							
Hydrocortisone (cortisol)	Cortef, Solu-Cortef[a]	5, 10, 20	1.0	1.0	20.0	80–160	
Cortisone		5, 10, 25	0.8	0.8	25.0	100–200	
Prednisone	Deltasone, Meticorten	1, 2.5, 5, 10, 20, 50	4.0	0.8	5.0	20–40	60–100
Prednisolone	Delta-Cortef, Meticortelone	5	4.0	0.8	5.0	20–40	60–100
Methylprednisolone	Medrol, Solu-Medrol[a]	2, 4, 8, 16, 24, 32	5.0	0.5	4.0	16–32	48–80 / 1000 pulse[b]
Intermediate-acting							
Triamcinolone	Aristocort, Kenacort	1, 2, 4, 8, 16	5.0	0	4.0	16–32	48–80
Paramethasone	Haldrone	1, 2	10.0	0	2.0	8–16	24–40
Long-acting							
Dexamethasone	Decadron, Hexadrol	0.25, 0.5, 0.75, 1.5, 4	25.0	0	0.75	3–6	9–15
Betamethasone	Celestone	0.6	25.0	0	0.6	2.4–4.8	7.2–12.0

[a]Parenteral forms: Dosages of oral and parenteral preparations are generally comparable.
[b]See Systemic Lupus Erythematosus, sec. **II.D.**

with active RA. A modification of this regimen utilizes a single dose of methylprednisolone, 1 gm IV monthly. The long-term complications of such therapy are unknown.

4. **Intraarticular administration** is useful for the temporary relief of pain when inflammation in only a few joints is present. The beneficial effects of intraarticular steroids can persist for days to months. The frequent use of injections is controversial, since animal models demonstrate accelerated cartilage destruction. Rarely, frequent injections can lead to systemic side effects. However, this therapy is often useful and may delay or negate the need for systemic glucocorticoid therapy.

   Triamcinolone hexacetonide (Aristospan) or **triamcinolone acetonide (Kenalog)** are effective intermediate-acting glucocorticoids well suited for intraarticular use. Doses vary from 2–5 mg in a finger joint to 25–50 mg in a knee. Up to 1 ml of 1% lidocaine (or its equivalent) may be administered simultaneously to promote immediate relief.

   The risk of introducing infections requires proper sterile technique. Synovial fluid should be removed from swollen joints during the arthrocentesis to relieve capsular swelling and to identify any potential infection that can mimic an acute monoarticular flare in RA. If the fluid does not look grossly purulent, the steroid can be injected immediately; however, if an infection is suspected when the fluid is seen, the steroid should not be injected unless cultures of the fluid are negative. An evanescent postinjection swelling may occur because of inflammation induced by microcrystallization of the steroid, but this usually subsides within a day. If it does not, the possibility of having introduced an infection must be considered.

5. **Contraindications and side effects.** See Systemic Lupus Erythematosus, sec. **II.E.**

G. **Cytotoxic drugs.** Three classes of immunosuppressive drugs have been studied in patients with RA: the purine antagonist **azathioprine (Imuran)**; the alkylating agents **cyclophosphamide (Cytoxan)** and **chlorambucil (Leukeran)**; and the folic acid antagonist **methotrexate**.

1. **Indications.** Cytotoxic drugs are indicated in patients with severe RA refractory to standard therapy, including salicylates, gold, penicillamine, and glucocorticoids, or in patients with severe disease who cannot tolerate standard drug therapy. Because of the toxicity of cytotoxic drugs, they should be reserved for patients who are significantly disabled by active synovitis or by systemic manifestations of rheumatoid disease. Patients must be well informed, cooperative, and willing to permit meticulous follow-up by the physician.

2. **Metabolism.** See Chap. 17.

3. **Administration and dosage.** With cytotoxic drugs, it is desirable to begin therapy with relatively small doses to minimize the chances of bone marrow suppression. **Peripheral blood counts must be monitored closely.**

   a. **Azathioprine** (25- or 50-mg tablets) is initiated at approximately 1.0 mg/ kg/day given as a single dose or in 2 divided doses. If GI toxicity occurs, a single bedtime dose may minimize this side effect. If there are no serious toxicities or if the initial response is unsatisfactory after 4–6 weeks, the dosage may be increased over a few weeks by increments of 0.5 mg/kg/ day, up to a maximum dosage of 2.5 mg/kg/day. **Since allopurinol (Zyloprim) decreases the metabolism of azathioprine, the concomitant administration of these two agents requires a 60–75% reduction in the dosage of azathioprine.**

   b. **Cyclophosphamide** (25- and 50-mg tablets) is started in relatively small, single oral dosages of 1.5–2.0 mg/kg/day. This dosage can be raised to

2.5–3.0 mg/kg/day over a few weeks if complete blood counts and platelet counts remain normal and no other toxicity appears. For patients with RA, a daily dosage of 3 mg/kg is considered maximal. Cyclophosphamide must be given in the morning with a large fluid load; patients should be encouraged to void frequently to minimize the chances of a toxic cystitis.

   c. **Chlorambucil** (2-mg tablets) is administered in an initial single oral dosage of 0.05 mg/kg/day. This dosage may be slowly increased over a few weeks to a maximum of 0.15 mg/kg/day if the initial response is poor and no serious toxicities are present.

   d. With **azathioprine, cyclophosphamide,** and **chlorambucil,** objective evidence of improvement may begin after 6–12 weeks of therapy. If there is no response after 16 weeks, the drug should be discontinued. After synovitis has been controlled for several months, it is desirable to taper slowly and then discontinue the agent. A flare may result, but this risk must be balanced by the increased risk of malignancy (lymphoma, leukemia) with long-term use.

   e. **Methotrexate** (2.5-mg tablets) is initiated at 2.5 mg PO q12h for 3 consecutive doses/week (total dosage, 7.5 mg/week). If no improvement is noted after 4–6 weeks of treatment, the dosage can be doubled to 5 mg q12h for 3 doses/week (total dosage of 15 mg/week). If no response has occurred within 10–12 weeks of therapy, the patient is considered a nonresponder, and the drug is discontinued. If the patient responds to the drug, it is continued for several months and then slowly tapered and eventually discontinued. Methotrexate administered in this manner has less hepatotoxicity than daily methotrexate therapy. In our experience, the total PO weekly dosage may be administered IM if oral ulcers occur; the basis for this phenomenon is not understood.

 4. **Contraindications and side effects.** See Chap. 17.

II. **Surgical treatment.** Corrective surgical procedures are sometimes indicated in patients with RA in an attempt to reduce pain and to improve function. Synovectomy may be tried if major involvement is limited to one or two joints and a 6-month trial of therapy with salicylates, NSAIDs, and a more specific remitting agent, such as gold or penicillamine, has failed. Usually, however, this procedure is only temporarily effective. Inability to extend one or more fingers suggests rupture of the extensor tendons requiring surgical repair as soon as possible. Other procedures that may be successful in restoring function and decreasing pain include total hip and knee replacements and resection of metatarsal heads in patients with bunion deformities and subluxation of the toes. Hand surgery to restore function of the metacarpophalangeal and the proximal interphalangeal joints may be useful in carefully selected patients. Surgical fusion of joints usually results in freedom from pain but total loss of motion. This is well tolerated in the wrist and thumb but may be disabling in the knee. When cartilage loss or joint deformity are contributing significantly to pain and disability, management by a team consisting of an internist, orthopedic surgeon, and rehabilitation expert is desirable.

III. **Adjunctive measures.** The physician must provide both medical and emotional support and educational information to RA patients. Tranquilizers or antidepressants may be used if necessary. Pamphlets about RA are available from the Arthritis Foundation.

Systemic and articular rest may be accomplished by the proper amount of bed rest and may be further enhanced by simple orthopedic supports, such as a splint used overnight.

Active-assistive exercises done within the limits of pain should be instituted early to maintain or to improve range of motion. Progressive resistive exercises are indicated to improve muscular function when the activity of the disease subsides.

Heat may be useful for its muscle-relaxing and mild analgesic effects when administered before the performance of exercises.

Physical and occupational therapists can instruct patients in work simplification, in joint positioning and protection, and in the performance of the activities of daily living.

Variants of Rheumatoid Arthritis

I. **Juvenile rheumatoid arthritis.** Juvenile rheumatoid arthritis can occur both in children and in adults. In children it has five modes of presentation: (1) **pauciarticular** (four or fewer joints), **early onset** (30%); (2) **pauciarticular, late onset** (15%); (3) **polyarticular** (five or more joints) **seropositive** (5%); (4) **polyarticular seronegative** (30%); and (5) **systemic onset,** or Still's disease (20%). In the adult, JRA usually presents as Still's disease, with high, spiking fevers, polyserositis, arthralgias, myalgias, evanescent macular rash, and polyarthritis. Laboratory abnormalities are nonspecific (elevated erythrocyte sedimentation rate, leukocytosis, mild anemia), and IgM rheumatoid factors by standard testing are usually absent.

Four major **medical therapies** are widely used in children: **salicylates, NSAIDs, gold salts,** and **glucocorticoids,** both systemic and intraarticular. In addition, topical steroids are useful for the treatment of iridocyclitis. Other drugs used with varying efficacy in the treatment of JRA include penicillamine and the immunosuppressives chlorambucil and azathioprine; these drugs should be reserved for the treatment of severe JRA refractory to more conservative management. The same drugs are used to treat Still's disease in adults (see Rheumatoid Arthritis for dosages).

II. **Sjögren's syndrome.** Sjögren's syndrome is a chronic disorder characterized by insufficient production of lacrimal and salivary secretions associated with autoantibodies or autoimmune diseases, usually RA. It may also be associated with polymyositis, SLE, or scleroderma. These patients are at higher risk of the development of B-cell lymphomas and vasculitis than the normal population. Peripheral neuropathies, defects of renal tubular function (e.g., renal tubular acidosis), pulmonary fibrosis, and diffuse lymphadenopathy can also develop in these patients. All these conditions are variably responsive to glucocorticoids. The use of artificial tears is essential for protection of the cornea. Gold salts can be used safely and effectively for the arthritis in RA patients with Sjögren's syndrome.

III. **Felty's syndrome.** Felty's syndrome is a triad of RA, splenomegaly, and granulocytopenia occurring in patients with severe, long-standing, and, in some cases, "burnt-out" arthritis. Hematologic abnormalities, including anemia and mild thrombocytopenia, may also be present. Frequent infections and chronic leg ulcers are common complications. The response of granulocytopenia to glucocorticoids is usually disappointing, since an elevated cell count is seldom sustained when glucocorticoids are tapered to lower dosages. Recurrent infections may be an indication for splenectomy, although granulocytopenia recurs in more than one-third of patients during long-term follow-up, and some patients continue to have frequent infections in spite of sustained improvement in granulocyte counts. A few reports suggest that the use of gold, penicillamine, and lithium may increase leukocyte counts and reduce the incidence of infections.

Ankylosing Spondylitis

Ankylosing spondylitis is a form of arthritis occurring predominantly in males. It is characterized by inflammation and ossification of the joints and ligaments of the spine and of the sacroiliac joints. The hips and shoulders are the most commonly involved peripheral joints. Approximately 95% of whites and 50% of blacks with ankylosing spondylitis are HLA-B27 positive.

Because progression of the spinal disease cannot be prevented at present, the therapeutic goal is to maximize the opportunity for the apophyseal joints of the spine to fuse in a straight line. Such fusion minimizes eventual postural and respiratory defects and helps to control pain. Patients should be instructed to sleep on their backs on a bed board without a pillow and to practice postural and deep-breathing exercises regularly. High-dose salicylate therapy is usually ineffective in controlling pain. However, other NSAIDs may provide symptomatic relief; indomethacin and phenylbutazone are the two NSAIDs most commonly used (see Rheumatoid Arthritis, sec. **I.B**). Glucocorticoid therapy may be tried in unusual patients who do not respond to other agents. Surgical procedures to correct some spine and hip deformities are available and can result in significant rehabilitation in carefully selected patients. Anterior uveitis occurs in up to 25% of patients with ankylosing spondylitis and can lead to glaucoma or blindness. Thus, regular ophthalmologic evaluations are advisable.

Reiter's Syndrome

Reiter's syndrome occurs predominantly in males and consists of asymmetric polyarthritis, urethritis, conjunctivitis, and characteristic skin and mucous membrane lesions. Since approximately 75% of whites and 40% of blacks with the disease are HLA-B27 positive, this marker can aid in diagnosis. The syndrome is usually a transient illness, lasting from one to several months; recurrences associated with varying degrees of disability are common.

In general, a conservative regimen is indicated to control pain and inflammation until a spontaneous remission occurs. High-dose salicylates are usually ineffective, but other NSAIDs are often useful (see Rheumatoid Arthritis, sec. **I.B**). Improvement is generally evident within a few days, and, as inflammation subsides, the drug can be tapered to the smallest dose necessary to control symptoms. In unusually severe cases, therapy with glucocorticoids or even cytotoxic agents may be required to prevent rapid joint destruction. Conjunctivitis is usually transient and benign, but if iritis occurs, treatment with topical or systemic glucocorticoids is indicated. Cutaneous and urethral inflammation usually subsides as the arthritis improves.

Systemic Lupus Erythematosus

Systemic lupus erythematosus is a multisystem disease of unknown etiology with a highly variable course. Women of childbearing age are affected primarily. Among its protean manifestations are fatigue, malaise, arthritis or arthralgia, fever, photosensitive skin eruptions, serositis, weight loss, nephritis, CNS involvement, pneumonitis, and myocarditis. Hematologic abnormalities include anemia, leukopenia (often present during flares), and thrombocytopenia (potentially life-threatening). Numerous autoantibodies are found in the serum; antinuclear antibodies are present in over 95% of patients. Hypocomplementemia and high level anti–native DNA antibodies are associated with disease flares (especially nephritis) in over half the patients. Treatment of this disorder is directed at the suppression of the disease manifestations, because no therapy is curative.

I. **Conservative therapy.** Conservative therapy should be used if the patient's manifestations are mild.

A. **General supportive measures.** Mild flares may subside after a few days of rest. Adequate sleep, midafternoon naps, and avoidance of fatigue are recommended. Although skin eruptions can be reduced by lotions of para-aminobenzoic acid (e.g., PreSun, Total Eclipse) with a minimum rating of 15, avoidance of sun exposure is best for photosensitivity. Isolated skin lesions can be treated with topical glucocorticoids.

B. The **NSAIDs** occasionally control arthritis, arthalgias, fever, and serositis, although they are less effective than glucocorticoids. Hepatic and renal toxicities of the NSAIDs must be monitored (see Rheumatoid Arthritis, sec. **I.B**). A few cases of aseptic meningitis have been reported with the use of ibuprofen in SLE patients. Fatigue, malaise, and major organ system involvement usually do not respond to NSAIDs.

C. Hydroxychloroquine may be effective in the treatment of skin lesions in discoid lupus and in the treatment of rashes, photosensitivity, arthalgias, pleuritis, and malaise associated with SLE. Skin lesions may begin to improve within a few days, but joint symptoms may take 6–10 weeks to subside. The drug is not effective in the treatment of fever or of renal, CNS, or hematologic problems in seriously ill patients (see Rheumatoid Arthritis, sec. **I.E**).

II. Glucocorticoid therapy

A. Indications for the use of systemic glucocorticoids are life-threatening or debilitating manifestations: diffuse glomerulonephritis, CNS involvement, hemolytic anemia, thrombocytopenia, myocarditis, systemic involvement unresponsive to conservative regimens, and vasculitis resulting in infarction of the skin, retina, or peripheral nerves.

B. Pharmacology. Glucocorticoids are both anti-inflammatory and immunosuppressive. Oral forms of hydrocortisone and its synthetic analogues are well absorbed by the intestine. The serum half-life of various synthetic glucocorticoids varies from a few minutes to several hours, but anti-inflammatory effects and adrenal suppression are not directly related to this half-life. Long-term administration of phenytoin or phenobarbital increases the metabolic clearance of glucocorticoids by induction of hepatic microsomal enzymes.

C. Preparations are listed in Table 21-2.

D. Dosage and routes of administration. The goal of glucocorticoid therapy is to suppress disease manifestations with a minimal amount of drug. Glucocorticoids should be given PO when possible, although parenteral preparations are available when needed. Long-acting depot glucocorticoid suspensions are erratically absorbed and should not be used in acute situations. Once-daily (A.M.) administration of a steroid is usually adequate for patients who are not acutely ill, but administration of prednisone in 2–4 divided doses/day may be necessary to control severe inflammatory disease. When the acute phase resolves, administration can be shifted to once in the morning.

Patients with life-threatening complications of SLE should be treated with 60–100 mg prednisone or the equivalent daily; some patients may require 200–300 mg/day initially. After the disease is controlled, the drug should be **slowly tapered,** e.g., by reducing the dosage by 10% every 5–7 days; a more rapid reduction may result in relapse. Maintenance dosage of prednisone is generally 10–20 mg daily or 20–40 mg every other day.

Intravenous "pulse" therapy has been utilized in SLE in such life-threatening situations as rapidly progressive renal failure, active CNS abnormalities, and severe thrombocytopenia. In this regimen, 500 mg of methylprednisolone is given by IV drip over 30 minutes q12h for 2–5 days. Patients who do not show improvement on this regimen are probably unresponsive to steroids, and other therapeutic alternatives must be considered. If improvement does occur, prednisone 100 mg/day PO is begun, and slow tapering is initiated as clinically permitted.

Alternate-day schedules (see Rheumatoid Arthritis, sec. **I.F.3**) markedly reduce the untoward effects of long-term glucocorticoid therapy but are usually ineffective in patients with severe, active disease.

E. Side effects. All glucocorticoid preparations have similar side effects, which are related to both dosage and duration of administration.

1. Different synthetic glucocorticoids **suppress the hypothalamic-pituitary-adrenal axis** for variable periods of time. It is thus desirable to control disease with short-acting preparations (24- –36-hour suppression), such as prednisone (least expensive) or methylprednisolone, rather than long-acting preparations (48-hour suppression), such as dexamethasone. For alternate-day use, a short-acting steroid is required and should be given in the morning to approximate more closely the normal morning cortisol surge.

   Hypoadrenalism may appear at times of severe stress (infection, major operations, serious intercurrent illnesses) in patients who are receiving glucocorticoid therapy. These patients should wear a Medic Alert bracelet or carry other identification to alert medical personnel that they would require supplemental glucocorticoids in an emergency situation. Also, patients who have received more than 10 mg of prednisone (or its equivalent) for more than several weeks may have some degree of axis suppression for months following cessation of therapy.

   To avoid possible adrenal insufficiency, hydrocortisone, 100 mg or equivalent, may be given IV or IM 6 hours before and immediately preceding an operation. During the surgery, 100–200 mg of hydrocortisone should be infused IV. Postoperatively, the dose should be tapered to the usual maintenance level over 2–5 days if no complications occur. Patients with acute medical illnesses should usually receive approximately double their maintenance dose of glucocorticoids for a few days, with rapid tapering to maintenance levels during recovery.

2. Resistance to **infections** is decreased by glucocorticoid therapy. Thus, minor infections may become systemic, quiescent infections may become activated, and organisms that are usually nonpathogenic may cause disease. Local and systemic signs of infection can be partially masked, although fever associated with infection is generally not completely suppressed by glucocorticoids. Regular immunizations with influenza and pneumococcal vaccines may be worthwhile as prophylactic measures.

3. **Changes in physical appearance,** including moon facies, redistribution of fat, acne, hirsutism, purplish striae, and easy bruisability can be emotionally disturbing. Most of these changes are at least partially reversible as the dosage is reduced.

4. **Mental reactions** to glucocorticoids can range from mild nervousness, euphoria, and insomnia to severe depression or psychosis (which can be confused with the CNS manifestations of SLE).

5. **Hyperglycemia** may be induced or aggravated by glucocorticoids, but it is usually not a contraindication to therapy, since ketoacidosis is rare. Insulin therapy may be required.

6. **Electrolyte abnormalities** include sodium retention and hypokalemia. Patients with congestive heart failure and peripheral edema should receive glucocorticoids with minimal mineralocorticoid properties (see Table 21-2). **Hypertension** may be induced or aggravated by glucocorticoids.

7. **Osteopenia** occurs in most patients receiving glucocorticoid therapy for several months; vertebral compression fractures occur in 10–15% of patients receiving long-term steroid therapy. Therapy with vitamin D, 50,000 units PO 2–3 times/week, or 25-OH vitamin D, 50 μg PO 5 times/week, and supplemental calcium (500–1000 mg/day PO) may reduce this osteopenia. If this therapy is used, serum and urine calcium levels must be monitored for drug-induced elevation (see Chap. 19).

8. Steroid-induced **myopathy** tends to involve the hip and shoulder girdle musculature. Although the patient is weak, the muscles are not tender, and

muscle enzymes are usually normal. Biopsy can sometimes differentiate steroid-induced myopathy from inflammatory myositis, but clinical judgment usually determines alterations in steroid dosage. Steroid-induced myopathy can be improved by a lower glucocorticoid dosage plus an aggressive exercise program.

9. **Ocular effects** include increased intraocular pressures (sometimes precipitating glaucoma) and the formation of posterior subcapsular cataracts.

10. **Ischemic bone necrosis** (aseptic necrosis, osteonecrosis, avascular necrosis) may be induced by glucocorticoids. Characteristic bone changes may be documented by plain radiographs; however, early changes may be demonstrated by bone scan alone. Surgical intervention with core decompression in early ischemic bone necrosis may be beneficial.

11. **Other undesirable effects** of glucocorticoid therapy include menstrual irregularities, increased perspiration with night sweats, hypercholesterolemia and type IV hyperlipoproteinemia, acute pancreatitis, and pseudotumor cerebri. Thrombophlebitis, necrotizing arteritis, and peptic ulcer disease have been attributed to glucocorticoid therapy, but evidence supporting these associations is controversial.

III. **Cytotoxic agents.** Cytotoxic agents used in patients with SLE include purine antagonists (azathioprine) and alkylating agents (chlorambucil, cyclophosphamide). Their use in SLE is controversial and should be restricted to patients with life-threatening disease uncontrolled by glucocorticoids or to patients who cannot tolerate steroid side effects. In such situations, **azathioprine,** 1.0–2.5 mg/kg/day, **cyclophosphamide,** 2–3 mg/kg/day, or **chlorambucil,** 0.05–0.15 mg/kg/day, may be added to the steroid regimen. They may provide a steroid-sparing effect. Cytotoxic drugs require several weeks to exert a beneficial effect; thus, immediate improvement should not be expected. Faster responses may be seen after administration of cyclophosphamide in a single "pulse" dose of 0.5–1.0 gm/M^2, which may be repeated if necessary after the nadir of bone marrow suppression (10–14 days) has occurred (see Chap. 17 for contraindications and side effects).

IV. **Plasmapheresis.** Plasmapheresis reduces the amount of circulating immune complexes, which sometimes corresponds to clinical improvement. However, the rebound of serologic and clinical parameters that occurs with discontinuance of plasmapheresis usually necessitates the addition of a cytotoxic drug to maintain stability. Because plasmapheresis is expensive and investigative, its use on a long-term basis is controversial.

V. **Transplantation and chronic hemodialysis.** Transplantation and chronic hemodialysis have been utilized in SLE patients with renal insufficiency. The survival rate in these patients is equivalent to that of patients with other forms of chronic renal disease; however, recurrence of nephritis in the allograft has been reported.

Scleroderma

Scleroderma (progressive systemic sclerosis) is a systemic illness of unknown cause characterized by Raynaud's phenomenon and sclerotic skin changes, especially sclerodactyly; in addition, multisystem disease can occur. Most of the manifestations of scleroderma have vascular features (Raynaud's phenomenon, telangiectasia, nephrosclerosis, nail-fold capillary changes, early edematous skin changes), but frank vasculitis is usually not seen. Progressive systemic sclerosis varies from a mild disease confined primarily to the skin and lasting for decades to a devastating systemic illness leading to death in a few months. No curative therapy is available. Therapy focuses on particular organ involvement.

I. **Raynaud's phenomenon.** Vasospasm in the digital arteries can result in ischemia of the digits. It is essential for the patient with Raynaud's phenomenon to avoid exposure of the entire body to cold and to protect the hands and feet from cold and trauma. Most therapeutic approaches to this disease have had limited success. Vasodilating drugs, such as phenoxybenzamine, reserpine, prazosin, calcium channel blocking agents, and ganglionic-blocking agents, are occasionally helpful, but significant side effects, especially orthostatic hypotension, may preclude their use. The efficacy of intraarterial reserpine has not been confirmed in most studies. Sympathectomy provides only transient benefit in most patients but should be considered when a patient has fingertip ulcers or gangrene that fails to improve after a conservative regimen of rest in a warm environment. Heat applied intermittently to the shoulder region may relieve symptoms in the ipsilateral fingers.

II. Skin and periarticular changes. No treatment for the skin changes of scleroderma is effective, although penicillamine may soften the skin and improve joint contractures. Moisturizing lotions can be somewhat useful, and physical therapy is important to retard and to reduce joint contractures. Secondary infections in digital ulcers should be treated with appropriate topical, and occasionally oral, antibiotics and debridement if necessary.

III. Myopathy. Muscle involvement in scleroderma usually consists of atrophy and fibrosis, for which exercise is the only therapy. A small proportion of patients have an inflammatory myopathy with enzyme elevations that may respond to glucocorticoid therapy.

IV. Gastrointestinal involvement. Reflux esophagitis resulting from lower esophageal abnormalities responds at least partially to a vigorous antacid regimen and elevation of the head of the bed during sleep. Cimetidine has also proved useful in some patients. Decreased motility can occur in bowel segments, leading to bacterial overgrowth, malabsorption, and weight loss. Treatment with broad-spectrum antibiotics, such as tetracycline or ampicillin, often eliminates the malabsorption.

V. Renal involvement. The appearance of hypertension and renal insufficiency signals a poor prognosis. A vigorous medical approach employing multiple antihypertensive agents in large doses may reverse renal insufficiency in a few patients. Dialysis and transplantation should be used when vigorous medical antihypertensive therapy fails to preserve renal function.

VI. Cardiopulmonary involvement. Patchy myocardial fibrosis can result in congestive heart failure or dysrhythmias and is usually associated with a poor prognosis. Standard therapies for these conditions are utilized. Pericarditis with an effusion that can lead to tamponade is often responsive to glucocorticoids. Pulmonary involvement can include pleurisy with effusion, interstitial fibrosis, pulmonary hypertension, and cor pulmonale. Glucocorticoids can be used to treat the pleurisy, but no therapy is effective for the other pulmonary lesions.

Necrotizing Vasculitis

Inflammation and necrosis of blood vessels define a clinicopathologic process called *necrotizing vasculitis*. This entity includes a broad spectrum of disorders involving vessels of different types, sizes, and locations, characterized by various clinical manifestations and having various causes. The immunopathogenic process often involves immune complexes.

The **clinical features** are diverse, including fever, weight loss, arthritis, myositis, neuropathies, CNS disturbances, renal disease, hypertension, cardiac failure, dysrhythmias, and GI catastrophies. **Hypersensitivity vasculitis** frequently manifests itself as small-vessel involvement of the skin. **Polyarteritis nodosa** usually attacks medium-sized vessels in major organs, such as the brain, heart, liver, and kidneys. **Wegener's granulomatosis** is typified by upper and lower airway involvement plus renal disease. **Rheumatoid vasculitis** occurs in approximately 5–10 percent of patients with RA and can be life-threatening. In its mildest form it is manifested as systemic fatigue, weight loss, fever, and peripheral neuropathy; in more severe forms, vasculitic purpuric skin lesions and digital gangrene can occur. Mortality is high if widespread vasculitis involves major organs, especially the GI or coronary vessels. Kidney involvement is rare.

There is evidence that glucocorticoids can be beneficial in most vasculitides, but the long-term prognosis is variable. Initial dosages should be high (60–100 mg prednisone/day), and a brief course of high-dose "pulse" therapy with 1000 mg of methylprednisolone/day for 3–5 days may be considered if life-threatening manifestations are present (see Systemic Lupus Erythematosus, sec. **II.D**). Cyclophosphamide (2–3 mg/kg/day) is the treatment of choice for Wegener's granulomatosis, with many patients entering long-term remissions with this agent alone. Since the prognosis of polyarteritis nodosa remains grave when treated with glucocorticoids alone, many physicians advocate the use of cytotoxic drugs such as cyclophosphamide (2–3 mg/kg/day) with steroids early in the course of this disease. High dosages of penicillamine (1000–1500 mg/day) may be helpful in rheumatoid vasculitis (see Rheumatoid Arthritis, sec. **I.D**). Rheumatoid arthritis patients who are unresponsive to steroids or in whom life-threatening steroid toxicity develops may require cytotoxic drugs. Plasmapheresis to remove presumed pathogenic immune complexes over a short period of time has been advocated in life-threatening vasculitic situations. It should be used in conjunction with a cytotoxic drug to prevent rebound production of the presumed offending complexes.

Temporal Arteritis and Polymyalgia Rheumatica

Patients with polymyalgia rheumatica (PMR) are elderly and have proximal limb girdle pain (without weakness or abnormal muscle enzymes), morning stiffness, fatigue, weight loss, low-grade fever, anemia, and an elevated ESR. Temporal arteritis is a form of giant-cell arteritis also seen primarily in the elderly. It can present with symptoms resembling PMR, as well as with headache, claudication of jaw muscles, abnormal taste sensations, visual disturbances including blindness, and even strokes. Rarely, it can affect major branches and portions of the thoracic and abdominal aorta. Up to 40% of patients with PMR also have temporal arteritis. The diagnosis of temporal arteritis is confirmed with a temporal artery biopsy.

Patients with temporal arteritis should receive 60–100 mg of prednisone/day in an attempt to control the disease and to prevent irreversible blindness. **Alternate-day dosage schedules should not be used in this disease.** When the ESR has returned to normal and symptoms have abated, the dosage should be gradually tapered by not more than 10%/week and continued for 1–2 years, with close monitoring of the ESR and clinical status. A maintenance dose of 10–20 mg of prednisone/day may be required for years.

If PMR is present without evidence of temporal arteritis, 10–15 mg of prednisone/day is often enough to produce a prompt, dramatic improvement in symptoms. We generally follow the ESR while the patient is receiving low dosages, to assess treatment efficacy. These low dosages of glucocorticoids are often required for 1–2 years, and some patients will require them indefinitely to control their musculoskeletal complaints and ESR.

Cryoglobulin Syndromes

Cryoglobulins are a group of serum proteins that share the property of reversibly precipitating in the cold. Over one-half of cryoglobulinemic patients have an underlying disease, such as immunoproliferative disease, autoimmune disorders, or underlying infections. About one-third of patients have no obvious underlying disease ("essential" or "idiopathic").

The **proper collection of serum** is essential for the detection of cryoglobulins; blood should be collected in prewarmed tubes and kept at 37°C while clotting occurs. Serum should be promptly harvested after centrifugation at 37°C and then incubated at 4°C for at least 72 hours. Normal values vary considerably among laboratories, but trace amounts of cryoblobulins may be found in normal persons.

Since there is no definitive therapy, treatment is generally directed at the underlying disease. Avoidance of cold exposure and minimizing prolonged standing are often helpful in relieving mild vasospastic symptoms. Prednisone, penicillamine, and cytotoxic agents have met with limited success. Plasmapheresis may be used in patients with severe cutaneous, renal, or CNS involvement.

Polymyositis and Dermatomyositis

Polymyositis (PM) is an inflammatory myopathy that produces tenderness, weakness, and ultimately wasting, primarily of the proximal hip and shoulder girdle musculature. A concomitant rash is present in dermatomyositis (DM). PM-DM can occur in five forms: (1) PM alone; (2) DM alone; (3) PM-DM in association with a variety of neoplasms (especially of the lung, prostate, ovary, uterus, breast, and colon); (4) DM in children; or (5) PM-DM in association with any other autoimmune disease (including Sjögren's syndrome). Patients in whom the onset of the disease occurs after the age of 50, particularly men with DM, may have up to a 40% risk of an associated malignancy. At least one of several muscle enzymes is usually elevated in PM-DM, and electromyographic patterns usually demonstrate the changes of a myopathy. The diagnosis is confirmed by muscle biopsy, although the disease is patchy, and a biopsy may miss involved areas or show nonspecific changes.

When PM-DM occurs without associated disease, it usually responds well to 40–80 mg of prednisone daily. Alternate-day therapy can also be successful and should be tried if the patient is not severely ill. As muscle strength improves and serum enzymes fall, the prednisone should be slowly reduced to maintenance levels of 10–20 mg daily or 20–40 mg every other day. The appearance of steroid-induced myopathy and hypokalemia must be monitored carefully. PM-DM associated with neoplasms tends to respond less well to glucocorticoid therapy. In a few patients, removal of an associated malignant tumor has resulted in complete remission of PM-DM.

Even in patients who have improved after the initiation of steroid administration, the disease is generally progressive, with flares of inflammation requiring frequent adjustments of steroid dosage. Patients who fail to respond to glucocorticoids or who cannot tolerate their side effects may respond to cytotoxic agents, such as methotrexate, azathioprine, cyclophosphamide, or chlorambucil (see Rheumatoid Arthritis, sec. **I.G**). Physical therapy to maintain muscular strength is very important.

Crystal-Induced Synovitis

Deposition of microcrystals in the joints and periarticular tissues results in the arthritis of **gout, pseudogout,** and **apatite disease.** Phagocytosis of the crystals by neutrophils, with subsequent release of enzymes into the joint fluid, leads to inflammation. In gout, the crystals are monosodium urate; in pseudogout, the crystals are calcium pyrophosphate dihydrate (CPPD); in apatite disease, the crystals are calcium hydroxyapatite. A definitive diagnosis of gout or pseudogout is made by examination of joint fluid using a compensated polarized light microscope and identification of neutrophils containing phagocytosed crystals: Urate crystals are needle shaped and strongly negatively birefringent; CPPD crystals are pleomorphic and weakly positively birefringent. A definitive diagnosis of hydroxy-apatite crystal disease is essentially one of exclusion, since the typical ultrastruc-tural appearance is determined only by electron microscopy or x-ray diffraction pattern techniques. In apatite disease, light microscopy of joint fluid after the addition of Wright's stain occasionally may reveal purple-stained cytoplasmic in-clusions within granulocytes.

I. Primary gout. Primary gout is an inherited metabolic disorder characterized by hyperuricemia that results from either overproduction or underexcretion of uric acid. Deposits of urate crystals (tophi) can form in the subcutaneous tissues, joints, and kidneys. Men are much more commonly affected than women; most pre-menopausal women with gout usually have a family history of the disease. The clinical phases of gout can be divided into asymptomatic hyperuricemia, acute arthritis, an interval phase, and chronic arthritis.

A. Asymptomatic hyperuricemia (uric acid levels >8 mg/dl in men and >7 mg/dl in women) is present in about 5% of the American male population, in 5–10% of whom acute gout will develop. The risk of gout is most significant in patients who have serum uric acid levels 2 or more standard deviations above the mean, and the risk seems to increase with increasing levels of serum urate. Never-theless, the treatment of asymptomatic hyperuricemia is controversial, since it is long term and exposes the patient both to the potential risks of the medication used and to an expensive prophylactic regimen whose benefit is not established. Since an attack of gouty arthritis is easily treated, long-term prophylaxis of arthritis in the asymptomatic hyperuricemic patient does not seem warranted.

On the other hand, renal calculi precede the arthritis in up to one-third of patients with gout. Very high urinary uric acid levels may also lead to renal damage that can be insidious and progressive. Therefore, we treat hy-peruricemic patients with allopurinol (see **C.1**) when their uric acid excretion is greater than 1000 mg/24 hours on a regular diet.

B. Acute gouty arthritis occurs as an attack of excruciating pain, usually in a single joint. Occasionally, a polyarticular form can mimic RA. These attacks are generally separated by months to years of pain-free intervals. Although the acute attacks subside spontaneously over several days, prompt medical atten-tion can abort the attack over hours. **Uric acid levels should not be manipu-lated until an acute attack has subsided.** If alteration of the uric acid level is planned after the acute attack subsides, maintenance oral colchicine should be used simultaneously to prevent a new attack.

   1. Colchicine is most effective if given in the first 12–24 hours of an acute attack and usually brings relief in 6–12 hours. It is available in PO and IV preparations.

   a. Oral administration is effective, but severe GI toxicity precludes its routine use. The dosage is 2 tablets (0.5 gm or 0.6 mg each), given im-mediately, followed by either 1 tablet q1–2h or 2 tablets q2h until symp-toms abate, GI toxicity develops, or the maximum dose of 16 tablets (8.0–9.6 mg) in a 24-hour period is reached. No more than 3 tablets/day should be used thereafter during that attack.

   b. The IV use of colchicine results in more rapid relief and fewer GI effects and is particularly useful when PO medication is containdicated. The drug should be diluted in 10–20 ml of sterile water or normal saline and given slowly over 3–5 minutes through a freely flowing IV route to avoid tissue irritation. Colchicine should not be diluted with, or injected into IV tubing containing, 5% dextrose or other fluid that could change the pH of the colchicine solution and lead to precipitation. The initial dose is 2 mg, followed by another 1–2 mg in 6 hours if necessary. The maximum IV dose during a given attack should not exceed 4 mg. Similar doses of IV colchicine should not be used again for several weeks, especially when oral colchicine has been subsequently added to the regimen.

    c. Toxicity includes abdominal pain, nausea, vomiting, and diarrhea. Rarely, long-term or high-dose administration has been associated with aplastic anemia, agranulocytosis, thrombocytopenia, myopathy, alopecia, neuropathy, respiratory depression, and hemorrhagic gastroenteritis. Extravasation of IV colchicine can lead to severe necrosis of the surrounding tissues. Anaphylaxis may occur with IV colchicine.

  2. The **NSAIDs** are as effective as colchicine, although 12–24 hours is usually required after their administration before an attack abates. Initial doses should be high, followed by rapid tapering over 2–8 days. For example, indomethacin is begun at 50 mg q6h for 2 days, followed by 50 mg q8h for 2 days, and then 25 mg q8h for 2–3 more days.

  3. Glucocorticoids are indicated for unusual attacks refractory to conventional therapy. Prednisone (40–60 mg/day) should be given until a response is obtained and then followed by rapid tapering.

C. Interval-phase gout. If a patient has infrequent attacks of gout with normal serum and urine uric acid levels between attacks, interval-phase medications other than prophylactic use of colchicine are often not needed. Avoidance of occasional aspirins (uricoretentive), most diuretics, a large alcohol intake, prolonged fasts, and foods high in purines (sweetbreads, anchovies, sardines, liver, kidney) will often prevent attacks. However, if arthritic attacks are frequent, if renal damage is present, or if serum or urine uric acid levels are consistently elevated, lowering of the uric acid level should be attempted.

Maintenance colchicine (0.5–0.6 mg PO bid) should be instituted a few days prior to manipulation of the uric acid level to prevent precipitation of an acute attack. Colchicine is the only drug that is prophylactic for acute gout; NSAIDs are not. If no attacks occur after the uric acid has been maintained in the normal range for several months, colchicine can be discontinued. Patients should be advised that gouty attacks might occur during this adjustment period.

  1. Allopurinol (Zyloprim), a xanthine oxidase inhibitor, is the drug of choice for controlling hyperuricemia in most patients. It is well absorbed orally without binding to plasma proteins and is rapidly metabolized to oxypurinol, an active form, which has a half-life of 30 hours. If an acute attack occurs while the patient is taking allopurinol, the drug should be continued at the same dosage while other agents are used to treat the attack. Allopurinol, available in 100- and 300-mg tablets, is given in a single daily dose, usually beginning at 300 mg/day. Dosages can be adjusted slightly every 2–4 weeks to arrive at a maintenance dose that will keep the uric acid level within the normal range. The drug must be used cautiously and in reduced dosage in patients with renal insufficiency or hepatic disease. The use of 6-mercaptopurine or azathioprine with allopurinol necessitates a 60–75% reduction in the cytotoxic drug dosages. The concomitant use of a uricosuric agent may hasten the mobilization of tophi but is rarely necessary.

Hypersensitivity reactions are the most common of the undesirable side effects of allopurinol therapy, occurring in up to 5% of patients. These can vary from a minor skin rash with fever to a diffuse exfoliative dermatitis or hypersensitivity angiitis. Such reactions often occur in patients with mild renal insufficiency who are taking diuretics. Ampicillin rashes may be more common in patients also taking allopurinol. Minor GI distress can occasionally occur, but bone marrow suppression, peripheral neuropathy, elevation of serum transaminases, and xanthine stones are rare. Allopurinol may potentiate the effect of oral anticoagulants.

  2. Uricosuric drugs lower serum uric acid levels by interfering with renal tubular resorption of uric acid. This increases urinary uric acid excretion but also increases the risk of urate stone formation. This danger can be minimized by maintaining a high fluid intake and alkalinizing the urine (impractical for long-term therapy). Uricosurics are ineffective if the glomerular filtration rate is less than 30 ml/minute and are contraindicated in patients with already high levels of urinary uric acid (>800 mg in 24 hours). These agents are generally indicated only when allopurinol cannot be used and when the 24-hour urinary uric acid is carefully monitored. If these drugs are being used when an acute gouty attack begins, they should be continued while other drugs are used to treat the acute attack.

    a. Probenecid (Benemid) is completely absorbed from the GI tract, has a half-life of 6–12 hours, and is excreted in the urine. The initial dosage is 500 mg daily (1 tablet), which can be raised by 500-mg increments every week until serum uric acid levels are normal. Most patients require a total of 1000–1500 mg daily in 3–4 divided doses. Salicylates and probenecid are antagonistic and thus should not be used together. Renal excretion of penicillin, indomethacin, and sulfonylureas is decreased when given with probenecid. **Side effects** are minimal: Hypersensitivity rashes, mild GI distress, flushing, and dizziness can occur. Hemolytic anemia in patients with G-6-PD deficiency and peptic ulcerations are rare complications.

    b. Sulfinpyrazone (Anturane) is a uricosuric agent chemically related to phenylbutazone and with similar toxicities. It is rarely indicated for the treatment of hyperuricemia.

  D. Chronic gouty arthritis results from continual inflammation in multiple joints in conjunction with frequent acute attacks. Tophaceous deposits in the joints lead to destructive erosions and to interference with joint motion. Colchicine (0.5–0.6 mg bid) can help prevent new attacks, NSAIDs can decrease existing inflammation, and allopurinol can help to mobilize tophi and decrease renal exposure to high levels of uric acid. Rehabilitation includes physical and occupational therapy as well as corrective surgery.

II. Secondary gout. Secondary gout occurs when the elevated uric acid level is a complication of another disease or of drugs. Hematologic malignancies can result in profound nucleoprotein breakdown and lead to hyperuricemia. Intrinsic renal disease itself can produce hyperuricemia, but articular manifestations of gout are uncommon in renal failure. Thiazide and furosemide diuretics can cause a mild elevation of serum uric acid levels that usually does not require therapy (see sec. **I.A**). Any cause of hyperlactacidemia, including preeclampsia, diabetic ketoacidosis, severe bouts of alcoholism, or starvation, can also induce hyperuricemia.

III. Pseudogout. Pseudogout results when CPPD crystals, presumably from cartilage, are deposited in the synovial fluid and induce acute inflammation. Associated diseases in some series include diabetes mellitus, hypertension, hyperparathyroidism, gout, and hyperuricemia. Despite an x-ray diagnosis of chondrocalcinosis, the diagnosis of pseudogout can be made only by identification of characteristic crystals on microscopic examination of synovial fluid. Pseudogout can present as acute intermittent attacks of arthritis resembling RA or as slowly progressive disease in weight-bearing joints (knees, hips) resembling osteoarthritis.

A brief, high-dose course of a NSAID (as discussed in sec. **I.B.2**) is the therapy of choice for most patients. However, colchicine (PO or IV) may also relieve symptoms promptly. The recommended colchicine dosage is the same as that used for acute gout. Maintenance colchicine may also diminish the number of recurrent attacks in some patients. Removal of the crystals by joint aspiration often results in prompt improvement. Glucocorticoids are rarely required to treat pseudogout.

IV. Apatite disease. The treatment of **apatite disease** is similar to that of pseudogout (see sec. **III**).

Osteoarthritis

Osteoarthritis, or degenerative joint disease, is a disorder of the joints characterized by deterioration and abrasion of articular cartilage, with concomitant formation of reactive new bone at the articular suface. The joints most commonly affected are the distal interphalangeal joints of the hands, weight-bearing joints such as the hips and knees, and the spine. The disease is more common in the elderly than in the younger age groups but may occur at any age, especially as a sequel to joint trauma or congenital malformations. Hydroxyapatite crystal deposition has been implicated in some acute flares. An erosive, polyarticular inflammatory variant, usually resulting in hand deformities, has a familial basis.

The objectives of **therapy** include relief of pain and prevention of disability. Full dosages of aspirin or one of the other NSAIDs are usually helpful. Intraarticular injections of glucocorticoids are sometimes beneficial. In combination with rest and physical therapy, such a regimen constitutes adequate management of most cases. Systemic steroids and addictive narcotic analgesics should be avoided.

When weight-bearing joints are affected, support in the form of crutches, canes, or walkers can be helpful. Since coexisting obesity may accelerate osteoarthritis in weight-bearing joints, weight reduction is advisable. Properly selected exercises are indicated to prevent or correct muscle atrophy. When serious disability results from severe pain or deformity, surgical procedures may be indicated. Total hip and knee replacement can relieve pain and increase function in selected patients. Prophylactic correction of childhood abnormalities will often prevent the development of osteoarthritis in later years.

Osteoarthritis of the spine can involve the intervertebral disks, the vertebral bodies, or the apophyseal joints. Local pain and spasm are caused by reactions in paraspinal soft tissues; radicular symptoms (sensory, reflex, or motor) result from pressure on neurologic structures by prolapsed disks or large osteophytes. Lumbosacral disease may cause low back pain and sciatica. The usefulness of NSAIDs, physical supports (cervical collars, lumbar corsets), muscle relaxants, exercises to strengthen abdominal and paravertebral musculature, and local heat is limited but may achieve relief in certain patients. Laminectomies and spinal fusions should be reserved for severe disease with intractable pain or neurologic complications.

Infectious Arthritis and Bursitis

I. **General principles of treatment** include hospitalization, joint fluid examination and culture, IV antimicrobials, and repeated joint aspirations if necessary.

   A. **Hospitalization** ensures drug compliance and careful monitoring of the clinical response.

   B. **When an infectious arthritis is suspected, joint fluid examination, including Gram stain and culture, is mandatory.** Aspirated fluid should be promptly cultured on a medium that will support the growth of a wide variety of microorganisms. A **joint fluid white cell count** is useful as a baseline for subsequent evaluations.

   C. **Intravenous antimicrobials** ensure good serum and synovial fluid concentrations of the drugs; intraarticular antimicrobials are rarely, if ever, needed.

   D. **Repeated arthrocenteses** (occasionally with saline lavage) are indicated for therapeutic removal of destructive by-products of inflammation and for decreasing intraarticular pressure to ensure good perfusion of antimicrobials. They enable one to repeat synovial fluid cultures (which should become negative) and to repeat synovial fluid white cell counts (which should decrease).

   E. **Surgical drainage** is indicated in the following situations: (1) septic hips that cannot be adequately evacuated with a needle; (2) joints in which large amounts of tissue debris or loculations of pus prevent adequate needle drainage; and (3) joints that do not respond in 5–7 days to appropriate antimicrobial therapy and needle aspirations. Splinting of the joint may relieve pain, but prolonged immobilization of the joint may result in stiffness. A NSAID is often useful in place of splints to reduce pain and to increase joint mobility.

II. **Gonococcal arthritis** accounts for one-third to one-half of all septic arthritides in otherwise healthy adults; **staphylococcal arthritis** accounts for another one-third of the cases.

    A. Gonococcal arthritis can be treated with aqueous penicillin G (10 million units IV/day) until improvement occurs followed by ampicillin (500 mg PO qid) or amoxicillin (500 mg PO qid) to complete at least 7 days of treatment; or amoxicillin (3.0 gm PO) or ampicillin (3.5 gm PO) plus probenecid (1.0 gm PO) followed by amoxicillin (500 mg PO qid) or ampicillin (500 mg PO qid) for at least 7 days. For nonpregnant patients allergic to penicillin, alternative therapy includes tetracycline (500 mg PO qid) or erythromycin (500 mg PO qid) for at least 7 days. Arthritis due to penicillinase-producing *Neisseria gonorrhoeae* can be treated with cefoxitin or cefotaxime (see Chap. 10).

    B. If *Staphylococcus aureus* is cultured, therapy with an appropriate β-lactamase–resistant penicillin (e.g., oxacillin, nafcillin) should be initiated and continued for at least 14 days.

    C. If the initial Gram stain of synovial fluid does not suggest the pathogen, pending culture results, adult patients should be treated empirically with antimicrobials that provide coverage for both organisms.

III. The incidence of **gram-negative bacillary arthritis** is increasing, especially in elderly patients with underlying chronic, debilitating diseases or in immunosuppressed hosts. When such patients present with a suspected septic joint, an aminoglycoside (pending susceptibility testing) should be chosen if gram-negative rods are seen on Gram stain. If no organisms are seen, an aminoglycoside plus a β-lactamase–resistant penicillin should be used, pending culture results. Therapy is continued for at least 14 days.

IV. Transient arthralgias and arthritis are common with many **viral infections,** especially rubella, mumps, infectious mononucleosis, and hepatitis. They are usually self-limited, last for less than 6 weeks, and respond well to a conservative regimen.

V. A number of **fungi** and **mycobacteria** can cause septic arthritis, particularly among patients presenting with a chronic monoarticular arthritis.

VI. **Septic bursitis,** usually involving the olecranon or prepatellar bursa, can be differentiated from septic arthritis by localized, fluctuant swelling and by generally painless joint motion (except with full flexion or extension). Most patients have a history of prior trauma to the area or an occupational predisposition ("housemaid's knee," "writer's elbow"). *S. aureus* is the pathogen in most patients. The principles of **management** are similar to those for septic arthritis. Preventive measures (e.g., knee pads) should be used in patients with occupational predispositions.

Tendinitis, Tenosynovitis, and Bursitis

Inflammation of paraarticular soft tissue structures can develop from trauma induced by strain or direct injury and from various rheumatic processes (e.g., RA, Reiter's syndrome, gout, infection). Common sites of inflammation include shoulder (supraspinatus or bicipital head tendinitis), elbow (epicondylitis—"tennis" or "golfer's" elbow), thumb (de Quervain's disease), hip (trochanteric bursitis), knee (prepatellar bursitis), and heel (Achilles or calcaneal bursitis). A sterile local injection of 20–40 mg of **triamcinolone (Aristospan, Kenalog),** plus 1 ml of 1% lidocaine, usually provides immediate relief that can last for months or more in some patients. Full-dose aspirin or other NSAIDs can be used if multiple areas are involved or if injections are required more frequently than every 2–3 months.

Dimethyl sulfoxide (DMSO), an industrial solvent, has been used in the treatment of arthritis, scleroderma, and other musculoskeletal disorders. Administered topically, it is rapidly absorbed from the skin. Toxicities include allergic reactions, garliclike taste and halitosis, local dermatitis, photophobia, headaches, nausea, and diarrhea. Animal studies demonstrate teratogenic effects, induction of cataracts, and changes of refractive index. Although it may prove effective in controlling soft tissue inflammation such as tendinitis, bursitis, and sprains, there are no convincing data to indicate that DMSO is effective in systemic rheumatic diseases. We do not recommend its use until its safety has been established and purified preparations are available for human use.

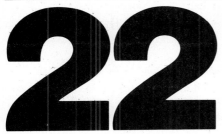

Neurologic Emergencies

Coma

Coma is a symptom rather than a specific disease. It has a wide variety of causes, ranging from metabolic to structural abnormalities. Coma requires urgent intervention, which is best accomplished by a systematic approach to the patient. For a complete discussion of coma, the reader is referred to F. Plum and J. B. Posner, *The Diagnosis of Stupor and Coma* (3rd ed.). Philadelphia: Davis, 1980.

I. **Pathophysiology.** To produce coma, a disease process must affect **both** cerebral hemispheres or the reticular formation from the pons to the diencephalon. Disease processes affecting **one** cerebral hemisphere do **not** usually cause stupor or coma. Tumors, infarcts, or hemorrhages in a single cerebral hemisphere cause stupor or coma by affecting the other cerebral hemisphere or the brainstem (e.g., by increasing intracranial pressure, causing compression of the other hemisphere or brainstem). Similarly a tumor, infarct, or hemorrhage in the cerebellum may cause stupor or coma by compression of the brainstem. Generally, stroke affecting a single cerebral hemisphere does not cause stupor or coma. The presence of stupor or coma in a patient with what is thought to be a single hemispheric lesion should alert the physician to the possibility of another process that may require urgent intervention, such as increased intracranial pressure (ICP).

II. **Assessment**

A. The **history** is critical to the establishment of a diagnosis. The nature, onset, and duration of the coma, past medical history, use of drugs and medicines, trauma, exposures to toxins, and history of seizures need to be determined. The circumstances in which the patient is found may suggest a diagnosis (e.g., the presence of empty pill bottles and a history of a change in mood or behavior suggest excessive drug ingestion). All those who had contact with the patient, such as friends, relatives, police, and ambulance drivers, should be questioned and should remain available for further questioning.

B. **A general examination** may reveal the presence of systemic illness associated with coma. For example, evidence of cirrhosis suggests hepatic failure, and a purpuric rash may suggest meningococcemia.

C. The **neurologic examination** must be as complete as possible and repeated at frequent intervals to evaluate the patient's course. Careful observation, particularly utilizing the criteria listed in **1–5**, may enable determination of the anatomic site of the lesion, which in turn suggests a differential diagnosis. An inability to identify a specific anatomic site strongly suggests a metabolic cause.

1. **Level of consciousness** is judged by the nature of the patient's response to various stimuli and the amount of stimulation required. Terms such as *semicomatose, stuporous,* and *obtunded* are vague, confusing, and lack reproducibility. It is best to avoid such terms and instead describe the patient's response. For example, is the patient aroused when called by name, or does

the patient require shouting, shaking, or painful stimulation to respond? Are the responses appropriate?

2. **Size and reactivity of the pupils**

   a. **Midposition (4–6 mm) and fixed pupil** implies a midbrain lesion.

   b. **Unilateral dilated and fixed pupil** implies a third cranial nerve lesion, as might be caused by uncal herniation.

   c. **Small but reactive pupils** are seen in metabolic encephalopathy, diencephalic or pontine lesions, or narcotic overdose.

   d. **Bilateral dilated and fixed pupils** are seen with severe anoxic encephalopathy or intoxication with scopolamine or glutethimide.

3. **Ocular position and movement**

   a. At rest, dysconjugate gaze may suggest a specific cranial nerve palsy. In a third nerve lesion the eye may be deviated laterally and inferiorly. With a sixth nerve lesion the eye will be deviated medially. When there is conjugate deviation of the eyes **away** from the hemiparetic side, the lesion is **above** the pons (usually in the cerebral hemisphere) **on the side** to which the eyes look. When there is conjugate deviation of the eyes **toward** the hemiparetic side, the lesion is **at** the pons **opposite the side** to which the eyes look.

   b. **Eye movements** can be evaluated by quick turning of the head (oculocephalic, or doll's-eye, maneuver). In comatose patients with an intact brainstem from pons to midbrain, the eyes move conjugately in a direction opposite to that of the head, to maintain the initial direction of gaze. Caloric stimulation can also be used to evaluate eye movement in the comatose patient. The intact tympanic membrane of a comatose patient is douched with 20–30 ml of ice water; the external auditory canals must first be checked to be sure they are free of obstruction, and the head should be elevated 30 degrees above the horizontal. In a comatose patient with an intact brainstem from pons to midbrain, the eyes will conjugately deviate **toward** the ear being stimulated. Failure of conjugate deviation to one side suggests a lesion in the pons on the side being stimulated. Dysconjugate gaze may indicate a third or sixth nerve lesion. In the conscious patient, nystagmus with the quick phase **away** from the stimulated ear will result.

4. **Motor response.** The position of the extremities at rest (e.g., external rotation of a lower extremity) may indicate weakness. One side of the face may puff out with expiration or grimace asymmetrically to pain. Spontaneous movements should be observed to see if they are purposeful or if one side is preferentially used. Painful stimulation may result in extensor (decerebrate) posturing or purposeful movement to ward off the stimulus. Deep tendon reflexes and the presence of pathologic reflexes (e.g., Babinski's sign) should be checked.

5. **Pattern of respiration.** Cheyne-Stokes respiration implies a bilateral cerebral hemispheric or diencephalic lesion. Central neurogenic hyperventilation in the absence of metabolic acidosis or hypoxia implies a midbrain or upper pontine lesion. A medullary lesion is suggested by irregular respirations or respiratory arrest. However, changes in respiratory patterns may not be specific, and caution is necessary in their interpretation.

III. **Treatment.** Certain measures should be initiated immediately as the patient is being assessed.

   A. **Ensure adequate respiration.** An airway or intubation may be necessary.

   B. **Ensure adequate circulation.** A large-bore IV catheter should be placed, since the administration of fluids or medicines may suddenly become necessary.

C. Maintain body temperature.

D. Draw blood specimens to determine glucose, electrolytes, arterial blood gases (ABGs), CBC, calcium, BUN, and creatinine. Urine and blood should be saved for possible toxicologic screening.

E. Administer 50 ml of a 50% dextrose solution IV if the cause of coma is not readily apparent.

F. If alcohol abuse is suspected, **thiamine** should be administered to prevent Wernicke's syndrome, which may be precipatated by a large carbohydrate load. The initial thiamine dose is 10 mg IV, plus 100 mg IM, then 100 mg IM qd for 3 days.

G. If narcotic overdose is suspected or the cause of coma is not immediately obvious, administer **naloxone hydrochloride** (Narcan), 0.4–0.8 mg IV. In the case of a narcotic overdose, the response should occur within minutes. Repeat doses may be necessary to treat deterioration following an initial improvement.

H. Increased intracranial pressure should be treated as outlined on p. 386.

I. The specific cause of coma should be defined and treated.

  1. Computed tomography (CT scan) should be perfomed when a CNS cause is suspected. Aneurysms, arteriovenous malformations, tumor, and infarctions may not be visualized unless an IV contrast medium is used.

  2. Skull and cervical spine radiographs should be obtained if there is a possibility of trauma.

  3. The use of **other diagnostic tests** (electroencephalography, radionuclide brain scan, lumbar puncture, and angiography) depends on the specific diagnosis suspected.

IV. General care of the comatose patient

  A. Prevent cutaneous pressure sores. The patient should be turned and positioned q2h. A soft mattress and sheepskin pads are recommended. Heels should be padded (*Ann. Intern. Med.* 94:661, 1981).

  B. Prevent corneal abrasions. Eyelids may be taped shut; methylcellulose eyedrops may be helpful.

  C. Change bed linen frequently. Condom catheters may be used in male patients, but penile maceration can result. **Indwelling urinary catheters** may be necessary but are a common source of infection.

  D. Maintain nutrition and hydration. Abnormalities of antidiuretic hormone secretion may occur in a variety of neurologic conditions.

  E. Maintain joint mobility by passive exercises. Footboards should be used to prevent heel contractures.

  F. Antacids and/or **cimetidine** may be useful in preventing GI hemorrhage associated with stress.

Delirium

Delirium is defined as a state characterized by any combination of confusion, disorientation, paranoia, irritability, hallucinations, delusions, combativeness, and autonomic nervous system overactivity. It may result from a great variety of diseases, including drug intoxication, drug or alcohol withdrawal, infections (particularly meningitis or encephalitis), hepatic failure, renal failure, electrolyte abnormalities, hypercalcemia, head trauma, superimposition of stress from any cause on dementia, porphyria, subarachnoid hemorrhage, hypoxia, thyrotoxicosis, or Cushing's syndrome. Particular problems are posed by evaluation and treatment.

I. **Evaluation.** Often, delirious patients are immediately thought to have psychotic illness. Psychotic illness, however, does not generally cause severe confusion, disorientation, or altered levels of consciousness, and this diagnosis should be made only by exclusion of the other possible causes. The physician should quickly work through the differential diagnosis. Electrolytes, ABGs, calcium, BUN, and creatinine should be determined. Urine and blood should be obtained for a toxicology screen. Where appropriate, CT scan of the head, skull radiographs, or lumbar puncture should be done. A radionuclide brain scan is very important in cases of suspected herpes simplex encelphalitis. An electroencephalogram (EEG) may also be helpful. Drug intoxication, encephalitis, and metabolic disturbances slow the EEG. In withdrawal states the EEG may show low-voltage fast activity.

II. **Treatment.** The physician is often tempted to sedate the delirious patient. This has many risks (e.g., hypotension), which are markedly increased in patients with drug-induced delirium. Often, a reassuring, well-lighted, and comfortable environment, free of dangerous objects, may be sufficient. When sedation is necessary, benzodiazepines may be used. If this appears insufficient, haloperidol or short-acting barbiturates may be used very cautiously. Phenothiazines should be avoided in possible drug intoxication, since hypotension may result. Rarely, restraints may be necessary.

Increased Intracranial Pressure

The treatment of choice for acute, life-threatening increased ICP is a rapid determination of the underlying cause, followed by specific therapeutic measures. Increased ICP may be due to an increase in any intracranial component, including the brain, blood, and cerebrospinal fluid (CSF). The differential diagnosis includes tumor, cerebral edema, hematoma, subarachnoid hemorrhage, and hydrocephalus.

I. **Presentation**

A. **Nonspecific changes** reflect a general response to increased ICP and are without localizing value. They include headache, nausea, vomiting, increased blood pressure, bradycardia, papilledema, sixth cranial nerve palsies, transient obscurations of vision, and alterations in the level of consciousness.

B. **Herniation** is usually due to a pressure gradient that shifts brain tissue. The location of the area of high pressure determines the nature of the herniation, which helps in localization of the lesion and guides therapeutic intervention. There are many types of herniation, but the following are of primary importance:

1. **Diencephalic herniation** is usually caused by a medial supratentorial lesion that forces the diencephalon through the tentorial notch. It results in (1) Cheyne-Stokes respiration, (2) small but reactive pupils, (3) paresis of upward gaze, and (4) altered mental status.

2. **Uncal herniation** usually is caused by a lateral supratentorial lesion that forces the medial portion of the temporal lobe (the uncus) through the tentorial notch. The subsequent pressure on midbrain structures results in (1) alterations of consciousness; (2) a dilated and fixed pupil from third nerve compression (eye movements may be intact), usually affecting the ipsilateral side; and (3) hemiparesis, which may affect either side.

3. **Tonsillar herniation** results from pressure that forces the inferior portion of the cerebellum (the cerebellar tonsils) through the foramen magnum, compressing the medulla. This usually results in (1) altered consciousness and (2) respiratory irregularity or arrest.

II. **Treatment.** Treatment is aimed at the specific cause as outlined in Coma, sec. **III.** Neurosurgical consultation should be obtained as soon as possible, since most causes of treatable increased ICP are neurosurgical. In the interim, the **nonspecific immediate measures** that follow can be initiated to gain needed time to obtain a specific diagnosis and treatment plan.

A. **Hyperventilation** to achieve a PCO_2 of 25–30 mm Hg. The effects are immediate.

B. **Mannitol,** 1.0–1.5 gm/kg of body weight, should be infused as a **20% solution** (100 gm of mannitol in 500 ml of 5% D/W) over 15–30 minutes. Mannitol should be given through a filter to eliminate crystals. Effects may take 1–2 hours to occur. The dose may be repeated once or twice q4–6h. Initially, this may result in intravascular volume overexpansion and pulmonary edema, but later there may be an osmotic diuresis with consequent dehydration. Fluid balance (consider a central venous line to measure pressures), electrolytes (especially sodium), and serum osmolality should be carefully monitored. There may be a **rebound increase in ICP** that may result in marked worsening of the patient's condition. The rebound is due to the retention of some mannitol in the brain tissue as the blood levels are falling. This reverses the desired osmotic gradient, with subsequent increase in brain fluid and, as a result, increased ICP several hours after administration. Therefore, mannitol should be used **only in emergency situations** as a temporary measure while other therapeutic modalities are being initiated.

C. **Glycerol** may be given PO or via a nasogastric tube in a dosage of 1–3 gm/kg/day in 4–6 divided doses. Complications include a large caloric load, hyperglycemia, hemolysis, and acute tubular necrosis. Careful monitoring of fluid balance, serum electrolytes, and serum glucose is necessary. Caution is necessary because a **rebound increase in ICP** (as with mannitol) has been reported with glycerol use.

D. **Glucocorticoids** may be used, but their effect may take 6–12 hours. **Dexamethasone (Decadron),** 10 mg IM or IV, followed by 4 mg q6h, may be used.

Cerebrovascular Disease

I. **Hemorrhages.** Intracranial hemorrhages are usually classified as subarachnoid, intracerebral, epidural hematoma, and subdural hematoma. The last two are discussed under Head Injury.

A. **Intracerebral hemorrhage** usually presents with a sudden onset of focal neurologic deficit that may be accompanied by alteration in mental status, headache, and vomiting. Other complications include rupture into the subarachnoid space and convulsion. Intracerebral hemorrhage may present as a rapidly expanding mass lesion with signs of increased ICP. Intracerebral hemorrhage secondary to hypertension (the most frequent cause) occurs in the basal ganglia (70%), brainstem (10%), cerebellum (10%), and cerebral white matter (10%). Other causes of hemorrhage include arteriovenous malformations, aneurysms, trauma, anticoagulation, blood dyscrasia, and tumor. These other causes should be considered when the history is suggestive or when the hematoma is not in a location that is usual for hypertension. **Computed tomography scans** have proved invaluable in the rapid diagnosis of intracerebral hematomas. **Treatment** is aimed at the cause (e.g., controlling hypertension, correcting blood dyscrasias) and the treatment of complications if they occur. Superficial cerebral hematomas, especially in the nondominant hemisphere, and cerebellar hematomas, causing life-threatening increased ICP, may require emergency surgical evacuation.

B. **Subarachnoid hemorrhage** can result from aneurysms, arteriovenous malformations, intracerebral hematomas, blood dyscrasia, head trauma, and tumor. The saccular or "berry" aneurysms may represent defects in the media and internal elastic membrane of arteries, which are prone to dilatation and rupture. Other types of aneurysm include fusiform aneurysm, thought to be secondary to atherosclerosis, and mycotic aneurysm. Aneurysms may present as a mass lesion, such as an aneurysm of the internal carotid and posterior communicating artery compressing the third nerve and resulting in a unilateral third nerve lesion (especially a dilated pupil). They may rupture into the brain parenchyma and present as an intracerebral hematoma, or into the subarachnoid space and present with sudden changes in mental status, headache, vomiting, nuchal rigidity, low back pain, focal neurologic deficits, and retinal hemorrhages. They may produce acute hydrocephalus or vasospasm with cerebral ischemia. Cardiac dysrhythmias may be seen.

1. **Diagnosis.** A CT scan may reveal an intracerebral or intraventricular hemorrhage. It may show blood in the subarachnoid space of the sulci and cisterna. Injection of contrast agents during the CT scan may reveal an aneurysm or arteriovenous malformation. **Lumbar puncture** may show a "bloody" CSF and should be performed if the CT scan does not show intracranial bleeding that is clinically suspected.

   a. Steps to **differentiate** a subarachnoid hemorrhage from a "traumatic" lumbar puncture include the following:

      (1) Immediately centrifuging a sample of CSF to determine whether or not the supernatant is xanthochromic. Xanthochromia indicates that the blood has been present in the CSF for several hours (suggesting a subarachnoid hemorrhage).

      (2) Performing a cell count on all collected specimens. If the cell count from the first specimen is the same as that of the last specimen, pathologic subarachnoid hemorrhage is indicated (*N. Engl. J. Med.* 290:225, 1974).

   b. **Angiography** should include both vertebral and carotid arteries, since multiple aneurysms are noted in approximately 20% of patients.

2. **Treatment.** Surgical repair of aneurysms is the treatment of choice but is dependent on the patient's level of consciousness, extent of the neurologic deficit, and nature of the aneurysm. Excision or embolic obliteration is the definitive treatment of arteriovenous malformations. Neurosurgical consultation should be obtained. Other **nonspecific therapy** includes the following:

   a. Bed rest and analgesia, as clinically indicated.

   b. Treatment of possible cerebral edema and increased ICP. Dexamethasone, 10 mg, followed by 4 mg q6h, may be given IV or IM.

   c. Laxatives to prevent straining at stool.

   d. Management of hypertension (see Chap. 7, sec. **IV**).

   e. **Aminocaproic acid (Amicar)** is an antifibrinolytic agent. The loading dose is 5 gm in 50 ml 5% D/W IV over 1 hour. The dosage is 24–36 gm in 500 ml 5% D/W by constant IV infusion daily for 10 days, followed by 3 gm PO q2h for 21 days or until surgical repair is performed. Aminocaproic acid is **contraindicated** in the presence of active disseminated intravascular coagulation. Complications include pulmonary embolism, deep vein thrombosis, and renal cortical necrosis (*Stroke* 6:622, 1975).

   f. Cardiac monitoring.

   g. There is currently no generally accepted means of treating vasospasm.

II. **Occlusive disease.** The **treatment** of occlusive disease is controversial. In addition to the direct treatment of stroke, the **underlying causes** (atherosclerosis, embolization from vegetations on heart valves, mitral valve prolapse, prosthetic valves, or mural thrombi from myocardial infarction, vasculitis, polycythemia, and thrombocytosis) and **risk factors** (hypertension, diabetes mellitus, and hyperlipidemia) should be treated.

A. Transient ischemic attack (TIA) is defined as a transient neurologic deficit of vascular origin that usually resolves within 24 hours. Roughly one-third of these patients subsequently will have a stroke; of these, approximately 20% will do so in the first month after the onset of the TIA. Other disorders that may be confused with TIAs include cardiac dysrhythmias, orthostatic hypotension, subclavian steal syndrome, anemia, polycythemia, mitral valve prolapse, cervical spondylosis, hypoglycemia, tumor, and subdural hematoma. The therapeutic approach to TIAs depends on whether the carotid or the vertebral-basilar circulatory system is involved (*Mayo Clin. Proc.* 53:665, 1978).

    1. Carotid circulation. The signs or symptoms are **referable** to the cerebral hemisphere and/or eye supplied by that carotid artery and most often include hemiplegia, hemisensory loss, and/or transient loss of vision in one eye (amaurosis fugax). When the dominant cerebral hemisphere is involved, aphasia may also result. The major significance of TIAs in the distribution of the carotid artery is the possibility for surgical intervention. **About 50%** of these TIAs may be attributable to lesions that are correctable, either with carotid endarterectomy or superficial temporal–middle cerebral artery bypass.

    A CT scan and CSF examination should be done on patients who present with TIAs. This is to rule out disorders that may present as TIAs and contraindicate the use of heparin (e.g., intracerebral or subarachnoid hemorrhage). In the absence of any contraindication, the patient should be placed on **heparin therapy,** especially if the TIAs are of less than 2 months' duration. Full anticoagulation dosages are required (see Chap. 16). If the patient is judged a surgical candidate, cerebral angiography should be performed, followed by surgery at centers experienced with these procedures. If the patient is judged not a surgical candidate, **sodium warfarin (Coumadin)** should be given (in the absence of specific contraindications, such as active peptic ulcer disease or severe hypertension) and the heparin discontinued. The patient's prothrombin time should be maintained at about 2 times control for a period of 3 months. At that time, warfarin should be stopped, and the patient should be placed on **aspirin.** (In most clinical studies, dosages of aspirin in the range of 650 mg bid have been used without dramatic benefit. However, experimental studies have suggested that lower a dosage, such as 325 mg qd, may be more appropriate [*N. Engl. J. Med.* 300:1142, 1979].) If TIAs recur, warfarin should be restarted in place of aspirin. Periodic attempts are then made every few months to switch to aspirin therapy.

    2. Vertebral-basilar TIA. The signs and symptoms of vertebral-basilar TIAs are referable to ischemia of the brainstem or occipital cerebral cortex. They usually include some combination of visual field loss, cortical blindness, diplopia, dysarthria, dysphagia, ataxia, generalized loss of muscular strength or tone without loss of consciousness, sensory changes (particularly circumoral numbness), deafness, tinnitus, or vertigo. Syncope, light-headedness, and vertigo, particularly when these appear alone, are not usually indicative of TIAs and strongly suggest disorders of the labyrinths or cardiovascular system (e.g., orthostatic hypotension or cardiac dysrhythmias).

    A CT scan and CSF examination are done (as in **1**). Angiography is not usually performed (unless to aid in the diagnosis), since the chances of a surgically correctable lesion are small. However, new surgical techniques are being devised, and their acceptance may alter this approach. If a candidate for long-term anticoagulation, the patient should be given heparin, followed by conversion to warfarin and, after 3 months, to aspirin (as described in **1**). If the patient is not a candidate for long-term anticoagulation, aspirin therapy should be considered.

B. Stroke in evolution refers to the progression of a neurologic deficit over 24 hours secondary to a stroke in the carotid artery distribution, or over 72 hours in the vertebral-basilar artery distribution. Evidence of progression may be obtained by history or by repeated examination. Thus, there is a need for close observation. A CT scan (if unavailable, angiography may be considered) and CSF examination should be done (for the reasons outlined in **A.1**). Barring any contraindication, the patient may be treated with heparin, followed by warfarin and aspirin (as described in **A.1**). Mortality from vertebral-basilar stroke in evolution has been shown to be significantly reduced with acute anticoagulation.

C. Completed stroke refers to a stable neurologic deficit for more than 24 hours with infarcts in the carotid artery distribution, or more than 72 hours with infarcts in the vertebral-basilar artery distribution. There is no evidence that anticoagulation is of any value in this situation. **Treatment** is aimed at identification and correction of the underlying causes, risk factors, and complications. Infarcts may swell, resulting in increased ICP. This is particularly true of cerebellar infarcts, which may then compress the brainstem and constitute a **neurologic emergency.** Overaggressive therapy of systemic hypertension is discouraged, and the maintenance of a diastolic blood pressure of 100–110 mm Hg may be appropriate. Supportive care should be given and efforts toward rehabilitation initiated. Patients with only a minimal fixed neurologic deficit in the carotid distribution constitute a difficult problem. Since a large percentage of strokes are due to proximal internal carotid artery disease, these patients are at risk of another stroke, with increasing neurologic deficit. Patients with stroke in the carotid distribution with a minimal deficit may be considered candidates for surgical intervention.

D. Lacunar infarcts are small infarcts (0.5–1.5 cm) that usually are multiple and associated with a history of hypertension. They characteristically occur in the basal ganglia, thalamus, ventral pons, internal capsule, corona radiata, and cerebellar white matter. They give rise to specific syndromes, including pure motor hemiplegia, pure hemisensory loss, clumsy hand dysarthria, and ataxic hemiparesis. The presence of aphasia, visual field deficits, and loss of cortical sensation (e.g., proprioception, astereognosis) with preserved primary sensation (e.g., pinprick, vibration) constitutes evidence against a lacunar infarct. **Treatment** consists of control of blood pressure. Anticoagulation generally is **not** used. Occasionally, large-vessel occlusive and/or embolic disease results in strokes or TIAs presenting as a pure motor hemiplegia or as pure hemisensory loss. These situations should be approached as outlined in **A** or **B** (particularly when the course is progressive, as in a stroke in evolution; or episodic, as in a TIA).

Weakness

Weakness is a common complaint and has a variety of causes, some of which are often overlooked. Weakness may be due to dysfunction at one or more of five levels: (1) muscle, (2) neuromuscular junction, (3) peripheral nerve, (4) lower motor neuron, and (5) upper motor neuron. Each level has its symptoms, signs, and differential diagnosis. Using this approach to the evaluation of weakness may serve to expand the differential diagnosis, so that specific diagnoses are not overlooked. Several specific disorders that may present as rapidly progressing generalized weakness will be discussed briefly. Common to management of all of these disorders is **maintenance of respiration** (see Chap. 8) and aggressive supportive measures similar to those described under Coma, sec. **IV.**

I. Polymyositis and dermatomyositis. Polymyositis and dermatomyositis may present with rapidly progressive proximal muscle weakness. Less than one-half of the patients with polymyositis have associated muscle pain, and approximately a third have elevated erythrocyte sedimentation rates (ESRs). (For a complete discussion of diagnosis and treatment see Chap. 21.) Other causes of acquired myopathies should be considered, although the list of possibilities is very extensive. In the initial evaluation it is especially important to measure electrolytes (particularly potassium, calcium, and phosphates), thyroid function, BUN, creatine kinase, ESR, and antinuclear antibodies. Complications of muscle breakdown must be anticipated (e.g., myoglobinuria).

II. Guillain-Barré syndrome. Guillain-Barré syndrome is a polyneuritis resulting in rapidly progressive motor paralysis, often following an acute febrile illness. Cranial nerves, especially the facial nerves, may be involved. Sensory symptoms may be present in the absence of objective sensory loss. Reflexes are usually hypoactive or absent. There is usually an elevated protein (especially IgG) in the CSF without a pleocytosis (occasionally lymphocytes, usually less than 20/μl, may be seen). The differential diagnosis includes arsenic exposure, acute porphyria, collagen vascular disease, tick paralysis, botulism, and postdiphtheritic paralysis.

Treatment is primarily supportive (especially respiratory support). Autonomic dysfunction, which may occur frequently, does not correlate with the amount of weakness and may be a leading cause of death. The dysfunction may result from overactivity or underactivity of either the sympathetic or parasympathetic nervous system. This results in paroxysmal episodes of hypertension, hypotension, cardiac dysrhythmias (tachycardia, bradycardia, or T-wave flattening or inversion in the ECG), increased pulmonary secretions, adynamic ileus, and urinary retention.

There is currently no generally accepted, organized approach to the treatment of the autonomic dysfunction. The use of various regimens has been anecdotal, and only general therapeutic guidelines can be given. In the treatment of the paroxysmal hypertension, short-acting agents that can be titrated against the patient's blood pressure should be used (see Chap. 7). The hypotension is usually due to decreased venous return secondary to peripheral vasodilatation. Patients on respirators, who already have compromised venous return, are particularly prone to hypotension. Treatment consists of intravascular volume expansion with IV fluids. Occasionally, this may not be sufficient, and vasopressors may be required (see Chap. 23). Cardiac monitoring is necessary, since cardiac dysrhythmias have been implicated as a significant cause of death in Guillain-Barré syndrome. The bradydysrhythmias respond to atropine, but caution is urged, since the bradydysrhythmias are usually transient, and atropine may worsen other aspects. Other possible causes of the cardiac dysrhythmias should be specifically excluded (e.g., hypoxia and electrolyte abnormalities). Supportive measures are carried out as outlined under Coma, sec. **IV.** The use of glucocorticoids is controversial, but it may be considered if the patient has not made any significant improvement after a few weeks of conservative therapy.

III. Myasthenia gravis. Myasthenia gravis is a disorder of the neuromuscular junction due to autoimmune mechanisms directed against the cholinergic receptor on the muscle membrane (*N. Engl. J. Med.* 298:135, 186, 1978). It is often associated with abnormalities of the thymus and is characterized by weakness and fatigability. The weakness is characteristically worse after exercise and improves with rest. A constant weakness, however, may occur. The pattern of muscle involvement determines its clinical presentation. It may present as ptosis, diplopia, dysarthria, dysphasia, extremity weakness, and/or respiratory difficulties. The clinical course is variable; spontaneous remissions or exacerbations may occur. The differential diagnosis includes botulism and the Eaton-Lambert (myasthenic) syndrome (neuromuscular defect associated with the remote effect of carcinoma).

A. Diagnosis

    1. Electromyogram. The response of the muscle action potential to repetitive nerve stimulation at 3 cps shows a decremental response in 95% of patients if affected muscles are tested. This decremental response is diagnostic. In botulism and the Eaton-Lambert syndrome there is an incremental response (at higher frequencies of 20 cps).

2. **Edrophonium (Tensilon) test.** Edrophonium inhibits the breakdown of acetylcholine released from nerves. This results in a marked improvement in strength in myasthenic patients. Patients with weakness from other causes, including hysteria, may also respond. Therefore, features that cannot be voluntarily produced by the patient should be checked, such as extraocular palsies or changes in the muscle action potential on repetitive nerve stimulation. A test dose of 2 mg is injected IV, and if no reaction occurs after 45 seconds, an additional 3 mg is injected. If no reaction occurs after 45 seconds, the remaining 5 mg is injected (a total dose of 10 mg). The response to edrophonium lasts approximately 5 minutes. Because of the possibility of severe bradycardia, atropine should be available.

B. **Treatment**

1. **Respiratory support** (see Chap. 8). Respiratory vital capacity should be checked frequently. Postural drainage and chest clapping should be done in patients with respiratory involvement. Suctioning of secretions may be necessary.

2. **Identify and treat precipitating factors,** such as thyroid abnormalities, pregnancy, infection, and drug reactions. Curare, ether, quinidine, quinine (in tonic water and some patent medicines), aminoglycosides, polymyxin, bacitracin, colistin, procainamide, phenytoin, and propranolol can worsen myasthenia.

3. **Anticholinesterase drugs** still constitute the symptomatic treatment of choice, particularly in ocular myasthenia, although this is controversial. These drugs function in a manner similar to edrophonium. The most commonly used ones are **pyridostigmine (Mestinon)** and **neostigmine (Prostigmin).** Sustained-release preparations **(Mestinon Timespan)** are available but should be used only at night if needed. **Pyridostigmine** can be started at 60 mg tid, and the dosage and timing of administration can be subsequently altered to anticipate the patient's needs. There is evidence to suggest that long-term anticholinesterase use may have an adverse effect on the neuromuscular junction. Excessive anticholinesterase use may cause marked weakness (see **C**). The dosage must be titrated to the **minimal amount** necessary to meet the individual patient's needs. In myasthenic crisis or in patients unable to tolerate oral medications, **neostigmine methylsulfate,** 0.5 mg IM q3–4h as needed, is available.

4. **Thymectomy** results in improvement in a majority of patients, particularly the young age group. In many centers, it is the treatment of choice. It is indicated in the young population (age <50 years), particularly in those who have not responded adequately to anticholinesterase therapy or who have a thymoma. Following thymectomy, the dosage of anticholinesterase drugs should be titrated to the **minimum necessary.**

5. **Glucocorticoids** are indicated for those who fail to respond adequately to anticholinesterase medications and thymectomy, or in whom thymectomy was not done. Prednisone therapy may be initiated at 25 mg qod and increased, if necessary, by 12.5 mg every third dose (up to 100 mg qod). Small doses of prednisone may be necessary on "off" days if the patient has many symptoms. Prednisone is continued until a maximal response is obtained and then is slowly tapered. At least a 3-month trial of prednisone is indicated. The **use of large initial doses may result in exacerbation of the myasthenia gravis.** Precautions must be taken regarding the complications of the long-term use of glucocorticoids (see Chap. 21, Systemic Lupus Erythematosus, sec. **II.E**). When glucocorticoids are used, the dosages of anticholinesterase drugs should be titrated down to the **minimum necessary.**

6. **Immunosuppressive drugs** may be used by experienced physicians in the unusual patients who are resistant to anticholinesterases, thymectomy, or glucocorticoids.

7. **Plasmapheresis** may result in remarkable symptomatic improvement but is impractical as maintenance therapy. It may be helpful during exacerbations of myasthenia gravis, particularly while other treatment modalities are being instituted.

C. **Cholinergic crisis** (rare) is increased weakness caused by excessive anticholinesterase. Other symptoms include abdominal cramps, diarrhea, increased lacrimation, increased salivation, excessive bronchial secretions, bradycardia, miosis, and muscle cramps and fasciculations. Differentiation from myasthenic crisis is often difficult. A **Tensilon test** may be of use. With excess anticholinesterase, no improvement occurs; indeed, the patient may worsen. When the differentiation from myasthenic crisis is **unclear,** or the crisis is caused by excess anticholinesterase administration, aggressive respiratory support and withholding anticholinesterase drugs is indicated. **Atropine,** 0.4 mg IM, may be used to counteract some of the muscarinic side effects.

IV. **Organophosphate poisoning.** Organophosphate poisoning results in symptoms as described in sec. **III.C** for cholinergic crisis. In addition, there may be tenesmus, pulmonary edema, and coma. Certain insecticides are the most common source. Since the poison can be absorbed through the skin, the patient's clothing should be removed, and the patient should be thoroughly washed. In adults, 1 gm of **pralidoxime chloride (Protopam, 2-PAM Chloride)** should be given IV. This should be done as soon as possible, since organophosphates may bind irreversibly to cholinesterases and become resistant to the effect of pralidoxime. The dose may be repeated, if needed, after 20 minutes. **Atropine,** 1 mg IV or IM (repeated q20–30min as needed), may be given to help control bradycardia and excess pulmonary secretions.

Head Injury

Two important points are often overlooked in the treatment of head trauma: (1) The reason for the head trauma may be secondary to some other illness, such as seizure, ataxia, or syncope; and (2) injury to other parts of the body is frequently associated. These oversights are especially likely to occur in evaluating the unresponsive patient.

I. **Types of head injury**

A. **Concussion** refers to a transient neurologic impairment not usually associated with any pathologically identifiable lesion. Deficits may include loss of consciousness or amnesia. The extent of retrograde amnesia may correlate with the severity of the head trauma.

B. **Contusion** usually refers to a longer-lasting neurologic deficit that may be associated with a pathologic alteration in the brain.

C. **Skull fractures** may be open or closed, and they may be linear, compound, or depressed. They signify significant head trauma and the need for close observation. A depressed skull fracture may require surgical elevation.

D. **Epidural hematoma** most commonly represents an accumulation of arterial blood between the dura and the inner table of the skull. With arterial bleeding there may be a rapid increase in ICP, with obtundation often following a lucid interval as long as several hours.

E. **Subdural hematoma** is a collection of venous blood between the dura and the arachnoid and can present as a mass lesion with focal neurologic deficits and increased ICP.

F. Intracerebral hematomas, lacerations, subarachnoid hemorrhage, and cerebral edema are other complications of head trauma.

II. Diagnosis

A. History. A detailed history should include events leading up to the injury, as well as the events immediately following it. The reason for the injury must be determined and may indicate the presence of another primary illness.

B. The **general physical examination** may provide evidence of other significant trauma. Careful examination of the head is important. Basilar skull fractures often cannot be seen on routine skull radiographs, and the presence of periorbital ecchymosis, ecchymosis over the mastoid process, hemotympanum, or CSF rhinorrhea or otorrhea may be the only sign of a basilar skull fracture.

C. The **neurologic examination** should be as complete as possible (see Coma, sec. **II.C**).

D. Skull and cervical spine radiographs should be obtained routinely (the head and neck should be stabilized until a cervical fracture has been excluded). One should specifically note the following in the review of the radiographs: (1) whether or not a fracture crosses the groove of the meningeal artery, thus placing the patient at risk of an epidural hematoma; (2) clouding of the sinuses, suggesting a basilar skull fracture; and (3) prevertebral soft tissue swelling on cervical spine radiographs as evidence of trauma when there are no obvious bony abnormalities.

E. Computed tomography scans and angiography may be needed. The CT scan has been a tremendous aid, since it enables easy recognition of acute collections of blood. A shift of midline structures suggests increased ICP and the danger of herniation.

III. Management

A. Maintenance of vital functions, such as respiration, blood pressure, and pulse, is the immediate concern. This is particularly true for patients with cervical and upper thoracic spinal cord lesions, since sudden and marked alteration in body temperature, blood pressure, or heart rate may develop in these patients. Hypertension and bradycardia may be a reflex response to some source of irritation that should be identified and treated (e.g., a distended urinary bladder). Hypotension usually results from a loss of venous return and usually responds to placing the patient supine with the legs elevated and the administration of IV isotonic fluids. However, other causes of hypotension should be considered (e.g., internal bleeding from a ruptured spleen).

B. In patients with altered mental status, especially in the presence of a focal neurologic deficit, one must consider the possibility of a surgically correctable, expanding mass lesion such as a hematoma (see Increased Intracranial Pressure).

C. Patients who are alert and without a neurologic deficit but with a history of loss of consciousness or amnesia (especially retrograde amnesia) should be considered for admission to the hospital for observation. Whether a patient with a less serious head trauma should be admitted to a hospital for observation may be dependent on other circumstances, such as proximity to a hospital and the availability of someone trustworthy to observe the patient and report untoward reactions. The patient should be admitted for a least 24–48 hours if there is any doubt.

D. Avoid medications that may alter mental status.

E. Avoid excessive hydration. Initially, the patient should be given nothing by mouth for 8–12 hours. Isotonic solutions at 75% of maintenance may be given IV, taking care to maintain good urine output, adequate blood pressure, and electrolyte balance.

F. Watch for complications, such as cerebral edema, diabetes insipidus, inappropriate antidiuretic hormone secretion, neurogenic pulmonary edema, or disseminated intravascular coagulation.

G. A **seizure** that occurs coincident with closed head trauma does not imply an increased risk of subsequent seizures, and anticonvulsant medications are not usually indicated. Seizures occurring after 1 week imply an increased risk of subsequent seizures and indicate the need for prolonged anticonvulsant therapy. The role of anticonvulsants in prophylaxis is unclear. Patients with injuries penetrating the dura should be considered for anticonvulsant prophylaxis.

H. Antibiotic prophylaxis for fractures that communicate with the scalp or sinuses is controversial. Generally, it is not recommended, since it may select out resistant organisms. Injuries penetrating the dura should be considered for antibiotic prophylaxis (especially against *Staphylococcus*).

Prolonged Seizures

For a general discussion of the treatment of seizures the reader is referred to G. Solomon and F. Plum, *Clinical Management of Seizures: A Guide for the Physician.* Philadelphia: Saunders, 1976. Discussed here is the treatment of the rare repeated generalized seizures between which the patient does not regain consciousness (i.e., **status epilepticus**). Patients who present with a single seizure should **not** be given IV anticonvulsants. Generally, the seizure will be over before the medication has any effect, and seizures usually will not immediately recur. In these situations, the patient is needlessly exposed to the risks of IV medication, and, in the case of drugs that cause sedation (e.g., diazepam and phenobarbital), the subsequent evaluation of the patient is made more difficult.

I. Treatment

A. Supportive measures. Vital functions such as respiration must be monitored and supported. Care should be taken to prevent aspiration. The patient must be protected from injury. A padded tongue depressor or plastic airway should be inserted between the teeth **if this can be done easily.** It does no good to damage teeth, gums, or tongue trying to force an object between tightly clenched teeth.

B. Rapid determination and treatment of the underlying cause. Seizures may be a manifestation of such underlying diseases as brain tumors, infarcts, meningitis, electrolyte abnormalities (including hyponatremia and hypocalcemia), uremia, anoxia, alcohol or drug withdrawal, inadequate anticonvulsant serum levels, and hypoglycemia. Unless the cause of the seizures is readily apparent, 50 ml of 50% D/W should be given IV after blood has been drawn for appropriate laboratory tests, including blood glucose. If alcohol abuse is suspected, thiamine, 10 mg given slowly IV and 100 mg IM, should also be administered, followed by 100 mg IM qd for 3 days.

C. Anticonvulsants

1. Diazepam (Valium), given IV, is often the drug of first choice in treating status epilepticus. It has a rapid onset of action. **It may stop the status epilepticus, but its use to prevent recurrence is impractical.** Once the seizures are controlled, longer-acting agents, such as phenytoin or phenobarbital, should be used. In adults, diazepam is given IV slowly and titrated to the dose that controls the seizures (usually up to 10 mg IV). This may be repeated once or twice at intervals of 10–15 minutes as necessary. Diazepam should **not** be given IM, since its absorption is erratic. Hypotension and respiratory suppression may occur, especially if diazepam is given concurrently with barbiturates. In some centers, IV phenytoin is the drug of first choice. However, many patients do not tolerate well the large loading dose of phenytoin that may be required for seizure control. Intravenous diazepam is usually well tolerated when used cautiously and, furthermore, allows the physician to administer phenytoin at a more cautious pace.

2. **Phenytoin** is used in the treatment of status epilepticus when diazepam has failed, or to prevent recurrence when diazepam has succeeded. Phenytoin must be given directly into the vein (when the patient cannot take it PO), since it does not mix with the usual IV solutions. It should be given at a rate not greater than 50 mg/minute, and vital signs should be monitored during administration. Hypotension, apnea, and cardiac dysrhythmias may occur. The usual loading dose is 750–1500 mg (i.e., 15–18 mg/kg body weight) and should be given in divided doses every few hours, depending on the patient's clinical status. Daily maintenance is 300–500 mg (i.e., 4–8 mg/kg body weight) PO or IV to maintain a therapeutic plasma level of 10–20 μg/ml (1.0–2.0 mg/dl). Phenytoin should not be given IM. It must be used with caution in patients with cardiac dysrhythmias.

3. **Phenobarbital** may be used when diazepam and phenytoin have failed. Care must be taken to avoid respiratory suppression, particularly in patients who have already received diazepam. The initial dose is 120–240 mg, given slowly IV. This may be repeated at intervals of 20–30 minutes with a total dosage up to 400–600 mg. Maintenance dosages are 1–5 mg/kg of body weight/day PO, IM, or IV to maintain a therapeutic plasma level of 15–40 μg/ml (1.5–4.0 mg/dl).

4. **Paraldehyde** may be used if the preceding measures fail. It should be given PR as 8–10 ml of paraldehyde mixed with an equal volume of **vegetable oil** in a retention enema (use a rubber catheter, since paraldehyde reacts with plastics). This may result in local irritation. Paraldehyde, 3–5 ml, may be given by deep IM injection, although this may result in sterile abscesses; 5 ml of paraldehyde in 500 ml of 5% D/W can be given as a constant IV infusion and titrated to control the seizures. Pulmonary edema and pulmonary hemorrhage may result from IV infusion, particularly from a bolus injection. Respiratory depression may occur. Glass syringes and containers must be used.

5. **Anesthesia.** If seizures persist despite the preceding measures, the patient should be intubated and placed under general anesthesia with large doses of short-acting barbiturates (e.g., sodium thiopental, 0.5–1.0 mg/kg body weight) under the supervision of an anesthesiologist. Rarely, neuromuscular blocking agents may be required.

II. **Complications.** Complications, such as cerebral edema, aspiration, rhabdomyolysis, myoglobinuria, and hyperthermia, must be anticipated and treated.

Alcohol Withdrawal

The disorders associated with alcohol withdrawal may occur in any walk of life. The diagnosis may be missed if a high index of suspicion is not maintained. The reason for the withdrawal from alcohol must be determined. Often, it is due to some illness that interferes with continued alcohol intake, such as trauma, infections, pancreatitis, and gastritis.

I. **Minor withdrawal.** Minor withdrawal is characterized by tremulousness, irritability, anorexia, nausea, and occasionally hallucinations. These symptoms usually appear in the first few hours and resolve within 48 hours after the last drink or marked reduction in intake. A well-lighted room, the presence of friends or relatives, and reassurance are important to the **treatment.** Many of the symptoms can be treated with benzodiazepines, including **chlordiazepoxide**, 25–100 mg PO q6h, or **diazepam**, 5–20 mg PO q6h. The **goal of therapy** is to calm the patient without causing stupor. The dosage must be titrated to the patient's clinical state. The patient should also be given thiamine and multivitamins and should be observed for the development of more severe withdrawal reactions. The social circumstances will dictate whether this should be done at home or in the hospital.

II. **Seizures.** Alcohol withdrawal seizures ordinarily occur 12–48 hours after cessation of drinking and are usually generalized motor seizures. They may occur several times, but status epilepticus is rare. Treatment of alcohol withdrawal seizures with anticonvulsants is usually **not** indicated. The seizures are usually few in number, and most drugs may be ineffective in preventing them. If seizures are frequent, the treatment approach outlined under Prolonged Seizures may be used. A major problem is that this population is prone to underlying seizure disorders other than those caused by alcohol withdrawal. Unless such disorders have been previously excluded, the patient should be evaluated (including CT scan, CSF examination, and EEG). Immediate causes of seizures should be investigated (e.g., meningitis, electrolyte abnormalities, hypoglycemia). Thiamine and multivitamins should be given.

III. **Delirium tremens.** Delirium tremens is characterized by tremulousness, hallucinations, agitation, confusion, disorientation, and **autonomic overactivity** (i.e., fever, tachycardia, and profuse perspiration). It usually occurs 72–96 hours after cessation of drinking and generally starts to resolve within 3–5 days. Other causes of delirium should be considered (see Delirium). This is a serious disorder with a significant risk of death. The major concern of **treatment** is to prevent patient injury. A well-lighted room, reassurance, and calm on the part of the physician are important. Drug sedation and physical restraints may be necessary. **Diazepam** may be used with dosages titrated to control the patient (5–10 mg IV initially, then 5 mg q5–10min until control is achieved, followed by 5–10 mg every few hours). After such large doses, subsequent doses must be tapered because of the accumulation of the parent compound or its active metabolites. **Chlordiazepoxide** may be used in an initial dose of 100 mg IV or PO and repeated q2–6h as needed, with a maximum dosage of 500 mg in the first 24 hours. One-half the total dosage may be administered over the next 24 hours and reduced by 25–50 mg/day each day thereafter. Neither diazepam nor chlordiazepoxide should be given IM, since absorption may be erratic. Thiamine, 100 mg IM, should be given and repeated daily for 3 days, then given PO. Multivitamins should also be given.

Maintenance of fluid and electrolyte balance is important, since these patients are susceptible to hypomagnesemia and hypoglycemia; fluid losses may be considerable because of fever, diaphoresis, and vomiting. Other medical complications should be anticipated and treated appropriately.

Tetanus

Tetanus is characterized by generalized (occasionally localized) muscle spasm (especially trismus), resulting from an intoxication of the nervous system by the exotoxin (tetenospasmin) of *Clostridium tetani*. The incubation period ranges from 2–54 days. In the majority of patients the date of onset is within 14 days from the time of injury. Tetanus often follows puncture wounds, lacerations, and crush injuries, but it may also occur without a demonstrable wound. Tetanus is also seen in the inadequately immunized parenteral drug abuser, particularly heroin addicts who "skin pop." Mortality may be as high as 50–60%, with most deaths occurring within 10 days.

I. **Prophylaxis.** Immunization is essential for prevention.

A. **Active immunization** is the most effective and preferred method of prophylaxis. School children (7 years of age or older) and adults not previously immunized should receive a primary immunization series of **tetanus and diphtheria toxoids (Td) for adult use:** One dose of Td (0.5 ml) is given IM, with the second dose

4–8 weeks after the first and the third dose 6–12 months after the second. Thereafter, periodic booster doses at 10-year intervals will maintain a protective level of immunity in the majority of patients. Patients who have sustained minor wounds are often given a single dose of Td (for adult use) if they have not received any immunization in the previous 10 years, or 5 years if the wound is "tetanus prone" (e.g., a severe deep puncture). The only contraindication to the use of Td is a neurologic or severe hypersensitivity reaction to a previous dose.

B. Passive immunization should be administered to unimmunized or inadequately immunized patients with other than clean, minor wounds. Human tetanus immune globulin, TIG(H), 250 units, is given IM. Equine or bovine antitoxin is not recommended if TIG(H) is available, because the animal antitoxins are associated with a considerable risk of anaphylactic reactions or serum sickness. The patient should be actively immunized (see **A**). A separate syringe and injection site should be used when both forms of immunization are administered concurrently.

II. Management. The goals of therapy are to prevent muscle spasm and respiratory complications, to remove the source of toxin, and to neutralize the toxin not yet fixed to the nervous system. The intensity of the muscle spasm begins to diminish slowly during the second week. Complete recovery may take several months.

A. General measures

1. The organism is usually noninvasive and produces its effect by systemic spread of its exotoxin. The wound must be thoroughly debrided and cleansed to remove the source of exotoxin.

2. **Antibiotics.** Penicillin G should be given IV in a dosage of 1 million units q6h for 10 days. In patients allergic to penicillin, tetracycline (2 gm/day) should be used.

3. Early endotracheal intubation or tracheostomy is indicated, since the severe muscle spasms may affect the larynx, resulting in suffocation.

4. General care is given as outlined under Coma, sec. **IV**.

5. **Analgesics** should be used to relieve the pain associated with the tonic contractions of tetanus.

6. Sympathetic nervous system involvement may occur, resulting in cardiac dysrhythmias and wide fluctuations in blood pressure.

B. For neutralization of toxin, 3000–10,000 units of TIG(H) should be given IM, distributed among several sites, including sites proximal to the suspected source of exotoxin. Active immunization with Td (adult dosage) is still necessary at the end of the illness (see sec. **I.A**).

C. Spasms are managed with diazepam, barbiturates, or chlorpromazine administration, with the patient kept in quiet isolation. The optimal level of continuous sedation is achieved when the patient remains sleepy but can be aroused to follow commands. Rarely, spasms may persist, and curariform drugs and ventilatory support of respirations may be indicated. **Convulsions** should be treated (see Prolonged Seizures).

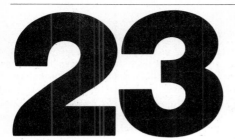

Medical Emergencies

Upper Airway Obstruction

Upper airway obstruction can be caused by infection, foreign body, tumor, trauma, laryngeal edema, laryngospasm, or, most commonly, the patient's own tongue (in the unconscious supine victim). In the awake patient, dyspnea, stridor, weak cough, inability to speak, and cyanosis may be present. In the unconscious victim, this condition may be recognized by inability to ventilate using the bag-valve-mask or mouth-to-mouth technique. It is essential to make the diagnosis early and establish an airway as soon as possible in order to prevent irreversible anoxic brain damage or cardiac arrest.

I. **Upper airway obstruction with adequate ventilation.** In adequately ventilated patients with upper airway obstruction, no emergency procedures are immediately necessary. Appropriate diagnostic tests, such as soft-tissue neck x rays, and specialty consultation are indicated.

II. **Upper airway obstruction with inadequate ventilation.** When ventilation is inadequate in upper airway obstruction, attempt to **open the airway** by properly positioning the patient and/or performing a standard airway maneuver, such as the head tilt–neck lift, head tilt–chin lift, or jaw thrust; the jaw thrust without head tilt is preferred in suspected neck injuries. These maneuvers are particularly useful in relieving soft tissue airway obstruction in patients with a depressed level of consciousness. If these procedures fail to establish an airway and attempts at ventilation with the bag-valve-mask or mouth-to-mouth technique are unsuccessful, proceed as described in **A** and **B**.

A. **Suspected foreign body**

1. **Four back blows** and then **four manual thrusts** (Heimlich maneuver) should be delivered immediately. This step may be omitted in the unconscious victim if proper equipment is readily available.

2. Next, if necessary, **manual removal** of the obstructing foreign body with a clamp or forceps under direct visualization with a laryngoscope should be attempted. If proper equipment is not available, removal should be attempted by sweeping the index finger across the posterior pharynx. The finger-sweep technique, however, should be used with caution, especially in awake patients, to avoid bite injuries or inadvertently pushing the foreign body deeper into the pharynx.

3. If these attempts fail, an airway must be established without delay distal to the site of obstruction by **transtracheal catheter ventilation, cricothyrotomy,** or, rarely, **tracheostomy.** Transtracheal catheter ventilation is performed by introducing a large-bore IV catheter through the cricothyroid membrane inferiorly into the trachea, attaching the catheter to a high-pressure oxygen source, and ventilating the patient with intermittent jets of oxygen 12–16 times/minute. In cricothyrotomy, the cricothyroid membrane is incised, and a small tracheostomy or endotracheal tube is inserted directly into the trachea.

B. Non-foreign-body obstruction

1. **Tracheal intubation** via the oral or nasal route should be attempted. The nasal route is preferred in suspected cervical spine injuries. Blind nasotracheal intubation, however, is not recommended in nonbreathing patients or in patients with laryngeal edema.

2. If tracheal intubation is not possible or unsuccessful, **transtracheal catheter ventilation, cricothyrotomy,** or, rarely, **tracheostomy** should be performed, preferably by personnel well trained in the technique.

Cardiac Arrest

Cardiac arrest is the cessation of breathing and circulation. It is recognized by pulselessness and absent breathing in an unconscious victim. The initial approach to the cardiac arrest victim is standardized with careful attention to the ABCs (*a*irway, *b*reathing, *c*irculation). Resuscitation efforts should follow the recommendations of the American Heart Association (*J.A.M.A.* 244:453, 1980).

I. Basic life support

A. Immediate response. Establish unresponsiveness, call for help, and place the victim in a supine position (taking care with suspected spinal injury).

B. ABCs

1. **Open the airway** with an appropriate airway maneuver (see Upper Airway Obstruction).

2. If spontaneous breathing does not occur, rescue **breathing** should be started with four quick ventilations. Oxygenation with mouth-to-mouth or bag-valve-mask technique should always precede attempts at endotracheal intubation.

3. **Circulation.** If no pulse is palpable, **external chest compression** is initiated with a 50% compression and 50% relaxation cycle. For a single rescuer, a compression-ventilation ratio of 15:2 with a compression rate of 80/minute is recommended. For two rescuers, a compression-ventilation ratio of 5:1 with a compression rate of 60/minute is indicated. It is essential not to stop cardiopulmonary resuscitation (CPR) for more than 5 seconds except under special circumstances, such as endotracheal intubation, and then cessation should not exceed 30 seconds.

II. Advanced life support

A. A **large-bore IV line** is essential. Initially, peripheral access is preferable if readily available. Later, a central venous catheter may be useful to deliver drugs directly into the central circulation and measure central venous pressure (CVP). Ideally, CPR should not be interrupted for central venous cannulation.

B. Drugs

1. Supplemental **oxygen** at 100% concentration should be delivered as soon as possible.

2. **Epinephrine,** an alpha- and beta-adrenergic agonist, stimulates spontaneous cardiac contractions, elevates perfusion pressure during CPR, and may convert fine ventricular fibrillation (VF) to a coarse pattern that is more amenable to electrical defibrillation. It is useful in **asystole, electromechanical dissociation,** and **VF** in dosages of 0.5–1.0 mg (5–10 ml of a 1:10,000 solution) given IV q5min as needed. Endotracheal administration is recommended when IV access is not readily available and an endotracheal tube is in place. **Intracardiac injections are not recommended.**

3. **Sodium bicarbonate** is indicated for correction of **metabolic acidosis.** Ideally, bicarbonate therapy should be guided by arterial blood gas (ABG) determinations. However, if blood gas results are unavailable, an initial bolus of 1 mEq/kg can be given IV, followed by half that dose q10–15min. Adequate ventilation is essential to eliminate the carbon dioxide generated. Complications of excess bicarbonate therapy include metabolic alkalosis, hyperosmolality, and fluid overload.

4. **Atropine,** a vagolytic drug, enhances the rate of discharge of the sinoatrial node and improves atrioventricular conduction. It is useful in treating **bradydysrhythmias** with associated hemodynamic compromise or ventricular premature depolarizations. Atropine may also be effective in restoring electrical activity in asystole. The recommended dosage is 0.5 mg IV (1 mg in asystole), repeated q5min as needed to a total dose of 2 mg.

5. **Isoproterenol** is a pure beta-adrenergic agonist with potent inotropic and chronotropic properties (at the expense of increased myocardial oxygen requirements). It is indicated for hemodynamically significant, atropine-resistant **bradydysrhythmias.** Isoproterenol may also be useful for asystole and electromechanical dissociation. An infusion is made by adding 1 or 2 mg of isoproterenol to 500 ml of 5% D/W (2 or 4 μg/ml) and titrating to the desired heart rate (usually 2–20 μg/minute).

6. **Calcium** ions play an important role in myocardial excitation-contraction coupling. Calcium increases myocardial contractility and may enhance ventricular automaticity. It is useful for **electromechanical dissociation** and **asystole** in a dose of 5 ml of a 10% solution of calcium chloride, given IV, repeated at 10-minute intervals as needed.

7. **Lidocaine** suppresses discharge from ventricular ectopic foci, increases the myocardial fibrillation threshold, and may terminate reentrant ventricular dysrhythmias. Lidocaine is the drug of choice for the treatment of **ventricular tachycardia** and may be useful as adjunctive therapy in the management of VF. It should also be used prophylactically following conversion of these dysrhythmias to a supraventricular rhythm. The dosage is 1.5 mg/kg IV initially, followed by 1 mg/kg q5–10min as needed, to a maximum of 225 mg. On dysrhythmia termination, an infusion of 1–4 mg/minute should be started. Maintenance dosages should be reduced in the presence of liver dysfunction or decreased hepatic blood flow (e.g., congestive heart failure, shock).

8. **Bretylium tosylate** produces adrenergic blockade, may terminate ventricular reentrant dysrhythmias, increases the VF threshold, facilitates electrical defibrillation, and may have direct defibrillatory activity. It is recommended in the treatment of **VF** and refractory ventricular tachycardia. The dosage is 5 mg/kg IV (by rapid injection if the patient is hemodynamically compromised but over 8–10 minutes if in a stable condition). Repeat doses of 10 mg/kg can be given at 15- –30-minute intervals to a total dosage of 30 mg/kg. For continued dysrhythmia suppression, a continuous infusion of 1–2 mg/minute may be used.

9. **Dopamine** is an alpha-, beta-, and dopamine-receptor stimulator. It differs from other vasopressors in its selective dose-related response. Dopamine is indicated for **hemodynamically significant hypotension not secondary to hypovolemia.** An infusion is made by adding 400 or 800 mg of dopamine to 500 ml of 5% D/W (800 or 1600 μg/ml) and titrating to the desired effect (usually 2–50 μg/kg/minute).

10. **Norepinephrine** has alpha- and beta-adrenergic properties and is useful in **nonhypovolemic hypotension.** Because of its potent vasoconstrictor activity, norepinephrine may increase coronary perfusion during CPR and thus be a beneficial adjunct in the treatment of cardiac arrest. An infusion is

prepared by adding 4 mg of norepinephrine (levarterenol) base to 500 ml of 5% D/W (8 µg/ml of base) and titrating to the desired blood pressure (initially 16–24 µg/minute).

C. Defibrillation, electrical cardioversion, and precordial thump

1. **Electrical defibrillation** is the termination of VF by an unsynchronized DC current. **Electrical cardioversion** is the termination of dysrhythmias other than VF, usually by a synchronized DC current. Emergency cardioversion is indicated for rapid ventricular or supraventricular rhythms in which dysrhythmia termination is essential to prevent clinical deterioration. **Blind defibrillation** is indicated when a defibrillator is immediately available in a witnessed, unmonitored cardiac arrest. It may be successful if VF is present and will not be harmful in the presence of asystole. **Countershock** is performed by placing one paddle to the right of the upper sternum and the other paddle to the left of the cardiac apex, or one paddle anteriorly over the sternum and the other posteriorly behind the heart. The energy dosage depends on the clinical setting (see **F.3** and **4**).

2. The **precordial thump** is accomplished by delivering a sharp blow to the midsternum. This produces a small electrical stimulus that may convert ventricular tachycardia or VF of recent onset or generate a beat in ventricular asystole secondary to complete heart block. Since this low-voltage stimulus may cause VF in an anoxic heart, the **precordial thump is recommended only in monitored patients** with these dysrhythmias.

D. The **MAST suit** (medical antishock trousers) appears to be a useful adjunct in cardiac arrest by increasing blood pressure, carotid blood flow, and possibly coronary perfusion during CPR (*Ann. Emerg. Med.* 10:560, 1981).

E. Transvenous or transthoracic pacemakers are indicated in hemodynamically significant, medically refractory **bradydysrhythmias** and **asystole**. During CPR, the subxiphoid transthoracic approach may be preferable, since it enables direct intracardiac electrode placement without interrupting CPR.

F. Dysrhythmia management. Successful management requires adequate coronary perfusion, correction of acidosis, hypoxia, and electrolyte disorders, and correct drug usage.

1. In **asystole, epinephrine** is the drug of choice and is given IV in doses of 0.5–1.0 mg q5min as needed. Calcium and atropine may also be useful. If this approach is unsuccessful, an infusion of a sympathomimetic agent may be tried; although isoproterenol is currently recommended, drugs with alpha-adrenergic properties (e.g., dopamine, norepinephrine) may be more beneficial (*Crit. Care Med.* 7:293, 1979). Early pacemaker insertion may also be helpful.

2. **Bradydysrhythmias.** For hemodynamically significant bradycardia (i.e., associated hypotension or ventricular ectopy), **atropine**, 0.5 mg IV q5min as needed to a total dosage of 2 mg, is the drug of choice. If this is unsuccessful, an **isoproterenol** infusion may be administered and followed by **pacemaker** insertion if necessary. In the presence of hypotension, epinephrine or dopamine may be preferable to isoproterenol.

3. **Ventricular tachycardia.** Initially, a precordial thump may be delivered in monitored patients. In **hemodynamically compromised** patients, immediate **countershock** (preferably with synchronized current) at 100–200 joules is indicated. If there is no response, additional countershocks at higher energy settings (up to 320–360 joules delivered energy) and concomitant lidocaine therapy (1.5 mg/kg IV, followed by 1 mg/kg q5–10min as needed, to a maximum of 225 mg) should be administered. If ventricular tachycardia is refractory to these measures, bretylium followed by additional countershocks is indicated. In patients in **stable condition**, pharmacologic conversion with

lidocaine should be attempted initially. If unsuccessful, synchronized DC cardioversion with 20–100 joules is recommended.

4. **Ventricular fibrillation.** In monitored patients a precordial thump may be attempted initially. Otherwise, an initial unsynchronized **countershock** at 200–300 joules should be administered and repeated immediately if unsuccessful. If this is ineffective, epinephrine and sodium bicarbonate should be given (and repeated as indicated). An attempt at electrical defibrillation with 320–360 joules delivered energy should follow and should be repeated if there is no response. If countershock is still unsuccessful, **lidocaine,** 1.5 mg/kg IV, should be administered and followed by countershock at 320–360 joules. If VF persists, **bretylium,** 5 mg/kg IV, should be given, repeated at 10 mg/kg q15min as needed, to a maximum dosage of 30 mg/kg, and followed by further attempts at electrical defibrillation.

5. **Electromechanical dissociation** (i.e., organized electrical activity without a pulse). **Epinephrine,** 0.5–1.0 mg IV q5min, and **calcium chloride,** 5 ml of a 10% solution IV q10min, are the mainstays of therapy. If they are unsuccessful, infusion of an adrenergic agent should be started. In addition, reversible causes, such as profound hypovolemia, tension pneumothorax, or cardiac tamponade, should be sought and corrected if present.

G. Continuous **monitoring** of cardiac arrest victims is essential to ensure adequate therapy. This includes cardiac monitoring, periodic blood gas determinations to evaluate oxygenation and acid-base status, and monitoring arterial pulsations to check the adequacy of chest compressions.

H. **Termination of CPR.** The decision to terminate CPR is difficult and controversial. In the emergency setting, it should be based on **cardiovascular unresponsiveness** rather than on suspected cerebral death.

Shock

Shock is a severe pathophysiologic syndrome due to a generalized **inadequacy of tissue perfusion** and characterized by impaired cellular metabolism. Clinical manifestations generally include altered sensorium, relative hypotension, tachycardia, tachypnea, oliguria, metabolic acidosis, weak or absent pulses, pallor, diaphoresis, and cool skin.

I. **Classification.** Shock may be classified according to the primary pathophysiologic mechanism involved as follows: **oligemic** (e.g., hemorrhage, fluid depletion or sequestration); **cardiogenic** (e.g., myocardial infarction, dysrhythmia, acute regurgitant lesions); **obstructive** (e.g., pericardial tamponade, pulmonary embolus); and **distributive,** characterized by maldistribution of vascular volume secondary to altered vasomotor tone (e.g., sepsis, anaphylaxis, spinal cord insult). (See the appropriate sections of the *Manual* for discussions of specific shock syndromes.)

II. **Assessment. Monitoring** vital signs, ECG, CBC, ABGs, serum electrolytes, creatinine, urinary output, and central venous or pulmonary artery occlusive (wedge) pressure is essential. Cardiac output determinations are also useful.

A. Decreased pulse pressure is often an early sign of shock, and **systolic pressures below 90 mm Hg are often associated with vital organ hypoperfusion.** It is important to remember, however, that blood pressure is not always a reliable indication of tissue perfusion, and cuff measurements are not always accurate in shock; accuracy, however, may be improved by the use of a Doppler device or preferably an arterial catheter.

B. A low **hematocrit** may indicate blood loss. In the acute setting, however, the hematocrit may not accurately reflect the amount of blood loss. A high hematocrit may indicate dehydration.

C. **Central venous pressure** (CVP) is a suboptimal method of assessing volume status, since it reflects only the right ventricular filling pressure. A low CVP (<5 cm H_2O), however, is usually a reliable sign of volume-responsive hypotension; a high CVP (>15 cm H_2O) suggests right ventricular dysfunction and/or volume overload. However, CVP measurements are most useful as a means of following trends in a patient's response to fluid therapy. In contrast, the **pulmonary artery occlusive pressure is usually a reliable indicator of left ventricular filling pressure and is the preferred method of monitoring volume status.** A low value (<6 mm Hg) indicates hypovolemia; an elevated measurement (>18 mm Hg) usually reflects left ventricular failure and/or fluid overload.

D. **Serum pH** and arterial lactate levels are useful indicators of the adequacy of tissue perfusion. Although respiratory alkalosis is frequently seen in early shock, metabolic acidosis secondary to accumulation of lactic acid is a sign of tissue hypoperfusion.

E. **Renal function** is a useful indicator of peripheral perfusion. Oliguria, increased urinary osmolarity, and decreased urinary sodium (<20 mEq/liter) are signs of peripheral hypoperfusion.

III. **Treatment.** The goal of therapy is **rapid achievement of adequate tissue perfusion.** This is generally indicated by a systolic blood pressure above 90 mm Hg, urinary output above 0.5 ml/kg/hour, correction of metabolic acidosis, and a cardiac index greater than 2.2. liters/M^2/minute. Specific therapy should be directed at correction of the underlying problem and tailored to the type of shock, which can often be determined by the history, physical examination, and appropriate diagnostic tests.

A. Supplemental **oxygen** should be administered to all patients in shock to enhance tissue oxygenation. Mechanical ventilation should be used as needed to maintain the PO$_2$ above 60 mm Hg.

B. Initially, rapid **volume expansion** with crystalloid (i.e., normal saline or Ringer's lactate) is indicated unless there is evidence of pulmonary congestion. If shock is accompanied by uncertain cardiac function and/or fluid status, a fluid challenge of 300 ml of crystalloid may be given over 15–20 minutes, followed by reevaluation of cardiopulmonary status. If there is no evidence of volume overload, similar infusions may be repeated as needed. In shock secondary to acute blood loss, persistent hypotension after infusion of 2 liters of crystalloid is an indication for immediate transfusion of whole blood (or packed cells).

C. The **MAST suit** minimizes venous capacitance in the lower half of the body, augments venous return, and elevates peripheral resistance, thus increasing perfusion pressure to vital organs. It is a useful adjunct in treating oligemic shock and may be useful in managing other types of shock in which an increase in afterload would not be detrimental.

D. **Sodium bicarbonate,** given IV, is indicated for correction of severe metabolic acidosis (i.e., pH <7.2).

E. **Vasoactive drugs** (inotropic drugs, vasopressors, vasodilators) may be needed to augment cardiac output and perfusion of vital organs but are **to be used only after an adequate circulating volume is established.** The choice of a given drug should be based on the underlying pathophysiologic features of the particular form of shock. (See other sections of the *Manual* for discussions of vasoactive drugs.)

Anaphylaxis and Anaphylactoid Reactions

Anaphylaxis is an acute allergic reaction following antigen exposure in a sensitized person. It is usually mediated by IgE antibodies and involves release of chemical mediators from mast cells and basophils. Anaphylactoid reactions are the result of direct release of these chemical mediators triggered by nonantigenic agents. Anaphylactic or anaphylactoid reactions may occur after exposure to extracts of pollen, drugs, foreign serum, insect stings, diagnostic agents such as iodinated contrast materials, vaccines, local anesthetics, and food products. A history of known sensitivity may not be elicited.

I. **Clinical features.** The clinical features span a wide spectrum, including apprehension, pruritus, urticaria, angioedema, respiratory distress, and hypotension. Respiratory embarrassment may be due to laryngeal edema, laryngospasm, or bronchospasm. Shock may be secondary to profound hypoxia, peripheral vasodilatation, or hypovolemia due to capillary leakage. Vascular collapse may develop in the absence of respiratory symptoms, and death may occur within minutes.

II. **Treatment**

A. **Epinephrine** is the drug of choice for initial treatment of anaphylactic or anaphylactoid reactions. For life-threatening reactions, 0.5 mg (5 ml of a 1 : 10,000 solution) should be given IV and repeated q5–10min as needed. Sublingual or endotracheal administration may be effective when an IV line cannot be established. For less severe reactions, 0.3–0.5 mg (0.3–0.5 ml of a 1 : 1000 solution) may be administered SQ q20–30min as needed, up to 3 doses.

B. **Maintaining a patent airway is essential.** Endotracheal intubation and assisted ventilation may be necessary for severe bronchospasm. In cases of severe laryngeal edema, transtracheal catheter ventilation, cricothyrotomy, or tracheostomy may be necessary (see Upper Airway Obstruction). **Oxygen** should be administered to all patients in respiratory distress.

C. **Aminophylline,** 6 mg/kg as a loading dose, may be infused IV over 20–30 minutes to treat bronchospasm. This should be followed by an initial maintenance infusion of 0.5–1.0 mg/kg/hour (*F.D.A. Drug Bull.* 10:4, 1980).

D. Rapid **volume expansion** with normal saline or Ringer's lactate solution may be needed to restore and maintain tissue perfusion. Large losses of fluid from the intravascular compartment are the rule and must be replaced, preferably with CVP monitoring.

E. A **vasopressor** is indicated to manage hypotension unresponsive to volume expansion. Dopamine, 2–50 µg/kg/minute, is the agent of choice.

F. **Hydrocortisone sodium succinate,** 500 mg IV q6h, or its equivalent should be administered for serious and life-threatening reactions. Corticosteroids are not first-line drugs; their major role is in preventing later redevelopment of the clinical syndrome. Their peak effect occurs in 6–12 hours.

G. **Antihistamines** are probably of little value in treating the acute episode. However, they may block further histamine binding to target tissues and thus shorten the duration of the reaction and prevent relapses. Diphenhydramine hydrochloride, 25–50 mg IV (or IM or PO) q6h, may be given.

H. To delay absorption of an injected antigen, place a tourniquet proximal to the injection site (if possible) to occlude lymphatic and venous drainage (but not arterial flow), and inject 0.3 mg of 1 : 1000 epinephrine SQ into the site. Forced emesis with syrup of ipecac, 30 ml PO, followed by administration of activated charcoal and a cathartic, may prevent continued absorption of an orally ingested antigen.

I. All patients with anaphylactic or anaphylactoid reactions should be observed for at least 6–12 hours.

Acute Adrenal Crisis

Acute adrenal crisis may be the initial presentation of occult adrenal insufficiency (Addison's disease) or the result of inadequate corticosteroid therapy in a patient with known adrenal insufficiency. Adrenal crisis may also occur following cessation of corticosteroid therapy or as a result of insufficient corticosteroid administration during a period of stress. Any patient who has been taking a daily dosage of hydrocortisone greater than 20–25 mg for more than 1–2 months has potentially undergone enough adrenal suppression to be at risk of the development of this syndrome. A crisis can be precipitated by a variety of stressful situations, including infection, hemorrhage, pregnancy, surgery, or trauma. Rarely, adrenal apoplexy may occur in a patient with overwhelming sepsis or receiving anticoagulant therapy.

I. Clinical features. The clinical features result from a deficiency of the adrenal glands' two primary hormones, aldosterone and cortisol. A **deficiency of aldosterone** leads to impaired salt retention and extracellular fluid volume depletion. This results in weakness, postural syncope, hypotension, azotemia, hyponatremia, and hyperkalemia. **Cortisol depletion** leads to impaired gluconeogenesis (which may result in symptomatic hypoglycemia), decreased vascular tone (which also contributes to hypotension), and GI upset (e.g., anorexia, nausea, vomiting, abdominal pain). Hyperpyrexia or hypothermia may also be present.

II. Treatment. Treatment requires prompt recognition of the disorder, based on its clinical features, and rapid administration of parenteral corticosteroids and fluids.

A. Although treatment should not be delayed to await the results of confirmatory laboratory tests, serum should be drawn for cortisol determination prior to initiating therapy.

B. Hydrocortisone sodium succinate, 100 mg, should be administered immediately by IV bolus and followed by a second 100-mg dose in the first liter of IV fluids (see sec. **C**). This should be followed by 100 mg IV q8h. Cortisone acetate, 50–100 mg IM, may also be given to provide a source of continuing hormone therapy should the IV infusion of hydrocortisone be interrupted. Mineralocorticoid administration is not necessary, because hydrocortisone in the doses employed has sufficient mineralocorticoid activity.

C. Intravenous fluids, initially 5% D/W in normal saline, should be administered rapidly, ideally with CVP monitoring, to correct hypovolemia. The average extracellular volume deficit is approximately 20%, or 3 liters.

D. A **vasopressor** (e.g., dopamine) may be required to manage hypotension unresponsive to IV corticosteroids and fluids.

E. Hypoglycemia, hyperkalemia, and hyperpyrexia or hypothermia should be treated appropriately.

F. The precipitating cause of the crisis requires identification and appropriate treatment. In particular, infection should be strongly suspected when adrenal crisis has developed without an obvious cause.

Heat Illness

I. Heat cramps. Heat cramps are painful skeletal muscle spasms resulting from sodium depletion secondary to sweat losses. Treatment involves rest in a cool environment and salt replacement.

II. Heat exhaustion. Heat exhaustion is due to salt and water depletion secondary to sweating. Manifestations include GI upset, mild CNS symptoms (e.g., headache, dizziness, lassitude, irritability), volume depletion (e.g., hypotension, tachycardia, syncope), and hyperventilation. Muscle cramps may also occur. Patients are sweating, and their body temperatures are usually normal or mildly elevated. Treatment consists of rest in a cool environment, rehydration, and salt replacement (e.g., administration of IV saline).

III. Heatstroke. Heatstroke is a life-threatening medical emergency due to excessive body heat secondary to overloading and/or impairment of the body's heat-dissipating mechanisms. Characteristic signs include **hyperpyrexia**, with a core temperature usually exceeding 41°C (106°F); severe **CNS dysfunction** manifested by delirium, psychosis, or coma; and often **anhidrosis** (sweating, however, may be present in exertional heatstroke of rapid onset). The diagnosis of heatstroke should be entertained in any patient in whom these manifestations develop under conditions of heat stress. Other common manifestations include sinus tachycardia, respiratory alkalosis, metabolic acidosis, and hypotension (secondary to hypovolemia, peripheral vasodilatation, and/or cardiac dysfunction).

A. Complications include dysfunction or failure of any organ system as a result of cellular damage due primarily to direct thermal injury. Morbidity and mortality are considerable and are principally related to the magnitude and duration of the hyperthermia.

B. Treatment is directed at immediate elimination of hyperpyrexia and support of vital organ systems.

    1. The hyperpyrexia must be reduced immediately. The best method is to immerse the patient in an **ice-water bath.** An alternative method of cooling involves continuous ice-water sponge baths. The extremities should be massaged during cooling to reduce cold-induced cutaneous vasoconstriction. To avoid hypothermia, active cooling should be discontinued when the core (rectal) temperature reaches 38.5°C (101°F). Chlorpromazine, 10–25 mg IM or IV at a rate of 1 mg/minute, may be administered as needed to stop shivering.

    2. Since convulsions and emesis are common, especially during cooling, **tracheal intubation** is indicated in comatose patients to secure a protected airway. **Oxygen** should be administered to supply the hypermetabolic tissue needs.

    3. Intravenous fluids (initially normal saline or Ringer's lactate) should be administered, preferably with CVP monitoring, to replace fluid losses, correct hypotension, and maintain an adequate urinary output. The average fluid requirement is 1200–1400 ml during the first 4 hours.

    4. Sodium bicarbonate should be given IV as needed to correct metabolic acidosis.

    5. Isoproterenol has been used successfully in managing the hypodynamic (cardiogenic shock) state in heatstroke, but **dobutamine,** 2–40 μg/kg/minute, may be preferable. Alpha-adrenergic vasocontrictors are contraindicated during the hyperthermic period because they impair heat dissipation.

    6. Mannitol, 12.5–25.0 gm IV, as needed to promote renal blood flow and urinary output, is beneficial in treating oliguria not responding to hydration and myoglobinuria secondary to rhabdomyolysis.

    7. The management of the bleeding diatheses of heatstroke is controversial. If treatment is required, most authorities recommend administration of clotting factors (e.g., fresh blood, fresh-frozen plasma, platelets) rather than heparin.

    8. Antibiotics should be reserved for definite infections and not used prophylactically. Corticosteroids are of no benefit in managing heatstroke.

Hypothermia

Hypothermia is a disorder in which the core or internal body temperature is less than 35°C (95°F). It is most often the result of exposure to cold. Associated or precipitating factors include alcohol or drug intoxication, acute and chronic incapacitating illnesses, metabolic disorders (e.g., hypoglycemia, hypothyroidism, hypoadrenalism), CNS disorders, dermal disorders, malnutrition, and sepsis. The diagnosis requires a high index of suspicion and a low-reading thermometer.

I. **Pathophysiology.** A fall in core temperature incites compensatory responses, primarily cutaneous vasoconstriction and shivering. Shivering, however, ceases at core temperatures below 32°C (90°F) and is replaced by muscular rigidity. Although cardiopulmonary stimulation occurs initially, a decline in core temperature below 32°C is associated with progressive decreases in respiratory minute volume, heart rate, and cardiac output. Hypotension may occur due to reduced cardiac output secondary to bradycardia and/or hypovolemia (resulting from intravascular fluid loss). A variety of dysrhythmias may be encountered secondary to increased myocardial irritability and depression of intracardiac conductivity and impulse formation. The ECG may also reveal the characteristic J or Osborn wave, an abnormal terminal deflection of the QRS complex. At core temperatures below 32°C (90°F), CNS depression occurs. Acidosis is common and is usually metabolic, secondary to tissue hypoxia. Hyperglycemia or hypoglycemia may be present. The state of profound hypothermia may be indistinguishable from death.

II. **Complications.** Complications include cardiac or respiratory arrest, dysrhythmias, aspiration or bronchopneumonia, pulmonary edema, pancreatitis, acute renal failure (acute tubular necrosis), intravascular thrombosis (e.g., cerebrovascular accident, myocardial infarction), and GI bleeding. Mortality in hypothermia is high and is primarily related to the presence of underlying disease.

III. **Management.** Treatment of hypothermia consists of careful monitoring, intensive supportive care, rewarming, and treatment of underlying and complicating disorders.

A. **Careful monitoring,** particularly of vital signs, cardiac rhythm, ABGs, and CVP, is vital. **Swan-Ganz catheterization should be avoided,** since in a cold, irritable heart it may precipitate VF. Arterial blood gases should be corrected to the patient's body temperature to avoid spurious results.

B. **Heated humidified oxygen** at 40°C (104°F) should be administered. **Tracheal intubation** is indicated in comatose patients and patients with respiratory insufficiency; intubation must be performed skillfully to avoid precipitating ventricular fibrillation. Positive pressure ventilation should be used as needed.

C. Because of the risk of precipitating VF, external cardiac massage generally should be avoided if there is organized electrical activity on the ECG.

D. **Intravenous fluids** should be heated to 40°C (104°F) and administered, with CVP monitoring, to correct the hypovolemia that is frequently present.

E. **Sodium bicarbonate** should be administered IV as needed to correct metabolic acidosis.

F. Since a cold heart is relatively unresponsive, cardiac drugs and electrical pacing generally should be avoided, except in the arrest situation. However, lidocaine should be used for suppression of ventricular irritability. Electrical cardioversion of VF is unlikely to be effective until the core temperature is greater than 28°C (82°F). Bretylium, however, may aid defibrillation. Maintenance dosages of all drugs must be reduced markedly because of the hypometabolic state.

G. Thyroid hormone should be reserved for patients strongly suspected of being hypothyroid. Corticosteroids and prophylactic antibiotics are not indicated.

H. **Rewarming** in hypothermia is controversial. Active external rewarming, although more effective than passive rewarming, appears to have a higher mortality and generally should be avoided. Active core rewarming or application of exogenous heat to the body's core is most physiologic but generally is technically difficult. It is recommended that the choice of a particular rewarming method be based on the clinical status of the patient. The following guidelines are suggested.

1. **Hypothermia with stable cardiovascular status. Passive rewarming** with blankets should suffice and is preferred.

2. **Hypothermia with cardiovascular insufficiency or instability** (i.e., persistent hypotension or serious dysrhythmias). Active core rewarming is indicated. **Peritoneal dialysis** with heated dialysate at 40–45°C (104–113°F) is effective. Hemodialysis or cardiopulmonary bypass may also be used.

3. **Hypothermia with cardiovascular collapse** (i.e., VF or asystole). Rapid core rewarming is indicated. **Cardiopulmonary bypass,** if available, is the method of choice. Otherwise, rewarming may be accomplished with peritoneal dialysis with CPR in progress. Hypothermic patients may tolerate prolonged CPR because of the protective effect of hypothermia on the CNS.

4. **Hypothermia with an associated toxic state** due to a dialyzable drug. **Hemodialysis or peritoneal dialysis** may be preferred, depending on the clinical status of the patient.

I. No patient should be pronounced dead while hypothermic. Such a determination can be made only after a patient fails to revive with rewarming to 32°C (90°F) and appropriate resuscitative measures.

J. Underlying and associated disorders must be actively sought and vigorously treated when present, since they contribute significantly to the high mortality associated with hypothermia.

Near-Drowning

Near-drowning refers to initial survival following submersion in a liquid medium. Death may ensue, however, primarily as a result of respiratory failure. Morbidity and mortality are principally related to the degree of pulmonary injury and hypoxic CNS insult.

I. **Freshwater versus saltwater near-drowning.** In theory, freshwater aspiration may result in hypervolemia, hemodilution, and hemolysis (with hemoglobinuria and hyperkalemia) as a result of absorption of water through alveoli into the circulation. In contrast, saltwater aspiration may lead to hypovolemia and increased serum concentrations of salts as a result of absorption of salts from seawater and a shift of fluid out of the circulation into the lungs. In reality, such volume and electrolyte abnormalities rarely occur, since aspiration of large volumes (>22 ml/kg) is required to produce such changes. On the other hand, both freshwater and saltwater near-drowning are characterized by **hypoxemia** and **acidosis.** Hypoxemia is due primarily to intrapulmonary shunting related to fluid-filled alveoli and alveolar collapse secondary to inactivation of surfactant. Acidosis is usually metabolic, secondary to tissue hypoxia, but there may be an associated respiratory component. Noncardiogenic **pulmonary edema** (adult respiratory distress syndrome) is common to both types of near-drowning, but its appearance may be delayed up to 3 days.

II. **Complications.** Complications of near-drowning are principally pulmonary (e.g., aspiration pneumonitis, bacterial pneumonia, pulmonary edema, respiratory failure) and neurologic (i.e., anoxic encephalopathy). Dysrhythmias and hypotension may occur and are usually due to hypoxia and acidosis. Hypothermia may be present as a result of cold exposure. Uncommon complications include hemolysis, acute renal failure (acute tubular necrosis), and disseminated intravascular coagulation.

III. **Treatment**

A. **Aggressive treatment of hypoxia** is the mainstay of management. Initially, 100% **oxygen** should be administered. Tracheal intubation and positive pressure ventilation are indicated in patients with respiratory insufficiency, and early use of **positive end-expiratory pressure** should be considered.

B. Initially, regardless of the type of near-drowning, normal saline or Ringer's lactate solution should be administered IV at a rate commensurate with the clinical situation. Monitoring of CVP or Swan-Ganz catheterization is useful in assessing fluid requirements.

C. Sodium bicarbonate should be administered IV as needed to reverse metabolic acidosis.

D. Gastric lavage, with prior protection of the airway if needed, is indicated to empty the stomach.

E. Bronchodilators may be useful in treating bronchospasm.

F. Corticosteroids generally are not effective in treating the pulmonary injury in near-drowning and are of questionable benefit in reducing cerebral edema secondary to anoxia. Antibiotics are recommended only for definite pulmonary infection.

G. Hypothermia must be considered and, if present, managed accordingly (see Hypothermia). Since hypothermia protects against anoxic encephalopathy, vigorous resuscitative efforts are indicated for all hypothermic immersion victims.

H. To lessen neurologic sequelae, **vigorous treatment of cerebral edema** is critical. Therapeutic modalities include fluid restriction, hyperventilation, and administration of corticosteroids, loop diuretics, and/or osmotic agents. Induced hypothermia and administration of barbiturates may also be beneficial. Intracranial pressure monitoring should be considered.

I. Due to the possible delayed appearance of pulmonary injury and respiratory insufficiency, all immersion victims with any suggestion of aspiration require hospitalization and careful observation for at least 24 hours.

Drug Overdosage and Poisoning

I. Management principles

A. Identification of the drug(s) is important, since knowledge of the toxic agent and dosage may influence therapy. Frequently, drug identification can be made from the history and physical findings. It should be remembered, however, that the history is notoriously unreliable regarding both the drug taken and the dosage, and clinical findings may be obscured by multiple ingestions. Specimens of urine, gastric contents, and blood should be obtained for definitive drug identification. Supportive therapy, however, should not be delayed while awaiting drug identification.

B. A knowledge of the drug's pharmacology and toxic effects is essential in guiding management. The regional **poison control center** should be contacted early for such information and specific therapeutic measures.

C. Intensive supportive care is the vanguard of poison management.

1. Maintenance of respirations

a. Assess the adequacy of ventilation and oxygenation. In general, ABGs should be monitored.

b. Establish and maintain a clear airway. Initially, the standard airway maneuvers (see Upper Airway Obstruction) should be performed as needed. Intoxicated patients, if not tracheally intubated, should be placed on the left side with the head down to protect against aspiration. **Orotracheal or nasotracheal intubation** should be performed in any patient with respiratory insufficiency, loss of consciousness, impaired or absent gag reflex, or status epilepticus. Supplemental **oxygen** and mechanical ventilation should be provided as indicated.

c. As a result of volume overload or pulmonary capillary endothelial damage, **pulmonary edema** may occur with drug overdosage. Appropriate management is indicated.

2. **Maintenance of circulation**

   a. **Assess the cardiovascular status** by following vital signs and the ECG. Monitoring of CVP or Swan-Ganz catheterization should be performed as needed. An IV line should be established in all patients with significant drug intoxication.

   b. **Hypotension** in drug overdosage may be due to multiple factors but is usually responsive to **volume expansion** with normal saline and correction of hypoxia and acidosis. Occasionally, hypotension is refractory to such measures, and a vasoactive drug is required. **Dopamine,** 2–50 µg/kg/minute, is the vasopressor of choice in most cases of drug overdose.

   c. **Hypertension** is uncommon, usually transient, and usually does not require treatment. Hypertensive crisis may occur, however, usually with sympathomimetic overdoses. **Sodium nitroprusside, sodium diazoxide,** and **propranolol** are useful therapeutic agents.

   d. **Dysrhythmias** may occur from autonomic and direct cardiac effects. Antidysrhythmic therapy may be needed, based on the clinical situation, and should be guided by the toxic mechanism involved.

3. **Central nervous system depression** is a common feature of many overdoses, particularly of the sedative-hypnotics and narcotics. Staging is as follows: O, asleep, arousable; I, comatose, withdrawal from painful stimuli; II, comatose, no withdrawal from painful stimuli, most reflexes intact; III, comatose, most reflexes absent, no respiratory or circulatory depression; IV, comatose, reflexes absent, respiratory and/or circulatory failure. Any patient with a depressed level of consciousness requires either immediate determination of the blood glucose (with Dextrostix) or administration of **50% dextrose.** In addition, **naloxone hydrochloride** may be used as a diagnostic agent or to reverse the depressant effects of narcotic overdosage. **Supportive care** is vital. Hemoperfusion or hemodialysis, however, is generally indicated in managing stage IV overdosage.

4. **Convulsions** may complicate poisonings. Repetitive seizures require treatment; **diazepam** is the anticonvulsant of choice.

5. Certain drugs (e.g., salicylates, methanol, ethylene glycol) may cause a **metabolic acidosis. Sodium bicarbonate,** given IV, is indicated for correction of significant acidosis (i.e., pH <7.2).

6. **Hyperpyrexia** (particularly with sympathomimetic and anticholinergic drug ingestions) and **hypothermia** (usually with sedative-hypnotic overdoses) may occur. Restoration of normothermia by appropriate means is indicated.

7. Analeptic agents are contraindicated. They have been associated with an increase in mortality.

D. **Prevention of drug absorption.** Methods to empty the stomach include **forced emesis** and **gastric lavage.** Since the history is often unreliable and many drugs delay gastric emptying, induced emesis or gastric lavage, unless contraindicated (see **1** and **2**), should be performed in all significant poisonings regardless of the time interval since ingestion.

   1. **Forced emesis** is the preferred means of emptying the stomach in awake patients. **Syrup of ipecac,** 30 ml PO, followed by at least 16 oz of water, may be given to induce vomiting. Syrup of ipecac is usually successful, but if emesis does not ensue in 20 minutes, the dose may be repeated. If there is still no response, gastric lavage must be performed to remove both the ingested drug(s) and the ipecac, which has cardiotoxic properties. **Contraindi-**

cations to forced emesis include CNS depression, impaired gag reflex, status epilepticus, caustic ingestions, and ingestion of certain hydrocarbons.

2. **Gastric lavage** is also an effective means of gastric emptying and is indicated for patients with a depressed level of consciousness after the airway has been protected as needed (see sec. **I.C.1.b**) by insertion of a cuffed nasotracheal or orotracheal tube. The gastric tube must be large bore (i.e., at least 28F); a 36F Ewald tube is ideal for removal of ingested pills. The tube may be inserted via the nasal or oral route. Isotonic saline is the preferred lavage solution, but tap water may be used. Copious quantities of fluid are used to lavage the stomach, but no more than 300–400 ml (300 ml is ideal) should be instilled at one time before withdrawing fluid, because larger volumes may wash toxic material into the duodenum. Lavage is continued until the return is clear. **Contraindications** to gastric lavage are generally the same as those for forced emesis, but in many cases can be overcome by prior endotracheal intubation.

3. **Activated charcoal,** an inert and nontoxic substance, effectively adsorbs most drugs and thus prevents their absorption from the GI tract. To inhibit absorption of drugs not removed by emesis or lavage, 50–100 gm of activated charcoal as a slurry should be administered PO or by gastric tube. Activated charcoal should not be administered if an oral antidote is to be given, since it will bind the antidote. Otherwise, there are no contraindications to its use.

4. **Cathartics** also should be administered PO or by gastric tube following emesis or lavage, to decrease the intestinal transit and absorptive times of ingested substances. Useful agents include magnesium citrate, 150–300 ml; 70% sorbitol, 50–150 ml; or magnesium or sodium sulfate, 15–30 gm. Oil-based cathartics (e.g., castor oil, mineral oil) are contraindicated because of the risk of aspiration lipoid pneumonia. Magnesium-containing cathartics should not be used in patients with renal failure.

E. **Removal of absorbed drugs**

1. **Forced diuresis** may enhance elimination of drugs that are distributed in plasma, not bound to tissue or plasma proteins, and excreted in the urine in active form. This technique, by itself, is rarely useful but may be of benefit for certain drugs when combined with altering the urinary pH to increase the ionized fraction, thereby decreasing renal tubular resorption by ion trapping. Forced diuresis should not be used unless specifically indicated because of the risk of causing electrolyte abnormalities and pulmonary and cerebral edema. The urinary output and pH, serum electrolytes, and, ideally, the CVP should be monitored. **Contraindications** to forced diuresis include renal insufficiency, cardiac disease, and hypokalemia.

   a. **Forced alkaline diuresis** is effective for certain drugs that are weak acids (e.g., salicylates, phenobarbital). Urinary alkalinization usually can be accomplished with sodium bicarbonate, 1 mEq/kg IV, as needed. Diuresis is achieved by administering saline IV along with a diuretic (mannitol or furosemide) as needed. A useful technique is to add 1 or 2 ampules of sodium bicarbonate to a liter of 0.45% saline and administer the solution at a rate of 250–500 ml/hour. Potassium should be given as needed. The goal of this therapy is to achieve a urinary output of 3–6 ml/kg/hour and a pH of 7.5–9.0.

   b. **Forced acid diuresis** may be achieved by administering saline IV, a diuretic, and ascorbic acid (0.5–2.0 gm IV or PO q4h) and/or ammonium chloride (1–2 gm IV or PO q6h) as needed. Ammonium chloride is more effective but also more toxic. A urinary pH of 4.5–5.5 and output of 3–6 ml/kg/hour are desired. Forced acid diuresis may be of benefit for certain drugs that are weak bases (e.g., amphetamines, phencyclidine).

2. **Dialysis** may be beneficial in removing drugs or toxins that are diffusible across a dialysis membrane (i.e., low-molecular-weight substances), distrib-

uted in plasma, not bound to tissue or plasma proteins, and have a slow body clearance, so that dialysis will significantly enhance their elimination (Table 23-1). Dialysis is indicated for: (1) management of **life-threatening poisonings** (i.e., potentially lethal dosage or blood level, clinical instability or deterioration, or severe electrolyte or acid-base abnormalities) due to dialyzable drugs; (2) removal of dialyzable drugs or toxins that have poor body clearances due to underlying hepatic or renal disease; and (3) management of renal failure. Hemodialysis is more effective than peritoneal dialysis. Dialysis with a lipid dialysate may be of benefit for fat-soluble drugs.

3. **Hemoperfusion** with either activated charcoal or resin columns may effectively remove a variety of drugs and toxins by adsorption (Table 23-1). This technique is indicated for **life-threatening poisonings** due to hemoperfusable agents.

4. Exchange transfusion can effectively remove drugs or toxins that remain in the circulation, but this technique is of limited use in adults.

F. **Administration of antidotes.** There are very few effective antidotes that can be used in treating overdoses (Table 23-2). Antidotes are indicated for specific poisonings as a diagnostic maneuver and to reverse or protect against life-threatening drug effects. They should not be used indiscriminately. Intensive supportive care remains the mainstay of poison management.

G. **Ancillary measures.** Psychiatric evaluation or drug abuse counseling should be obtained for patients with intentional overdoses and substance abuse.

II. Specific agents

A. **Acetaminophen** is a common ingredient in many analgesic and antipyretic preparations. A toxic dose is generally greater than 10 gm. Determination of toxicity, however, should be made by plotting a plasma acetaminophen level on a nomogram (Fig. 23-1). Toxicity is primarily hepatic and is related to accumulation of a toxic intermediate metabolite secondary to depletion of hepatic glutathione during overdosage. Uncommonly, renal or cardiac toxicity also occurs.

1. The **clinical course** involves four stages. During the first 24 hours after ingestion, patients may experience anorexia, nausea, vomiting, and malaise. During the next 24–48 hours, there is clinical improvement, but liver function tests become abnormal. After 48–72 hours, frank hepatic necrosis may occur, followed by recovery or death.

2. **Treatment**

a. **Gastric lavage** or forced emesis with ipecac should be performed. Activated charcoal and a cathartic should not be administered, since they impair absorption of the antidote.

b. **Acetylcysteine** (Mucomyst) is a specific antidote, presumably acting as a glutathione substitute or precursor. To be effective, acetylcysteine therapy must be initiated within 16 hours of ingestion (ideally within 10 hours). Thus, it is recommended that treatment with acetylcysteine be started, pending determination of a plasma acetaminophen level drawn 4 or more hours after ingestion. The dosage is 140 mg/kg PO initially, followed by 70 mg/kg q4h for 17 doses (*Arch. Intern. Med.* 141:380, 1981). If the plasma level is found to be in the toxic range (see Fig. 23-1), acetylcysteine therapy is continued for 17 doses; if the level is nontoxic, antidote therapy is discontinued.

c. Charcoal hemoperfusion or hemodialysis is not indicated. Effective treatment of acetaminophen poisoning is early administration of the antidote.

B. **Amphetamines** are potent CNS and sympathetic stimulants. Ingestion of 20–25 mg/kg is potentially lethal, but blood levels may correlate poorly with clinical status.

Table 23-1. Substances removed by hemodialysis and hemoperfusion[a]

Hemodialyzable		Hemoperfusable
Acetaminophen	Iodide[b]	Acetaminophen
Aluminum	Iron deferoxamine[b]	*Amanita* toxins[b]
Amanita toxins[b]	Isoniazid	Ammonia[b]
Amikacin	Isopropyl alcohol	Amobarbital
Ammonia	Kanamycin	Bromide[b]
Amobarbital	Lactate[b]	Butabarbital
Amoxicillin	Lead edetate[b]	Carbon tetrachloride[b]
Amphetamines[b]	Lithium	Chloral hydrate
Ampicillin	Magnesium	Creatinine
Aniline[b]	Mannitol[b]	Demeton
Arsenic	Meprobamate	Digoxin
Azathioprine	Methanol	Dimethoate
Barbital	Methaqualone	Ethanol
Borate[b]	Methotrexate	Ethchlorvynol
Bromide	Methyldopa	Glutethimide
Calcium	Methylprednisolone[b]	Meprobamate
Camphor[b]	Methyprylon	Methaqualone
Carbenicillin	Metronidazole	Methotrexate[b]
Carbon tetrachloride[b]	Monoamine oxidase	Methyprylon
Cephalosporins (most)	inhibitors[b]	Nitrostigmine
Chloral hydrate	Neomycin	Paraquat
Chloramphenicol	Nitrofurantoin	Parathion[b]
Chlorate[b]	Nitroprusside	Pentobarbital
Chromate[b]	Ouabain	Phenobarbital
Cimetidine	Paraquat[b]	Salicylate
Cisplatin	Penicillin	Secobarbital
Citrate	Phenobarbital	Theophylline
Creatinine	Potassium	Thyroxine[b]
Cyclophosphamide	Primidone	Uric acid
Demeton	Procainamide	
Diazoxide	Quinidine	
Dimethoate	Quinine[b]	
Disopyramide	Salicylate	
Ethambutol	Sodium	
Ethanol	Streptomycin	
Ethchlorvynol	Sulfonamides	
Ethinamate[b]	Theophylline	
Ethylene glycol	Thiocyanate	
Flucytosine	Ticarcillin	
Fluoride	Tobramycin	
5-Fluorouracil	Urea	
Gallamine	Uric acid	
Gentamicin	Water	
Hydrogen ions		

[a]This table is only a guide. The need for hemodialysis or hemoperfusion should be based on the toxicity of the substance, the effectiveness of the procedure, and the clinical state.
[b]Possibly effectively removed (but insufficient data).
Source: Data from J. R. Winchester et al., Dialysis and hemoperfusion of poisons and drugs-update. *Trans. Am. Soc. Artif. Intern. Organs* 23:762, 1977; and W. M. Bennett et al., Drug therapy in renal failure: Dosing guidelines for adults. *Ann. Intern. Med.* 93:62, 286, 1980.

Table 23-2. Antidotes*

Antidote	Adult dosage	Usage
Acetylcysteine	140 mg/kg PO, followed by 70 mg/kg q4h for 17 doses	Acetaminophen
Atropine sulfate	1–5 mg IV (IM) q15min as needed	Cholinergics Organophosphates
Benztropine mesylate	1–2 mg IV (IM, PO) as needed	Extrapyramidal signs
Calcium disodium edetate	1 gm IV (IM) over 1 hr q12h	Lead
Deferoxamine mesylate	1 gm IM (IV at a rate ≤ 15 mg/ kg/hr if shock or coma) followed by 0.5 gm q4h	Iron
Dimercaprol	2.5–5.0 mg/kg IM q4–6h	Arsenic Gold Mercury Lead
Diphenhydramine hydrochloride	25–50 mg IV (IM, PO) as needed	Extrapyramidal signs
Ethanol	1 ml/kg of absolute (100%) ethanol in 5% D/W IV over 15 min, followed by 0.1–0.2 ml/kg/hr to maintain a blood level of 100 mg/dl	Ethylene glycol Methanol
Methylene blue	1–2 mg/kg IV (0.1–0.2 ml/kg of 1% solution) over 5 min	Methemoglobinemia
Naloxone hydrochloride	0.4–2.0 mg IV (IM, SQ) q30–60min as needed	Opiates Diphenoxylate Pentazocine Propoxyphene
Nitrites		Cyanide
Amyl nitrite	Inhalation pearls q1min	
Sodium nitrite	300 mg IV (10 ml of 3% solution) over 3 min	
Oxygen	100%, hyperbaric	Carbon monoxide
Penicillamine	250–500 mg PO q6h	Copper Mercury
Physostigmine salicylate	0.5–2.0 mg IV (IM) over 2 min q30–60min as needed	Anticholinergics
Pralidoxime chloride	1–2 gm IV (PO) over 15–30 min as needed (usually q8–12h × 3)	Organophosphates Anticholinesterases

*Dosages may require adjustment according to specific clinical situations.

1. **Clinical manifestations** include hyperactivity, irritability, delirium, psychosis, mydriasis, hypertension, dysrhythmias, hyperpyrexia, vomiting, and diarrhea. Coagulopathies, rhabdomyolysis, acute renal failure, convulsions, CNS hemorrhage, coma, and circulatory collapse may also occur.

2. **Treatment**

   a. **Gastric emptying,** followed by administration of activated charcoal and a cathartic, is indicated.

   b. **Forced acid diuresis** (see sec. I.E.1.b) increases renal excretion.

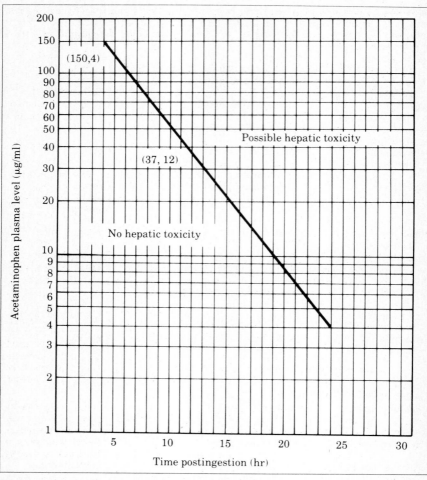

Fig. 23-1. Nomogram for acetaminophen toxicity. (Adapted, with permission, from B. H. Rumack and H. Matthew, Acetaminophen poisoning and toxicity. *Pediatrics* 55:871, 1975. Copyright American Academy of Pediatrics 1975.)

    c. Agitation or psychosis may be treated with **chlorpromazine** or **haloperidol;** diazepam may also be used.

    d. Diazepam is the drug of choice for managing convulsions.

    e. Amphetamine-induced dysrhythmias are secondary to increased sympathetic stimulation and are often responsive to **propanolol.**

    f. Chlorpromazine is useful in treating hypertension; **sodium nitroprusside, diazoxide,** or phentolamine, however, may be required to manage severe sustained hypertension.

    g. Hemodialysis may be beneficial for life-threatening overdosage.

C. Barbiturates may be divided into (1) long-acting drugs (e.g., phenobarbital, barbital) that are primarily cleared by the kidneys and (2) short-acting drugs (e.g., amobarbital, secobarbital, pentobarbital) that are principally metabolized in the liver. Ingestion of more than 6 gm of the long-acting barbiturates and 3 gm of the short-acting drugs may be fatal; potentially lethal blood levels are 8 mg/dl and 3 mg/dl respectively.

1. **Clinical manifestations.** Although excitement and hallucinations may be seen initially, progressive CNS depression leading to coma may ensue. In severe overdoses, respiratory depression, hypotension, areflexia, hypothermia, rhabdomyolysis, and bullous skin lesions may occur.

2. **Treatment.** Routine overdose measures are indicated; intensive **supportive care** is the mainstay of management.

   a. **Dopamine** or levarterenol may be used to manage fluid-resistant hypotension.

   b. **Forced alkaline diuresis** (see sec. **I.E.1.a**) enhances renal excretion of the long-acting barbiturates but is ineffective for the short-acting drugs.

   c. Hemodialysis is ineffective in removing short-acting barbiturates but may be useful in long-acting barbiturate overdoses. **Charcoal hemoperfusion,** however, is the preferred procedure for both long- and short-acting, life-threatening barbiturate overdoses not responding to intensive supportive measures.

D. **Benzodiazepines** (e.g., chlordiazepoxide, diazepam, flurazepam, oxazepam) commonly produce sedation but are generally safe and have minimal serious side effects even after ingestions of 50-100 times the usual daily dosage. General management principles for overdosage should be followed.

E. **Caustics** include acids and alkalis. The latter are common ingredients in cleaning agents, washing powders, and paint removers. Substances with pH less than 2 or more than 12.5 are particularly prone to cause tissue injury to the GI tract. Acids produce a coagulation necrosis and most frequently involve the stomach; in contrast, alkalis cause a liquefaction necrosis and principally affect the esophagus. Oropharyngeal burns do not necessarily correlate with the presence of esophageal or gastric burns.

1. **Clinical manifestations** include pain in the oropharynx, chest, or abdomen, dysphagia, and drooling. Respiratory distress secondary to upper airway edema or tracheal aspiration may occur. Gastrointestinal hemorrhage, perforation with mediastinitis or peritonitis, sepsis, and shock are other serious complications. Death is usually due to circulatory collapse or airway obstruction.

2. **Treatment**

   a. If tolerated, **dilution** of the ingested acid or alkali with 6–8 oz of milk or water is probably beneficial. This should be followed by having the patient take nothing by mouth. **Induced emesis, gastric lavage, and charcoal and cathartic administration should not be performed.**

   b. Although controversial, early endoscopy is a means to document injury.

   c. Airway management, adequate fluid replacement, and careful monitoring for perforation and hemorrhage are essential. Steroids and prophylactic antibiotics are controversial and of questionable benefit.

F. **Cocaine** is a powerful CNS and sympathetic stimulant. It is most commonly administered by nasal insufflation, but it may be smoked or injected IV; oral absorption is poor as a result of gastric hydrolysis.

1. **Clinical manifestations** vary from excitability, mydriasis, tachycardia, and hypertension to severe complications, including hyperthermia, seizures, dysrhythmias, coma, respiratory arrest, and circulatory failure. Blood and urine determinations may be useful in confirming the diagnosis.

2. Treatment consists of **supportive care. Diazepam** may be used to treat severely anxious patients, and **propranolol** may be used to manage adrenergic phenomena.

G. Ethanol is a CNS depressant. Blood levels above 100 mg/dl are generally regarded as defining legal intoxication. Lethal levels vary widely but are usually between 350–700 mg/dl.

1. Clinical manifestations include vomiting, ataxia, nystagmus, slurred speech, altered sensorium, and acute psychosis. Shock, cardiac dysfunction, hypothermia, hypoglycemia, and lactic acidosis or ketoacidosis may complicate acute intoxication. Death, when it occurs, is usually due to respiratory arrest.

2. Treatment is primarily **supportive.** Thiamine, 100 mg IM, should be administered. If hypoglycemia is suspected, 25–50 gm of dextrose should be given IV. For uncomplicated intoxication, observation is all that is necessary. For comatose patients, gastric lavage (with the airway protected by tracheal intubation), followed by charcoal and cathartic administration, is indicated. Hemodialysis is rarely necessary, but it may be helpful in life-threatening intoxications.

H. Ethchlorvynol, glutethimide, methaqualone, and methyprylon

1. Clinical manifestations of overdosage with these sedative-hypnotics commonly include coma, respiratory depression, and hypotension. Pulmonary edema, convulsions, and hypothermia may also occur. Unique features include anticholinergic effects and cyclic coma with glutethimide poisoning and pyramidal signs (e.g., hypertonicity, hyperreflexia, myoclonus) with methaqualone intoxication.

2. Management. Routine overdose measures are indicated. Intensive **supportive care** is the mainstay of management.

a. Diazepam is the drug of choice for terminating seizures.

b. Dopamine or norepinephrine may be used to treat hypotension unresponsive to fluid administration.

c. Hemoperfusion is more effective than hemodialysis and is preferred for life-threatening overdosage.

I. In **hydrocarbon** ingestions, the principal effects are GI upset, pulmonary aspiration, and CNS alterations. Less frequently, myocardial, renal, hepatic, and hematologic complications occur. Morbidity and mortality are usually due to pulmonary aspiration, with low-viscosity hydrocarbons (e.g., gasoline, turpentine, kerosene, petroleum ether, petroleum naphtha, mineral spirits, mineral seal oil) commonly involved.

1. Clinical features are usually apparent within the first 6 hours after ingestion and include vomiting, chest or abdominal pain, cough, dyspnea, low-grade fever, dysrhythmias, convulsions, altered sensorium, and radiographic changes of aspiration pneumonitis or pulmonary edema. Bacterial pneumonia, hematologic abnormalities, and hepatic or renal injury may be late effects.

2. Treatment

a. To prevent dermatitis and percutaneous absorption, remove all contaminated clothing and wash affected skin.

b. Supplemental oxygen is indicated in all significant aspiration injuries.

c. Although controversial, gastric emptying followed by catharsis is recommended for ingestion of **toxic hydrocarbons**: halogenated hydrocarbons (e.g., carbon tetrachloride, trichloroethane); aromatic hydrocarbons (e.g., benzene, xylene, toluene, turpentine); certain petroleum products (e.g., petroleum ether, petroleum naphtha, naphtha paint thinner, mineral spirits); and petroleum distillates with toxic additives (e.g., insecticides, heavy metals). In awake patients, **gastric emptying** should be performed by induced emesis with ipecac; gastric lavage should not be used because of the associated increased incidence of aspiration. However, in patients with CNS depression, a depressed gag reflex, or convulsions, gastric lavage with a cuffed endotracheal tube in place is indicated. Ingestions of **nontoxic hydrocarbons** generally can be treated with **catharsis** alone. It is important, however, to contact the regional **poison control center** for specific therapeutic guidelines.

   d. Epinephrine generally should be avoided because of the risk of inducing dysrhythmias. Corticosteroids and prophylactic antibiotics should not be used.

   e. Observation for at least 6 hours is required for all patients who have ingested hydrocarbons. Hospital admission is recommended for patients who are symptomatic or have pulmonary findings or an abnormal chest x ray.

J. Methemoglobinemia may be caused by many oxidizing agents, including nitrites, nitroglycerin, chlorates, sulfonamides, aniline dyes, nitrobenzene, and phenazopyridine. These substances oxidize hemoglobin to its ferric state, thereby limiting its oxygen-carrying capacity and producing symptoms of anemia. The diagnosis is suggested in patients with generalized **cyanosis** (unrelieved with oxygen) and a normal PaO_2. Blood levels greater than 50% are indicative of severe toxicity, and levels greater than 70% are often fatal. **Treatment** is with supplemental **oxygen. Methylene blue,** 1–2 mg/kg IV over 5 minutes, is indicated if there are signs of hypoxia or the methemoglobin level exceeds 30%.

K. Narcotics are substances that have a morphinelike pharmacologic action. Overdoses may occur with true narcotics (e.g., heroin, morphine, meperidine, codeine) or drugs that have similar properties (e.g., propoxyphene, pentazocine).

   1. Clinical manifestations. The triad of a depressed mental status, respiratory depression, and miosis is characteristic of narcotic overdosage. Bradycardia and hypotension are also common.

   2. Treatment of narcotic overdoses consists of routine measures to prevent drug absorption (when dealing with suspected ingestions), **intensive supportive care,** and administration of **naloxone hydrochloride** for diagnostic and therapeutic purposes. Naloxone is a specific narcotic antagonist effective in reversing the CNS and respiratory depression of narcotics; it also reverses narcotic-induced peripheral vasodilatation (*Clin. Pharmacol. Ther.* 28:541, 1980). The initial dose is 0.4–0.8 mg IV (IM or SQ if IV access is not readily available); if there is no response in 5 minutes, a second dose of 2 mg should be given. Large doses of naloxone may be needed to reverse the effects of propoxyphene, pentazocine, and large overdoses of other narcotics. Since the half-life of naloxone is short (i.e., approximately 60 minutes), careful observation of patients for at least 24 hours is essential, and repetitive doses may be needed for reversal of life-threatening manifestations.

   3. Complications

   a. Pulmonary edema is an uncommon but serious complication that often occurs immediately after narcotic injection but may be delayed for up to 48 hours. Treatment consists of **respiratory support** with oxygen, mechanical ventilation, and positive end-expiratory pressure as needed and administration of naloxone to reverse respiratory depression.

   b. Infections, including hepatitis, tetanus, cutaneous abscesses, cellulitis, thrombophlebitis, endocarditis, and pneumonia, are common among parenteral drug abusers. Cultures are essential, because unusual organisms may be involved; appropriate antibiotic therapy is indicated.

L. Pentazocine (Talwin) and the antihistamine **tripelennamine (Pyribenzamine)** in combination form an abused substance known as **"Ts and Blues."** These drugs, when dissolved into solution and injected IV, may produce an altered mental status, seizures, and sclerosed vessels. Serious **complications** may result from the parenteral injection of unsterile and insoluble materials and include infections and pulmonary microembolization. **Treatment** consists of **supportive care. Naloxone** may be used to reverse the CNS depression of pentazocine. **Aminophylline** is useful in treating bronchospasm (secondary to pulmonary microembolization).

M. Phencyclidine (PCP), an illicit drug, produces CNS stimulation or depression, depending on the dose, has potent sympathomimetic and psychotomimetic properties and is a dissociative anesthetic. It is commonly smoked but may be snorted, ingested, or injected IV.

1. Cardinal signs of PCP intoxication are altered mental status, hypertension, and horizontal and vertical nystagmus. Ataxia and generalized anesthesia are also common. Low-dose intoxications usually result from smoking or snorting the drug and are characterized primarily by behavioral disturbances, including agitation, confusion, psychosis, catatonia, and violent and bizarre behavior. Moderate and high-dose intoxications (i.e., >5 mg) are often associated with ingestion and are characterized by physiologic disturbances: stupor or coma, tachycardia, hypertension, myoclonus, hypertonicity, hyperpyrexia, convulsions, hypersalivation, and bronchorrhea. With massive overdoses, hypotension, apnea, areflexia, and status epilepticus may occur. Rhabdomyolysis and secondary renal failure are common complications of severe overdosage.

2. Treatment

a. In conscious patients, induced emesis or gastric lavage is generally not recommended. For severe poisoning resulting in coma, gastric lavage should be performed after the airway is protected by tracheal intubation. This should be followed by administration of activated charcoal and a cathartic. Tracheal intubation, however, must be skillful to avoid inducing laryngospasm.

b. The behavior induced by PCP is best managed by providing a **quiet, nonthreatening, protective environment** and minimizing sensory input. **Haloperidol** is the drug of choice for managing psychotomimetic effects; **diazepam** may be used for sedation.

c. Since PCP is a weak base excreted by the kidneys, **acid diuresis** (see sec. **I.E.1.b**) is beneficial. In awake patients, ascorbic acid and cranberry juice PO may be used to acidify the urine.

d. Appropriate supportive and ancillary measures should be instituted as needed. **Propranolol** may be used to reverse adrenergic effects. **Diazoxide, sodium nitroprusside,** or phentolamine may be used to treat severe hypertension. **Diazepam** is the agent of choice for managing seizures. Pancuronium bromide may be required to manage uncontrollable motor activity.

e. Patients with low-dose intoxications (characterized by behavioral disturbances) usually can be discharged from the emergency department after symptoms subside; patients with more severe intoxications, however, generally require hospitalization.

N. Phenothiazines (e.g., chlorpromazine, fluphenazine, prochlorperazine, thioridazine)

1. **Clinical manifestations** of overdosage include a spectrum from confusion, agitation, and delirium to CNS depression and coma. Hypotension (primarily due to alpha-adrenergic blockade), anticholinergic signs, and extrapyramidal effects are also common. Less commonly, convulsions and loss of thermoregulation may occur. Cardiac toxicity is related to a quinidinelike effect; dysrhythmias and prolongation of the P–R, Q–Tc, and QRS intervals may occur.

2. **Treatment**

   a. **Gastric emptying** by lavage is preferred because of the drugs' antiemetic properties and risk of aspiration if extrapyramidal signs develop during induced emesis.

   b. Extrapyramidal reactions may be treated with **diphenhydramine hydrochloride,** 25–50 mg IV (IM or PO), or **benztropine mesylate,** 1–2 mg IV (IM or PO), as needed.

   c. Hypotension should be treated with saline IV. If a vasopressor is needed, **norepinephrine** is recommended.

   d. Because of the potential for cardiac dysrhythmias, patients with significant phenothiazine overdoses, especially those with acute ECG changes, should be monitored for at least 48 hours. **Lidocaine** and **phenytoin** are the agents of choice for treating ventricular dysrhythmias; quindine and procainamide, however, are contraindicated. Cardiac pacing may be useful in managing high-degree atrioventricular block or refractory ventricular tachycardia.

O. **Salicylate** overdosage is most commonly due to ingestion of acetylsalicylic acid. Toxic effects are manifested at plasma levels exceeding 30 mg/dl and are generally associated with ingestions of 10 gm or more.

   1. The major **toxic manifestations** of salicylates result from initial stimulation and terminal depression of the CNS and include altered mental status (confusion, agitation, delirium, lassitude, coma), convulsions, emesis, tinnitus, and decreased auditory acuity. Initially, a respiratory alkalosis (hyperpnea) occurs as a result of direct stimulation of the medullary respiratory center. Later—although this is uncommon in adults—a metabolic acidosis may intervene, primarily as a result of altered metabolism. Hyperpyrexia, hypovolemia, hyper- or hypoglycemia, and hypokalemia may be encountered. Coagulation abnormalities may be present due to inhibition of prothrombin production and platelet aggregation. Gastrointestinal bleeding and, uncommonly, pulmonary edema and renal failure may occur. Death is usually due to respiratory failure or cardiovascular collapse; acid-base and metabolic disturbances, however, may contribute to a fatal outcome.

   2. **Specific therapeutic measures**

      a. **Gastric emptying,** charcoal administration, and catharsis are indicated.

      b. **Correction of systemic acidosis,** if present, with IV sodium bicarbonate is particularly important to increase the ionized fraction of salicylic acid and thus decrease CNS levels and the CNS toxicity of the drug. In addition, hypovolemia, hyperpyrexia, hypoglycemia, hypokalemia, and hypoprothrombinemia, if present, require correction.

      c. **Forced alkaline diuresis** (see sec. I.E.1.a) is indicated, since it accelerates elimination of salicylic acid. Urinary alkalinization should be attempted with sodium bicarbonate; acetazolamide is contraindicated because it produces systemic acidosis, which increases salicylate toxicity. Potassium repletion is usually required.

      d. **Dialysis or hemoperfusion** is indicated in the following situations: **life-threatening intoxication** (i.e., coma, respiratory or cardiovascular insufficiency, severe unresponsive acidosis, or plasma salicylate level >100 mg/dl), renal failure, or inability to induce an alkaline diuresis when essential.

P. Tricyclic antidepressants include amitriptyline, imipramine, desipramine, nortriptyline, doxepin, and protriptyline. These drugs have a low therapeutic index. Their toxic effects are due to three mechanisms: inhibition of acetylcholine at neuroreceptor sites (anticholinergic effect); blockade of norepinephrine reuptake by adrenergic nerve terminals (sympathomimetic effect); and a direct, quinidinelike myocardial effect. Major overdosages are associated with acute prolongation of the QRS interval to 0.10 seconds or more and plasma levels greater than 1000 ng/ml. Ingestions exceeding 10 mg/kg may be lethal.

1. The **clinical manifestations** of tricyclic antidepressant overdoses result from central and peripheral anticholinergic effects and the direct and indirect (autonomic) cardiac effects. The CNS manifestations include agitation, confusion, delirium, myoclonus, convulsions, coma, and respiratory depression. Mydriasis, dry mucous membranes, ileus, urinary retention, and hyperpyrexia are peripheral anticholinergic signs. Cardiovascular effects include supraventricular tachydysrhythmias, ventricular dysrhythmias, conduction blocks, and hyper- or hypotension.

2. **Treatment** includes routine overdose management, cardiac monitoring, intensive supportive care, and the specific measures that follow.

   a. **Sodium bicarbonate**, given IV, is the drug of choice for reversing the cardiovascular complications of tricyclic antidepressant intoxication. Alkalinization of the blood to a pH of 7.5 has been shown to be effective in correcting hypotension, dysrhythmias, and conduction disturbances; the mechanism of action is unknown (*J.A.C.E.P.* 8:413, 1979). For hypotension unresponsive to alkalinization and a fluid challenge, norepinephrine is considered the vasopressor of choice. **Physostigmine salicylate**, 1–2 mg given slowly IV q30–60min as needed, or **propranolol** may be used to treat serious supraventricular tachydysrhythmias but generally should be avoided in the presence of conduction disturbances or hypotension. **Lidocaine** or **phenytoin** may be used to manage ventricular dysrhythmias. Procainamide and quinidine, however, are contraindicated, and electrical cardioversion of dysrhythmias is usually ineffective. Phenytoin is also effective in reversing the conduction blocks of tricyclic antidepressant overdoses. **Isoprotenenol** or **cardiac pacing** may be required to manage bradycardia and high-degree heart block.

   b. **Diazepam** and **physostigmine** are effective in managing convulsions. Phenobarbital and phenytoin, however, are less effective.

   c. **Physostigmine salicylate** will effectively reverse the coma and delirium of tricyclic antidepressant overdosage but should be used only if these manifestations become life-threatening to the patient.

   d. Since the tricyclic antidepressants are highly protein bound and tissue bound, with a large volume of distribution, dialysis and hemoperfusion are generally not considered to be useful. Repetitive administration of activated charcoal PO q4h may be beneficial in eliminating the tricyclic antidepressants because of their gastric and biliary excretion.

   e. Since cardiotoxicity is the primary mechanism of death in tricyclic antidepressant poisonings, all patients with dysrhythmias (including sinus tachycardia) and conduction blocks require cardiac monitoring until disturbance free for 24 hours.

Appendixes

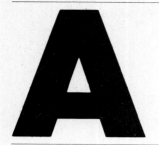

A

Nomogram for Calculating the Body Surface Area of Adults*

*From Eugene F. DuBois, *Basal Metabolism in Health and Disease*. Philadelphia: Lea & Febiger, 1936. Copyright 1920 by W. M. Boothby and R. B. Sandiford.

425

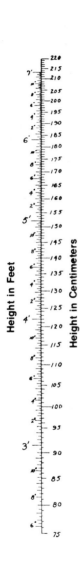

Height in Feet

Height in Centimeters

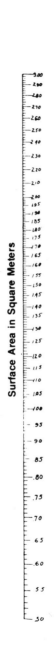

Surface Area in Square Meters

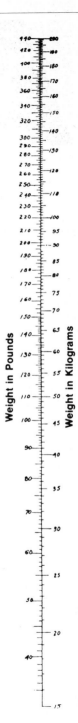

Weight in Pounds

Weight in Kilograms

B

Immunizations

Immunization Information[a]

Disease	Vaccine	Administration	Recommendations	Contraindications	Major adverse reactions	Passive immunization
DTP (diphtheria, tetanus, pertussis)	Toxoid[b] (tetanus and diphtheria) Killed vaccine (pertussis)	A. **Primary** immunization <7 yr 1. One dose IM q4–8wk × 3 2. 4th dose 1 yr later B. ≥7 yr: 1. Two doses IM separated by one period of 4–8 wk 2. 3rd dose 6–12 mo later *Booster:* 1. School entry (DTP) 2. Every 10 yr (Td)	<7 yr: DTP (or DT if pertussis contraindicated) ≥7 yr: Td Ideally, begin immunization at 6–8 wk of age See footnote c for guide to prophylaxis in wound management	Postpone use in those with serious febrile illnesses Do **not** give pertussis vaccine to those >7 yr or with history of major adverse reaction or of bacteriologically confirmed pertussis or in the presense of an evolving neurologic picture Do **not** give Td if history of major adverse reaction	Diphtheria and tetanus toxoid: rare neurologic or severe hypersensitivity reaction Pertussis vaccine: Collapse or shocklike state, persistent screaming episodes, temperature ≥40.5°C, seizures, encephalopathy, thrombocytopenia, hemolytic anemia, or systemic allergic reactions	See footnote c and Chap. 22, Tetanus secs. I and II
Influenza	Multivalent antigen[d] (inactivated virus)	Annual SQ or IM injection, usually in the fall	Annual vaccination for those at risk of serious complications	1. Anaphylactic hypersensitivity to eggs 2. History of	Increased risk of Guillain-Barré syndrome noted during	None

Immunization Information[a] (Continued)

Disease	Vaccine	Administration	Recommendations	Contraindications	Major adverse reactions	Passive immunization
Influenza (cont.)		Number of doses as per package insert	from influenza[e] Consider for medical personnel and those providing essential services (e.g., military personnel)	Guillain-Barré syndrome	1976; no significant association noted during subsequent 3 influenza seasons	
Measles	Live, attenuated[f]	Single SQ dose	All persons ≥15 months of age (born after 1957 without a documented history of infection or vaccination after age 1 yr or without laboratory evidence of immunity or prior vaccination with inactivated vaccine available in USA from 1963–1967)	1. Pregnancy (Caution: avoid pregnancy for at least 3 mo after vaccination) 2. Compromised immune response (immunodeficiency states, malignancy, immunosuppressive therapy) 3. Febrile illness 4. Allergy to antibiotics in vaccine (see package insert) 5. Anaphylactic hypersensitivity to eggs	CNS (including encephalopathy or encephalitis): 1 case/1 million doses given	When live virus vaccine is contraindicated in a person exposed to measles, or when close exposure has occurred >72 hr previously, give immune globulin (IG), 0.25 ml/kg, with a maximum dose of 15 ml

			Indications	Contraindications	Side effects	Gamma globulin
				6. Immune globulin (IG) or other source of antibodies in previous 3 months 7. Tuberculosis		
Meningococcus	Purified capsular polysaccharide[g]	Single SQ dose	1. To control outbreaks following isolation of organism (use group-specific monovalent vaccine) 2. For those traveling to countries experiencing meningococcal outbreaks 3. As an adjunct to antibiotic prophylaxis for household contacts in cases caused by serogroups A or C	Pregnancy (unless substantial risk of infection exists)	None known	None
Mumps	Live, attenuated[h]	Single SQ dose	All persons ≥12 mo without a history of mumps and born since 1957	See Measles	Very rare central nervous system involvement	Not recommended

Immunization Information[a] (Continued)

Disease	Vaccine	Administration	Recommendations[a]	Contraindications	Major adverse reactions	Passive immunization
Pneumococcus	Purified capsular polysaccharide[1] (**Pneumovax**)	Single SQ dose	1. For those >2 yr with anatomic or functional asplenism (e.g., sickle cell disease; chronic cardiorespiratory, renal, and/or hepatic disease; diabetes mellitus 2. Closed community outbreaks	1. <2 yr 2. Sensitivity to phenol 3. Pregnancy (unless substantial risk of infection exists)	Rare: Anaphylactic reactions	None
Poliomyelitis	Oral polio vaccine (OPV), attenuated live virus vaccine	OPV: 1 dose q6–8 wk × 2; 1 dose 8–12 mo after 2nd dose; additional dose on entering school	≤18 yr of age: OPV is preferred. Ideally, begin immunization at 6–12 wk of age >18 yr: Vaccination not routinely recommended	1. Compromised immune states or contact with such patients 2. Allergy to antibiotics in vaccine (see package insert)	Vaccine-associated paralysis (1 case/3–4 million doses) in recipients and contacts	None
	Inactivated polio vaccine (IPV)	IPV: 1 dose every 1–2 mo × 3; 4th dose 6–12 mo after 3rd; booster every 5 yr until 18 yr old	In epidemics OPV is preferred. Recommend IPV for unimmunized adults who travel to endemic areas or are members of specific high-	None	None known	None

		risk population groups or for health care workers or high-risk laboratory workers Consider IPV for unimmunized adults where children are receiving OPV			
Rabies	Human diploid cell rabies vaccine (HDCV); inactivated virus	*Postexposure*: 5 1-ml doses of HDCV IM; rabies immune globulin (RIG) and first dose of HDCV given simultaneously as soon as possible. Additional doses of HDCV on days 3, 7, 14, and 28 after the first dose. If serologically documented adequate prior rabies immunization, then give booster doses on days 0 and 3. Serologic testing to document a satisfactory anti-	Combined passive (RIG) and active (HDCV) treatment is recommended for all exposures to animals suspected of being rabid[i]	None if the situation warrants its use	1. HDCV: One reported case of Guillain-Barré syndrome 2. RIG: Same as for IG	1. RIG[j] preferred: 20 IU/kg (one-half dose IM and one-half infiltrated around the wound)

Immunization Information[a] (Continued)

Disease	Vaccine	Administration	Recommendations	Contraindications	Major adverse reactions	Passive immunization
Rabies (*cont.*)		body response is recommended for persons suspected of being immunocompromised. *Preexposure:* 3 0.1-ml doses of HDCV intradermal (ID) on days 0, 7, and 21 or 28. Booster vaccination (0.1 ml ID) should be given every 2 years to persons at continuing risk, e.g., veterinarians		Preexposure treatment: Allergy to the vaccine (HDCV) or its components		
Rubella	Live, attenuated[k]	Single SQ dose	All persons >12 mo of age who have not received rubella vaccine or who do not have laboratory evidence of immunity	See Measles	1. Arthralgias (40%; lower rate in children) 2. Arthritis (<1%)	Not routinely recommended

[a]Obtaining a vaccination history from adults should be a routine part of the history. With present vaccines, interruption of a course of immunization does not require starting the series over again. The vaccination schedule can be resumed where it was stopped. No vaccine is perfect in conferring protection; and all vaccines have some side effects. The reader is referred to "General recommendations on immunization," Morbid. Mortal. Weekly Rep. 32:1, 1983.

[b]Available as DTP (diphtheria, tetanus, pertussis), DT (diphtheria, tetanus, pediatric use), Td (tetanus, diphtheria, adult type), and T (tetanus toxoid).

[c]Guide to tetanus prophylaxis in wound management:

History of Tetanus Immunization (Doses)	Clean Minor Wounds		All Other Wounds	
	Td	TIG	Td	TIG*
Uncertain	Yes	No	Yes	Yes
0–1	Yes	No	Yes	Yes
2	Yes	No	Yes	No†
3 or more	No**	No	No††	No

*TIG (tetanus immune globulin) given concurrently with toxoid at separate sites, 250 units.
†Unless wound is more than 24 hours old.
**Unless it is more than 10 years since the last dose.
††Unless it is more than 5 years since the last dose.

[d]Antigen components and concentrations may vary yearly.

[e]The population at risk includes those with (1) acquired or congenital heart disease; (2) chronic disorders with impaired pulmonary function; (3) chronic renal disease or nephrotic syndrome; (4) chronic, severe anemia, e.g., sickle cell; (5) diabetes mellitus; (6) immunocompromised states; and (7) all >65 years of age.

[f]Available as a monovalent (measles only) form and in combinations: measles-rubella (MR) and measles-mumps-rubella (MMR) vaccines.

[g]Available in the following forms: monovalent A, monovalent C, and bivalent A-C.

[h]Available as a monovalent (mumps only) form and in combinations: mumps-rubella and measles-mumps-rubella (MMR) vaccines. MMR should be used at ≥15 months of age.

[i]Includes 14 of the 83 capsular antigen types; immunity specific only to those 14 types. Only general guidelines for vaccine use can be offered.

[j]Exposure antirabies treatment guide: This guide should be applied in conjunction with knowledge of the animal species involved, circumstances of the bite or other exposure vaccination status of the animal, and presence of rabies in the region.

Species	Condition of the Animal at Time of Attack	Treatment In Exposed Human
Wild		
Skunk		
Fox		
Coyote	Regard as rabid	RIG + HDCV*
Raccoon		
Bat		

*Discontinue vaccine if fluorescent antibody test results in the animal killed at the time of attack are negative.
†Begin RIG + HDCV at first sign of rabies in biting dog or cat during holding period (10 days).

Species	Condition of the Animal at Time of Attack	Treatment In Exposed Human
Domestic		
Cat	Healthy	None†
Dog	Unknown (escaped)	RIG + HDCV
	Rabid or suspected rabid	RIG + HDCV*

[k]Available as a monovalent (rubella only) form and in combinations: measles-rubella (MR) and measles-mumps-rubella (MMR) vaccines. MR and MMR should be used at ≥15 months of age.

Source: Adapted from materials provided by the Immunization Division, Centers for Disease Control (Department of HEW), Atlanta, Ga.

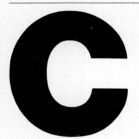

Dopamine

Dopamine
400 mg (2 vials)/500 ml = 0.8 mg/ml

Weight		Dosage (μg/kg/min)							
lb	kg	1.0	2.5	5.0	7.5	10.0	12.5	15.0	20.0
88	40	3	8	15	22	30	37	45	60
99	45	4	9	17	25	34	42	50	67
110	50	4	9	19	28	38	47	56	75
121	55	5	10	21	31	42	51	62	82
132	60	5	11	23	34	45	56	68	90
143	65	5	12	24	36	49	61	74	97
154	70	6	13	26	39	52	66	79	104
165	75	6	14	28	42	56	70	84	112
176	80	7	15	30	44	60	75	90	120
187	85	7	16	32	47	64	80	96	128
198	90	8	17	34	51	68	84	101	136
209	95	8	18	36	53	72	90	107	143
220	100	8	19	37	56	75	94	113	150

Flow rate in drops/min

Based on a microdrip:
60 drops = 1 ml

Dopamine
800 mg (4 vials)/500 ml (1.6 mg/ml)

Weight		Dosage (μg/kg/min)							
lb	kg	1.0	2.5	5.0	7.5	10.0	12.5	15.0	20.0
88	40	2	4	7	11	15	19	22	30
99	45	2	4	8	12	17	20	25	34
110	50	2	5	9	14	19	23	28	38
121	55	2	5	10	15	22	25	31	42
132	60	3	6	11	17	23	28	34	46
143	65	3	6	12	18	25	30	36	49
154	70	4	7	13	20	26	33	39	52
165	75	4	7	14	21	28	35	42	57
176	80	4	8	15	22	30	38	45	60
187	85	4	8	16	23	32	40	48	64
198	90	4	9	17	25	34	42	51	68
209	95	5	9	18	26	36	45	53	72
220	100	5	10	18	27	38	47	57	76

Flow rate in drops/min

Based on a microdrip:
60 drops = 1 ml

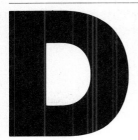

Dobutamine

Dobutamine
250 mg (1 vial)/500 ml = 0.5 mg/ml

Weight		Dosage (μg/kg/min)							
lb	kg	1.0	2.5	5.0	7.5	10.0	12.5	15.0	20.0
88	40	4	13	24	36	48	60	70	96
99	45	5	14	27	41	54	68	81	108
110	50	6	15	30	45	60	75	90	120
121	55	7	17	33	50	66	83	99	132
132	60	7	18	36	54	72	90	108	144
143	65	8	20	39	59	78	98	117	156
154	70	8	21	42	63	84	105	126	168
165	75	9	23	45	68	90	113	135	180
176	80	10	24	48	72	96	120	144	192
187	85	10	26	51	77	102	128	153	204
198	90	11	27	54	81	108	135	162	216
209	95	11	29	57	86	114	143	171	228
220	100	12	30	60	90	120	150	180	240
242	110	13	33	66	99	133	165	198	264

Flow rate in drops/min

Based on a microdrip: 60 drops = 1 ml

Dobutamine
500 mg (2 vials)/500 ml = 1.0 mg/ml

Weight		Dosage (μg/kg/min)							
lb	kg	1.0	2.5	5.0	7.5	10.0	12.5	15.0	20.0
88	40	2	5	11	16	22	29	36	45
99	45	3	7	14	20	27	34	41	54
110	50	3	8	15	23	30	38	45	60
121	55	3	8	17	25	33	41	50	66
132	60	4	9	18	27	36	45	54	72
143	65	4	10	20	29	39	49	59	78
154	70	4	11	21	32	42	53	63	84
165	75	5	11	23	34	45	56	68	90
176	80	5	12	24	36	48	60	72	96
187	85	5	13	26	38	51	64	77	102
198	90	5	14	27	41	54	68	81	108
209	95	6	14	29	43	57	71	86	114
220	100	6	15	30	45	60	75	90	120
242	110	7	17	33	50	66	83	99	132

Flow rate in drops/min

Based on a microdrip: 60 drops = 1 ml

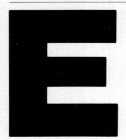

Barnes Hospital Laboratory Reference Values[a]

Reference values for the more commonly employed laboratory tests are given in the following tables. The reference values are given in the units currently used at Barnes Hospital and in the International System (SI) of Units that is being adopted in some areas of the world. The footnotes and a key to the abbreviations appear on pages 441–442.

Common Serum Chemistries

Test	Current units	Factor[b]	SI units
Albumin	3.5–4.8 gm/dl	.154	0.54–0.74 mmol/L
Ammonia (plasma)	18–48 µg/dl	.587	10.6–28.2 µmol/L
Bilirubin			
Total	.25–1.5 mg/dl[c]	17.1	4.3–25.6 µmol/L
Direct	0–.2 mg/dl		0–3.4 µmol/L
Blood gases (arterial, whole blood)			
pH	7.35–7.45	1	7.35–7.45
PO_2	80–105 mm Hg	.133	10.6–14.0 kPa
PCO_2	35–45 mm Hg	.133	4.7–6.0 kPa
Calcium			
Total	9.0–10.3 mg/dl	.25	2.25–2.57 mmol/L
Free[d]	4.5–5.0 mg/dl	.25	1.12–1.25 mmol/L
Carbon dioxide content	24–32 mEq/L	1	24–32 mmol/L
β-Carotene	70–250 µg/dl	.0186	1.3–4.7 µmol/L
Ceruloplasmin	15–60 mg/dl	.067	1.0–4.0 µmol/L
Chloride	95–105 mEq/L	1	95–105 mmol/L
Copper[c]			
Male	70–140 µg/dl	.157	11.0–22 µmol/L
Female	85–155 µg/dl		
Complement (total)[e]	150–250 CH50	1	13.3–24.3 µmol/L
C3	690–1470 mg/L	.001	0.7–1.5 gm/L
C4	105–305 mg/L	.001	0.10–0.30 gm/L
Creatinine			
Male	.8–1.3 mg/dl	88.4	71–115 µmol/L
Female	.6–1.1 mg/dl		53–97 µmol/L
Fibrinogen[f]	1.5–3.6 gm/L	1	1.5–3.6 gm/L
Folate			
Plasma[g]	2.5–17.5 ng/ml	2.27	5.7–39.7 nmol/L
Red cell	225–600 ng/ml		511–1362 nmol/L

Common Serum Chemistries (Continued)

Test	Current units	Factor[b]	SI units
Glucose, fasting (plasma)	65–110 mg/dl	.055	3.57–6.05 mmol/L
Haptoglobin	100–300 mg/dl	.01	1.10–3.00 gm/L
Immunoglobulin[h]			
IgA	39–358 mg/dl	.01	0.39–3.58 gm/L
IgM	33–229 mg/dl	.01	0.33–2.29 gm/L
IgG	679–1537 mg/dl	.01	6.79–15.37 gm/L
Iron			
Male	80–160 µg/dl	.179	14.3–28.6 µmol/L
Female	60–135 µg/dl		10.7–24.2 µmol/L
Binding capacity	250–350 µg/dl		44.7–62.6 µmol/L
Lactate (plasma)	.3–1.3 mmol/L	1	0.3–1.3 mmol/L
Lipids			
Cholesterol[c]	150–270 mg/dl	.0259	3.9–7.0 mmol/L
Triglyceride[c,i]	55–320 mg/dl		
Magnesium	1.5–2.1 mEq/L	.5	0.7–1.1 mmol/L
Osmolality	270–290 mOsm/kg	1	270–290 mOsm/kg
Phosphorus, inorganic[c]	2.5–4.5 mg/dl	.323	0.8–1.5 mmol/L
Potassium (plasma)	3.5–4.5 mEq/L	1	3.5–4.5 mmol/L
Protein electrophoresis[j]			
Albumin	3.5–4.8 gm/dl	10	35–48 gm/L
Alpha-1-globulin	0.1–0.5 gm/dl	10	1–5 gm/L
Alpha-2-globulin	0.3–1.2 gm/dl	10	3–12 gm/L
Beta globulin	0.7–1.7 gm/dl	10	7–17 gm/L
Gamma globulin	0.7–1.7 gm/dl	10	7–17 gm/L
Protein total	6.5–8.5 gm/dl	10	65–85 gm/L
Pyruvate (whole blood)	30–70 µmol/L	1	30–70 µmol/L
Sodium	135–145 mEq/L	1	135–145 mmol/L
Urea nitrogen[c]	8–25 mg/dl	.357	2.9–8.9 mmol/L
Uric acid[c]	3.5–8.0 mg/dl	.059	0.21–0.47 mmol/L
Vitamin A	30–65 µg/dl	.035	1.05–2.27 µmol/L
Vitamin B_{12}	250–1000 pg/ml	.739	185–739 pmol/L

Common Serum Enzymatic Activities

Aldolase[k]	1.5–8.1 mU/ml	16.67	25.0–135.0 nmol/L • s
Amylase[l]	23–85 IU/L	1	23–85 IU/L
Creatine phosphokinase[m]	25–145 IU/ml	.0167	.42–2.42 µmol/L • s
Lactic dehydrogenase[c]	90–250 mU/ml	.0167	1.50–4.17 µmol/L • s
Lipase	4–24 IU/dl	10	40–240 IU/L
Phosphatase, acid[n]	Up to 0.7 IU/L	1	Up to 0.7 U/L
Phosphatase, alkaline[o]	45–115 mU/ml	.0167	0.75–1.90 µmol/L • s

Common Serum Chemistries (Continued)

Common Serum Enzymatic Activities (Continued)

Test	Current units	Factor[b]	SI units
Transaminase			
Alanine amino (SGPT)	5–35 IU/ml	16.67	83–583 nmol/L · s
Aspartate amino[c] (SGOT)	5–40 mU/ml	16.67	83–667 nmol/L · s

Common Serum Hormone Values[p]

ACTH	10–100 pg/ml	1	10–100 ng/L
Aldosterone[q]	10–160 pg/ml	2.77	28–443 mmol/L
Cortisol (plasma)	8–21 µg/dl	.027	0.22–0.57 µmol/L
FSH, male[r]	<5–19 mIU/ml	1	<5–19 IU/L
Gastrin, fasting[s]	25–190 pg/ml	1	25–190 ng/L
Growth hormone, fasting	<5 ng/ml	1	<5 µg/L
Insulin, fasting (72 hr)	<10 mU/L	1	<10 mU/L
LH, male	7–24 mIU/L	1	7–24 IU/L
Parathyroid hormone	2–10 U/ml	1	0–10 arb units
Prolactin			
Male	<20 ng/ml	1	<20 µg/L
Female	<25 ng/ml	1	<25 µg/L
Renin activity (plasma)[t]	0.9–3.3 ng/ml/hr	.278	0.2–0.9 ng/L · s
Testosterone			
Male	280–1000 ng/dl	.0346	10–35 nmol/L
Female	20–120 ng/dl		1–4 nmol/L
Thyroxine, total (T$_4$)	5.0–11.0 µg/dl	12.9	64–142 nmol/L
T$_3$ resin uptake	35–45%	.01	0.35–0.45 arb units
Triiodothyronine (T$_3$)	125–245 ng/dl	.0154	1.93–3.77 nmol/L
TSH	Up to 8 µU/ml	1	Up to 8 mU/L

Common Urinary Chemistries

Calcium	50–250 mg/day	.025	1.25–6.25 nmol/day
Catecholamines	Up to 135 µg/day	1	Up to 135 µg/day
Epinephrine	Up to 20 µg/day	5.5	Up to 110 nmol/day
Norepinephrine	10–80 µg/day	5.9	59–472 nmol/day
Copper	15–60 µg/day	.0157	0.24–0.94 µmol/day
Cortisol	20–90 µg/day	2.76	55–248 nmol/day
Creatine	15–25 mg/kg/day	.0088	0.13–0.22 nmol/kg/day

Common Serum Chemistries (Continued)

Common Urinary Chemistries (Continued)

Test	Current units	Factor[b]	SI units
17-Hydroxycortico- steroids			
Male	4.5–12 mg/day	2.76	12–33 μmol/day
Female	2.5–10 mg/day		7–28 μmol/day
5-Hydroxyindole- acetic acid	1–7 mg/day	5.3	5.3–37.1 μmol/day
17-Ketosteroids			
Male	2–12 mg/day	3.46	7–42 μmol/day
Female	2–10 mg/day		7–35 μmol/day
Protein	Up to 150 mg/day	.001	Up to 0.150 gm/day
Vanillylmandelic acid (VMA)	.5–7 mg/day	5.05	2.5–35.3 μmol/day

Common Hematologic Studies

Test	Current units	Factor[b]	SI units
Coagulation studies			
Bleeding time[u]	2.5–9.5 min	60	150–570 sec
Partial thrombo- plastin time	24–36 sec	1	24–36 sec
Prothrombin time	70–100%	.01	.7–1.0 arb units
Thrombin time	11.3–18.5 sec	1	11.3–8.5 sec
Complete blood count			
Hematocrit			
Male	42–52%	.01	0.42–0.52 arb units
Female	37–47%		0.37–0.47 arb units
Hemoglobin			
Male	14.0–18.0 gm/dl	.620[v]	8.7–11.2 mmol/L
Female	12.0–16.0 gm/dl		7.4–9.9 mmol/L
Erythrocyte count			
Male	$4.6–6.2 \times 10^6$/cu mm	10^6	$4.6–6.2 \times 10^{12}$/L
Female	$4.2–5.4 \times 10^6$/cu mm		$4.2–5.4 \times 10^{12}$/L
Leukocyte count	$4.8–10.8 \times 10^3$/cu mm	10^6	$4.8–10.8 \times 10^9$/L
Platelet count	$159–400 \times 10^3$/cu mm	10^6	$150–400 \times 10^9$/L
Erythrocyte indices			
Mean corpuscular hemoglobin	26–34 pg/cell	.062[v]	1.6–2.1 fmol/cell
Mean corpuscular hemoglobin conc.	31–37%	.620[v]	19.2–22.9 mmol/L
Mean corpuscular volume	80–100 cu μ	1.0	80–100 fl
Sedimentation rate[w]			
Male	Up to 15 mm/hr	1	Up to 15 mm/hour
Female	Up to 20 mm/hr	1	Up to 20 mm/hour

Common Serum Chemistries (Continued)

Therapeutic Agents

Test	Current units	Factor[b]	SI units
Digitoxin	10–30 µg/L	1.30	13–39 nmol/L
Digoxin	0.5–2.0 µg/L	1.28	0.6–2.6 nmol/L
Lithium	0.6–1.2 mEq/L	1	0.6–1.2 nmol/L
Phenobarbital	15–40 mg/L	4.30	64–172 µmol/L
Phenytoin (diphenyl-hydantoin)	10–20 mg/L	3.95	39–79 µmol/L
Quinidine	1.3–5.0 mg/L	3.08	4.0–15.4 µmol/L
Salicylate[x]	30–290 mg/L	.0072	0.22–2.1 mmol/L
Theophylline	10–20 mg/L	5.5	55–110 µmol/L

[a]We would like to thank Dr. Michael A. Pfaller, Department of Laboratory Medicine, for reviewing and updating the laboratory values listed in this Appendix.
[b]A complete list of multiplication factors for converting conventional units to SI units can be found in *N. Engl. J. Med.* 292:795, 1975.
[c]Variation with age and sex occurs. This range includes both sexes and persons >13 years old.
[d]Performed by an ion-selective electrode technique.
[e]Reported as CH50: the reciprocal of the dilution of sera required to lyse 50% of sheep erythrocytes.
[f]Determined by the Clauss method.
[g]Competitive protein binding assay using β-lactoglobulin.
[h]The units for quantitating immunoglobulins are not agreed on. They are arbitrarily expressed here as grams per liter as determined by radial immunodiffusion. The normal ranges for blacks include substantially higher values.
[i]Because of the variable composition of serum triglycerides, their concentration is expressed here as grams rather than moles per liter. A mean molecular weight of 875 gm has also been used. Varies with age (see Chap. 20).
[j]In the International System, serum protein concentrations determined by electrophoresis are expressed as g/L.
[k]For conversion from international units to mass of enzymatic activity, 1 IU = 16.7 nmol/sec.
[l]The substrate employed is maltopentose.
[m]SMA-12 value.
[n]The substrate employed is thymolphthalein monophosphate.
[o]Much higher values (up to 250 mU/ml) can be normal in persons <20 years of age.
[p]Since most hormones are measured by immunologic techniques and because the hormones may vary in molecular weight (e.g., gastrin), most are expressed as mass per liter.
[q]The range of values given is for supine patients on a normal salt diet; in the upright position, the reference range is 40–310 pg/ml.
[r]Range given is for males <60. For males >60, range is <5–102 mIU/ml.
[s]Antibody-dependent determinations. Normal values may vary 1–2 times from laboratory to laboratory.
[t]The range of values given is for patients on high-sodium diet, supplemented with 3 gm sodium/day; for patients on 0.5 gm sodium/day, the reference range is >5.1 ng/ml/hr. These are method-dependent determinations. Normal values may vary 2–4 times from laboratory to laboratory.
[u]Template modified after Ivy.
[v]This factor assumes a unit molecular weight of 16,000; assuming a unit molecular weight of 64,500, the multiplication factor is 0.155.
[w]Westergren technique, not corrected for hematocrit.
[x]Therapeutic range for treatment of rheumatoid arthritis.

Key to abbreviations
        ACTH = adrenocorticotropic hormone
  arb units = arbitrary units
       cu µ = cubic microns
     cu mm = cubic millimeter
           d = day (24 hours)

Key to abbreviations (Cont.)

fl	= femtoliter
fmol	= femtomole
g, gm	= gram
h, hr	= hour
IU	= international unit
kPa	= kilopascal
kg	= kilogram
L	= liter
LH	= luteinizing hormone
µg	= microgram
µmol	= micromole
µU	= microunit
mEq	= milliequivalent
mg	= milligram
mm	= millimeter
mmol	= millimole
mOsm	= milliosmole
mIU	= milliInternational unit
ng	= nanogram
nmol	= nanomole
pg	= picogram
pmol	= picomole
s, sec	= second
SGOT	= serum glutamic oxaloacetic transaminase
SGPT	= serum glutamic pyruvic transaminase
TSH	= thyroid-stimulating hormone

Index